# LIVER BIOPSY

Edited by **Hirokazu Takahashi**

**Liver Biopsy**
Edited by Hirokazu Takahashi

**Published by InTech**

Janeza Trdine 9, 51000 Rijeka, Croatia



**Publishing Process Manager** Mirna Cvijic

**Technical Editor** Teodora Smiljanic

**Cover Designer** InTech Design Team

Additional hard copies can be obtained from orders@intechopen.com

Liver Biopsy, Edited by Hirokazu Takahashi
p. cm.
ISBN 978-953-307-644-7

For EU product safety concerns:
IN TECH d.o.o., Prolaz Marije Krucifikse Kozulić 3, 51000 Rijeka, Croatia, info@intechopen.com or visit our website at intechopen.com.

# Meet the editor

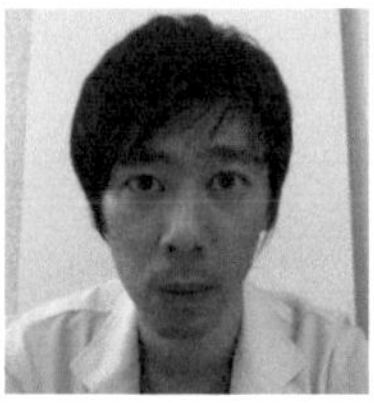

Dr. Takahashi is a graduate of Saga Medical School, in Saga, Japan. He is a Hepatology specialist and is currently working as an Assistant Professor in the Department of Hepatology, Diabetes, Metabolism and Endocrinology at Saga Medical School.
In 2008, dr. Takahashi received a Travel Award for the 18th Annual Meeting of United European Gastroenterology. He was 2009 the recipient of the Young Investigator's Award from The Japan Society of Ultrasonics in Medicine at their 19th Annual Meeting.
Dr. Takahashi is an active board member of Japanese Society of Gastroenterology, Japan Society of Hepatology and Japan Society of Ultrasonics in Medicine. Dr. Takahashi has featured as a guest editor for numerous journals and has been a reviewer for the Journal of Gastroenterology, Liver International, the European Journal of Ultrasound and Hepatology International.

# Contents

# Preface

Liver biopsy is recommended as the gold standard method to determine diagnosis, fibrosis staging, prognosis and therapeutic indications in patients with chronic liver disease. This book covers the whole clinical field of liver biopsy including the basic principles of the procedure, protocol, indications, pathohistological evaluation, and complications. The book covers special evaluation procedures such as electron microscopy, immunostochimistry and flow cytometry. Non-invasive methods, especially the elastography, which is the new procedure in hot topics, are all here frequently reported. One of the reasons for the progress of non-invasive technologies is that liver biopsy is an invasive procedure with a risk of complications- which can be very serious. This book provides the references for the non-invasive procedures including elastography, imaging methods and blood panels which could present the alternatives to liver biopsy. In this book, the professionals of elastography show the mechanism, availability and how to use it in a clinical field. The comprehension of elastography could be a great help for dealing and for understanding for liver biopsy.

**Hirokazu Takahashi, M.D, PhD**
Department of Internal Medicine,
Saga Medical School,
Nabeshima, Saga,
Japan

# Part 1

## Procedure, Techniques and Comprehension of Liver Biopsy

1

# The Role of Liver Biopsy in the Non-Invasive Methods Era and Liver Stiffness Measurement Using Transient Elastography

C. Rinaldi A. Lesmana and Laurentius A. Lesmana
*Division of Hepatology, Department of Internal Medicine,*
*Cipto Mangunkusumo Hospital, University of Indonesia*
*Digestive Disease Centre, Medistra Hospital, Jakarta*
*Indonesia*

## 1. Introduction

Liver biopsy is still the most accurate tool to assess liver histopathology in chronic liver disease (CLD), especially in patients with chronic active hepatitis who need a treatment decision. Nowadays, there are many non-invasive methods are being used to assess liver fibrosis and might replace liver biopsy. One of the new methods is transient elastography (TE/Fibroscan) which has been widely used to predict liver fibrosis in chronic active hepatitis B and C. However, whether TE is ready to replace the liver biopsy is still controversial.

In cases like chronic hepatitis B infection (CHB), autoimmune hepatitis (AIH), non-alcoholic steatohepatitis (NASH), drug induced liver injury (DILI), and cholestatic liver diseases, the role of liver biopsy is very important to make the whole information of liver histopathology (not only about liver fibrosis). On the other hand, to make a diagnosis of liver cirrhosis, we have some parameters that can be used, such as clinical stigmata of advanced chronic liver disease (jaundice, hyper pigmentation, spider nevi, palmar erythema, ascites, edema, and others), low level of platelet count, and low level of albumin, prolonged protombin time, and picture of liver cirrhosis based on ultrasound examination.

In chronic active hepatitis B infection, the treatment decision is usually based on the increase level of alanine aminotransferase (ALT), high HBV-DNA serum level, and the presence of HBeAg status. In patients with normal ALT level or less than 2x ULN, the liver biopsy is needed to decide whether the antiviral therapy should be started or not. In this group, not only liver fibrosis assessment is important, but also the degree of necroinflammation will influence the decision of antiviral therapy. From the point of view of liver fibrosis itself when using TE, it is not always accurate to differentiate between fibrosis 1 or 2, since this differentiation is also important to start antiviral therapy.

Despite the etiology of liver injury, TE itself has problem with overweight and obese patients, and patients with narrowed intercostals space. TE also cannot be performed in ascitic patient because the interposed fluid blocks the shear wave. The increase of liver stiffness cut off is also can be influenced by metabolic syndrome, age, BMI, and the increase of ALT level.

The liver biopsy still has the most important role in assessing liver histopathology but we might reduce the need of liver biopsy examination in some patients. At this moment, TE can

be used as a predictor tool in assessing liver fibrosis in chronic active hepatitis with regard to clinical and laboratory parameters.
A lot of study is still needed to validate the usefulness of TE in assessing liver fibrosis in chronic active hepatitis.

## 2. Liver biopsy

### 2.1 History and definition

In 1883, the first liver biopsy was performed by Ehrlich to assess hepatic glycogen content in a diabetic patient, followed by Lucatello who performed liver biopsy to analyze a tropical abscess of the liver 12 years later. In 1907, Schuper is the one who published a series number of liver biopsy which are performed in humans and rats. The liver biopsy technique has been evolved for many years, and in 1958 Menghini technique of liver biopsy has been introduced and widely used in the clinical practice. This technique can be easily performed by experienced and well-trained clinicians and especially hepatologists. Liver biopsy is a technique to obtain, view, and assess the liver histology, either by cutting or aspiration. This technique can be done via transcutaneous route, or transjugular. (1)

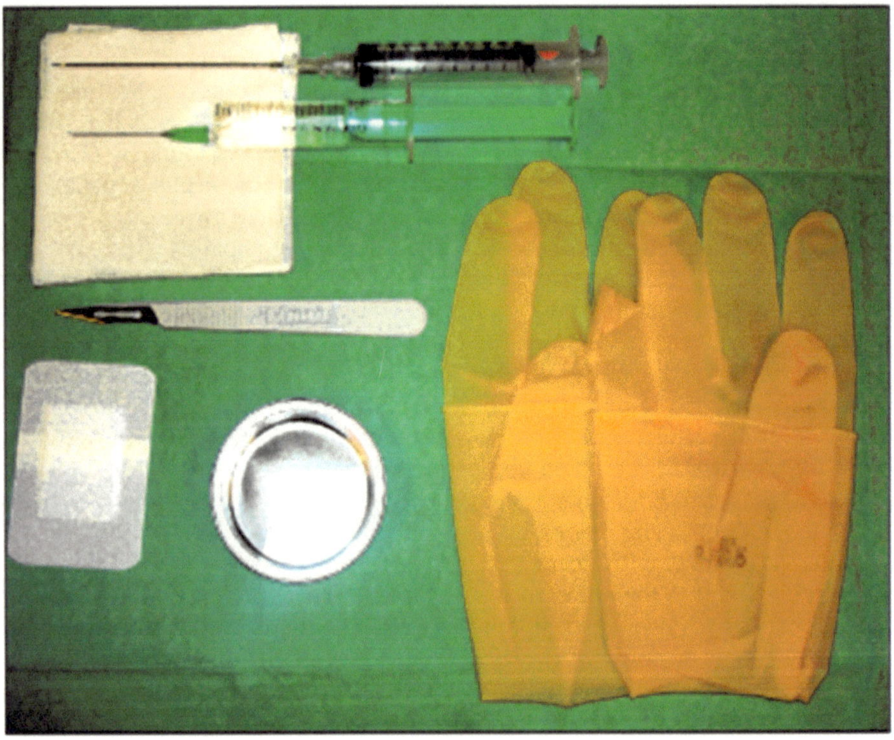



Fig. 1. Typical set-up of materials required for an aspiration transcutaneous liver biopsy. The syringe is already connected to an aspiration needle (Menghini) biopsy set. The other syringe is used for local anesthesia. Adapted from Zakim and Boyer's Hepatology 2006.

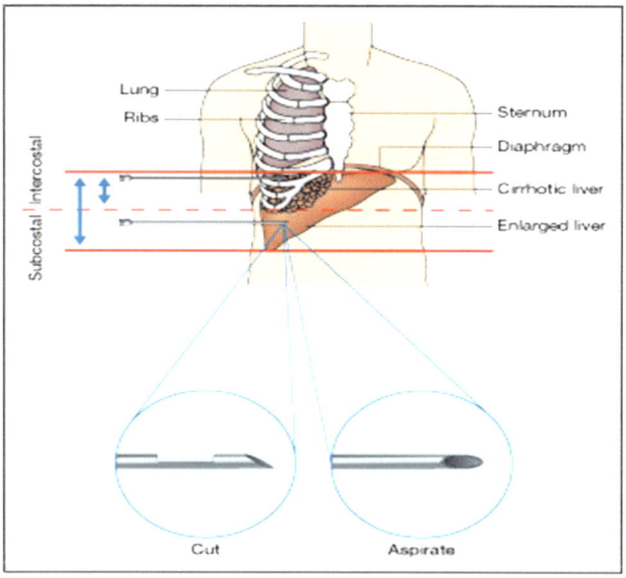




Fig. 2. The approach to transcutaneous liver biopsy. A transcutaneous biopsy of the liver is performed in complete expiration to limit accidental pulmonary injury. As the liver is frequently cirrhotic and therefore small, an intercostal approach is necessary. However, in large livers a subcostal route is preferred as a safer route. The schematic illustrates the two principal types of needle used: cutting needles and aspiration needles, for which several models are commercially available and which should be chosen according to the patient's risk profile and the clinical indication for the biopsy. Adapted from Zakim and Boyer's Hepatology 2006.

### 2.2 The clinical importance of liver biopsy: Its use, risk and assessment

Liver biopsy is an important examination in assessing the progression of liver disease, establish the diagnosis when there is no clear etiology, and to make a decision of therapy. We know that the risks of liver disease progression are liver cirrhosis (LC) and liver cancer/hepatocellular carcinoma (HCC). These could be due to chronic active hepatitis virus infection (such as hepatitis B (HBV) and C (HCV) virus), drug induced liver injury (DILI), alcoholic liver disease (ALD), non-alcoholic steatohepatitis (NASH), autoimmune hepatitis (AIH), etc. In chronic active hepatitis virus infection, of course we need to do liver biopsy in special circumstances (based on the guidelines). However, the disease such as AIH, DILI, and NASH, liver biopsy examination could be a mandatory since we need to see clearly the histology picture to establish the diagnosis. Even sometimes, patient with unknown etiology of hepatomegaly with abnormality liver biochemistry test, we do need a liver biopsy. Liver biopsy in Non-Alcoholic Fatty Liver Disease (NAFLD) can become a dilemma since we know that not all patients with fatty liver will develop NASH. There were some contrarily about doing liver biopsy since there are side effects that could happen, such as bleeding/hemorrhage and pain. The frequency of complications was 3.2% in physicians with a history of less than 20 biopsies, compared to 1.1% when over 100 had been performed. Recently, the use of ultrasound as a guide to liver biopsy has been used widely among the hepatologists. Many recommendations has also been made regarding to liver biopsy preparation but there is still lack of evidence. The only thing is that really matters are anticoagulant use and hemostase examination. Sampling error is that something that could happened because we only use small needle and probably we could only assess small area of the liver tissue even though we have the preconditions for liver tissue sampling so it can be assessed very well by the pathologist. However, until now liver biopsy is still a gold standard to obtain information about what happened in the progression of liver diseases and of course to see the improvement of liver histology after the patients received treatment. In Advanced liver disease, we have clinical (chronic liver disease stigmata such as icteric, spider nevi, hyper pigmentation, palmar erythema, splenomegaly, ascites, caput Medusa, and leg edema), biochemical parameters (low platelet count, albumin globulin ratio, hyperbilirubinemia, abnormal hemostase, etc), and imaging studies (ultrasound, CT-scan, MRI) to confirm the diagnosis so we don't have to perform any liver biopsy. (2,3,4,5)

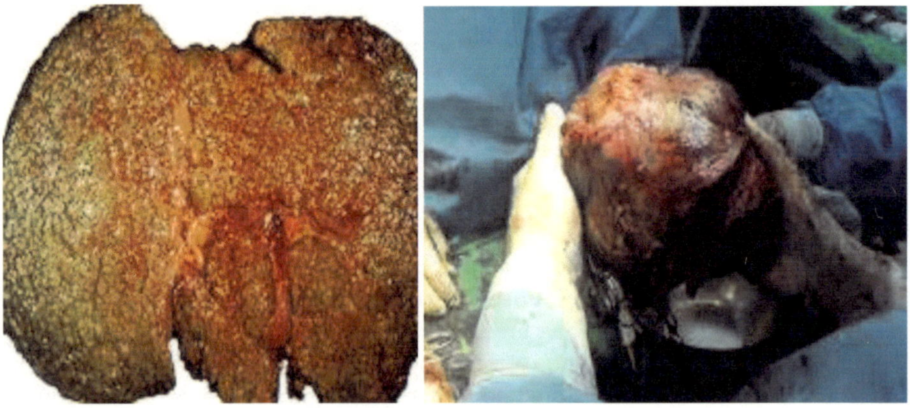

Fig. 3. Liver Cirrhosis and Hepatocellular Carcinoma Illustrations.

### 2.3 Non invasive methods in assessing liver fibrosis

The ideal non invasive methods in assessing liver fibrosis should be highly sensitive and specific, technically easy to measure, inexpensive, minimal or no side effect, and can be used easily to monitor the progression or regression of liver disease during the treatment. There are several direct and indirect serum markers that have been studied for long time to assess liver fibrosis. The direct markers such as collagens (procollagen I C peptide/PICP, procollagen III N peptide/PIIINP, type IV collagen and its fragments (NC1 and PIVNP), glycoproteins and polysaccharides (hyaluronic acid/HA, laminin, tenascin, YKL-40/chondrex), collagenase and their inhibitors (metalloproteinases/MMPs, tissue inhibitors of metalloproteinases/TIMPs), and cytokines (TGF-$\beta$1 and PDGF) are related to matrix deposition since we know that the activation process of stellate cell which is the key event of liver fibrosis is related to the increase production of MMP-1, MMP-2, and TIMPs, and leading to replacement by interstitial collagen. However, most of the studies showed the significant difference between no or mild fibrosis group (F0-F1) and moderate-severe liver fibrosis group (F2-F4) or between F0-F2 vs. F3-F4 group. (6,7,8,9,10) When it comes to differentiate between F1 and F2, most of the studies showed unsatisfied result. Mostly have not very high sensitivity when it is used to differentiate between F1 and F2. In a large cohort study, nine different markers have been evaluated in HCV, ALD, and NAFLD patients, and it is found that HA, TIMP-1, and PIIINP were selected as having the best accuracy in diagnosing F2-F4 with the AUROC were 0.77, 0.94, and 0.87. Another large study in 696 HCV patients has shown that HA, TIMP-1 and α-2-macroglobulin were having 75% accuracy in diagnosing F2-F4 with AUROC 0.82-0.83. Zhang BB et al also showed very good results of the direct serum markers such as PDGF-BB, TIMP-1, TIMP-1/MMP-1, and TIMP-1mRNA when diagnosing hepatic inflammation and fibrosis in CHB patients compared to normal control. It showed good correlations (r=0.239-0.565; *p*=0.000-0.0033), but in this study didn't show any differences between fibrosis stages. Study by Oberti et al, showed that the best diagnostic accuracy was found for HA, laminin, PIIINP, and TGF-β1, but it didn't show any diagnostic advantage when those markers were taken together. All of these markers are not liver specific as it might be influenced by some other conditions, such as inflammation at any other organs. The value of these markers in diagnosing the liver condition also can be questionable whether due to the progression of matrix deposition or recovery process after inflammation process. (6,11,12) The cost-effectiveness of the non-invasive markers is still debatable since in most countries in Asia, the price of non-invasive markers can become a problem when it comes to the market.

The indirect markers such as serum ALT levels, AST/ALT ratio, platelet count (PT), prothrombin index, and multi-combination indirect fibrosis test (Forns index, Fibro Test, APRI, PGA, PGAA, FIB-4, Hepascore and Acti Test) also have been studied for many years whether it could be used to replace liver biopsy or not. The simple indirect marker test such as ALT level seemed that is not really a good marker in hepatic fibrosis prediction since there have been many studies showed that even though patients with normal ALT could possibly have advance liver fibrosis. (8,13,14,15,16) The AST/ALT ratio showed a good predictive value in advanced liver disease, especially when combined with platelet count which has been reported mostly in CHC patients. A retrospective study by Yilmaz et al showed statistically significance for the correlation between APRI score and hepatic fibrosis in CHC (r=0.2634, *p*=0.0059) and NAFLD (r=0.2273, *p*=0.0069) patients but not in CHB (r=0.1005, *p*=0.1495) patients even though the r values showed not very strong correlation. This study also found that APRI has sensitivity 55.0% and specificity 75.4% for CHC, 60.0% and 73.3% for NAFLD, and 55% and 75.4% for CHB. (17) Another retrospective study comparing 6 non-invasive liver fibrosis markers (APRI, Fibrometer, FIB-4, Hepascore, Forns index, and Shanghai Liver Fibrosis Group/SLFG's index) showed that better correlation were found in Fibrometer (r=0.69), Hepascore (r=0.62), and SLFG (r=0.68) with METAVIR score (*p*< 0.001) of liver histopathology compared with others. Fibrometer, Hepascore, and SLFG are more representing direct markers while APRI, FIB-4, and Forns index are indirect markers. However, in this study only showed the AUROCs were better when these markers are used to differentiate between F0-F2 and F3-4 compared to F0-1 and F2-4 group. (18)

### 2.4 Imaging studies in assessing liver fibrosis

There are some imaging studies that can be used to assess the liver morphology such as ultrasound, CT-scan, and Magnetic Resonance Imaging (MRI). However, none of these modalities can be used when the differentiation between mild and early significant liver fibrosis is needed. In chronic active hepatitis, the only finding that can be found with these imaging modalities is the cirrhotic liver. (7,19) On the other side the imaging studies like CT-scan and MRI will cost a lot of money. A retrospective cross sectional study looking at comparative MR imaging studies with superparamagnetic iron oxide (SPIO)-enhanced and double-enhanced spoiled gradient echo (SPGR) sequences in 101 patients (HCV, HBV, AIH, NASH, PBC, PSC, alcoholic hepatitis, and cryptogenic) showed that qualitative and quantitative image scores were significantly higher for patients with METAVIR fibrosis scores of 3 or higher than for those with scores of 2 or lower ($p < .001$). Diagnostic performance for detection of grade 3 or more severe fibrosis was better with the doubled-enhanced sequence than with the SPIO-enhanced sequences. This study showed a good performance only when it comes to assess advanced liver fibrosis. The limitations of this study were retrospective study and only have a small number patient with mild fibrosis.(20) During the development of imaging studies, a modified phase contrast magnetic resonance (MR) imaging sequence to assess liver tissue shear waves, which is called MR elastography, also has been studied. In twelve patients with chronic liver disease (HCV, AIH, NASH, liver cirrhosis due to sarcoidosis) who underwent MR elastography, there were 11 patients with liver fibrosis (stage 1 in four patients, stage 2 in three patients, stage 3 in three patients, and stage 4 in one patient) based on histopathology results and from the imaging result showed that the mean liver stiffness was significantly higher than was found in healthy control group ($p < .001$). This preliminary study has shown that MR elastography can be used to differentiate between normal and fibrotic liver but still it needs a lot of sample to confirm these findings especially when it will be used to differentiate between mild and advance liver fibrosis. (21)

### 2.5 Transient elastography (Fibroscan) in assessing liver fibrosis

Transient Elastography (TE/Fibroscan, Echosens, Paris, France) has been introduced recently as a new tool for liver fibrosis assessment. It is an easy and user friendly technique for clinicians and very comfortable examination for the patients. The non-fasting patients lying flat on their back, with the right arm tucked behind the head to facilitate access to the right upper quadrant. The ultrasound transducer probe is mounted on the axis of a vibrator and the elastic shear wave induced by the vibrations will propagates through the liver tissue. The examination will takes only less than 5 minutes in experienced and well trained clinicians or nurses (after 100 examinations). Liver stiffness values range from 2.5 to 7.5 kPa. The validity of this examination depends on the interquartile range (IQR), which reflects the variability of the validated measures, and should not exceed 30% of the median value. The success rate should be at least 60%. The limitations of this examination are when dealing with obese patients, patients with ascites, and high ALT level. Failure rates to perform this examination in high BMI patients have been showed in several studies and the range was showed between 2.4% and 9.4%. (22,23) The level of ALT has become a major issue since many studies have shown that higher ALT will make the higher liver stiffness value. (24,25,26) Most of the TE studies in Western countries were done in CHC patients since we know that CHC is more prevalent. On the other side, most Asian countries tried to look this new tool for liver fibrosis assessment in CHB patients. There are several major issues when we look two sides of the world's perspective about this examination. First, the different etiology of the liver disease could make the difference of liver stiffness value even though there were some studies in CHB patients done in Western countries and showed the similar proposed cut off with CHC for F2. In Asian countries, many factors have been known can influence the progression of liver disease such as metabolic factors, medicines, genetic polymorphism, and viral genotype. These factors could contribute differently when compare to Western countries. Second, the liver stiffness value impact between CHC and CHB is still debatable in liver fibrosis measurement. When diagnosing the liver fibrosis progression to consider for antiviral therapy, in CHC patients probably is simpler than in CHB patients because in CHB not only the fibrosis is important but also the necroinflammation of the liver. Third, the AUROCs for F2 prediction in CHB which were reported in Asian studies found lower value than it found in Western studies. Beyond this point, study by Chan et al has showed there was a grey area in CHB patients with normal ALT between LSM 6.0-9.0 kPa, where a LSM 5.0-6.0 kPa would indicate insignificant fibrosis, a LSM >9.0 kPa had a high chance of bridging fibrosis, and that >12.0 kPa had a high chance of cirrhosis. It means in this grey zone the liver biopsy might be needed. (24,27,28) The use of TE in liver cirrhosis (LC) patients is still controversies since we have a lot of non-invasive parameters that can be used to diagnose LC. In some special conditions such as hemophilia, aplastic anemia, thrombocytopenia not related to liver disease, etc, TE might be a good consideration when those patients suffered from chronic active hepatitis virus infection (B & C).

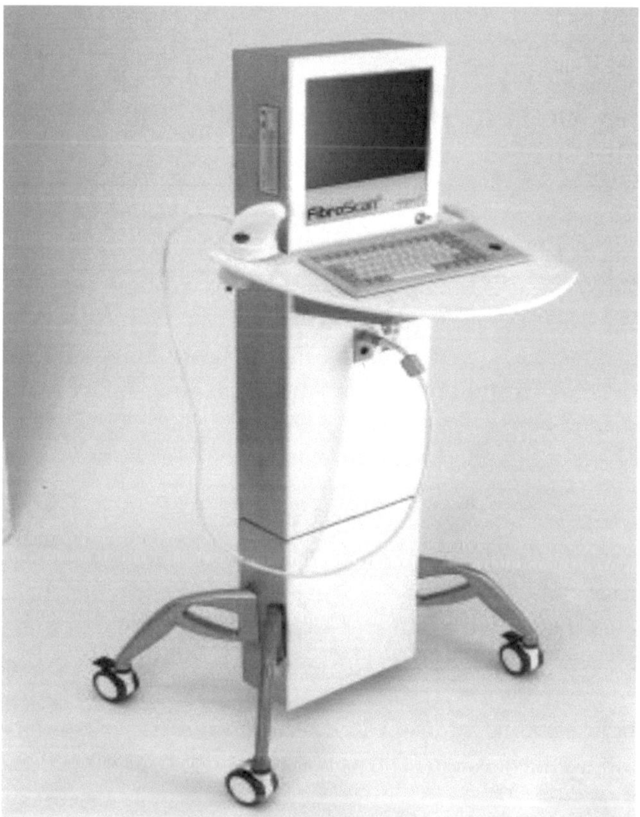


Fig. 4. Fibroscan.

### 2.6 Liver biopsy or non invasive method in clinical practice

In clinical practice, it is not about which one is better to another method in liver fibrosis assessment but it is more important to see patient to patient's problem based. The final purpose of all these is to make a better clinical decision for the patient but not for the doctor because most patients would like to know whether they have advanced fibrosis or not. Overall, we need to give more concern in patient's safety, cost-effectiveness, and of course what advantage that the patient will have from each examination for disease management.

## 3. Conclusions

Liver biopsy still has an important role in the non-invasive methods era even though the need of liver biopsy could be reduced with many kinds of non-invasive methods in liver fibrosis prediction. Further development of non-invasive methods is still needed since we haven't found the perfect non-invasive method that can entirely replace liver biopsy examination.

## 4. References

[1] Strassburg CP, Manns MP. Liver biopsy techniques in: Boyer TD, Wright TL, Manns MP, editors. Zakim and Boyer's Hepatology. A textbook of liver disease. Saunders Elsevier, Canada 2006; 5th ed; vol.1: p 195-203.

[2] Rockey DC, Caldwell SH, Goodman ZD, Nelson RC, Smith AD. Liver biopsy. Hepatol 2009; 49(3): p 1017-44.

[3] Liauw YF, Leung N, Kao JH, Piratvisuth T, Gane E, Han KH, et al. Asian pacific consensus statement on the management of chronic hepatitis B: a 2008 update. Hepatol Int 2008; 2: 263-83.

[4] Lok ASF, McMahon BJ. AASLD practice guidelines. Chronic hepatitis B: update 2009. Hepatol 2009; 50(3): 1-36.

[5] Rockey DC, Friedman SL. Hepatic fibrosis and cirrhosis in: Boyer TD, Wright TL, Manns MP, editors. Zakim and Boyer's Hepatology. A textbook of liver disease. Saunders Elsevier, Canada 2006; 5th ed; vol.1: p 87-109.

[6] Grigorescu M. Noninvasive biochemical markers of liver fibrosis. J Gastrointestin Liver Dis 2006; 15(2): 149-59.

[7] Carey E, Carey WD. Noninvasive tests for liver disease, fibrosis, and cirrhosis: is liver biopsy obsolete? CCJM 2010; 77(8): 519-27.

[8] Castera L, Pinzani M. Biopsy and non-invasive methods for the diagnosis of liver fibrosis: does it take two to tango? Gut 2010; 59: 861-88.

[9] Lesmana CRA, Hasan I, Budihusodo U, Gani RA, Krisnuhoni E, Akbar N, Lesmana LA. Diagnostic value of a group of biochemical markers of liver fibrosis in patients with non-alcoholic steatohepatitis. J Dig Dis 2009; 10: 201-6.

[10] Geramizadeh B, Janfeshan K, Saberfiroozi M. Serum hyaluronic acid as a noninvasive marker of hepatic fibrosis in chronic hepatitis B. Saudi J Gastro 2008; 14(4): 174-7.

[11] Rosenberg WMC, Voelker M, Thiel R, et al. Serum markers detect the presence of liver fibrosis: a cohort study. Gastroenterol 2004; 127: 1704-13.

[12] Patel K, Gordon SC, Jacobson I, et al. Evaluation of a panel of non-invasive serum markers to differentiate mild from moderate-to-advanced liver fibrosis in chronic hepatitis C patients. J Hepatol 2004; 41: 935-42.

[13] Lai CL, Yuen MF. The natural history and treatment of chronic hepatitis B: A critical and evaluation of standard treatment criteria and end points. Ann Intern Med 2007; 147: 58-61.

[14] Lai M, Hyatt BJ, Nasser I, Curry M, Afdhal NH. The clinical significance of persistently normal ALT in chronic hepatitis B infection. J Hepatol 2007; 47: 760-7.

[15] Nguyen MH, Garcia RT, Trinh HM, Lam KD, Weiss G, Nguyen HA, et al. Histological disease in Asian-Americans with chronic hepatitis B, high hepatitis virus DNA, and normal alanine aminotransferase levels. Am J Gastroenterol 2009; doi: 10.1038/ajg.2009.48.

[16] Lesmana CRA, Gani RA, Simadibrata M, Lesmana LA, Pakasi LS, Hasan I, et al. Histopathological findings in chronic hepatitis B patients with ALT less than 2x ULN and its correlation with various clinical variables. J Gastroenterol Hepatol 2010; 25(suppl.2): A140.

[17] Yilmaz Y, Yonal O, Kurt R, Bayrak M, Aktas B, Ozdogan O. Noninvasive assessment of liver fibrosis with the aspartate transaminase to platelet ratio index (APRI): usefulness in patients with chronic liver disease. Hepat Mon 2011; 11(2): 103-7.

[18] Wu SD, Wang JY, Li L. Staging of liver fibrosis in chronic hepatitis B patients with a composite predictive model: a comparative study. World J Gastroenterol 2010; 16(4): 501-7.

[19] Martinez SM, Crespo G, Navasa M, Forns X. Noninvasive assessment of liver fibrosis. Hepatol 2011; 53: 325-35.

[20] Aguirre DA, Behling CA, Alpert E, Hassanein TI, Sirlin CB. Liver fibrosis: noninvasive diagnosis with double contrast material-enhanced MR imaging. Radiology 2006; 239(2): 425-37.

[21] Rouviere O, Yin M, Dresner MA, Rossman PJ, Burgart LJ, Fidler JL, Ehman RL. MR elastography of the liver: preliminary results. Radiology 2006; 240(2): 440-8.

[22] Castera L, Forns X, Alberti A. Non-invasive evaluation of liver fibrosis using transient elastography. J Hepatol 2008; 48: 835-47.

[23] Sirli R, Sporea I, Deleanu A, Tudora A, Bota S, Popescu A, Danila M. Factors associated with failure of liver stiffness measurement using transient elastography. TMJ 2009; 59(1): 34-8.

[24] Chan HLY, Wong GLH, Choi PCL, Chan AWH, Chim AML, Yiu KKL, et al. Alanine aminotransferase-based algorithms of liver stiffness measurement by transient elastography (Fibroscan) for liver fibrosis in chronic hepatitis B. JVH 2009; 16: 36-44.

[25] Fung J, Lai CL, Cheng C, Wu R, Wo DKH, Yuen MF. Mild-to-moderate elevation of alanine aminotransferase increases liver stiffness measurement by transient elastography in patients with chronic hepatitis B patients. Am J Gastroenterol 2011; 106: 492-6.

[26] Myers RP, Crotty P, Layrargues, Ma M, Urbanski SJ, Elkashab M. Prevalence, risk factors and causes of discordance in fibrosis staging by transient elastography and liver biopsy. Liver Int 2010; DOI: 10.1111/j.1478-3231.2010.02331.x.

[27] Cobbold JFL, Morin S, Taylor-Robinson SD. Transient elastography for the assessment of chronic liver disease: ready for the clinic? World J Gastroenterol 2007; 13(36): 4791-7.

[28] Poggio PD, Colombo S. Is transient elastography a usefull tool for screening liver disease? World J Gastroenterol 2009; 15(12): 1409-14.

# 2

# Proposed Protocol for Histopathological Examination of Liver Specimen in Diagnosing Chronic Hepatitis

Andrzej Gabriel and Michał Kukla
*Medical University of Silesia in Katowice*
*Poland*

## 1. Introduction

The most common histopathological classification of chronic hepatitis was determined by descriptive terms, which included a subjective factor of histopathological description. It might have caused a lot of interpretative discrepancies among diagnosticians dealing with chronic liver inflammation. These difficulties led sometimes to inappropriate treatment protocol, such as the use of interferon, or caused discrepancies in the morphological rating of treatment efficiency. The first attempt of rating liver specimens in an objective way was Histological Activity Index (HAI), reported in 1981 by Knodell et al. Subsequently, many locally used modifications have been created (Lindh, Scheuer, Batts&Ludwig, Ishak, Gabriel, METAVIR). It made chronic hepatitis classification much more objective and helped in statistical analysis of research results. New diagnostic criteria of chronic liver diseases prepared in 1984 by the World Congress of Gastroenterology and International Association for the Study of the Liver (IASL) prompted authors to update previously used classifications (International Working Party, 1994). The purpose of this study is to optimize the clinical data necessary in proper diagnosis, taking into account the new criteria of inflammatory activity, process of fibrosis and steatosis.

### 2.1 Clinical part of the protocol

The points of the protocol relating to the anamnesis are to determine the nature of the disease - acute or chronic - in accordance with definition based on time criterion proposed by Leevy in 1976 (Leevy et al., 1976). Additionally, anamnesis should lead to the detection of two or more coexisting etiologic factors, for example infection with two hepatitis viruses. The protocol also considers the source of infection, as this factor may be important in determining prognostic significance, such as perinatal HBV/HCV infection, which leads to chronic state and increases the probability of developing primary liver cancer in adulthood.

The authors propose to include five hepatotrophic viruses into the protocol. Knowledge and description of the viruses will help in development of serological and immunological tests. Viral factors can be detected using:

- Indication of viral markers by immunoassay and radioimmunoassay methods (EIA and RIA),

- Polymerase Chain Reaction (PCR) in the serum,
- Fluorescence in situ hybridisation (FISH) or chromogenic in situ hybridization (CISH)
- Measurement of viral genetic material (RNA, DNA) in the serum (RT-PCR).

A large number of liver lesions are caused by toxic agents such as alcohol and long-term drug use. This aspect requires special attention in anamnesis. Less common etiologic factors in adults, but more common in children are congenital metabolic disorders such as: α1-antiprotease (α1-antitrypsin) deficiency, storage diseases, galactose intolerance or abnormal metabolism of copper and iron.

Laboratory test are divided into three groups:

- non-specific tests of liver parenchymal necrosis,
- tests to assess liver viability,
- general tests of the inflammatory process.

Radiological procedures, such us abdominal ultrasonography, bile ducts X-ray (cholecystography, cholangiography), magnetic resonance imaging (MRI) and computed tomography (CT) are the main sources of knowledge relating to the size of the liver, presence of focal lesions and some of the extrahepatic bile ducts malfunctions. If liver biopsy is performed earlier, its results should be attached. This knowledge simplifies proper diagnosis and enables assessment of the dynamics of the inflammatory and fibrotic process. The summary of the clinical part of the protocol is to establish preliminary diagnosis causing liver dysfunction. If the diagnostician is unable to establish the etiology of the disease it is possible to conduct research with additional selective histopathological techniques, such as immunohistochemical analysis of liver tissue performed using sera containing monoclonal antibodies to detect viral antigens. It is possible to use other specific techniques, PCR or hybridization *in situ*, to detect viral nucleic acids. If the clinical data is not complete and morphological picture is not characteristic, descriptive morphological diagnosis should be used. When there is the suspicion of morphological abnormalities the test for the presence of iron or copper can be performed.

## 2.2 Morphological part of the protocol

Morphological protocol describes necro-inflammatory activity, fibrosis and degenerative alteration of hepatocytes.

*Grading* for necro-inflammatory activity is based on a 4-point scale assessing the intensity of inflammatory and necrotic process - piecemeal necrosis including bridging necrosis, focal lobular necrosis and portal inflammation. The primary grading scoring system for necro-inflammatory activity proposed by Batts (Table 1) was modified by a group of Polish hepatologists and introduced to the protocol (Batts&Ludwig 1995, Gabriel et al., 1999). Piecemeal necrosis is a specific morphological change produced by a cytotoxic reaction of lymphocytes to hepatocytes. It is the death of hepatocytes at the margin of the lobule which is associated with the destruction of the limiting plate. The process extends piecemeal towards the centre of the lobule. Lymphocytes are seen adjacent to the damaged hepatocytes. The severity of lobular necrosis may encompass changes from a single foci of lymphocytic or lymphocytic-granulocytic infiltration (without hepatocyte death), through inflammatory-cell infiltration with single hepatocyte destruction to advanced confluent bridging necrosis involving a considerable portion of lobular surface with the associated collapse of the lobular stroma or perivenular confluent necrosis. The assessment of the intensity of inflammatory infiltration in portal spaces was not taken into consideration due to less prognostic significance and difficulties in objective assessment. This category of portal inflammation, according to Theise, is inappropriate for clinical evaluation as it is a defining lesion for chronic hepatitis. Furthermore, prominent lymohoid aggregates or follicles of hepatitis C might falsely inflate the severity of necroinflammatory activity compared to conditions where such lymphoid follicles are much less typical (chronic hepatitis B, autoimmune cholangitis, primary biliary cirrhosis) (Theise 2007). The presence of degenerative and regenerative changes in hepatocytes is an additional element accompanying inflammatory infiltrations and/or necrosis. It seems that these changes are of minor importance in determining the inflammatory activity and are secondary to necrosis and inflammation.

| **Grading Terminology** | | **Criteria** | |
|---|---|---|---|
| **Semiquantitative** | **Descriptive** | **Lymphocytic piecemeal necrosis** | **Lobular inflammation and necrosis** |
| 0 | Portal inflammatory only, no activity | None | None |
| 1 | Minimal | Minimal, patchy | Minimal; occasional spotty necrosis |
| 2 | Mild | Mild; involving some or all portal tracts | Mild; little hepatocellular damage |
| 3 | Moderate | Moderate; involving all portal tracts | Moderate; noticeable hepatocellular damage |
| 4 | Severe | Severe; may here bridging necrosis | Severe; prominent diffuse hepatocellular damage |

Table 1. Grading of disease activity in chronic hepatitis (Batts&Ludwig)

Another part of the protocol is the assessment of the intensity of fibrotic process - *staging*. The evaluation of fibrosis staging is based on a 4-point scale proposed by Batts&Ludwig. There are also other semi-quantitative scoring systems by METAVIR, Knodel, Desmet or Scheuer used to assess hepatitis activity but of local significance and usage. The comparison of scoring systems used by different authors for staging of chronic hepatitis is presented in Table 2. This parameter can be accurately assessed in histopathological sections after additional histochemical staining techniques for the detection of collagen fibers, such as Azan and Masson's trichrome. When pathological fibrosis is present in the liver tissue, both the number of actively formed collagen fibres and their location should be determined to assess its severity. The term 'portal fibrosis' refers to the involvement in the process of collagen fibroplasia of portal tracts alone. Periportal fibrosis means the presence of collagen fibres in portal tracts and their extension into the lobules or formation of single fibrous bridges which connect the adjacent portal tracts (portal portal fibrosis). Bridging fibrosis is the presence of fibrous bridges which connect the adjacent portal tracts or portal tracts and the central venule, which leads to architectural distortion. Bridging fibrosis and nodular regeneration correspond to stage 4 of histopathological severity. Proposed protocol does not include the scoring system proposed by Desmet, which differentiated the occurrence of porto-portal and porto-central septa as separate stages. The latter was attributed as playing a greater importance in the development of cirrhosis (Desmet 1994). The authors have added the description of advanced vascular changes to this point after consideration of the submitted proposals. It is of great importance in describing specimens of transplanted liver, especially during chronic graft rejection process. It is also useful in the evaluation of portal hypertension.

| Score | **Description** | **Knodell et al. (1981)** | **Desmet et al. (1994)** | **Scheuer (1991)** |
|---|---|---|---|---|
| **0** | No fibrosis | No fibrosis | None | None |
| **1** | Mild fibrosis | Fibrosis portal expansion | Periportal fibrous expansion | Enlarged, fibrotic portal tracts |
| **2** | Moderate fibrosis | | Porto-portal septa ( ≥ 1 septum) | Periportal or portal-portal septa, but intact architecture |
| **3** | Severe fibrosis | Bridging fibrosis (portal-portal or portal-central linkage) | Porto-central septa ( ≥ 1 septum) | Fibrosis with architectural distortion, but no obvious cirrhosis |
| **4** | Cirrhosis | Cirrhosis | Cirrhosis | Probable or definite cirrhosis |

Table 2. Scoring systems for staging of chronic hepatitis.

Additional morphological features of lesser importance are ballooning degeneration, steatosis, cholestasis, bilirubinostasis, state of bile in ducts and ductules. The presence of ballooning degeneration and steatosis may indicate toxic damage or metabolic disorders such as non-alcoholic fatty liver disease/non-alcoholic steatohepatitis (NAFLD/NASH). Determining the degree of steatosis is important in liver transplant eligibility. 70% of cases of infections with HCV (mostly genotype 3a HCV) is associated with the presence of steatosis. Hepatic steatosis in the course of chronic hepatitis C is one of the risk factors for

fibrosis progression. Moreover, steatosis decreases the rate of sustained response for antiviral therapy.
Estimation of steatosis extent with numerical semi-quantitative assessment is commonly used in NAFLD. Many scoring scales were proposed. Currently the most widely used are the scales proposed by Brunt, Kleiner, Mendler and Dixon. The scoring system proposed by Kleiner et al. estimating NAFLD activity score (NAS) seems to be most suitable due to its simple and clear grading of steatosis and ballooning degeneration. The scoring scale proposed by Kleiner et al. is presented in Table 3.

| **NAFLD Activity Score (NAS) (0-8)** | | |
|---|---|---|
| Sum of scores for steatosis, lobular inflammation and hepatocellular ballooning. | | |
| **Steatosis (0-3)** | **Hepatocyte ballooning (0-2)** | **Lobular inflammation (0-3)** |
| **0** - 5% hepatocytes involved | **0** – none | **0** – none |
| **1** – 5-33% of hepatocytes involved | **1** – few ballooned cells | **1** - <2 foci per x 200 field |
| **2** - 33-66% hepatocytes involved | **2** – many cells / prominent ballooning | **2** – 2-4 foci per x 200 field |
| **3** - >66% hepatocytes involved | | **3** - >4 foci per x 200 field |
| **Correlation between total NAFLD activity scores and an overall histological diagnosis of steatohepatitis** | | |
| NAFLD activity score | Histological diagnosis of steatohepatitis | |
| **≥5** | Probable or define NASH | |
| **3-4** | Uncertain NASH | |
| **≤2** | Not NASH | |

Table 3. Scoring system according to Kleiner et al.

Cholestasis is usually observed in chronic biliary diseases such as primary liver cirrhosis, primary sclerosing cholangitis and autoimmune cholangitis. Cholestasis in acute phase of infection is typical for viral infections, but it occurs rarely during chronic and autoimmune hepatitis. Accurate assessment of biliary tracts within portal spaces is important for determining the stage of primary biliary cirrhosis, primary sclerosing cholangitis and autoimmune processes of destruction of the bile ducts during chronic graft rejection. Regenerative proliferation of bile ductules is accompanied by advanced changes in organ architecture in cases of chronic inflammations with high activity and in the course of cirrhosis.
The last point of the morphological protocol is biopsy-point rating, which seems to be useful for statistical evaluation of process activity. A justified criticism of the approach proposed by Knodell et al. is that it incorporates necro-inflammatory activity and fibrosis into an overall grade (Knodell et al., 1981). This implies that these two histological features increase in parallel to each other. The morphological component of the protocol involves a detailed description of the specimen, which helps for proper interpretation by the clinician. The last point of the protocol is to establish a final diagnosis with the use of descriptive terminology

(hepatitis with minimal, mild, moderate, severe inflammatory activity [grade], portal, periportal, septal fibrosis, cirrhosis [stage]).

There are several possibilities as to how to compose the final conclusion:

a. The unequivocal histopathological picture is indictive for…
b. The histopathological picture, aside from the clinical data, can lead to diagnosis.
c. The unequivocal diagnosis is not possible due to i.e. disintegrated material, improper fixing of material, non-representative material.

If the etiology is unknown, the pathologist may propose additional tests. When the clinical data is not complete, the morphological picture is not characteristic or specimen is insufficient for certain diagnosis – the biopsy specimen is shorter than 25 mm or includes less than 11 portal tracts – delineation of morphological features and alterations should be carried out. *Staging* and *grading* is allowed only for the assessment of biopsy specimens which fulfill all of the above mentioned criteria.

Additional tests can be performed in the case of morphological abnormalities - the Prussian blue reaction in Perl's test for iron presence, rhodamine according to Lindqvist for copper deposits, PAS following digestion with diastase for α1-antiprotease.

Results of prior biopsy should be attached. This allows for the assessment of the dynamics of the inflammatory or fibrotic process.

The summary of the clinical part of the protocol is to establish preliminary diagnosis of liver dysfunction.

If the diagnostician is unable to establish the etiology of the disease, it is possible to conduct research with additional selective histopathological techniques, such as immunohistochemical analysis of liver tissue performed using sera containing monoclonal antibodies to detect viral antigens. It is possible to use other specific techniques, PCR or hybridization *in situ*, FISH and CISH to detect viral nucleic acids.

## 2.3 Difficulties in the differential diagnosis of chronic hepatitis

So far, pathologists have generally determined the degree and extent of hepatitis activity or progression of disease. Lobular inflammatory cell infiltration tends to predominate in acute phases of hepatitis, while portal and periportal inflammation is characteristic of chronic state. Portal hepatitis is a frequent form of chronic inflammation, consisting of infiltrations which comprise lymphocytes, plasma cells and macrophages. Plasma cells are predominant in autoimmune hepatitis alongside destruction of bile ducts with lymphocytic infiltration. Aggregates of lymphocytes or lymph follicles are observed in approximately 50% of chronic hepatitis C patients. When portal hepatitis is not accompanied by periportal or lobular infiltrations, the process is described as non-active. When periportal hepatitis is associated with focal hepatocyte destruction, the process is termed piecemeal necrosis. Mild inflammation, involving portal tracts is known as portal hepatitis. It is difficult to differentiate between true chronic hepatitis and non-specific hepatitis, or reactive chronic hepatitis, which accompanies a number of systemic diseases. When piecemeal necrosis or marked lobular necrosis coexists with inflammatory cells infiltrations, chronic hepatitis should be suspected. Marked fibrosis (septal fibrosis/cirrhosis) suggests chronic hepatitis or chronic biliary disease. If mild inflammatory infiltration in portal tracts exists as separate alteration, the condition is described as chronic reactive hepatitis. The diagnosis of chronic liver disease cannot be stated only on the basis of histopathological assessment and must be supported by clinical data (disease duration at least 6 months).

## 2.4 Proposed protocol for histopathological examination of liver biopsy specimen

**ID History**

| | | |
|---|---|---|
| **First Name** | | **Address:** |
| **Last name** | | |
| **Date of birth** | | |

| | |
|---|---|
| (Preliminary) **Clinical diagnosis** | |
| **Since when has he/she been ill?** *(month, year)* | |
| **Has he/she ever suffered from hepatitis?** *(year)* | |
| **What type**? *(if documented)* | |
| **The way of infection** | |
| **Completed hepatitis vaccination** | |

| | | |
|---|---|---|
| **Other diseases** | *metabolic diseases* | |
| | *other* | |

| | | | |
|---|---|---|---|
| **BMI** | *kg/m²* | **Height** | *cm* |
| **Body weight** | *kg* | **Waist circumference** | *cm* |
| | | **Hip circumference** | *cm* |

| | | |
|---|---|---|
| **Drugs used:** | *Actually* | |
| | *Formerly* | |
| **Alcohol** *(average amount per week)* | | |

**Etiological factors examined**
*(serological methods and molecular biology)*

| **HBV** | **HCV** | **HDV** | **Others** |
|---|---|---|---|
| HBsAG ...<br>Anty HBs...<br>HBeAg ...<br>Anty HBe...<br>Anty HBc...<br>DNA-HBV (*PCR)* ...<br>HBV-DNA *(pg/ml)* ... | Anty HCV ...<br>RNA HCV*(PCR)* ...<br>Viral genotype ...<br>Viral load (IU/ml) ... | Anty HDV ...<br><br>RNA-HDV*(pg/ml)* .... | HAV ...<br>HGV ...<br><br>HIV ...<br>CMV ...<br>HSV ... |

**Radiology** *(USG, CT, MRI, bile ducts X-ray)*

**Laboratory tests**

| | | | |
|---|---|---|---|
| pANCA | | Total protein | ........................... |
| ANA | ............... | Albumin: | ........................... |
| SMA | ............... | Globulin: | |
| LKM-1 | ............... | *α1* | ........................... |
| AMA | ............... | *α2* | ........................... |
| IgG | ............... | *β* | ........................... |
| α1 AT level | ............... | *γ* | ........................... |

**a) parenchymal necrosis tests:**

| | | | |
|---|---|---|---|
| ALT | .................. | AST | .................. |

**b)**

| | | | | | |
|---|---|---|---|---|---|
| alkaline phosphatase | ............ | GGTP | ............ | bilirubin | ............... |
| TIBC | ............ | Fe | ............ | ferritin | ............... |
| cholesterol | ............ | HDL | ............ | LDL | ................ |
| triglycerides | ............ | ceruloplasmin | ............ | glucose | ................ |

**c) blood morphology**

| | | | | | |
|---|---|---|---|---|---|
| RBC | ............ | WBC | ............ | Neutrophils | ............... |
| HGB | ............ | | | Lymphocytes | ............... |
| HCT | ............ | | | Monocytes | ............... |
| MCV | ............ | PLT | ............ | Eosynophils | ............... |

**d) inflammatory process test**

| | | | |
|---|---|---|---|
| CRP | .................. | Erythrocyte sedimentation rate | .................. |

**e) coagulation**

| | | | | | |
|---|---|---|---|---|---|
| INR | .................. | prothrombin index | .................. | fibrinogen | .................. |

**Short course of the disease: results of the former liver biopsy (Nr... Date...)**

date and signature of physician

## Histopathology

**Immunohistochemical and in situ hybridisation tissue tests:**

Etiologic factors.......................................................................

HBsAg...... HCVAg................. HBV DNA (PCR/CISH or FISH)

HBcAg......... HDVAg................. HCV RNA (PCR/CISH or FISH)

HBeAg.........

Staining for the presence of: Fe........... Cu.............. α1- antiprotease.................

| **Inflammatory activity grade**<br>*Criteria* | | |
|---|---|---|
| **Score *** | **piecemeal necrosis-range** | **lobular inflammation and necrosis** |
| **0** | none | none |
| **1** minimal | single | minimal grade inflammation, single focal necrosis |
| **2** mild | occupying single portal areas | low grade inflammation, slight destruction of hepatocytes |
| **3** moderate | occupying all portal areas | moderate grade inflammation, noticeable destruction of hepatocytes |
| **4** severe | occupying all portal areas | high grade inflammation, prominent diffuse hepatocellular damage, the presence of bridging or perivenular necrosis |

| **Regressive changes in hepatocytes** | |
|---|---|
| Ballooning degeneration grade..............<br>Score** | Steatosis grade..............<br>Score** |
| 0 – none | 0 – <5% hepatocytes involved |
| 1 – few ballooned cells | 1 – 5-33% hepatocytes involved |
| 2 – many cells or prominent ballooning | 2 – 33-66% hepatocytes involved |
| | 3 – >66% hepatocytes involved |

**Regenerative changes in hepatocytes** (dysplasia).........................................

| Stage of fibrosis | | |
|---|---|---|
| **Score *** | **Fibrosis** | **Criteria** |
| **0** | no fibrosis | normal amount of connective tissue |
| **1** | fibrosis of portal area | occupation of portal areas by fibrosis |
| **2** | periportal fibrosis | periportal fibrosis or single bridges portal-portal |
| **3** | bridging fibrosis | many fibrous bridges with distortion of hepatic architecture |
| **4** | cirrhosis | cirrhosis |

**Cholestasis and bilirubinostasis**………………………………………
Changes in vessels……………………………

**Scoring**

inflammation … steatosis … ballooning … fibrosis …

Histopathological description:

Additional studies proposed ………………………………………………

**Final diagnosis** ……………………………………………………….

**In descriptive terminology** ……………………………………………………….

**Proposed differentiation** ……………………………………………………….

date and signature of physician

*According to modified Batts & Ludwig scoring system
** According to Kleiner scoring system

## 3. Conclusion

A standardized universal protocol of liver biopsy such as the proposed scheme will facilitate the diagnosis of patients with suspected chronic liver disease. Obtaining complete and accurate clinical data by pathologists will allow more precise interpretation of observed

histological findings and will point to the necessity of additional tests. The histopathological picture should be assessed independently by two experienced pathologists in the case of research. In normal practice assessment by one experienced hepato-pathologist is accurate. In the future, in the final version of the protocol, histopathological data should be stored in a database especially prepared for pathologists.
The prevalence of this protocol will unify the terminology used so far and will reduce differences in interpretation between the various centers. Modern treatment of chronic liver diseases is very expensive, especially in the case of viral infections. It requires a strict eligibility of patients for therapy. We hope that application of this protocol will assist in the proper use of financial resources thus leading to an increase in the number of complete recoveries.

## 4. Acknowledgment

The authors would like to thank professors Adam Nowosławski and Julian Stolarczyk for their helpful suggestions and remarks. The authors would also like to thank the group of Polish hepato-pathology experts (Adam Ziółkowski, Wojciech Szczepański, Bożena Walewska-Zielecka, Janusz Miętkiewski) who prepared the recommendations for morphological assessment of liver biopsy specimens. Also many thanks to Dr. Krzysztof Tomaszek for helping prepare the final manuscript.

## 5. References

Batts, T. & Ludwig, J. (1995). *Chronic hepatitis. An update on terminology and reporting*. Am J Surg Pathol ,Vol.19, pp. 1409-1419

Desmet, V.J. et al. (1994). *Classification of chronic hepatitis: diagnosis, grading and staging*. Hepatology, Vol.19, pp.1513–1520.

Gabriel, A. et al., (1999). *Podsumowanie wstępne dotyczące wypracowania standardu oceny histopatologicznej bioptatów w przebiegu przewlekłych zapaleń wątroby* - Katowice 15.04.1999 Pol J Pathol ,Vol.50, No 4, supp.1, pp.31-32 (in Polish).

International Working Party (1994). Terminology of chronic hepatitis. Am J Gastroenterol, Vol.90 pp.181

Kleiner, D.E. et al. (2005) Design and validation of histological scoring system for non-alcoholic fatty liver disease. Hepatology, Vol. 41, pp.1313-1321.

Knodell, R.G. et al. (1981). *Formulation and application of a numerical scoring system for assessing histological activity in asymptomatic chronic active hepatitis*. Hepatology, Vol.1, pp.431–43

Theise, N.D.(2007). *Liver biopsy assesment in chronic viral hepatitis: a personal, practical approach.* Modern Pathology, Vol.20, pp.3-14

# 3

# Principles of the Biopsy Procedure

Anna Piekarska
*Medical University of Łódź*
*Poland*

## 1. Introduction

A liver biopsy is a procedure where a small piece of liver tissue or liver cells are removed for microscopic examination. Taking a liver biopsy specimen for a microscopic examination can be performed in two ways: blind and guided liver biopsy.

### 2.1 Blind biopsy

The first, most common type of biopsy is a **core-needle, blind biopsy**.

In this procedure a small piece of liver tissue is taken from the organ with the use of needle which diameter is 1.2 - 1.6 mm. The principle of this procedure is that the morphology of the liver specimen is the same as the morphology of whole organ. The size of the tissue sample taken from the liver enables the pathologist to evaluate the cell composition and to describe the location of particular cells in relation to other cells.

Indications for a core-needle liver biopsy are presented in Table1.

A core-biopsy can be performed as: a percutaneous core -needle biopsy, a transvenous (transjugular) core-needle biopsy, laparoscopic liver biopsy, open wedge (surgical) biopsy.

#### 2.1.1 A percutaneous core -needle biopsy

This type of biopsy is the most frequent. Indications are presented in Table 1. Percutaneous core-needle biopsy can be performed relatively easy. It can be performed in local anesthesia with the use of basic equipment.

#### 2.1.2 A transvenous (transjugular) core-needle biopsy

This technique of performing a liver biopsy is indicated in patients with the increased risk of bleeding (e.g. thrombocytopenia), since in case of bleeding from biopsy site, liver blood directly flows to the lumen of hepatic vein and therefore it does not cause a subcapsular hematoma or bleeding into body cavities. However, the transvenous biopsy is a more invasive technique than the percutaneous biopsy. It requires technical resources (imaging equipment) and is more expensive.

#### 2.1.3 Laparoscopic liver biopsy

The laparoscopic surgery in the upper abdomen enables to take a liver tissue for pathological examination. However, the necessity to make a liver biopsy is hardly ever an indication for performing a laparoscopic surgery. Liver biopsy made with the use of this technique most frequently accompanies other medical procedures (e.g. cholecystectomy).

| Disease entity | Reason for performing biopsy | Comments |
|---|---|---|
| Chronic viral hepatitis B and C | 1. Confirmation of clinical diagnosis<br>2. Assessment of grading of inflammation and staging of fibrosis | In many cases – necessary to qualify a patient for antiviral treatment |
| Alcoholic hepatitis<br>Non-alcoholic fatty liver disease<br>Autoimmune hepatitis | 1. Confirmation of clinical diagnosis<br>2. Assessment of progression of disease | Most often it serves as a tool for differential diagnosis |
| Hemochromatosis | 1.Setting a diagnosis<br>2. Quantitative evaluation of liver iron level | |
| Wilson's disease | | |
| Primary biliary cirrhosis | 1. Confirmation of clinical diagnosis<br>2. Assessment of progression of disease | |
| Primary sclerosing cholangitis | 1.Setting a diagnosis<br>2. Differential diagnosis of cholestasis | Liver biopsy is indicated when diagnosis is not possible on the basis of imaging |
| Drug-induced liver disease | 1. Confirmation of clinical diagnosis<br>2. Assessment of progression of disease | |
| Evaluation of transplanted liver in a recipient | 1. Diagnosis of acute or chronic transplant rejection<br>2. Post – transplant viral hepatitis | |
| Fever of unknown origin | 1.Setting a diagnosis | |
| Anomalous levels of liver enzymes of unknown origin | 1.Setting a diagnosis | |

Table 1. Indications for a core-needle blind liver biopsy

### 2.1.4 Open wedge (surgical) liver biopsy

A small piece of subcapsular liver tissue can be obtained during laparotomy.

The piece of tissue taken during open surgery is usually bigger than the specimen taken percutaneously. However, the tissue is often damaged due to the technique of excision and handling of specimen during surgery. Moreover the subcapsular specimen may not be fully representative for morphology of liver diease.

### 2.2 Guided liver biopsy

The second type of biopsy is a core-needle or fine-needle-aspiration biopsy.
Guided biopsy is aimed at diagnostics of focal lesions in liver and must be performed under visual control. In most cases ultrasonography is used for this purpose. Computed tomography is used less frequently.
The use of a fine needle allows for aspiration of liver cells only. The obtained biological material consists of liver cell which are not bound to each other and immersed in liquid material. This type of biopsy is used for diagnostics of focal changes in liver - filled with liquid or hypoechogenic (e.g. cysts).
However, for diagnostics of solid focal changes in liver (tumour metastasis, hepato-cellular carcinoma) core needle biopsy is recommended. This technique allows for obtaining a tumour tissue, which considerably facilitates setting a diagnosis.

## 3. A place of liver biopsy in diagnostic workup in liver disease

It should be underlined that a decision to make a biopsy is one of the last steps taken in diagnostics of liver diseases. In view of the fact that the method is invasive and has its limitations, it should be performed only when it is supposed to provide information necessary for treatment of the patient. Below there is a list of information about the patient and additional examinations which should be made before taking a decision of performing a biopsy.

### 3.1 Hepatological diagnostics before taking a liver biopsy

Before performing a biopsy one should try to establish the cause of the liver disease on the basis of non-invasive examinations so as to gather as much information as possible for the pathologist examining the specimen referring to etiology, progression of the liver disease. Following tests should be made in each patient:

- blood cell count (pancytopenia might imply portal hypertension)
- biochemical (ALT, AST, ALP, GTP, bilirubin), indicating the presence of hepatocyte necrosis and cholestasis
- viral markers (anti-HAV IgM, HBsAg, HBeAg, anti-HBc-total, anti-HCV, anti-delta)
- molecular examinations - depending on the results received above. (HBV-DNA quantitatively, HCV-RNA quantitatively)
- antibody analysis (ANA, AMA, ASMA, anti-LKM, anti-SLA)
- proteinogram
- *in justified cases* - examination for presence of Wilson's disease (plasma ceruloplasmin level, plasma copper level, copper excretion via urine), hemochromatosis (plasma ferritin level, plasma iron level, possibly analysis of mutation of C282Y and H63D genes)
- ultrasonography examination of a liver and evaluation with the use of Doppler analysis of potential presence of portal hypertension

**The age of the patient** is often a determining factor as for the decision about performing a liver biopsy and the way in which it should be performed. In case of children and young adults (younger than 16 years old) parents often do not give consent to a liver biopsy and they demand less invasive diagnostic methods. Moreover, children who are subjected to a percutaneous biopsy, should undergo a short-term general anesthesia. In the case of elderly patients the doctor should decide whether the information gathered after taking a liver biopsy specimen will considerably influence further treatment. For example: elderly patients suffering from chronic hepatitis C very often have numerous contraindications for interferon and ribavirin therapy. Therefore, a liver biopsy as a tool for qualification to antiviral treatment is useless in this setting.

**A free consent** to liver biopsy.

In every case the written consent for the procedure should be obtained from the patient or his committee. The patient should achieve complete information about indications for the procedure, diagnostic benefits and potential complications.

**Cooperation of the patient** is a crucial element qualifying him for liver biopsy.

The procedure performed in local anesthesia involves inserting a needle when the patient has exhaled the air. Inhaling or moving the body when the doctor inserts a needle might lead to liver rupture and massive hemorrhage. The patient must be informed about such possibility and should be taught to control his breathing. If, in the doctor's opinion, it is not possible (small children, patients with mental or behavioral disorders), the patient should be given short-term general anesthesia. Otherwise the procedure should be abandoned. Moreover, the patient is then asked to stay in bed for 3 hours following the procedure.

**Body mass (BMI).** In obese patients (>30 BMI) it might be difficult to take a liver biopsy specimen percutaneously because of thick subcutaneous fatty tissue.

**Concomitant diseases** (e.g. circulatory insufficiency, scoliosis) might hamper performing a liver biopsy as it might be difficult to put the patient in the appropriate position and make him stay in that position for more than 10 minutes. Those suffering from hemophilia are usually disqualified from this kind of procedure because of the increased risk of bleeding.

**Allergy to medicaments** used for local anesthesia (e.g. lidocaine) might make the percutaneous biopsy impossible to perform.

The information on **medicaments taken** by the patient for a longer period, especially anticoagulant medications (salicylic acid, acenocumarol) is crucial when the liver biopsy is planned. Patient should stop taking salicylic acid for one week before the liver biopsy. Administering of acenocumarol should be stopped two days before the liver biopsy. If it is not possible the doctor should perform transvenous biopsy or should not perform the biopsy at all.

**Menstrual cycle** phase should be considered in female patients. Biopsy should not be made during menstruation (1 – 5 day) because of the increased risk of liver bleeding.

## 4. Answers a liver biopsy can give

- In majority cases of acute viral hepatitis liver biopsy is not performed. The diagnosis can be set on the base of biochemical and serologic examinations. The exceptions are the patients in whom on the base of other examinations and anamnesis it is not possible to determine whether they suffer from chronic or acute hepatitis. Since pathomorphological findings in these two kinds of hepatitis are different, liver biopsy might be helpful in setting the right diagnosis and qualifying for treatment. It is important as the treatment of these diseases differ a lot.
- In case of chronic viral hepatitis B and C morphological evaluation of a liver biopsy specimen helps to assess the grade and stage of the diasease (according to one of

assessment scales). In routine diagnostics the pathological examination of specimen does not help to discover etiology. The results of assessment of grade of inflammation and stage of fibrosis serve as a tool for qualification for treatment. Besides, morphological analysis facilitates diagnosing other liver diseases which accompany viral hepatitis (fatty liver disease, alcoholic liver disease, autoimmune hepatitis). Morphological analysis also helps to evaluate remission of changes after antiviral treatment.

- Alcoholic liver disease (ALD) can be diagnosed without an analysis of the specimen in most cases. In any doubts, biopsy helps to set the right diagnosis, evaluate the fibrosis and presence of other inflammatory processes (e.g. AIH).
- Biopsy specimen analysis is crucial in the case of non-alcoholic fatty liver disease (NAFLD) since additional analysis (biochemical and serologic) allow to exclude existence of other liver diseases. Morphological analysis helps to differentiate NAFLD and non-alcoholic steatohepatitis (NASH), evaluate accumulation of fat in hepatocytes in Dixon's scale as well as consequences of the disease manifested by progression of fibrosis.
- Suspicion of the presence of autoimmune hepatitis (AIH) is an indication for liver biopsy. Morphological analysis helps to set a diagnosis in the case of unclear results of autoantibodies, differentiate e.g. AIH and ALD and evaluate the progression of the disease and its consequences - fibrosis and cirrhosis. Morphological analysis also proves how effective the applied treatment is.
- Diagnosing liver metabolic diseases (Wilson's disease, hemochromatosis) without morphological analysis might be impossible to do. Morphological analysis not only enables to set the right diagnosis and differentiate with other liver diseases but also helps to make a quantitative evaluation of iron in the liver biopsy specimen, which is significant for further therapy.

## 5. Answers a liver biopsy cannot give

Liver biopsy should not be made:

- if the diagnosis can be established with the use of non-invasive methods,
- if the information gathered does not change decisions as for the therapy,
- if biopsy might be a health hazard.

Therefore, the biopsy should not be performed in patients with decompensated liver cirrhosis. When the clinical diagnosis is obvious (ascites, oedema, jaundice, symptoms of portal hypertension) the liver biopsy will not give more diagnostic information and will not influence on the choice of treatment method. Besides, in the case of hemorrhagic diathesis which accompanies cirrhosis, the liver biopsy may lead to hemorrhage. As medical practice shows, in patients suffering from cirrhosis, it is difficult or even impossible to obtain a representative liver biopsy specimen. Moreover, the specimen is often small and dismembered, which makes the pathologic examination almost impossible.

## 6. Diagnostic workup before commencing a liver biopsy

Set of tests which should be performed during last 24 hours before core biopsy is presented in Table 2.

| Analysis | Comments |
|---|---|
| Blood cell count | The number of platelets should exceed 60,000/μl, to avoid bleeding |
| Blood group | Identifying blood group before the biopsy allows for faster blood transfusion in the event of possible hemorrhage |
| Coagulogical analysis | Prothrombin time should not exceed the reference value by more than 4 seconds (INR>1.4)<br>Activated partial thromboplastic time (APTT) should not exceed the reference value by 1.5 times |
| Image examination (e.g. USG, CT) | Excluding focal lesions in the liver |

Table 2. Set of tests which should be made directly before blind liver biopsy.

## 7. The choice of type of liver biopsy

Focal changes discovered in ultrasound examination or computed tomography are indications for an image-controlled biopsy.

In patient with chronic hepatitis in whom a solid focal change is diagnosed two USG-guided core biopsies should be made. The first specimen should be obtain from the solid lesion. The other should be obtained from other part of liver (with the avoidance of lesion volume).

## 8. How to prepare a patient to liver biopsy

On the day of biopsy the patients is advised to remain fast. He should be examined by the physician performing the procedure. Fever, cough, bleeding or circulatory insufficiency diagnosed prior to the biopsy should be temporary contraindications for it. Thirty minutes before the surgery the patient is sedated with 5 mg of diazepam administered intramuscularly.

## 9. Anesthesia

In adults and children who can cooperate during the procedure (usually above 15 years of age) liver biopsy is made in local anesthesia. To do it one should use 8-10 ml of 1% lidocaine solution. The technique of anesthesia is described below (Point 10). When the patient is not willing to cooperate, the procedure should be performed in short-term general anesthesia.

## 10. Technique of core biopsy

### 10.1 The position of the patient

The patient should be in supine position, with his right upper limb placed behind the head, the left one - along the body. Intercostals spaces should be as wide as possible (middle armpit line should be in the shape of arch).

### 10.2 Determining the area of biopsy

Upper and lower limits of liver dullness should be established with the use of percussion. Next, the physician should mark the area of biopsy in the intercostals space, in the middle of liver dullness, on the middle armpit line or anterior armpit line.

### 10.3 Antiseptics

After putting on sterile gloves the area of biopsy should be cleansed twice with antiseptic substance and the skin should be left to dry.

### 10.4 Local anesthesia

The anesthesia should be done in the place selected beforehand. Lidocaine solution should be injected subcutaneously and later on, the needle must be inserted deeper, inside the intercostals space, continuously injecting a solution. Once the needle touches the capsule the needle should be slowly withdrawn and the solution – administered.

### 10.5 Liver biopsy

After application of anesthetic, the assisting nurse opens a set for liver biopsy. It consists of a blockage controlled syringe, a biopsy needle, a hypodermic needle and a blade.
The first activity involves putting a hypodermic needle for on the blockage controlled syringe and then aspiration of 4 ml of aseptic solution of isotonic salt in such a way that the "brake" in the syringe remains in the unblocked position. Next, the hypodermic needle should be taken off and replaced with the biopsy needle. The syringe with the biopsy needle should be put aside in a sterile place and with the use of scalpel the doctor should make an incision - 2 to 3 mm long - in the intercostals space skin. Then the needle biopsy should be placed inside the incision as deep as to the liver capsule. At this moment the needle should be moved a few milimetres backwards. The patient should inhale air, exhale it to the end and then hold his breath. At the moment the patients does not breathe the doctor should inject about 2 ml of isotonic salt and then, pull the piston to block the "brake" and quickly move the needle in the direction of liver to the depth of about 3 cm and take it out immediately. After removing the needle from the intercostals space the patient should be allowed to breathe freely. With a sterile gauze pad one should press the area where the liver specimen has been taken since the skin might start bleeding a little. After putting a sterile dressing on the biopsy area the biopsy needle should be emptied , which should be done by unblocking the "brake" of the syringe. The content of the needle should be put in a prepared container with formalin solution. Then the doctor performing the biopsy should macroscopically evaluate the size of the taken specimen. If it is too small or dismembered too much, the procedure should be repeated.

## 11. References

[1] Scheuer PJ & Lefkowitch JH. *Liver Biopsy Interpretation*. 7th Edition. Edinburgh: Elsevier

[2] Sherlock S & Dooley J. (2002). *Diseases of the Liver and Biliary System*. 11th ed. Oxford: Blackwell Science

[3] Bruno MA, Rodríguez Fuchs C, Gallo J, González Boix J. (1990) *Percutaneous hepatic biopsy puncture in patients with hemostasis disorders. A new technique. Acta Gastroenterol Latinoam,* Vol.20, No1, pp. 25-30

[4] M Horejsová & F Koukolík (1989). *Thin-needle aspiration biopsy under ultrasonic control. The examination technic.* Casopis Lekaru Ceskych, Volume: 128, Issue: 49.

[5] Gutkowski K. *Percutaneous liver biopsy - indications, contraindications and possible complications.* (2004) Nether J Med, Vol. 62, pp. 441-5

# 4

# Immunological Analysis of Liver Diseases with Liver Biopsy Specimens

Kazuto Tajiri[1] and Yukihiro Shimizu[2]
[1]*The Third Department of Internal Medicine, University of Toyama, Toyama*
[2]*Gastoenterology Unit, Takaoka City Hospital, Toyama*
*Japan*

## 1. Introduction

Most liver diseases are caused by host immune responses, and there have been many studies on the analysis of circulating lymphocyte subsets and their production of cytokines in patients with liver diseases. Although circulating lymphocytes are relatively easy to obtain and analyze, analysis of intrahepatic lymphocytes would be more important for understanding the immunopathogenesis of liver diseases, especially, viral hepatitis and autoimmune liver diseases.

Two approaches are currently available to analyze intrahepatic lymphocytes in liver biopsy specimens, an immunohistochemical approach and a flow cytomeric analysis of isolated lymphocytes from liver tissues. Although use of an immunohistochemical approach would allow the distribution of particular lymphocyte subsets to be determined, quantitative estimation of infiltrating lymphocyte populations may be incorrect. In contrast, flow cytometry can determine the precise percentages of each lymphocyte population, but it does not provide any information on their intrahepatic distribution. The use of multiple antibodies to identify lymphocyte subsets can enable multi color flow cytometric analysis, revealing the precise percentages of each subset, even those constituting an extremely minor subset of lymphocytes. Moreover, molecular biological approaches have been used to analyze the immunopathogenesis of liver diseases.

This chapter summarizes findings obtained from the immunological analyses of biopsied liver tissues and how immunological analyses of liver biopsy specimens have contributed to the understanding of the immunopathogenesis of liver diseases. We also describe recent technical advances in the immunological analyses of liver biopsy specimens that can further enhance our understanding of the pathogenesis of liver diseases.

## 2. Methods for analyzing immunological responses in the liver

### 2.1 Immunohistochemical approach (Luttmann et al., 2006)

Immunohistochemical methods can be used to characterize and localize liver-infiltrating cells and proteins such as cytokines, as well as quantitate their degree of infiltration, information essential for the analysis of local immune responses. Paraffin-fixed and frozen liver biopsy specimens, as well as specimens fixed by other methods, can be analyzed, although the immunogenicity of some antigens can be usually better preserved by cryofixation than by chemical fixation. The underlying principle of the immunohistochemical approach is the binding of an antigen by a specific antibody (the first antibody). The first antibody is usually labeled with a fluorochrome, enzyme, or particle. If an unlabeled antibody is used, the secondary antibody must be labeled. Staining with labeled primary antibodies results in better detection of antigens, with less nonspecific background staining. Although high concentrations of antibodies can detect small amounts of antigens, higher antibody concentrations are associated with increased nonspecific binding. Therefore, the specific detection of each antigen requires the optimal dilution of each antibody as well as an optimal incubation period and temperature. As an example, we describe the immunohistochemical detection of antigen, using both a primary and a secondary antibody, in paraffin-fixed tissue samples.

Paraffin-fixed tissue samples must firstly be deparaffinized and rehydrated. Sections are then immersed in 10 mM citrate buffer, pH 6.0, and heated in a microwave oven for antigen retrieval. Alternatively, sections can be heated in a water bath, autoclave, or steam pot, or incubated with proteolytic enzymes, for antigen retrieval. After quenching endogenous peroxidase activity with 0.3% $H_2O_2$ in methanol, the sections are incubated with non-specific proteins, such as normal horse serum or bovine serum albumin, to inhibit non-specific finding. The sections are subsequently incubated with primary antibodies, either for 30 min at room temperature or overnight at 4˚C, with shorter incubation periods usually effective for the detection of specific antigen-antibody binding. After rinsing in PBS three times, the sections are incubated with biotinylated secondary antibody for 60 min at room temperature, followed by treatment with peroxidase-labeled streptavidin for 20 min. Peroxidase activity is developed with 0.25 mg/ml 3,3'-diaminobenzidine tetrahydrochloride in the presence of 0.003% hydrogen peroxide in 0.05 M Tris-buffered saline, pH 7.4, and the sections are counterstained for nuclei in hematoxylin.

### 2.2 Gene expression associated with immune responses in liver biopsy specimen

In situ hybridization can be used to analyze the expression of specific genes in liver biopsy specimens. In addition, the distribution of expression of specific genes in these samples can be analyzed by in situ hybridization followed by counter staining for cells and organelles.

In situ hybridization can be performed using both isotope-labeled and non-isotope-labeled probes. We briefly describe a non-isotope-labeled method. Tissue samples are digested with proteinase and incubated overnight with digoxigenin-labeled riboprobes at 55°C. The slides are then washed in sodium dodecyl sulphate in saline sodium citrate and finally in Tris buffered saline containing 0.1% Tween 20 and 1% fetal calf serum (FCS). The tissue samples are subsequently incubated with an alkaline phosphatase conjugated antibody against digoxigenin. Signal is detected using 5-bromo-4-chloro-3-indoyl phosphatase as a substrate and nitro blue tetrazolium as a coupler.

### 2.3 Characterization of the phenotypes of isolated intrahepatic lymphocytes (IHLs)

IHLs can be isolated from liver biopsy specimens by enzymatic digestion and density gradient centrifugation (Hata et al., 1990, Doherty et al., 1999). Briefly, tissue samples are minced into 1 $mm^2$ pieces and incubated while rotating for 20 min at 37°C in Hank's Balanced Salt Solution (HBSS) containing 0.5 mg/ml collagenase, 0.02 mg/ml DNase, 2% FCS and 0.6% bovine serum albumin (BSA). Undigested tissue is removed by filtration through a 100 µm diameter mesh and the cells are washed twice with HBSS. Hepatocytes are removed by centrifugation at 30 × *g* for 1 min and the remaining cells are collected and resuspended in RPMI medium containing 10% FCS. Cell yields and viabilities are determined by microscopic examination of ethidium bromide/acridine orange stained preparations. Yields are usually about 1–2 × $10^6$ mononuclear cells per 200 mg tissue sample, a sufficient number of cells for further analyses.

The phenotype, cytotoxicity (Hata et al., 1990) and cytokine production (Doherty et al., 1999) of isolated IHLs can be analyzed by flow cytometry. Moreover, multi-color flow cytometric analyses can identify minor populations of lymphocytes and intracytoplasmic cytokines. The function of IHLs present in liver biopsy specimens can therefore be analyzed in detail, resulting in a comprehensive understanding of intrahepatic immune responses in liver diseases.

### 2.4 Further application of immunological analysis

RNA and DNA in liver biopsy specimens can be isolated using commercial kits, followed by PCR or RT-PCR for the quantitative evaluation of DNA or RNA encoding proteins associated with the immune system.

Recent advances in microarray technology can be also applied to liver biopsy samples. Tissue microarrays are constructed by transferring cores of paraffin-embedded tissue to precored holes in a recipient paraffin block (Kononen et al., 1998). Microarray analysis enables the evaluation of the expression of multiple genes in liver biopsy specimens in a high throughput manner.

## 3. Immunological analysis in liver diseases

Intrahepatic immune responses have been analyzed in liver biopsy specimens, enhancing our understanding of the immunopathogenesis of liver diseases.

### 3.1 Acute viral hepatitis

Immunological analysis has been extensively performed in transgenic mouse and chimpanzee models of acute infection. In one model, transgenic mice, in which infectious HBV virions replicate in the livers with all HBV-related antigens expressed, were injected with HBsAg-specific cytotoxic T lymphocytes (CTLs) that had been induced in nontransgenic mice. The transgenic mice produced interferon (IFN)-γ and tumor necrosis factor (TNF)-α, which purged viral RNA and DNA without destroying infected hepatocytes (Guidotti et al., 1996, Chisari, 1997, Guidotti et al., 2001). Importantly, this noncytolytic clearance of intracellular HBV is more efficient at controlling HBV replication than the killing of infected hepatocytes. In this sense, hepatitis is not only a harmful event but also represents an effective mechanism by which CTLs suppress HBV. Noncytolytic viral eradication can account for recovery from acute HBV infection, in that most HBV is cleared from hepatocytes with only a fraction of the hepatocytes being destroyed. This phenomenon was confirmed using a chimpanzee infection model. HBV-DNA was profoundly decreased in the liver and blood of acutely infected chimpanzees before peak serum alanine aminotransferase (ALT) concentrations were reached (Guidotti et al., 1999), suggesting that this noncytopathic T cell effector mechanism results in early viral inhibition or eradication, whereas a cytopathic T cell effector mechanism would be required to eliminate the remaining virus by destroying infected hepatocytes.

There have been a limited number of immunological analyses of local immune responses in the liver of patients with acute viral hepatitis, due primarily to relative contraindications for liver biopsy in these patients. Moreover, the kinetics of local immune response cannot be analyzed in humans, because repeated liver biopsies are not usually required and are ethically not allowed during the course of acute hepatitis.

The CD4/CD8 ratio of liver-derived T cell clones was found to be 0.3-0.5 during the acute phase of HAV infection, indicating a CD8+ T cell predominance, but 1.2 during the recovery phase, indicating a CD4+ T cell predominance (Fleischer et al., 1990). Half of the T cell clones showed cytotoxicity against HAV-infected autologous fibroblasts, further suggesting that the intrahepatic HAV-specific T cell response has an important role in the pathogenesis of acute hepatitis A and in viral eradication.

Immunohistochemical analysis of intrahepatic lymphocyte populations in patients with acute hepatitis A, B and C showed that CD45RO+ memory T cells were the most prominent cell population in all 3 types of acute hepatitis, and that the numbers of these cells were significantly higher in portal areas of patients with acute hepatitis C than in those with acute hepatitis B (Hashimoto et al., 1996). In addition, the ratio of CD20+ B cells to CD45RO+ memory T cells was significantly lower in acute hepatitis B than in the two other types of acute hepatitis (Hashimoto et al., 1996). These data indicate that memory T cells are involved in the immunopathogenesis of all types of acute viral hepatitis. However, the clinical significance of the differences among acute hepatitis A, B and C remains unclear.

Recently, the signal delivered by a CD28 superfamily, programmed death-1 (PD-1) protein, was shown to impair virus-specific CD8+ T-cell responses during chronic viral infection (Watanabe et al., 2010), suggesting that this protein plays an important role in insufficient T cell responses against hepatitis viral antigen, leading to persistent viral infection. In patients with acute hepatitis C, PD-1 expression was higher on CD4+ than on CD8+ T cells in the liver, with expression more prominent on intrahepatic than on peripheral blood lymphocytes. However, no correlation was observed between PD-1 expression on T cells and clinical outcomes in patients with acute viral hepatitis (Kasprowicz et al., 2008).

PD-1 expression is thought to be regulated during acute hepatitis, with PD-1 up-regulated on CD8+ T cells during the early phase of acute hepatitis B (Zhang et al., 2008). Successful viral clearance correlated with a subsequent decrease in PD-1 expression, and the delayed PD-1 expression on HBV-specific CD8+ T cells was associated with acute liver failure (Zhang et al., 2008), suggesting that impaired regulation of PD-1 expression may lead to enhanced immune response and severe hepatitis.

In summary, intrahepatic viral-specific memory T cells are directly involved in the immunopathogenesis of acute viral hepatitis, and the kinetics of PD-1 expression in the liver may determine patient outcomes. However, there is limited information on the characterization of intrahepatic lymphocytes and on local immune responses in the liver in patients with acute viral hepatitis.

### 3.2 Chronic hepatitis

There are few animal models of chronic hepatitis, and most of our knowledge regarding its immunopathogenesis is derived from analyses of human liver tissues. Because local immune responses cannot be analyzed over time in patients, however, findings obtained from animal models may help enhance our understanding of the kinetics of immune responses in the liver.

Many studies have analyzed intrahepatic lymphocytes in patients with chronic hepatitis, both immunohistochemically and by flow cytometry. Most of these studies analyzed the makeup of infiltrating cells, the expression of costimulatory molecules in the liver and the antigen specificity of infiltrating T cells. These results have greatly contributed to understanding the immunopathogenesis of various chronic liver diseases.

### 3.2.1 Composition of infiltrating cells

Chronic hepatitis is characterized by lymphoid cell infiltration mainly in portal tracts. Most infiltrating cells are CD3+ T cells, with most of the latter being CD45RO+ memory cells. The CD4/CD8 ratio is similar in patients with hepatitis B and C; 50-60% of infiltrating cells are CD4+ helper T lymphocytes, around 25% are CD8+ CTLs and 15% are B lymphocytes. CD8+ T lymphocytes are located in the peripheral part of portal tracts and intralobular necrotic foci (Walewska-Zielecka et al., 2008). Natural killer cells are also involved in the immunopathogenesis of chronic hepatitis, with CD3-CD56$^{bright}$NKG2A+ cells associated with necroinflammation of the liver and CD3-CD56$^{dim}$NKG2A+ cells associated with low viral load (Bonorino et al., 2009).
The percentages of virus-specific T lymphocytes in the liver have been clarified by immunohistochemical staining with peptide-MHC tetramer. The proportion of CD8+T lymphocytes in the livers of patients with chronic HBV specific for HBc18-27, a major HBV epitope, has been found to range from 0.18% to 1.28% (Shimada et al., 2003). In patients with chronic hepatitis C, 1-2% of CTLs in the liver were found to be HCV NS3-specific, compared with 0.01% to 1.2% of PBLs (He et al., 1999). Due to the low percentages of lymphocyte populations specific for viral epitopes, most intrahepatic lymphocytes are thought to be antigen-nonspecific. The contribution of virus-specific and -nonspecific cells to hepatocyte damage and viral control in chronic viral hepatitis in humans remains unclear. However, in the HBV transgenic mouse model of acute hepatitis, administration of antibodies against the chemokines, IFN-gamma inducible protein (IP-10) and monokine induced by interferon-gamma (Mig) reduced the recruitment of mostly Ag-nonspecific mononuclear cells into the liver that had been induced by cytokines and chemokines produced by injected CTLs, leading to a reduction in the severity of hepatitis without affecting the antiviral activity of the CTLs (Kakimi et al., 2001). The findings indicate that CTLs can suppress virus without damaging hepatocytes, whereas secondarily recruited mononuclear cells, with little antiviral activity, destroy hepatocytes in an Ag-nonspecific manner.
In humans, several cytokines and chemokines are thought to be involved in the recruitment of T lymphocytes into the liver. For example, intrahepatic levels of IP-10/CXCL10 and Mig/CXCL19 have been reported to correlate with liver inflammation and fibrosis in the livers of patients with chronic hepatitis C (Zeremski et al., 2008). Moreover, their receptor, CXCR3, is expressed on most intrahepatic T lymphocytes, indicating that chemokine/receptor systems have an important role in T cell recruitment into inflamed livers. We have reported that Mip3α produced by DCs after phagocytosis of apoptotic cells is chemotactic for CCR6-expressing CD4+ T lymphocytes, but not for CD8+ T lymphocytes (Shimizu et al., 2001). A complex chemokine/chemokine receptor network is therefore present in the livers of patients with chronic hepatitis, and manipulation of this network may control the magnitude of liver inflammation.

### 3.2.2 Chronic hepatitis B

Several studies have characterized CD4+ T lymphocytes in patients with chronic hepatitis B. For example, these livers have been found to contain Th0 cells, which produce not only IFN-γ, but also IL-4 and IL-5, thus differing from cells in the livers of patients with chronic hepatitis C, which are mostly Th1 cells (Bertoletti et al., 1997). CD4+ T lymphocytes that produce TNF-α and IL-17 infiltrate into the livers of patients with chronic hepatitis B and are involved in liver inflammation (Zhang et al., 2010). IL-17 producing CD4+ T lymphocytes, called Th17 cells, are a third distinct subset of T helper cells and play an important role in innate and adoptive immunity and in autoimmunity. In a transgenic mouse model, CD4+ T lymphocytes, as well as CD8+ T lymphocytes, have been shown effective for noncytolytic viral purge by secreting TNF-α and IFN-γ (Franco et al., 1997).

Although noncytolytic antiviral mechanism mediated by T lymphocytes was first described in a transgenic mouse model (Guidotti et al., 1996), a similar phenomenon was recently observed in the livers of patients with chronic hepatitis B.

The natural history of chronic HBV infection is somewhat complex. Most people infected at birth are asymptomatic during their first 20-30 years, called the immune tolerant phase. This tolerant phase later breaks down, resulting in ALT flare-ups due to activation of the immune response against HBV. After an ALT flare, 80-90% of chronically infected patients experience a great reduction, but not a diminishing, of HBV replication, these patients seroconvert, from HBeAg to anti-HBe antibody, and become inactive carriers. In the other 10-20% of chronically infected patients, ALT remains elevated and active HBV replication persists, resulting in disease progression to chronic hepatitis, liver cirrhosis and hepatocellular carcinoma. Although the precise pathogenetic mechanisms differentiating inactive carriers from chronic hepatitis patients are unclear, recent immunological analyses have provided new insights into the understanding of these mechanisms.

Livers of patients with low HBV replication contain intralobular CD8+ T lymphocytes (Tang et al., 2003), suggesting that the host immune system recognizes viral antigens and may carry out immune surveillance in the livers of inactive carriers. Moreover, the same numbers of HBcAg-specific CD8+ T lymphocytes are present in the livers of individuals with high viral replication/elevated serum ALT and low viral load/normal ALT (Maini et al., 2000), suggesting that HBV-specific CD8+ T cells effectively control viral replication without damaging infected hepatocytes in inactive carriers, but fails to do so in patients with chronic hepatitis. Although the mechanism underlying this failure of viral control remains unclear, two possible mechanisms have been hypothesized, one involving regulatory T cells and the other involving the costimulatory molecule, PD-1. Regulatory T cells (Tregs) expressing the transcription factor Foxp3 are specialized cells that exert negative control on a variety of physiological and pathological immune responses, resulting in maintenance of immunological self-tolerance (Miyara et al., 2011). Circulating and intrahepatic Tregs are involved in persistent infection by hepatitis virus. CD4+CD25+ cells and Foxp3+ cells are increased in the livers of patients with chronic hepatitis B (Xu et al., 2006), and patients with high viral load have a higher proportion of Tregs in the liver (Stoop et al., 2008), suggesting that intrahepatic Tregs suppress antiviral immune responses in the liver.

PD-1 is a surface receptor critical for the regulation of T cell function (Francisco et al., 2010, Fife BT et al., 2011). The binding to PD-1 by its ligands PD-L1 and PD-L2 results in the antigen-specific inhibition of T-cell proliferation, cytokine production, and cytolytic function. In the liver, PD-1 is expressed on lymphocytes; PD-L1 is expressed on lymphocytes, hepatocytes and sinusoidal endothelial cell; and PD-L2 is expressed on Kupffer cells and DCs (Chen et al., 2010). Intrahepatic HBV-specific CD8+ T cells express higher levels of PD-1, and upregulation of intrahepatic PD-1/PD-L1 is associated with liver inflammation and ALT elevation (Fisicaro et al., 2010, Xie et al., 2009). Although the mechanism underlying the upregulation of PD-1 on CD8+ T cells in inflamed livers is unknown, signals from PD-1 inhibit HBV-specific T cells, resulting in insufficient antiviral responses and liver inflammation. Importantly, PD-1/PD-L1 blockade increased CD8+ T cell proliferation and enhanced IFN-γ and IL-2 production by intrahepatic lymphocytes (Fisicaro et al., 2010). These findings suggest that inhibiting PD-1/PD-L1 may have therapeutic potential for the control of hepatitis B.

Local immune response is also regarded as important during the treatment of hepatitis B. The numbers of pretreatment intrahepatic CD8+ T cells has been shown to predict better responses to IFN-α and lamivudine (Tang et al., 2004, 2005).

### 3.2.3 Chronic hepatitis C

The local immune response occurring in the livers of patients with chronic hepatitis C is similar to that in chronic hepatitis B. Intrahepatic CD4+ T cells, most of which are Th1 cells producing IFN-γ but not IL-4 and IL-5 (Bertoletti et al., 1997), are located in portal and periportal areas, with the proportions of these cells correlating with histological activity index (Fiore et al., 1997). However, no correlation has been found between the proportion of intrahepatic CD4+ T cells and viremia or serum ALT levels (Tran et al., 1997). Most intrahepatic CD4+ T cells in the livers of patients with chronic hepatitis C are CD45RO+, but the percentages of CD4+CD27+ and CD4+CD28+ T cells are lower (Wang et al., 2006), suggesting that memory T cells at relatively early stages of differentiation are involved in liver inflammation.

In patients with chronic hepatitis C, CD8+ T cells are located in the lobules within areas of inflammation and spotty necrosis, with the proportion correlating with histological activity index (Fiore et al., 1997). Intrahepatic CD8+ T cells show higher percentages of CCR7+L-selectin- cells, which are distinct from central memory and effector memory cells (Heydtmann et al., 2006). The CCR7 ligands CCL19 and CCL21 are expressed on sinusoidal endothelial cells, suggesting a mechanism of CD8+ T cell recruitment to the inflamed liver. Other chemokine receptors that mediate T cell recruitment are CCR5 and CXCR3 (Larrubia et al., 2007). Although the numbers of intrahepatic CD8+ T cells were reported to correlate with serum enzyme concentrations, and intralobular CD8+ T cells showed weak correlation with serum ALT concentrations (Freeman et al., 2003), intrahepatic HCV-specific CD8+ T cells do not secrete IFN-γ but secrete IL-10, an immunosuppressive cytokine (Spangenberg et al., 2005). The presence of these IL-10 secreting T cells is associated with low levels of hepatocyte apoptosis, ALT and fibrosis (Abel et al., 2006). Increased production of IL-10, but not IFN-γ, may result in an insufficient anti-HCV response in the liver.

Similar to intrahepatic T cells in patients with chronic hepatitis B, intrahepatic HCV-specific cells were found to express high levels of PD-1 (Radziewicz et al. 2007), which may be responsible for the absence of IFN-γ production, as well as poor proliferation and low cytolytic activity. Moreover, large numbers of Foxp3+ cells, mostly CD4+ T cells, are present in the portal tracts of the livers of patients with chronic hepatitis C (Ward et al., 2007, Claassen et al., 2010, Sturm et al., 2010). These cells are also in contact with CD8+ T cells in necro-inflammatory areas, suggesting that CD8+ T cells are inhibited by cell-cell contact with Tregs (Sturm et al., 2010). These immunosuppressive mechanisms present in the livers of patients with chronic hepatitis C may be responsible for persistent HCV infection despite the presence of HCV-specific T cells in the liver.

In addition to T cells, livers of patients with chronic hepatitis C often contain lymphoid follicles in portal tracts, a characteristic of HCV-infected livers. We previously reported that functional and clonal expansion of B cells occurs in lymphoid follicles with germinal centers in HCV-infected livers (Murakami et al., 1999), although the antigen specificity of these B cells is unclear.

Local immune responses may be involved in viral eradication during patient treatment with IFN. The numbers of pretreatment CD8+ T cells in portal tracts and intrahepatic HCV-specific CD8+ CTLs have been reported associated with a better response to IFN-α or a sustained virological response (Nelson et al., 1998, Vrolijk et al., 2003). Therefore, upregulation of intrahepatic T cell response may enhance the effectiveness of antiviral treatment.

### 3.3 Autoimmune liver disease

The dominant population of intrahepatic T cells in patients with primary biliary cirrhosis has been reported to be CD4+TCRαβ+ T cells, whereas the dominant population in patients with chronic hepatitis B and C has been reported to be CD8+TCRαβ+ T cells (Löhr et al., 1994). This finding, however, remains controversial and it does not help distinguish autoimmune liver disease from viral hepatitis.

#### 3.3.1 Primary biliary cirrhosis (PBC) and primary sclerosing cholangitis (PSC)

The liver histology of patients with PBC has been extensively analyzed. A characteristic early stage histologic feature in these patients is nonsuppurative destructive cholangitis. Although the biliary epithelium is thought to be the target for host immune responses, the mechanism underlying epithelial destruction is unclear. CD8+ T cells are present within the bile duct epithelial layer of patients with chronic nonsuppurative destructive cholangitis, suggesting that CTLs destroy the bile duct epithelium. B7-2 (CD86), but not B7-1 (CD80), expression has been observed in bile duct epithelium during early stages of PBC and PSC (Tsuneyama et al., 1998), suggesting that bile duct epithelium may act as antigen-presenting cells. Immunopathologically important target antigens have not been determined. Although the generation of anti-mitochondrial antibodies is important for the diagnosis of PBC, mitochondrial antigens are not thought to be the pathogenetic target for immune cells. Livers of patients with PBC have been reported to contain more Tregs than livers of patients with autoimmune hepatitis (Sasaki et al., 2008), with Tregs infiltrating into the biliary epithelial layer during chronic nonsuppurative destructive cholangitis (Sasaki et al., 2007). Moreover, the numbers of Foxp3+ Tregs were found to parallel the degree of portal inflammation. These results, showing the presence of Tregs in the livers of patients with PBC and that their regulatory functions are not reduced in the livers of patients with PBC and PSC, suggest that autoimmunity in PBC is not due to a reduction in Treg function.

PD-1 expression has also been assayed in livers of patients with PBC. PD-1 is expressed on more than 50% of intrahepatic T lymphocytes in the portal tracts, but their levels of expression are lower than in patients with autoimmune hepatitis (Oikawa et al., 2007).

#### 3.3.2 Autoimmune hepatitis (AIH)

CD4+ T cells and CD20+ B cells have been reported to be located in the center of portal areas, with CD8+ T cells at the periphery of the portal area (De Biasio et al., 2006). Although

CD4+ T cells constitute the major population of intrahepatic lymphocytes, many CD80+, CD86+ and CD152+ cells are present in the livers of patients with autoimmune hepatitis (Kurokochi et al., 2006). Moreover, patients with high levels of intrahepatic CD86+ cells showed good responses to corticosteroids (Kurokochi et al., 2006).
One of the putative target antigens in the immunopathogenesis of autoimmune hepatitis is asialoglycoprotein receptor, and antibodies against this receptor are often present in patients with autoimmune hepatitis. Although the mechanism of antibody production is unknown, intrahepatic T helper cells in patients with autoimmune hepatitis can stimulate the production of the autoantibody. Few Tregs are observed in these livers, with those present having impaired function (Longhi et al., 2010), suggesting that decreased functional activity of Tregs may predispose to enhanced autoimmune reactions.

### 3.4 Nonalcoholic fatty liver disease

Nonalcoholic fatty liver disease (NAFLD) is a frequently occurring chronic liver disease and can range in intensity from simple steatosis to nonalcoholic steatohepatitis (NASH). Due to chronic necro-inflammatory changes, patients with NASH may develop cirrhosis or hepatocellular carcinoma, although these are rare in patients with simple steatosis. Histologically, steatosis (usually >5% per liver tissue section), cellular injury such as ballooned hepatocytes or Mallory-Denk bodies, and accompanying lobular inflammation are observed in the livers of patients with NAFLD. Inflammatory infiltrates in these livers consist predominantly of lymphocytes, as well as plasma cells and polymorphonuclear leucocytes in portal tracts of the liver (Brunt et al., 2010). The 'two-hit theory' is widely accepted in the pathogenesis of NAFLD, and patients with simple steatosis are regarded as not showing disease progression because of the absence of the second hit (Day et al., 1998). Adipocytokines from adipose tissue and gut-derived factors (i.e. endotoxin) are regarded as the principal pathogenetic factors, the second hits, in the disease progression of NAFLD (Tilg et al., 2010), but recent reports have revealed that immunological mechanisms are directly involved in its pathogenesis. An immunohistochemical analysis of liver biopsy specimens showed that cells of the innate immune system, including neutrophils, macrophages (Kupffer cells) and NKT cells, are involved in the pathogenesis of NAFLD. Livers of patients with NASH showed increased hepatic neutrophil infiltration and increased hepatic expression of mRNAs coding for proinflammatory cytokines, as determined by quantitative RT-PCR. Furthermore, activation of the complement system in the liver is associated with the severity of NAFLD (Rensen et al., 2009). In rodent models of NAFLD, activation of Kupffer cells and proinflammatory cytokines are involved in disease progression (Maher et al., 2008, Syn et al., 2009). Kupffer cells are thought to be activated by gut-derived factors, adipocytokines and apoptotic cells, and to produce proinflammatory cytokines and reactive oxygen species (ROS). Proinflammatory cytokines and ROS may induce insulin resistance, which is regarded as important in the development of NAFLD. In addition, recent studies by our group and others have found that accumulation of NKT cells in the liver is associated with disease progression to NASH (Fig. 1), suggesting that NKT cells may contribute to disease progression in NAFLD (Tajiri et al., 2009, Syn et al., 2010). CD1d, a molecule essential for the activation and maintenance of NKT cells (Godfrey et al., 2004), is highly expressed on activated macrophages in the livers of NASH patients (Tajiri et al., 2009), suggesting that NKT and Kupffer cells may interact during the pathogenesis of NAFLD (Fig. 2).

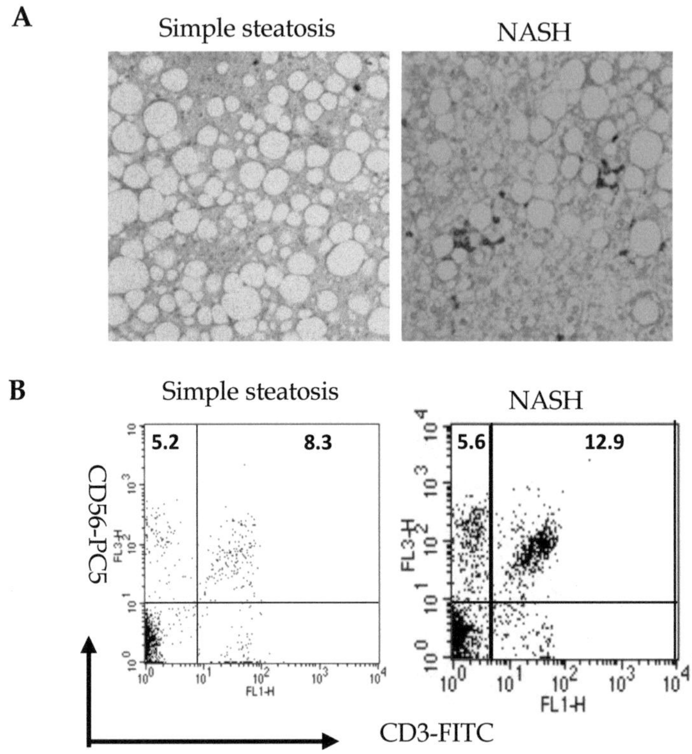


Fig. 1. Immunological analysis of liver biopsy specimens in patients with NAFLD. (A) Samples were stained with monoclonal antibody against CD56 in patients with (left panel) simple steatosis and (right panel) NASH. (B) Flow cytometric analysis of mononuclear cells isolated from livers of patients with (left panel) simple steatosis and (right panel) NASH. The numbers in each quadrant represent the percentages of mononuclear cells. Right-upper quadrant represents NKT (CD3+CD56+) cells.

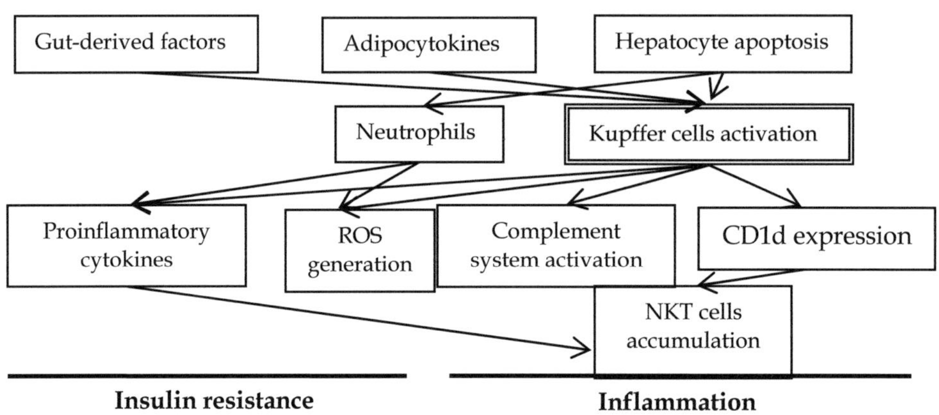


ROS: reactive oxygen species

Fig. 2. Hypothesis of the pathogenesis of NAFLD.

## 4. Conclusion

Although analysis of intrahepatic immune response is difficult to be performed, valuable information on the immunopathogenesis of liver diseases could be obtained. Accumulation of the findings would finally lead to a novel immunotherapeutic approach for the management of various liver diseases.

## 5. References

Abel, M; Sène, D; Pol, S; Bourlière, M; Poynard, T; Charlotte, F; Cacoub, P & Caillat-Zucman, S. (2006). Intrahepatic virus-specific IL-10-producing CD8 T cells prevent liver damage during chronic hepatitis C virus infection. *Hepatology*, Vol.44, No.6, (December 2006), pp. 1607-1616.

Bertoletti, A; D'Elios, MM; Boni, C; De Carli, M; Zignego, AL; Durazzo, M; Missale, G; Penna, A; Fiaccadori, F; Del Prete, G & Ferrari, C. (1997). Different cytokine profiles of intraphepatic T cells in chronic hepatitis B and hepatitis C virus infections. *Gastroenterology*, Vol.112, No.1, (January 1997), pp. 193-199.

Bonorino, P; Ramzan, M; Camous, X; Dufeu-Duchesne, T; Thélu, MA; Sturm, N; Dariz, A; Guillermet, C; Pernollet, M; Zarski, JP; Marche, PN; Leroy, V & Jouvin-Marche, E. (2009). Fine characterization of intrahepatic NK cells expressing natural killer receptors in chronic hepatitis B and C. *J Hepatol*, Vol.51, No.3, (June 2009), pp. 458-467.

Brunt, EM & Tiniakos, DG. Histopathology of nonalcoholic fatty liver disease. (2010). *World J Gastroenterol*, Vol.16, No.42, (November 2010), pp. 5286-5496.

Chen, J; Wang, XM; Wu, XJ; Wang, Y; Zhao, H; Shen, B & Wang, GQ. (2010). Intrahepatic levels of PD-1/PD-L correlate with liver inflammation in chronic hepatitis B. *Inflamm Res*, 2010 Jul 27. [Epub ahead of print]

Chisari FV. (1997). Cytotoxic T cells and viral hepatitis. *J Clin Invest*, Vol.99, No.7, (April 1997), pp. 1472-1477.

Claassen, MA; de Knegt, RJ; Tilanus, HW; Janssen, HL & Boonstra, A. (2010). Abundant numbers of regulatory T cells localize to the liver of chronic hepatitis C infected patients and limit the extent of fibrosis. *J Hepatol*, Vol.52, No.3, (December 2009), pp. 315-321.

Day, CP & James, OF. (1998). Steatohepatitis: a tale of two "hit"? *Gastroenterology*, Vol.114, No.4, (April 1998), pp. 842-845.

De Biasio, MB; Periolo, N; Avagnina, A; García de Dávila, MT; Ciocca, M; Goñi, J; de Matteo, E, Galoppo, C; Cañero-Velasco, MC; Fainboim, H; Muñoz, AE; Fainboim, L & Cherñavsky, AC. (2006). Liver infiltrating mononuclear cells in children with type 1 autoimmune hepatitis. *J Clin Pathol*, Vol.59, No.4, (February 2006), pp. 417-423.

Doherty, DG; Norris, S; Madrigal-Estebas, L; McEntee, G; Traynor, O; Hegarty, JE, & O'Farrelly, C. (1999). The human liver contains multiple populations of NK cells, T cells, and CD3+CD56+ natural T cells with distinct cytotoxic activities and Th1, Th2, and Th0 cytokine secretion patterns. *J Immunol*, Vol.163, No.4, (August 1999), pp. 2314-2321.

Fife, BT & Pauken, KE. (2011). The role of the PD-1 pathway in autoimmunity and peripheral tolerance. *Ann N Y Acad Sci*, Vol.1217, (January 2011), pp. 45-59.

Fiore, G; Angarano, I; Caccetta, L; Serrone, M; Jirillo, E; Schiraldi, O & Antonaci, S. (1997). In-situ immunophenotyping study of hepatic-infiltrating cytotoxic cells in chronic active hepatitis C. *Eur J Gastroenterol Hepatol*,Vol.9, No.5, (May 1997), pp, 491-496.

Fisicaro, P; Valdatta, C; Massari, M; Loggi, E; Biasini, E; Sacchelli, L; Cavallo, MC; Silini, EM; Andreone, P; Missale, G & Ferrari, C. (2010). Antiviral intrahepatic T-cell responses can be restored by blocking programmed death-1 pathway in chronic hepatitis B. *Gastroenterology*. Vol.138, No.2, (September 2009), pp. 682-693, 693.e1-4.

Fleischer, B; Fleischer, S; Maier, K; Wiedmann, KH; Sacher, M; Thaler, H & Vallbracht, A. (1990). Clonal analysis of infiltrating T lymphocytes in liver tissue in viral hepatitis A. *Immunology*, Vol.69, No.1, (January 1990), pp. 14-19.

Francisco, LM; Sage, PT & Sharpe, AH. (2010). The PD-1 pathway in tolerance and autoimmunity. *Immunol Rev*, Vol.236, (July 2010), pp. 219-242.

Franco, A; Guidotti, LG; Hobbs, MV; Pasquetto, V & Chisari, FV. (1997). Pathogenetic effector function of CD4-positive T helper 1 cells in hepatitis B virus transgenic mice. *J Immunol*,Vol.159, No.4, (August 1997), pp. 2001-2008.

Freeman, A;, Pan, Y; Harvey, CE; Post, JJ; Law, MG; White, PA; Rawlinson, WD; Lloyd, AR; Marinos, G & Ffrench, RA. (2003). The presence of an intrahepatic cytotoxic T lymphocyte response is associated with low viral load in patients with chronic hepatitis C virus infection. *J Hepatol*,Vol.38, No.3, (March 2003), pp. 349-356.

Godfrey, DI & Kronenberg, M. (2004). Going both ways: immune regulation via CD1d-dependent NKT cells. *J Clin Invest*, Vol114, Vol.10, (November 2004), pp. 1379-1388.

Guidotti, LG; Ishikawa, T; Hobbs, MV; Matzke, B; Schreiber, R & Chisari, FV. (1996). Intracellular inactivation of the hepatitis B virus by cytotoxic T lymphocytes. *Immunity*, Vol.4, No.1, (January 1996), pp. 25-36.

Guidotti, LG; Rochford, R; Chung, J; Shapiro, M; Purcell, R & Chisari, FV. (1999). Viral clearance without destruction of infected cells during acute HBV infection. *Science*, Vol.284, No.5415, (April 1999), pp. 825-829.

Guidotti, LG & Chisari, FV. (2001). Noncytolytic control of viral infections by the innate and adaptive immune response. *Annu Rev Immunol*, Vol.19, pp. 65-91.

Hashimoto, E; Kojimahara, N; Noguchi, S; Taniai, M; Ishiguro, N & Hayashi, N. (1996). Immunohistochemical characterization of hepatic lymphocytes in acute hepatitis A, B, and C. *J Clin Gastroenterol*, Vol.23, No.3, (October 1996), pp. 199-202.

Hata, K; Zhang, XR; Iwatsuki, S; Van Thiel, DH; Herberman, RB & Whiteside, TL. (1990). Isolation, phenotyping, and functional analysis of lymphocytes from human liver. *Clin Immunol Immunopathol*,Vol.56, No.3, (September 1990), pp. 401-419.

He, XS; Rehermann, B; López-Labrador, FX; Boisvert, J; Cheung, R; Mumm, J; Wedemeyer, H; Berenguer, M; Wright, TL; Davis, MM & Greenberg, HB. (1999). Quantitative analysis of hepatitis C virus-specific CD8(+) T cells in peripheral blood and liver using peptide-MHC tetramers. *Proc Natl Acad Sci U S A*, Vol.96, No.10, (May 1999), pp. 5692-5697.

Heydtmann, M; Hardie, D; Shields, PL; Faint, J; Buckley, CD; Campbell, JJ; Salmon, M & Adams, DH. (2006). Detailed analysis of intrahepatic CD8 T cells in the normal and hepatitis C-infected liver reveals differences in specific populations of memory cells with distinct homing phenotypes. *J Immunol*, Vol.177, No.1, (July 2006), pp. 729-738.

Kakimi, K; Lane, TE; Wieland, S; Asensio, VC; Campbell, IL; Chisari, FV & Guidotti, LG. (2001). Blocking chemokine responsive to gamma-2/interferon (IFN)-gamma inducible protein and monokine induced by IFN-gamma activity in vivo reduces the pathogenetic but not the antiviral potential of hepatitis B virus-specific cytotoxic T lymphocytes. *J Exp Med,* Vol.194, No.12, (December 2001), pp. 1755-1766.

Kasprowicz, V; Schulze Zur Wiesch, J; Kuntzen, T; Nolan, BE; Longworth, S; Berical, A; Blum, J; McMahon, C; Reyor, LL; Elias, N; Kwok, WW; McGovern, BG; Freeman, G; Chung, RT; Klenerman, P; Lewis-Ximenez, L; Walker, BD; Allen, TM; Kim, AY & Lauer, GM. (2008). High level of PD-1 expression on hepatitis C virus (HCV)-specific CD8+ and CD4+ T cells during acute HCV infection, irrespective of clinical outcome. *J Virol,* Vol.82, No.6, (December 2007), pp. 3154-3160.

Kononen, J; Bubendorf, L; Kallioniemi, A; Bärlund, M; Schraml, P; Leighton, ;, Torhorst, J; Mihatsch, MJ; Sauter, G & Kallioniemi, OP. (1998) Tissue microarrays for high-throughput molecular profiling of tumor specimens. *Nat Med,* Vol.4, No.7, (July 1998), pp. 844-847.

Kurokohchi, K; Masaki, T; Himoto, T; Deguchi, A; Nakai, S; Morishita, A; Yoneyama, H; Kimura, Y; Watanab, S & Kuriyama, S. (2006). Usefulness of liver infiltrating CD86-positive mononuclear cells for diagnosis of autoimmune hepatitis. *World J Gastroenterol,* Vol.12, No.16, (April 2006), pp. 2523-2529.

Larrubia, JR; Calvino, M; Benito, S; Sanz-de-Villalobos, E; Perna, C; Pérez-Hornedo, J; González-Mateos, F; García-Garzón, S; Bienvenido, A & Parra, T. (2007). The role of CCR5/CXCR3 expressing CD8+ cells in liver damage and viral control during persistent hepatitis C virus infection. *J Hepatol,* Vol.47, No.5, (May 2007), pp. 632-641.

Löhr, HF; Schlaak, JF; Gerken, G; Fleischer, B; Dienes, HP & Meyer zum Büschenfelde, KH. (1994). Phenotypical analysis and cytokine release of liver-infiltrating and peripheral blood T lymphocytes from patients with chronic hepatitis of different etiology. *Liver,* Vol.14, No.3, (June 1994), pp. 161-166.

Longhi, MS; Ma, Y; Mieli-Vergani, G; & Vergani, D. (2010). Aetiopathogenesis of autoimmune hepatitis. *J Autoimmu,.* Vol. 34, No. 1, (September 2009), pp.7-14.

Luttmann, W; Bratke, K; Kupper, M & Mytrek, D. (2006). *Immunology.* In situ Immunolocalization pp. 127-151, Elsevier.

Maher, JJ; Leon, P & Ryan, JC. (2008). Beyond insulin resistance: innate immunity in nonalcoholic steatohepatitis. *Hepatology,* Vol.48, No.2, (August 2008), pp. 670-678.

Maini, MK; Boni, C; Lee, CK; Larrubia, JR; Reignat, S; Ogg, GS; King, AS; Herberg, J; Gilson, R; Alisa, A; Williams, R; Vergani, D; Naoumov, NV; Ferrari, C & Bertoletti, A. (2000) The role of virus-specific CD8(+) cells in liver damage and viral control during persistent hepatitis B virus infection. *J Exp Med,* Vol.191, No.8, (April 2000), pp. 1269-1280.

Miyara, M & Sakaguchi, S. (2011). Human FoxP3(+)CD4(+) regulatory T cells: their knowns and unknowns. *Immunol Cell Biol,* Vol.89, No.3, (February 2011), pp. 346-351.

Murakami, J; Shimizu, Y; Kashii, Y; Kato, T; Minemura, M; Okada, K; Nambu, S; Takahara, T; Higuchi. K; Maeda, Y; Kumada, T & Watanabe, A. (1999). Functional B-cell response in intrahepatic lymphoid follicles in chronic hepatitis C. *Hepatology,* Vol.30, No.1, (July 1999), pp. 143-150.

Nelson, DR; Marousis, CG; Ohno, T; Davis, GL & Lau, JY. (1998). Intrahepatic hepatitis C virus-specific cytotoxic T lymphocyte activity and response to interferon alfa therapy in chronic hepatitis C. *Hepatology,* Vol.28, No.1, (July 1998), pp. 225-230.

Oikawa, T; Takahashi, H; Ishikawa, T; Hokari, A; Otsuki, N; Azuma, M; Zeniya, M & Tajiri H. (2007). Intrahepatic expression of the co-stimulatory molecules programmed death-1, and its ligands in autoimmune liver disease. *Pathol Int,* Vol.57, No.8, (August 2007), pp. 485-492.

Radziewicz, H; Ibegbu, CC; Fernandez, ML; Workowski, KA; Obideen, K; Wehbi, M; Hanson, HL; Steinberg, JP; Masopust, D; Wherry, EJ; Altman, JD; Rouse, BT; Freeman, GJ; Ahmed, R & Grakoui, A. (2007). Liver-infiltrating lymphocytes in chronic human hepatitis C virus infection display an exhausted phenotype with high levels of PD-1 and low levels of CD127 expression. *J Virol,* Vol.81, No.6, (December 2006), pp. 2545-2553.

Rensen, SS; Slaats, Y; Driessen, A; Peutz-Kootstra, CJ; Nijhuis, J; Steffensen, R; Greve, JW & Buurman, WA. (2009). Activation of the complement system in human nonalcoholic fatty liver disease. *Hepatology,* Vol.50, No.6, (December 2009), pp. 1809-1817.

Sasaki M; Ikeda, H; Sawada, S; Sato, Y & Nakanuma, Y. (2007). Naturally-occurring regulatory T cells are increased in inflamed portal tracts with cholangiopathy in primary biliary cirrhosis. *J Clin Pathol,* Vol.60, No.19, (December 2006), pp. 1102-1107.

Sakaki, M; Hiroishi, K; Baba, T; Ito, T; Hirayama, Y; Saito, K; Tonoike, T; Kushima, M & Imawari, M. (2008). Intrahepatic status of regulatory T cells in autoimmune liver diseases and chronic viral hepatitis. *Hepatol Res,* Vol38, No.4, (November 2007), pp. 354-361.

Shimizu, Y; Murata, H; Kashii, Y; Hirano, K; Kunitani, H; Higuchi, K & Watanabe, A. (2001). CC-chemokine receptor 6 and its ligand macrophage inflammatory protein 3alpha might be involved in the amplification of local necroinflammatory response in the liver. *Hepatology,* Vol.34, No.2, (August 2001), pp. 311-319.

Spangenberg, HC; Viazov, S; Kersting, N; Neumann-Haefelin, C; McKinney, D; Roggendorf, M; von Weizsäcker, F; Blum, HE & Thimme, R. (2005). Intrahepatic CD8+ T-cell failure during chronic hepatitis C virus infection. *Hepatology,* Vol.42, No.4, (October 2005), pp. 828-837.

Sturm, N; Thélu, MA; Camous, X; Dimitrov, G; Ramzan, M; Dufeu-Duchesne, T; Bonorino, P; Guillermet, C; Brambilla, E; Arvers, P; Pernollet, M; Leroy, V; Zarski, JP; Marche, PN & Jouvin-Marche, E. (2010). Characterization and role of intra-hepatic regulatory T cells in chronic hepatitis C pathogenesis. *J Hepatol,* Vol.53, No.1, (April 2010), pp. 25-35.

Stoop, JN; Claassen, MA; Woltman, AM; Binda, RS; Kuipers, EJ; Janssen, HL; van der Molen, RG & Boonstra, A. (2008) Intrahepatic regulatory T cells are phenotypically distinct from their peripheral counterparts in chronic HBV patients. *Clin Immunol,* Vol.129, No.3, (September 2008), pp. 419-427.

Syn, WK; Oo, YH; Pereira, TA; Karaca, GF; Jung, Y; Omenetti, A; Witek, RP; Choi, SS; Guy, CD; Fearing, CM; Teaberry, V; Pereira, FE; Adams, DH & Diehl, AM. (2010). Accumulation of natural killer T cells in progressive nonalcoholic fatty liver disease. *Hepatology,* Vol.51, No.1, (June 2010), pp. 1998-2007.

Syn, WK; Choi, SS & Diehl, AM. (2009). Apoptosis and cytokines in nonalcoholic steatohepatitis. *Clin Liver Dis,*Vol.13, No.4, (November 2009), pp. 565-580.

Tang, TJ; Kwekkeboom, J; Laman, JD; Niesters, HG; Zondervan, PE; de Man, RA; Schalm, SW & Janssen, HL. (2003). The role of intrahepatic immune effector cells in inflammatory liver injury and viral control during chronic hepatitis B infection. *J Viral Hepat,* Vol.10, No.3, (May 2003), pp. 159-167.

Tang, TJ; de Man, RA; Kusters, JG; Kwekkeboom, J; Hop, WC; van der Molen, RG; Schalm, SW & Janssen, HL. (2004). Intrahepatic CD8 T-lymphocytes and HBV core expression in relation to response to antiviral therapy for chronic hepatitis B patients. *J Med Virol,*Vol.72, No.2, (February 2004), pp. 215-222.

Tang, TJ; Kwekkeboom, J; Mancham, S; Binda, RS; de Man, RA; Schalm, SW; Kusters, JG & Janssen, HL. (2005). Intrahepatic CD8+ T-lymphocyte response is important for therapy-induced viral clearance in chronic hepatitis B infection. *J Hepatol,* Vol.43, No.1, (Apriel 2005), pp. 45-52.

Tajiri, K; Shimizu, Y; Tsuneyama, K & Sugiyama, T. (2009). The role of liver-infiltrating CD3+CD56+ NKT cells in the pathogenesis of nonalcoholic fatty liver disease. *Eur J Gastroenterol Hepatol,* Vol.21, No.6, (June 2009), pp. 673-680.

Tilg, H & Moschen, AR. (2010). Evolution of inflammation in nonalcoholic fatty liver disease: the multiple parallel hits hypothesis. *Hepatology,* Vol. 52, No.5, (November 2010), pp. 1836-1846.

Tsuneyama, K; Harada, K; Yasoshima, M; Kaji, K; Gershwin, ME & Nakanuma, Y. (1998). Expression of co-stimulatory factor B7-2 on the intrahepatic bile ducts in primary biliary cirrhosis and primary sclerosing cholangitis: an immunohistochemical study. *J Pathol,* Vol.186, No.2, (October 1998), pp. 126-130.

Tran, A; Yang, G; Doglio, A; Ticchioni, M; Laffont, C; Durant, J; Bernard, JL; Gugenheim, J; Saint-Paul, MC; Bernard, A; Rampal, P & Benzaken, S. (1997). Phenotyping of intrahepatic and peripheral blood lymphocytes in patients with chronic hepatitis C. *Dig Dis Sci,* Vol.42, No.12, (December 1997), pp. 2495-2500.

Vrolijk, JM; Kwekkeboom, J; Janssen, HL; Hansen, BE; Zondervan, PE; Osterhaus, AD; Schalm, SW & Haagmans, BL. (2003). Pretreatment intrahepatic CD8+ cell count correlates with virological response to antiviral therapy in chronic hepatitis C virus infection. *J Infect Dis,* Vol.188, No.15, (October 2003), pp. 1528-1532.

Walewska-Zielecka, B; Madalinski, K; Jablonska, J; Godzik, P; Cielecka-Kuszyk, J & Litwinska, B. (2008). Composition of inflammatory infiltrate and its correlation with HBV/HCV antigen expression. *World J Gastroenterol,* Vol.14, No.7, (July 2008), pp. 4040-4046.

Watanabe, T; Bertoletti, A & Tanoto, TA. (2010). PD-1/PD-L1 pathway and T-cell exhaustion in chronic hepatitis virus infection. *J Viral Hepat,* Vo.17, No.7, (July 2010), pp. 453-458.

Xie, Z; Chen, Y; Zhao, S; Yang, Z; Yao, X; Guo, S; Yang, C; Fei, L; Zeng, X; Ni, B & Wu, Y. (2009). Intrahepatic PD-1/PD-L1 up-regulation closely correlates with inflammation and virus replication in patients with chronic HBV infection. *Immunol Invest,* Vol.38, No.7, pp. 624-638.

Xu, D; Fu, J; Jin, L; Zhang, H; Zhou, C; Zou, Z; Zhao, JM; Zhang, B; Shi, M; Ding, X; Tang, Z; Fu, YX & Wang, FS. (2006). Circulating and liver resident CD4+CD25+ regulatory T cells actively influence the antiviral immune response and disease progression in patients with hepatitis B. *J Immunol,* Vol.177, No.1, (July 2006), pp. 739-747.

Ward, SM; Fox, BC; Brown, PJ; Worthington, J; Fox, SB; Chapman, RW; Fleming, KA; Banham, AH & Klenerman, P. (2007). Quantification and localisation of FOXP3+ T lymphocytes and relation to hepatic inflammation during chronic HCV infection. *J Hepatol,* Vol.47, No.3, (April 2007), pp. 316-324.

Zeremski, M; Petrovic, LM; Chiriboga, L; Brown, QB; Yee, HT; Kinkhabwala, M; Jacobson, IM; Dimova, R; Markatou, M & Talal, AH. (2008). Intrahepatic levels of CXCR3-associated chemokines correlate with liver inflammation and fibrosis in chronic hepatitis C. *Hepatology,* Vol.48, No.5, (November 2008), pp. 1440-1450.

Zhang, Z; Zhang, JY; Wherry, EJ; Jin, B; Xu, B; Zou, ZS; Zhang, SY; Li, BS; Wang, HF; Wu, H; Lau, GK; Fu, YX & Wang, FS. (2008). Dynamic programmed death 1 expression by virus-specific CD8 T cells correlates with the outcome of acute hepatitis B. *Gastroenterology,* Vol.134, No.7, (March 2008), pp. 1938-1949.

Zhang, JY; Zhang, Z; Lin, F; Zou, ZS; Xu, RN; Jin, L; Fu, JL; Shi, F; Shi, M; Wang, HF & Wang, FS. (2010). Interleukin-17-producing CD4(+) T cells increase with severity of liver damage in patients with chronic hepatitis B. *Hepatology,* Vol.51, No.1, (January 2010), pp. 81-91.

5

# Immunostochimistry as a Tool for Chronic Hepatitis Diagnosis

P Chevallier-Queyron[1] and I Chemin[2]
[1]*Virology Laboratory, Hospices civils de Lyon, Croix Rousse Hospital and Université Lyon 1, Lyon,*
[2]*Université Lyon 1, Lyon, Centre de Recherche en Cancérologie de Lyon, Lyon, France*

## 1. Introduction

Detection and localization of hepatitis viruses in liver tissue are vital for diagnostic purposes and clinical management of infected patients, as well as for the elucidation of viropathological mechanisms. The fragility of RNA and/or the low levels of viral expression in infected tissues are a constant limitation in molecular assays for viral characterization. Viral antigen detection, by immunochemistry, in liver biopsies is an attractive option for precise localization and quantification of viral proteins with direct access to histological patterns. We will describe studies using immunohistochemical methods effective on fixed, archived specimens, including liver biopsies and surgical resection samples.

### 1.1 Chronic hepatitis B

Natural course of type B hepatitis is now well established and the different phases of the disease are clearly defined. Briefly, after contamination early in life, there is a first phase of *immune tolerance*. During this phase, the virus is highly replicative, HBV DNA, HBs and HBe antigen are at high level in the serum, but clinical, biological, and histological signs are more or less normal. These patients are highly contagious, and most of them are going to be HBV carriers for the rest of their life. This model if frequent in highly endemic countries where a high rate of mother-to-baby transmission exists (especially in Asia); This phase is absent when people are infected as adults, their immune system being mature. They present an acute hepatitis and only a few of them (10%) will remain carrier with chronic hepatitis B. The phase of tolerance lasts for about 15 to 20 years. Nowadays very few people are having liver biopsy during that period. When it was done in the 70's/80's HBV antigens immunostaining were quite impressive: HBs antigen was present in a diffuse aspect grade associated with a strong expression for HBc antigen on more than 50% of nuclei (Table 1).

During the second phase of *the immune clearance phase,* hepatitis activity increase with fluctuating high level of ALT, necrosis, inflammatory cells infiltrates, fibrosis and decrease HBV viraemia. This period of high activity is associated sometimes with severe hepatic failure. At the end of this phase occurs HBe seroconversion which is often associated with clinical remission. The expression of HBV antigens detected by immunostaining is varying according to the time from infection when the biopsy was performed. The large number of HBs diffuse positive hepatocytes is decreasing with time. Many small clusters of cytoplasmic or sub membranous cells are gathering in the liver tissue the nuclear expression of HBc antigen is progressively changed in cytoplasmic expression and finally HBc antigen is undetectable. This stage corresponds to a very low viral replication (HBV DNA from 1000 UI/ml to null.).

| Phases of natural history | HBs diffuse | HBs cluster | | | HBc nuclear | HBc cytoplasmic |
|---|---|---|---|---|---|---|
| | | membranous | Sub membranous | cytoplasmic | | |
| Immune tolerance | ++ to +++ | unusual | unusual | unusual | very frequent | unusual |
| Immune clearance | 0 to +++ | frequent | emerging | rare | frequent | emerging |
| Inactive phase early period | 0 to + | rare | frequent | frequent | unusual | frequent |
| Inactive phase late period | 0 to + | absent | frequent | Very frequent | absent | rare or absent |
| Reactivation | + to +++ | frequent | frequent | frequent | frequent | frequent |

Table 1. Summary of the aspects and patterns of HBV antigen along the natural course of chronic type B hepatitis.

*During the third phase called the inactive carrier phase,* clinical remission may occur earlier in life if infection had occurred in adulthood ; Usually liver biopsy is done at that period to graduate residual inflammatory activity and over all staging the fibrosis. HBs Ag can be detected by immunostaining :

- on very few hepatocytes; this can be seen after a very long carriage of HBV; it is correlated with a low level of HBs antigen in the serum.
- on very large clusters of cytoplasmic pattern including almost all the hepatocytes. These patients have a very high level of HBs antigen in serum, exclusively made of spherical and tubular empty particles.

HBc antigen is usually undetectable. In very low replicative patients some cytoplamic expression can be detected in rare hepatocytes.

*During this inactive phase, reactivations may occur.* If liver biopsy is done during this period, expression of viral antigens is similar to the clearance period, associated in many cases with intense expression of HBs antigen in the diffuse or cluster like pattern. If the patient is not treated for this reactivation, HBs antigen will decrease and HBc antigen will appear in some nuclei.

### 1.2 Liver transplantation

In the vast majority of the cases, histological examination is able to explain if a flare of activity (cytolysis) is associated with graft rejection or re-infection of the graft by HBV. In case of re-infection, diffuse HBs antigen is weakly present in its cytoplasmic pattern and nuclear HBc is detected.

### 1.3 Occult HBV hepatitis

In some cases of occult hepatitis infection (HBV DNA detectable in the liver and possibly in the serum in the absence of the landmark of HBV infection, the HBsAg in the serum).
In those cases, few hepatocytes may be weakly positive for either HBs or HBc antigen. It can be helpful for the diagnosis of these very peculiar forms of HBV infections.

### 1.4 Hepatitis C hepatitis

The Hepatitis C virus (HCV) genome is a single stranded RNA molecule of about 9500 bp. This RNA encodes for a large poly-protein that is processed by host and virus proteases into several structural and non structural viral proteins (Envelope, Capsid and NS2a/b NS3a/b NS4a/b NS5a/b respectively). The detection of HCV replicative intermediates or virus antigen may be helpful for diagnosis or clinical management of patients with HCV infection and it is of crucial importance for monitoring patients prior and post- HCV-related liver transplantation. In a general point of view, HCV replication level seems to be relatively low in infected liver, hampering the detection of HCV particles directly in the liver (Shimizu *et al.*, 1996, Negro, 1998). Detection methods based on HCV RNA amplification as *in situ* PCR or *in situ* hybridization are not completely efficient for HCV detection and can lead to conflicting results concerning viral particles localization (Lau *et al.*, 1996). However they remain an interesting tool when used in complement of classical method (Biagini *et al.*, 2001, Comar *et al.*, 2006). Limitation of these methods is probably due to RNA rapid degradation in tissues and difficulty to design efficient probes to overcome high variability of HCV genomes.
Detection of HCV antigens by immunochemistry in liver biopsies constitutes therefore an interesting option that allows both localization and quantification of viral proteins (Galy et al, 2006).

## 2. Methods

### 2.1 Hepatitis B antigens

Slides are deparaffinized in methylcyclohexane (two baths for 10 minutes) then re-hydrated through 4 baths of ethanol and soaked for half an hour in PBS pH 7.2; and endogenous peroxidase blocked by $H_2O_2$.
Slides are then incubated in a humid chamber for 30 minutes at room temperature with diluted anti-HBs antibody, and then rinsed 4 times in PBS pH 7.2. A second incubation in same conditions is made with the secondary antibody (anti rabbit or mouse immunoglobulin, according to the primary antibody) labelled with peroxydase. Commercial kit with DAB substrate (Dako USA) are used to develop the final reaction.
Counterstaining with Harris haematoxylin is added on slides for HBs antigen search. Usually no counterstaining is performed on slides tested for HBc antigen as it might interact with the nuclear expression of this viral antigen.
Reagents:

- Anti-Hbs monoclonal mouse antibody Dako USA (clone 3E7) or Argene F( ref:11-086)
- Polyclonal rabbit Anti –Hbc ready to use Dako USA
- Antibody diluent Dako USA
- Envision dual link kit Dako USA
- Hematoxylin Biomedia USA

### 2.2 Hepatitis C antigen

First tissue sections are deparaffinized in xylene for 10 minutes (twice). Then Rehydrate in graded ethanol concentrations (100% and 95% for 5 min each) and proceed immediately to Block endogenous peroxidase activities with incubation in methanol (0.3% hydrogen peroxide) for 30 minutes at room temperature. The unmasking procedure includes a microwave treatment. The slides are placed in microwave for 15min in antigen unmasking solution (Vector H3300 - Vector Laboratories, Burlingame, CA, USA). Keep slides to cool down for 30 min in the same unmasking solution. Incubate with PBS solution (5% skimmed milk and 0,1% BSA) for 1 hour at room temperature. Sections are incubated overnight with the primary mAb (For $D_{4.12.9}$: concentration 0.2µg/ml) at 4°C. Sections without primary antibody can be used as controls. Wash in PBS (3x5 min). Incubate 30 min with Secondary antibody at 5µl/ml (Elite Kit- Vector Laboratories, Burlingame, CA, USA) in PBS solution (0,1% BSA). Wash again in PBS (3x5 min). Amplify signal at 37°C for 45min with VECTASTAIN ABC Kit (Vector Laboratories, Burlingame, CA, USA) - Use 0,1%BSA PBS solution. Wash in PBS (3x5 min).Incubate tissue sections with the DAB substrate (Vector kit SK 4100, Vector Laboratories, Burlingame, CA, USA) at room temperature for 5 minutes.Wash in PBS (3x5 min). Counterstain the sections with Mayer's haematoxylin. Dehydrate through a successive ethanol baths (95% Ethanol, absolute ethanol and xylene -5 min in each solution). Mount slides using standard microscope cover glass and mounting medium.

### 2.3 Hepatitis delta antigen

Direct immunostaining in fluorescence may be used for delta antigen. Once deparaffinized as above, slides are at first incubated for 30 minutes with a solution of proteinase K(21 mg/ml in Tris EDTA buffer) then rinsed in PBS for 15 minutes . Incubation with the FITC labelled anti-delta antibody is performed in humid chamber for half an hour. Slides are rinsed in two baths of PBS for 15 minutes and mounted.

Reagents:

- Proteinase K recombinant Roche USA
- Tris EDTA buffer Sigma Aldrich USA
- Polyclonal rabbit anti delta antibody labelled with FITC is kindly provided by Dr Alan Kay INSERM unit 1052, Lyon, France.

## 3. Examples of viral hepatitis antigens detection

### 3.1 Hepatitis B

#### 3.1.1 Cytological patterns of HBs antigen

Three different patterns are seen on liver biopsies:

i. *Cytoplasmic* : this is the most common pattern , consisting in a large vacuole made of the Golgi reticulum full of viral envelopes. In light microscopy it is usually called "ground glass" hepatocytes. The intensity of the staining is closely correlated with the amount of viral envelope in the cell (Figure 1).

ii. *Submembranous* : This pattern is not frequent ; it is associated with a strong production of viral envelope and might be a former stage of the cytoplasmic pattern (Figure 2).

iii. *Membranous*: This is a less common pattern. It is often seen on a few hepatocytes; it is mostly associated with strong viral expression and is rather present in active periportal zone. Staining underlines the cell membrane in a perfect straight line. (Figure 3)

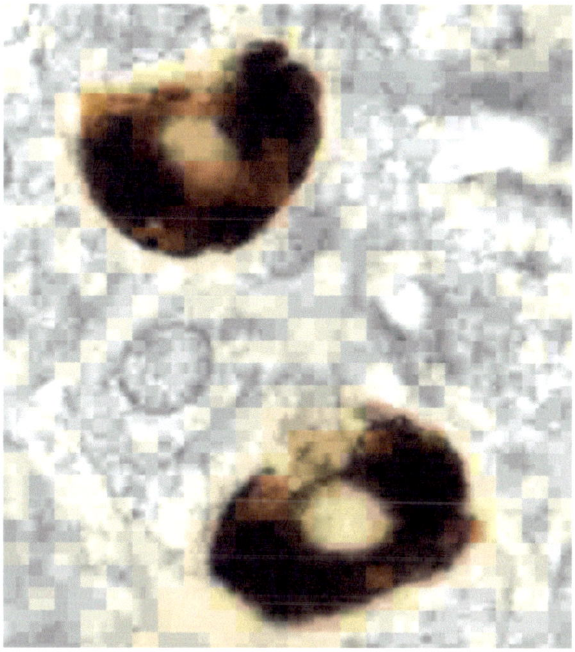

Fig. 1. Two typical ground glass hepatocytes stained with immunoperoxydase for HBs antigen.( magnification x 600)

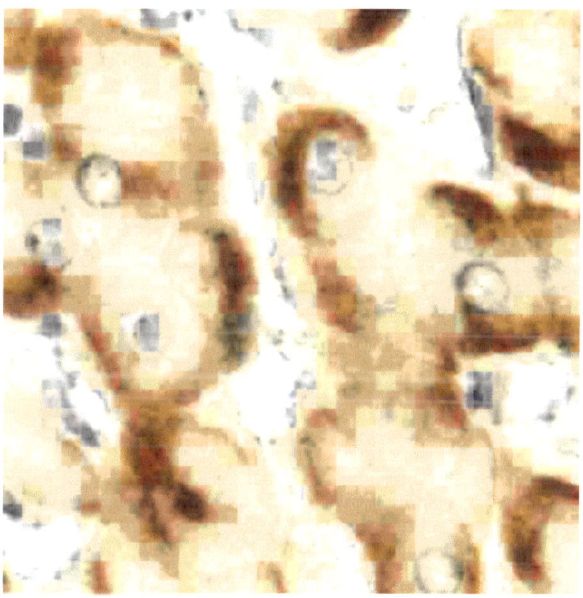

Fig. 2. Submembranous expression of HBs antigen in hepatocytes ( immunoproxydase magnification x 600).

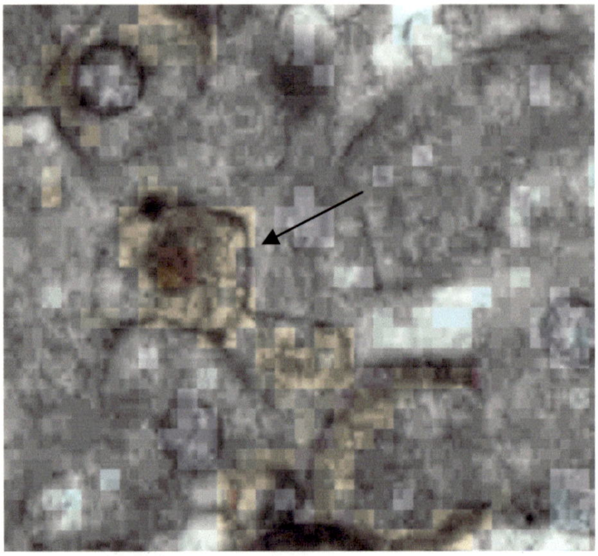

Fig. 3. Membranous expression of HBs antigen: arrow shows the perfectly straight pattern of the cell membrane (immunoperoxydase magnification x 600).

### 3.1.2 Cytological patterns of HBc antigen

i. *Nuclear*: This is the most common expression pattern of this antigen in liver cells (Figure 4).
ii. *Cytoplasmic* : The design is different from the HBs Antigen one as it is not gathered in a part of the cell but more or less diffuse in the whole cytoplasmic area (Figure 5).
iii. In many cases, cells can express both of these patterns (Figure 6).

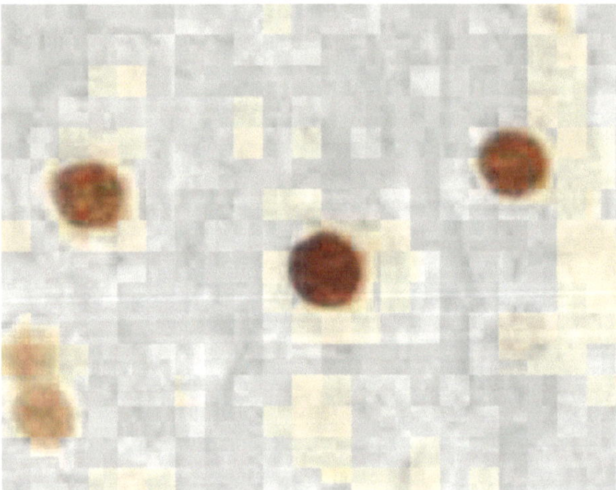

Fig. 4. Nuclear expression of HBc antigen. Note the large scale of intensity of the staining (immunoproxydase, magnification x 600).

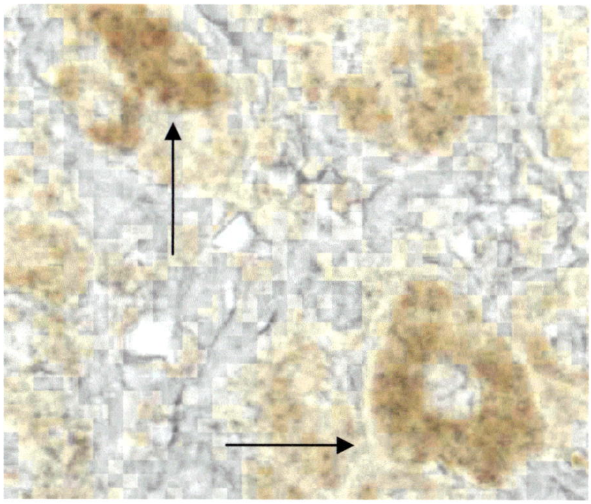

Fig. 5. Cytoplasmic expression of HBc antigen (immunoperoxydase, magnification x 600).

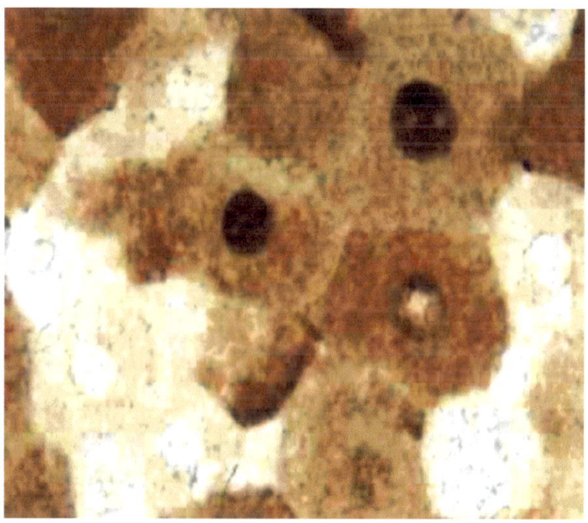

Fig. 6. Double expression of HBc antigen: cytoplasmic and nuclear, sometimes in the same hepatocyte (immunoperoxydase magnification x 600).

### 3.1.3 Antigen expression in liver tissue

The antigen expression in liver tissue is important to observe as it correlates to the stage of replication and natural history of the disease.

**HBs antigen**

Two main patterns can be observed:

i. *Diffuse or dotted*: Positive liver cells are non confluent, diffuse in the lobule. It can be useful to estimate the number of positive cells in the biopsy. This can be done semi quantitatively as an amount grade +, ++, +++ (Figures 7, 8, 9).

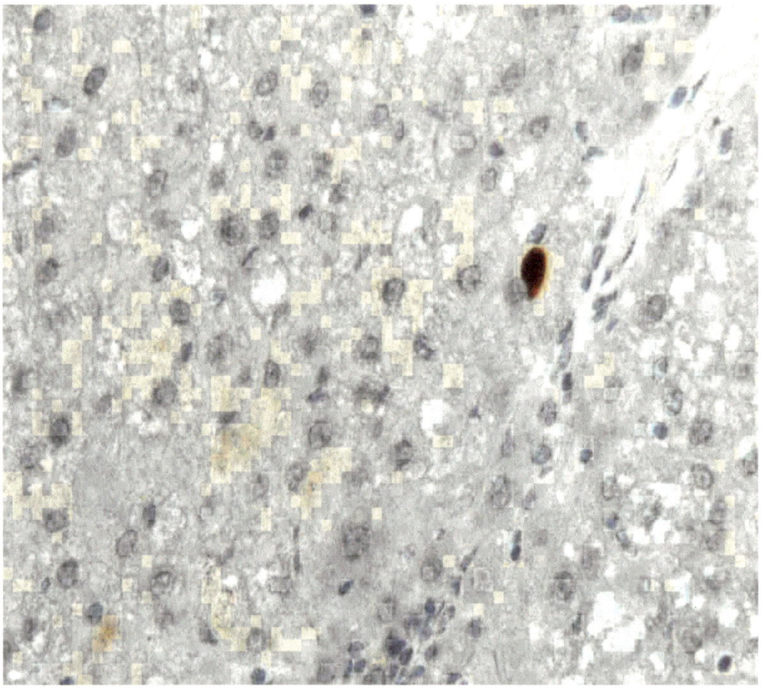

Fig. 7. Diffuse expression of cytoplasmic HBs antigen: amount grade: + , the only strong positive cell out of a 15 mm length needle biopsy (immunoperoxydase magnification x 100).

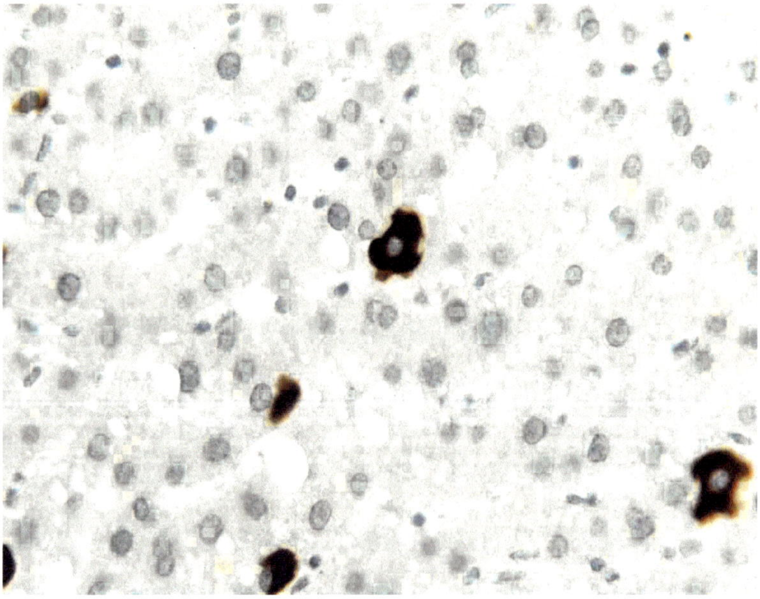

Fig. 8. Diffuse expression of cytoplasmic HBs antigen in strongly stained hepatocytes, amount grade: ++ (immunoperoxydase magnification x 100)

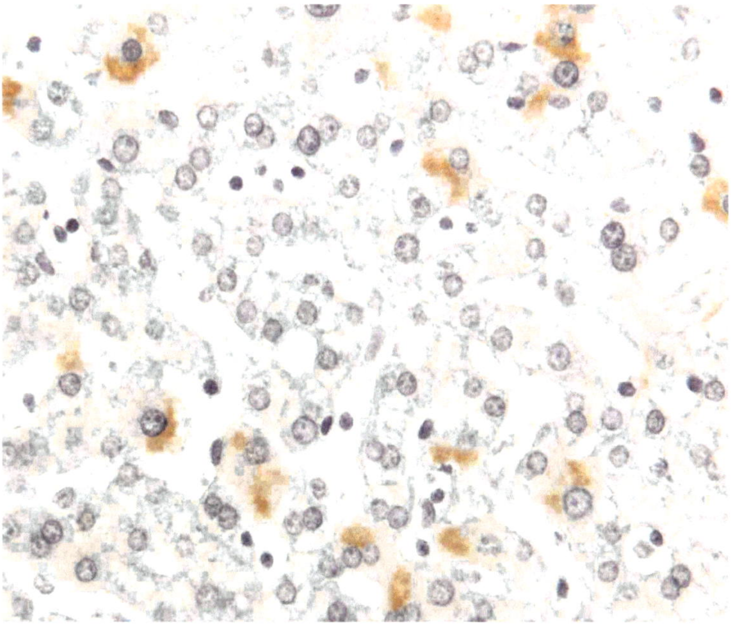

Fig. 9. Diffuse expression of cytoplasmic HBs antigen, light staining, amount grade +++ (immunoperoxydase, magnification x 100)

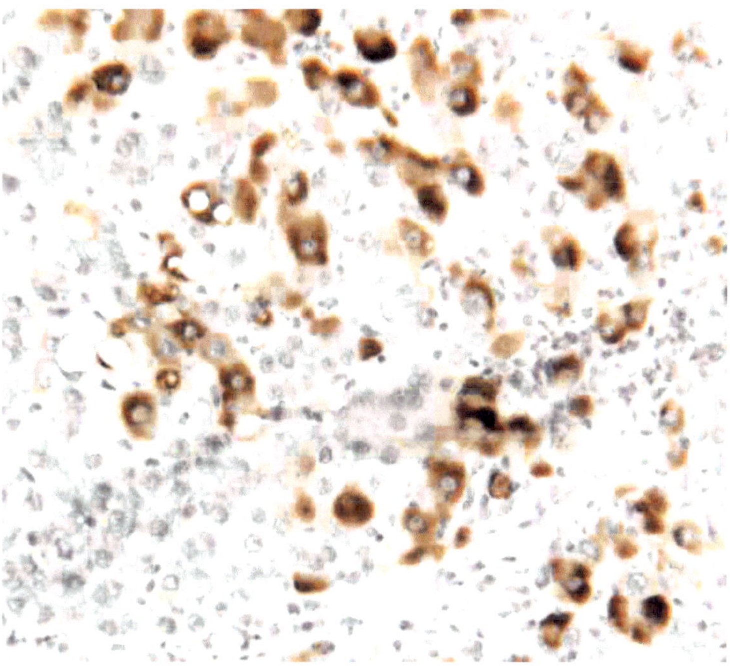

Fig. 10. Diffuse expression of cytoplasmic HBs antigen, strong staining, amount grade +++ (immunoproxydase, magnification x 75).

ii. *Confluent or cluster-like pattern*: Positive cells are closely gathered inside the lobule can be detected on contiguous lobules (Figures 11, 12, 13). Sometimes, this pattern can be associated with the diffuse pattern on the external zone of the cluster (around the cluster). The distribution of these clusters of positive cells is not homogenous in the whole liver. False negative of the immunochemistry staining is possible if the needle doesn't reach a positive zone (See Figure 12) with a strong contrast between positive and negative area on a surgical biopsy);

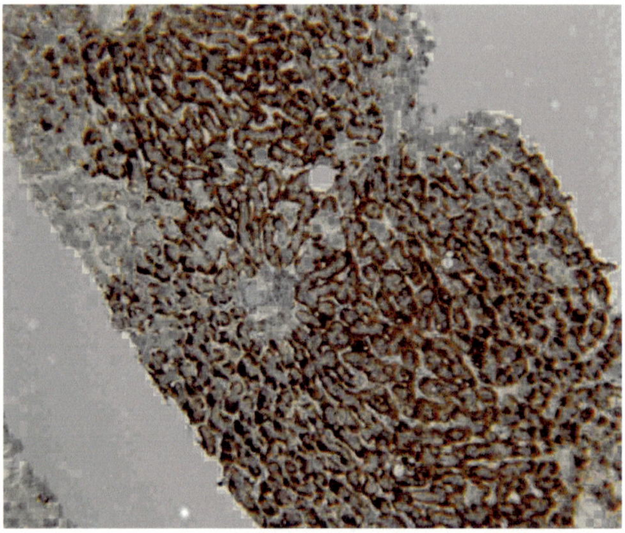

Fig. 11. Large cluster of sub membranous HBs antigen positive hepatocytes (immunoperoxydase, magnification x 40).

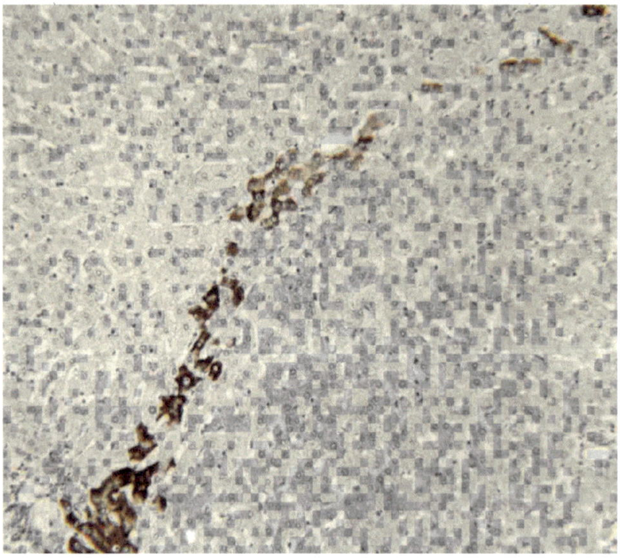

Fig. 12. Cluster of HBs antigen positive cells crossing a lobule from portal tract to Centro lobular vein. ( immunoperoxydase, magnification x 75

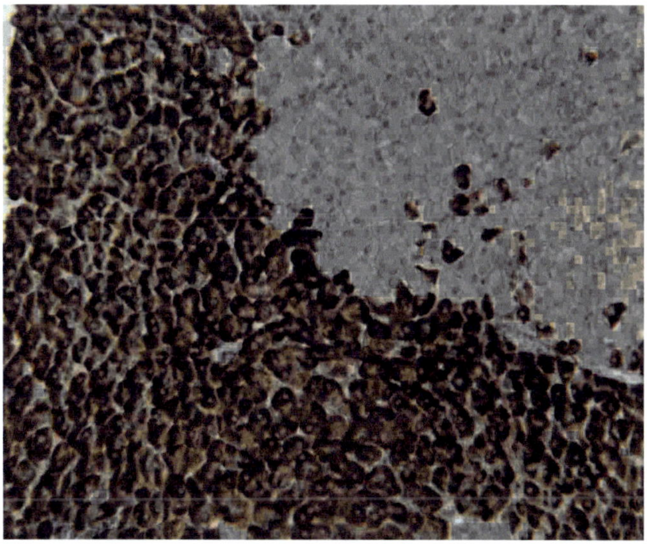

Fig. 13. Large cluster of HBs antigen positive hepatocytes with a cytoplasmic pattern. Note the strong contrast between positive and a very weak positive area (immunoproxydase, magnification x 40).

Sub membranous and membranous pattern are always expressed in the liver tissue as a cluster like pattern (Figure 14)

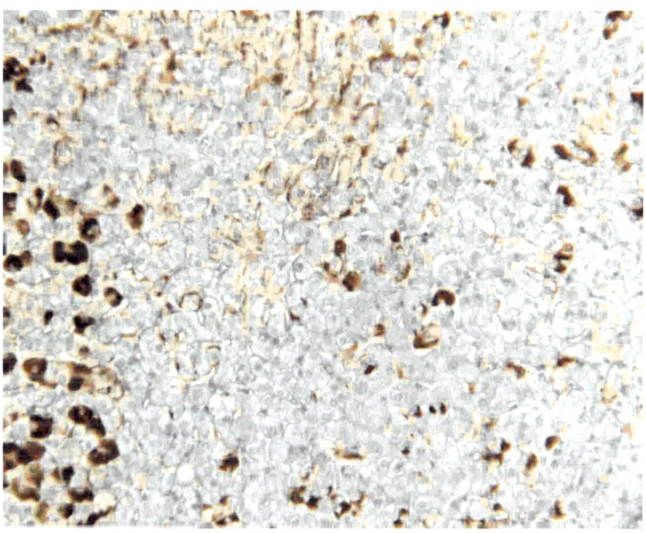

Fig. 14. Presence of three patterns of HBs antigen:
top : sub membranous, centre: membranous and left: cytoplasmic. (immunoperoxydase, magnification x 40)

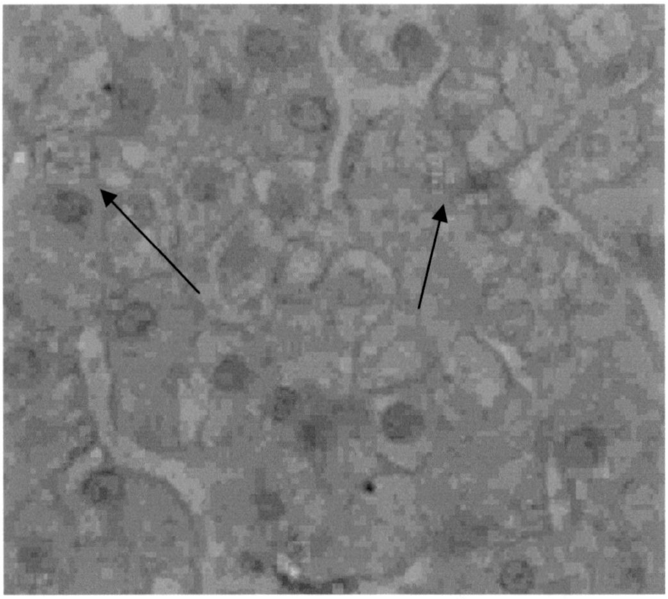

Fig. 15. Very weak expression of HBs antigen in a liver biopsy of an occult carrier of HBV (immunoperoxydase, magnification x 400).

**HBc antigen**

As the presence of HBc antigen in the liver is correlated with the amount of invective whole Dane particles, quantification is possible. For the nuclear pattern it is usual to calculate the percentage of positive cells in the biopsy.

Five classes of percentage are described: less than 1%, from 1 to 5%, from 5 to 20%, from 20% to 50% and over 50%.

The cyoplasmic pattern is more difficult to quantify as it might be very weakly expressed in some cells. We usually describe 4 classes: rare positive cells, positive +, positive ++, positive +++.

### 3.2 Hepatitis C

In our personal experience (Galy *et al.*, 2006), the staining location for Anti-E2 immunostaining is mainly cytoplasmic with occasional perimembranous staining (including cytoplasmic and nuclear membrane). Staining pattern is mainly coarse granular with microvesicular pattern (Figure 16 ). HCV staining patterns appears to differ slightly according to the pathological status of the liver tissue. We observed a very strong staining of hepatocyte membrane, cytoplasm and perinuclear regions in liver from patient with active HCV-related cirrhosis (Intense plasma and nuclear membrane staining was observed in cases with high inflammatory activity). In non-cirrhotic and non-tumoral tissues Anti-E2 staining intensity increases with hepatitis fibrosis state. In HCV-related tumors, staining was exclusively detected within regeneration nodules and confined to hepatocytes whose morphology remains unchanged. Staining pattern appeared with two distinct patterns: trabecular throughout the hepatic parenchyma or concerning isolated cells.

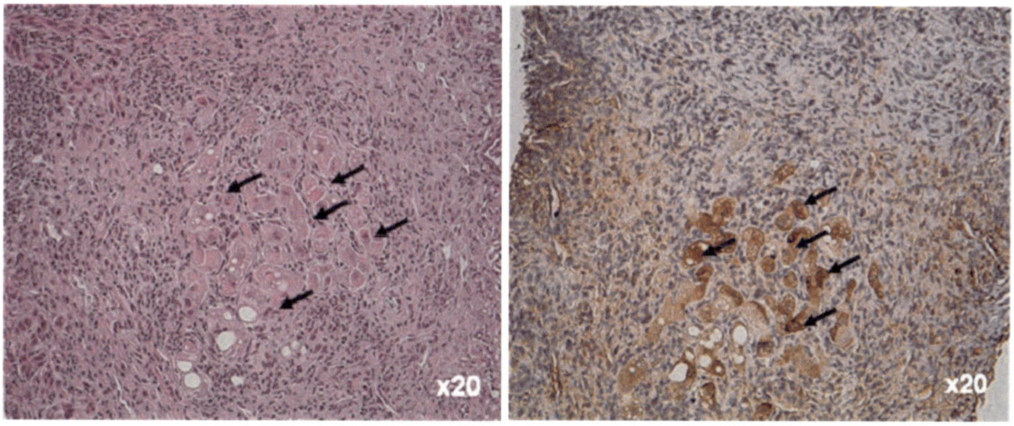


Fig. 16. Expression of HCV E2 antigen in a liver biopsy of cirrhotic liver of an HCV chronic carriers. Arrows: Few remaining hepatocytes strongly positive with anti-E2 antibody. Immunoperoxydase magnification X 200

### 3.3 Hepatitis delta

Antigen delta is expressed mainly in the nucleus of the hepatocyte and in rare cases can also be expressed in the cytoplasm; it depends on the stage of the replication and the production of antigen. The nuclear expression seems to be more correlated with a period of stoking of viral core. The result of the test is qualitative: negative or positive (Figure 17).

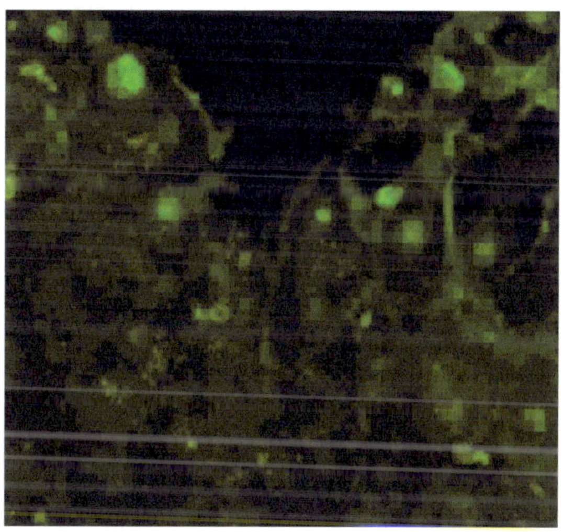

Fig. 17. Intranuclear expression of Delta (HDV) antigen. FITC labelling, magnification x 100

## 4. Conclusion

Concerning Hepatitis B virus (HBV) detection of HBs and HBc antigens are informative and provide different patterns providing elements in correlation with the natural history of HBV infection including viral load. In the specific case of occult HBV infection (HBV DNA

detected in the absence of HBsAg in the serum) it may help to confirm the diagnosis. For Hepatitis C virus (HCV) antigen detection it exists antibodies that are able to successfully detected HCV on paraffin-embedded sections from fresh as well as archived-frozen, material. It should be noted that HCV detection in archived serum may be problematic due to delicate extraction and stability of RNA and this is the same for hepatitis delta virus diagnosis (HDV). Thus, IHC represents a very stable diagnostic tool as compared to RNA-based approaches. We found important differences in the localization of HCV between tumor and non-involved, adjacent tissue in HCC cases.
These protocols offer easy, precise and strong staining resolution with distinct patterns consistent with the liver pathology, irrespective of the hepatitis viruses examined. This approach provides applications for diagnosis as well as for exploratory pathological studies. Thus, IHC to detect viral hepatitis antigens may have a number of important applications for clinical diagnostic, research on the mechanisms of pathogenesis of viral hepatitis-containing lesions, and retrospective evaluation of the contribution of hepatitis viruses to liver diseases using archives of paraffin-embedded material not suitable for molecular analysis.

## 5. Acknowledgements

Thanks to Dr M. Chevallier , J.Y. Scoazec, B. Bancel and F. Berger who kindly provide us with liver sections.

## 6. References

[1] Shimizu, Y.K., et al., *Hepatitis C virus: detection of intracellular virus particles by electron microscopy. Hepatology,* 1996. 23(2): p. 205-9.
[2] Negro, F., *Detection of hepatitis C virus RNA in liver tissue: an overview.* Ital J Gastroenterol Hepatol, 1998. 30(2): p. 205-10.
[3] Lau, J.Y., et al., *In situ detection of hepatitis C virus--a critical appraisal.* J Hepatol, 1996. 24(2 Suppl): p. 43-51.
[4] Biagini, P., et al., *Hepatitis C virus RNA detection by in situ RT-PCR in formalin-fixed paraffin-embedded liver tissue. Comparison with serum and tissue results.* Cell Mol Biol (Noisy-le-grand), 2001. 47 Online Pub: p. OL167-71.
[5] Comar, M., et al., *HBV, HCV, and TTV detection by in situ polymerase chain reaction could reveal occult infection in hepatocellular carcinoma: comparison with blood markers.* J Clin Pathol, 2006. 59(5): p. 526-9.
[6] Galy, O., et al., *Efficient hepatitis C antigen immunohistological staining in sections of normal, cirrhotic and tumoral liver using a new monoclonal antibody directed against serum-derived HCV E2 glycoproteins.* Cancer Lett, 2006.

# Microanalytical Determination of Trace Elements from Liver Biopsy Materials of Patients with Chronic Diffuse Liver Diseases with Different Ultrasound Attenuation

Szebeni A.[1], Varga I.[2], Kovács B.[3], Tolvaj Gy.[4] and Zalatnai A.[5]
[1]*MI Central Hospital, Ultrasonic Laboratory*
[2]*L. Eotvos University, Institute of Chemistry, Department of Analytical Chemistry*
[3]*University of Debrecen - Centre for Agricultural and Applied Economic Sciences, Institute of Food Science, Quality Assurance and Microbiology*
[4]*MI Central Hospital, 1st Internal Department*
[5]*Semmelweis University, Faculty of Medicine, 1st Department of Pathology and Experimental Cancer Research*
*Hungary*

## 1. Introduction

Liver biopsy remained the gold standard in the diagnostics of chronic diffuse liver diseases despite the effectivity of some recent noninvasive diagnostic tools for the detection of fatty liver (Amacher, 2011; Copel, 2003; Germani et al, 2011; Karamashi, 2008; Lewindon, 2011; Sporea, et al., 2008; Strauss, 2010; Talwalkar, 2002).This means, that liver biopsy is applied in the diagnostic procedure of almost every patient with suggested chronic diffuse liver disease. Beside establishment of the diagnosis, liver biopsy specimens can be used also for research projects, aiming to obtain knowledge from the pathophysiological background of these conditions.

Trace element contamination is growing with the great progress of industry. Consequently, the trace element load of living organisms is also increasing. Some elements can play a role in the formation of malignant tumors. (Boffetta, 1993; Hayes, 1997; Navarro Silvera, 2007; Sky-Peck, 1986; Wingren & Axelson, 1993). It is well known that the liver is involved in the metabolism of compounds containing also certain trace elements. Thus, determination of these elements in biopsy samples and searching for correlations between element content and some liver diseases seems to be promising.

Ultrasonography is widely used in the diagnostic procedure of patients with liver diseases. Chronic diffuse liver diseases produce the characteristic ultrasound image of bright liver (Lonardo et al., 1997; Joseph et al., 1979). On the basis of in vivo measurements of liver ultrasound attenuation (α), two major appearances of bright liver were differentiated, the low (DI type) and the high (DII type) attenuation types. It was proved previously that low (DI type) bright liver shows increase of connective tissue content, while high (DII) attenuation type bright liver is associated with fatty liver, correlating with subcutaneous fat thickness (SCF) and body mass index (BMI). (Szebeni et al., 1999; Szebeni et al., 2006).

## 2. Objectives

The main objective was to determine the trace element content of the liver from biopsy samples. It was also studied that the trace element content is similar or differing from each other in patients with normal ultrasound liver pattern as well as in patients with chronic diffuse liver diseases showing low attenuation (DI) type or high attenuation (DII) type bright liver. Another objective of the present study was the determination of possible contamination of biopsy samples by steel-metals during sample collection using a porcine liver model. Additional objective was the determination and comparison of intra-individual variability of element concentrations in a porcine liver as well as in a human liver obtained from cadaveric donor with liver steatosis. The choice of analytical methods was a key question. An appropriate method should be capable of measuring very low concentrations simultaneously and sample consumption should be restricted to the possible minimum. The suitability of histochemical staining methods and two microanalytical methods were studied. Inductively coupled plasma mass spectrometry (ICP-MS) has favourable detection limits and was selected for simultaneous determination of micro and trace elements (Labat, et al., 2003; Millos, et al., 2008). Total reflection X-ray fluorescence spectrometry (TXRF) is also a suitable and powerful technique for analysis of small-mass biopsy samples, because it requires small amount of substance (Marco, et al., 2004).

## 3. Material and methods

### 3.1 Material

183 patients (110 males, age 26-80; and 73 females, age 23-70) were examined because of the suggestion of chronic diffuse liver disease. After clinical (history, physical examination, BMI, abdominal circumference, waist/hip ratio), laboratory (liver function tests, total se cholesterol, low density and high density cholesterol, trigliceride, INR, platelet count, etc...) and ultrasound examinations, liver biopsy was performed for establishing the correct diagnosis. Semiquantitative histopathological analysis was also done in these patients. Biopsy materials were used retrospectively for research purposes, namely for analysis of the concentration of the following trace elements: Cr, Mn, Fe, Ni, Cu, Zn, Rb, Mo and Pb.

### 3.2 Methods

#### 3.2.1 Ultrasound examinations

Ultrasound scanning of the liver - as part of a general abdominal ultrasound examination - and subcutaneous fat thickness determinations were made by a B-K Medical Hawk 2102 EXL scanner. For liver scanning 5 MHz curved transducer, for subcutaneous fat thickness measurements 12 MHz linear transcducer was used. Attenuation of the liver was measured with the aid of a homogeneous tissue equivalent reference phantom with known attenuation. After scanning of the phantom and the patient's liver with the same equipment setting, a special software was applied, capable to digitizing the image, as well as obtain and compare their brightness diagrams and evaluate attenuation of the patient's liver (Szebeni et al., 2006).

#### 3.2.2 Percutaneous liver biopsy

Before the intervention, detailed information was given to the patient about the procedure and importance of percutaneous liver biopsy. Thereafter a statement of permission was subscribed by the patient. 30 minutes before the biopsy slight sedation was applied (0,07 mg/kg midazolam was given intramuscularly). 15 minutes before the intervention

0,5 mg atropin was injected subcutaneously. The biopsy was made in the left decubitus position using generally applied disposable Braun Hepafix needle. The site of the biopsy was determined by percussion between the anterior and median axillary line according to the hepatic dullness. 1% Lidocain injection was used for local anaesthesia. The puncture was made in deep outbreath in most cases blindly, but sometimes under ultrasonic guidance. The obtained biopsy specimen was fixed in 4% neutral formalin solution for histological examination. For trace element determination a small part of the material was deep-freezed and stored on -20° C till the analytical process.

### 3.2.3 Semiquantitative histopathologic evaluation

Histopathological studies have been performed in formalin-fixed, paraffin-embedded biopsy materials. In addition to the routine hematoxylin-eosin (H&E), periodic acid-Schiff (PAS) stains, the specimens were also stained by picrosirius red (Szendrői et al., 1984), a 1% alcoholic solution of rubeanic acid (dithiooxamide) counterstained with Nuclear Fast Red (Vacca, 1985). The amount and distribution of connective tissue was visualized by the picrosirius red stain. Fibrosis was diagnosed when the retained lobular architecture was surrounded by the collagen fibers, and it was semiquantitatively graded as mild, intermediate and severe. In cirrhotic livers the lobular architecture has been distorted. Rubeanic acid method is principally used for identification of copper in histological preparates, but other metals are also identifiable: while the copper granules are characteristically greenish-black, the nickel is bluish-violet, and the cobalt is yellowish-brown (Quicke,1979, Vacca, 1985).

The severity of the fatty change was semiquantitatively scored in H&E stained samples. Mild form was diagnosed when the lipid droplets occupied up to 25% of the liver, intermediate between 25-65%, and severe when they exceeded 65%. The necroinflammatory reaction was evaluated in at least 20 portal of intralobular areas, and graded as mild (1-5 portal tracts involved), intermediate (6-10 portal tracts) or severe (over 10 portal tracts affected).

### 3.2.4 Trace element analysis

#### 3.2.4.1 Sample collection and preparation

For reference measurement twelve porcine liver portions (different size, in the range from 7 mg to 545 mg wet weight) were cut by a quartz blade, immediately weighed on a microbalance and freeze-dried. Time relationship of element release from biopsy needles was investigated applying 0.1, 1 and $24^h$ contact time. Disposable Braun-Hepafix liver biopsy needles were used for sampling porcine and human cadaver liver and the same sample preparation was applied. The sample preparation was performed in a clean bench and the porcine liver was stored at 4°C during the exposure intervals. Suprapure nitric acid (Merck, Darmstadt, Germany) and high-purity water from a Milli-Q system were used throughout the work. Polypropylene microvials (used for sample storage) were cleaned with 0.5 mol/l nitric acid for $1^h$ then rinsed with high-purity water and dried in a clean bench. The samples were digested in a laboratory microwave system according to the method described in our previous work (Varga et al., 2005). Distribution of the elements within the liver was investigated taking biopsy samples from different localizations of a cadaveric liver with steatosis with the same technique described before.

### 3.2.4.2 Instrumentation and technique

Total reflection X-ray fluorescence (TXRF) analysis was performed using an Atomika EXTRA IIA spectrometer equipped with line focused X-ray tubes and an energy dispersive Si(Li) detector. Mo K$\alpha$ 17.4 keV, W continuum (Bremsstrahlung) 35 keV excitation and 1000 s data acquisition live time were applied. K lines were used for Cr, Mn, Fe, Ni, Cu, Zn, Rb and Mo, L line was used for Pb determination. 100 μl of sample solution was used to prepare specimens for the TXRF analysis in the following manner. 25 μl of sample solution was pipetted onto a previously siliconized quartz glass carrier and allowed to dry in a clean bench at 40°C. This procedure was repeated until 100 μl total volume of sample solution was reached. Finally, 10 μl yttrium chloride solution containing 0.1 mg/dm$^3$ yttrium was added as an internal standard for the quantification of TXRF measurements. Biopsy samples were analyzed by TXRF spectrometry after nitric acid digestion. Small volume microwave digestion was developed especially for biopsy samples and proved to be applicable for liver biopsies having sample size as small as only 1 mg or less. An efficient XRF method was developed for autopsy samples having sample mass of about 500 mg without digestion. Samples were analyzed by a benchtop XRF spectrometer -PANalytical MiniPal2 (Almelo, the Netherlands)- equipped with low power, Rh anode X-ray tube and a Si-PIN semiconductor detector (Fig. 1).

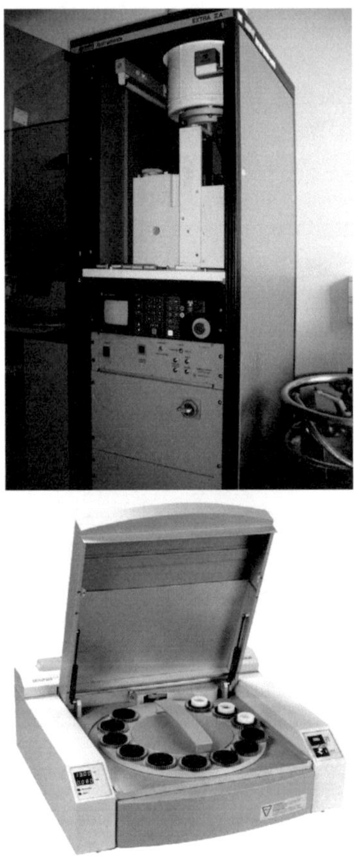

Fig. 1. Atomika Extra IIA TXRF Spectometer and PANalytical MiniPal2 benchtop XRF Spectrometer

TXRF analytical method was validated applying NIST 1577a Bovine Liver Certified Reference Material (Table 1.)

| | *Certified values* (*µg/g*) | *Measured values* (*µg/g*) | *SD* | *Recovery* (*%*) |
|---|---|---|---|---|
| P | 11100 ± 400 | 11780 | 880 | 106.1 |
| S | 7800 ± 100 | 7290 | 550 | 93.5 |
| K | 9260 ± 70 | 11300 | 830 | 113.5 |
| Mn | 9.9 ± 0.8 | 11.8 | 0.9 | 119.2 |
| Fe | 194 ± 20 | 193 | 14 | 99.5 |
| Pb | 0.135 ± 0.015 | n.d. | - | - |
| Cu | 158 ± 7 | 156 | 11 | 98.5 |
| Se | 0.71 ± 0.07 | 0.56 | 0.21 | 78.9 |
| Zn | 123 ± 8 | 127 | 9 | 103.3 |
| Rb | 12.5 ± 0.1 | 11.9 | 0.8 | 94.8 |
| Sr | 0.138 ± 0.003 | n.d. | - | - |
| Mo | 3.5 ± 0.5 | 3.7 | 0.4 | 105.7 |

(4 independent replicate, concentrations in µg/g corresponding to dry weight)
n.d. signifies concentration under the limit of detection (LOD)

Table 1. TXRF analysis results of NIST 1577a Bovine Liver CRM.

An inductively coupled plasma mass spectrometer (ICP-MS) is capable for analysis of 70-80 elements in multielemental mode, from 1-5 $cm^3$ volume of a sample, moreover the detection limits of elements are in µg/kg-ng/kg (ppb-ppt) concentration range. Nowadays there is very important to analyze growingly smaller concentrations of elements. An ICP-MS has different physical and chemical interfering effects analyzing various samples. The smaller the concentration of an analyte and the larger the concentration of the matrix the larger the interfering effects (Kovács et al., 2006). From the spectroscopic analytical instruments generally the inductively coupled plasma mass spectrometer is capable of analyzing the smallest concentration of elements.

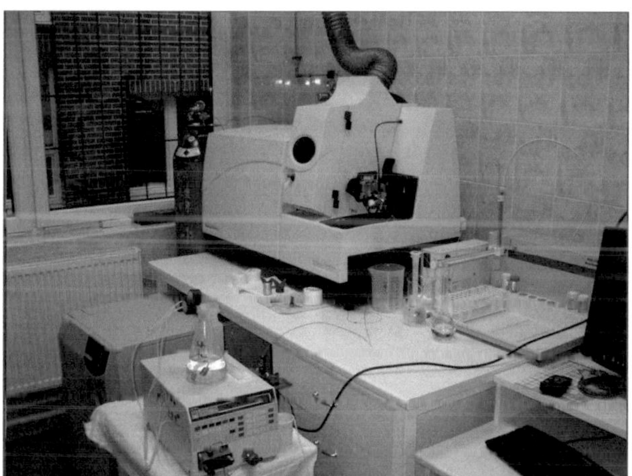

Fig. 2. The applied inductively coupled plasma mass spectrometer

As the human origin samples (e.g. human liver) contain small enough concentration of elements so an inductively coupled plasma mass spectrometer (Fig. 2.) was applied to analyze the various elements.
An X7 type (Thermo Elemental, Winsford, UK) inductively coupled plasma quadrupole mass spectrometer was used to detect the elements.
The instrument was operated with a Peltier cooled impact bead spray chamber, single piece quartz torch (1.5 mm i.d. injector) and a conventional glass concentric nebulizer.
The following isotopes were measured during the research work: $^{25}$Mg, $^{52}$Cr, $^{53}$Cr, $^{55}$Mn, $^{54}$Fe, $^{56}$Fe, $^{58}$Ni, $^{59}$Co, $^{60}$Ni, $^{65}$Cu, $^{64}$Zn, $^{66}$Zn, $^{75}$As, $^{78}$Se, $^{80}$Se, $^{82}$Se, $^{111}$Cd, $^{114}$Cd and $^{208}$Pb.Table 2. shows the applied operating instrumental parameters.

| | |
|---|---|
| **ICP-MS system:** | X7 type (Thermo Elemental, Winsford, UK) |
| RF power: | 1400 W |
| Nebulizer gas flow: | 0.80 L/min |
| Auxiliary gas flow: | 0.95 L/min |
| Cool gas flow: | 15.0 L/min |
| Sample uptake rate: | 0.88 mL/min |
| Interface: | Xi interface cones (Ni) |
| **Data acquisition:** | |
| Dwell time per isotope: | 20 ms |
| Number of sweeps: | 21 |
| Number of replicates: | 3 |
| Sample uptake and wash time: | 35 s |
| Calibration mode: | Peak jump |
| Number of integration: | 3/sample<br>5/blank |

Table 2. ICP-MS operating and data acquisition parameters

### 3.2.4.3 Intra-individual variability of element concentrations in human liver

A small liver biopsy specimen does not represent the liver as a whole. In order to be able to draw conclusions regarding differences of trace element contents of liver samples, we have to assume uniform trace element distributions throughout the whole organ. This assumption should be checked by comparison of samples taken from different lobes of the same liver. The latter study can be performed only on autopsy samples.
Intra-individual variability of elemental concentrations was investigated by the analysis of multiple human liver biopsy samples obtained from cadaveric donor with liver steatosis. The purpose of these investigations was the high hepatic Ni concentration observed in the human liver and its uneven distribution. Similar sampling was made on porcine liver for comparison. Concentrations of Fe, Ni, Cu, Zn, Rb, and Mo determined by total reflection X-ray fluorescence spectrometry are listed in Table 3. Cr, Mn, Co and Pb were measured only by inductively coupled plasma-atomic emission spectrometry. Element concentrations determined by both techniques were in good agreement and not presented in Table 3. as a repetition. The variability of element concentrations was between 8.7 and 17.6 % RSD. Exceptions were Pb, Ni and Cr having variability of 27.8, 73.0 and 68.6 % RSD, respectively. In case of porcine liver the intra-individual variability was less than 13.5 % RSD for each element. It can be also emphasized, that nickel distribution was quite even in porcine liver and average Ni concentration (0.16 μg/g dry weight) was two orders of magnitude lower compared to the value measured in the investigated human liver.

| | Cr[b] | Mn[b] | Fe[a] | Co[b] | Ni[a] | Cu[a] | Zn[a] | Rb[a] | Mo[a] | Pb[b] |
|---|---|---|---|---|---|---|---|---|---|---|
| 1 | 1.80 ±0.09 | 6.2 ±0.4 | 789 ±106 | 0.20 ±0.03 | 45.2 ±1.7 | 21.0 ±1.5 | 402 ±44 | 9.7 ±0.7 | 3.50 ±0.12 | 2.53 ±0.14 |
| 2 | 1.15 ±0.16 | 7.3 ±0.5 | 910 ±81 | 0.17 ±0.02 | 26.3 ±1.4 | 15.3 ±1.6 | 401 ±32 | 9.3 ±1.1 | 3.66 ±0.17 | 1.54 ±0.11 |
| 3 | 0.82 ±0.08 | 6.5 ±0.5 | 843 ±77 | 0.13 ±0.02 | 12.9 ±1.7 | 14.5 ±1.2 | 395 ±40 | 6.8 ±1.0 | 6.16 ±0.18 | 1.23 ±0.12 |
| 4 | 2.28 ±0.15 | 6.8 ±0.4 | 865 ±99 | 0.23 ±0.02 | 20.8 ±1.1 | 17.2 ±1.4 | 397 ±36 | 9.4 ±0.9 | 2.98 ±0.21 | 1.81 ±0.09 |
| 5 | 1.42 ±0.15 | 6.8 ±0.6 | 790 ±92 | 0.20 ±0.01 | 37.9 ±2.1 | 19.5 ±1.4 | 349 ±38 | 7.2 ±0.6 | 3.18 ±0.13 | 2.52 ±0.10 |
| 6 | 3.66 ±0.18 | 7.7 ±0.7 | 980 ±68 | 0.15 ±0.03 | 34.7 ±1.5 | 19.5 ±1.8 | 425 ±28 | 8.9 ±0.6 | 3.23 ±0.14 | 1.51 ±0.11 |
| 7 | 0.65 ±0.10 | 7.0 ±0.5 | 1205 ±88 | 0.13 ±0.02 | 15.5 ±0.9 | 18.0 ±1.4 | 523 ±44 | 10.9 ±0.7 | 3.00 ±0.18 | 1.22 ±0.10 |
| 8 | 4.08 ±0.22 | 7.4 ±0.5 | 944 ±76 | 0.19 ±0.02 | 30.8 ±1.5 | 17.6 ±1.5 | 480 ±39 | 9.2 ±0.8 | 3.15 ±0.11 | 1.89 ±0.12 |
| 9 | 0.76 ±0.11 | 5.6 ±0.5 | 842 ±53 | 0.19 ±0.03 | 99.1 ±2.4 | 15.0 ±1.2 | 384 ±30 | 9.9 ±0.7 | 2.73 ±0.16 | 2.27 ±0.10 |
| mean | 1.85 | 6.8 | 906 | 0.18 | 35.6 | 17.5 | 417 | 9.0 | 3.18 | 1.84 |
| RSD% | 68.6 | 9.5 | 14.4 | 17.6 | 73.0 | 12.9 | 12.7 | 14.3 | 8.7 | 27.8 |

Table 3. Intra-individual variation of element concentrations in a human liver obtained from cadaveric donor. (concentrations in µg/g dry weight, a: measured by TXRF, b: measured by ICP-MS)

## 4. Results

### 4.1 Investigation of possible contamination from biopsy needles

Percutaneous human liver biopsies taken from living patients could not be repeated frequently; therefore considerable contamination was indirectly disproved. In the present study, the possible contamination of biopsy samples during sample collection was determined using a porcine liver model. Availability in large amount was the purpose of using porcine liver for the method development. Twelve portions from a porcine liver were freeze-dried. Portions of porcine liver were cut by a quartz blade and treated as same as the steel needle biopsy samples. Concentrations determined in samples taken by a quartz device represented the non-contaminated values and were used to determine reproducibility of measurement and intra-individual variations. The precision of the drying process, the sample preparation and the analytical measurements was tested by the analysis of porcine liver. Calculated mean dry/wet mass ratio was 0.347 with an acceptable low relative standard deviation (RSD) of 2.2 %. Freeze-dried samples were subjected to microwave digestion in concentrated nitric acid (Suprapure, Merck). The precision of the concentration determination was found to be better than 14.2 % RSD by TXRF and 13.9 %RSD by ICP-MS for Mn, Fe, Cu, Zn, Rb and Mo (Cr, Co and Ni in the porcine liver was below the detection limit of TXRF in the given conditions: LODs of TXRF measurement were 0.92, 0.89 and 0.85 µg / g d.w. for Cr, Co and Ni).

All materials, solutions and tools used during the sample collection and preparation were tested for possible contamination: Analysis of repeated procedural blank samples showed that no measurable contamination of steel-metals originates from labware or reagents. Biopsy needles and scalpels were digested and analyzed previously. The material of biopsy needles was found to be a standard stainless steel with a main composition of Cr:Fe:Ni / 18:72:9 and Mn content of 0.1 % w/w. These four metals would be expected as possible contaminants. To investigate the possible release of elements from the steel needle biopsies the samples were allowed to contact with the needle for different time in a refrigerator at 4°C. According to the present data no observable contamination could be determined after 6 minutes contact of the porcine liver tissue and the biopsy needle. After 1 hour contact the tissue concentration of Cr and Ni was significantly higher than those measured in the samples taken by a quartz blade (0.41 and 0.29 μg/g instead of 0.06 and 0.15 μg/g d.w., respectively). The change of Mn and Fe concentration was in the range of measurement uncertainty.

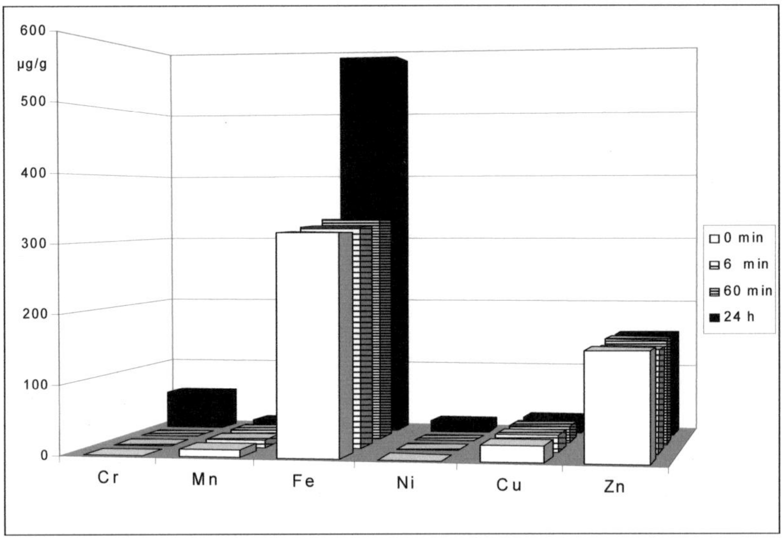


Fig. 3. Concentration of different elements in porcine liver samples after increasing contact time with biopsy needle.

The analysis of biopsy samples having $24^h$ contact with the needle showed considerable increase of chromium, manganese, iron and nickel concentration: the increments were 54.9 for Cr, 269 for Fe 15.6 for Ni and 2.1 for Mn in μg/g d.w. The results are demonstrated in Fig. 3. In contrast of steel metals, concentration of essential elements, such as copper and zinc remained constant as expected. Although the steel needles in the present study could not be substituted by polypropylene or Teflon utensils, it was demonstrated that the application of needle biopsy sampling in the reported analysis does not involve measurable contamination if contact time is kept to several minutes as usual in the clinical practice.

### 4.2 Intra-individual variability of element concentrations in human liver

A small specimen from liver biopsy does not represent the liver as a whole. In order to able to draw conclusions regarding differences of trace element contents of liver samples, we have to assume uniform trace element distributions throughout the whole organ. This

assumption should be checked by comparison of samples taken from different lobes of the same liver. The latter study can be performed only on autopsy samples.
Intra-individual variability of elemental concentrations was investigated by the analysis of multiple human liver biopsy samples obtained from cadaveric donor with liver steatosis. The purpose of these investigations was the high hepatic Ni concentration observed in the human liver and its uneven distribution. Similar sampling was made on porcine liver for comparison. Concentrations of Fe, Ni, Cu, Zn, Rb, and Mo determined by total reflection X-ray fluorescence spectrometry are listed in Table 3. Cr, Mn, Co and Pb were measured only by inductively coupled plasma-atomic emission spectrometry. Element concentrations determined by both techniques were in good agreement and not presented in Table 3. as a repetition. The variability of element concentrations was between 8.7 and 17.6 % relative standard deviation (RSD). Exceptions were Pb, Ni and Cr having variability of 27.8, 73.0 and 68.6 % RSD, respectively. In case of porcine liver the intra-individual variability was less than 13.5 % RSD for each element. It can be also emphasized, that nickel distribution was quite even in porcine liver and average Ni concentration (0.16 µg/g d.w.) was two orders of magnitude lower compared to the value measured in the investigated human liver.

### 4.3 Correlation between ultrasound data and trace element concentration

From the 183 examined patients 54 normal liver pattern was found (Fig. 4.), 53 showed low attenuation type (DI) (Fig. 5.) and 76 had high attenuation type (DII) bright liver (Fig. 6.). Average attenuation in the normal group was 0,61 ± 0,07 dB/cm/MHz, in the DI group 0,75 ± 0,12 dB/cm/MHz and in the DII group 1,34 ± 0,28 dB/cm/MHz. SCF values proved to be 6,8 ± 3,8 mm in the normal group, 8,4 ± 3,9 mm in the DI type, and 14,5 ± 5,5 mm in DII type bright liver.

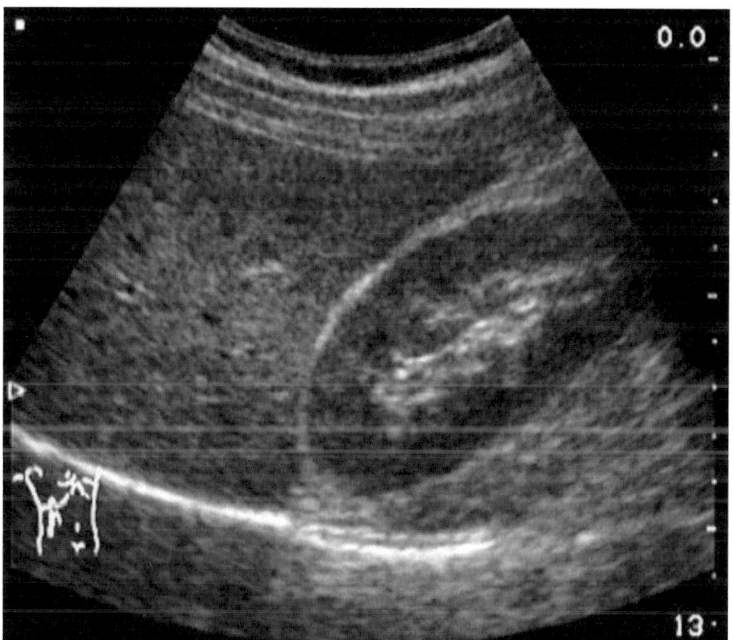


Fig. 4. Normal ultrasound liver pattern. Echogenicity and echodensity of the liver and the kidney are similar.

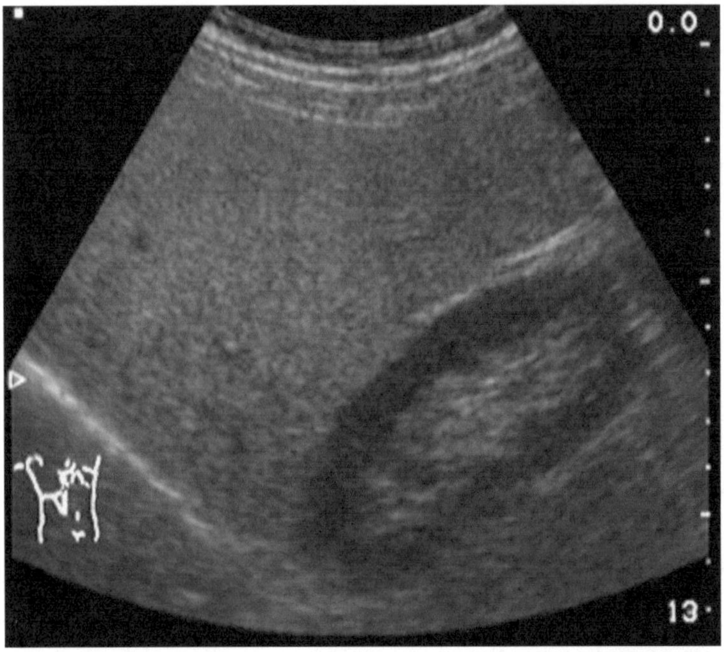

Fig. 5. Low attenuation (DI) type bright liver pattern. Echogenicity and echodensity of the liver and the kidney are different. The bright liver pattern is seen throughout the whole depth of the liver.

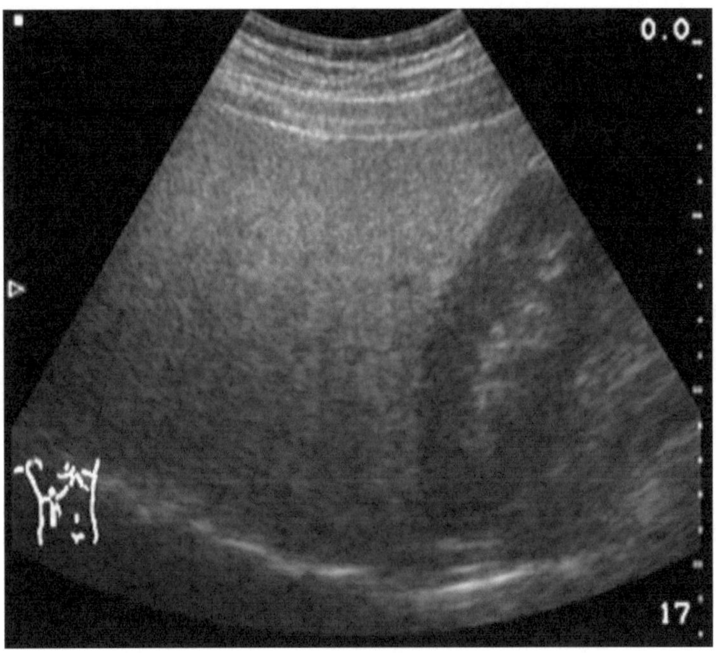

Fig. 6. High attenuation (DII) type bright liver pattern. Echogenicity and echodensity of the liver and the kidney are different. The bright liver pattern is seen mainly superficially, toward the depth of the liver gradually decreasing.

Mild fatty degeneration did not alter the ultrasonic reflectivity and echodensity, but the DII type bright liver pattern was always accompanied by severe fatty change (Fig. 7.). In hepatic samples from patients with normal ultrasound pattern, the amount of connective tissue was either normal, or just a slight fibrosis was seen (5/54 cases). In DI type bright liver pattern the typical histopathological alteration was the moderate or severe accumulation of connective tissue (Fig. 8.), accompanied by necroinflammation (Fig. 9.), but in DII type bright liver there typical morphological finding was just a slight portal fibrosis (37 samples).

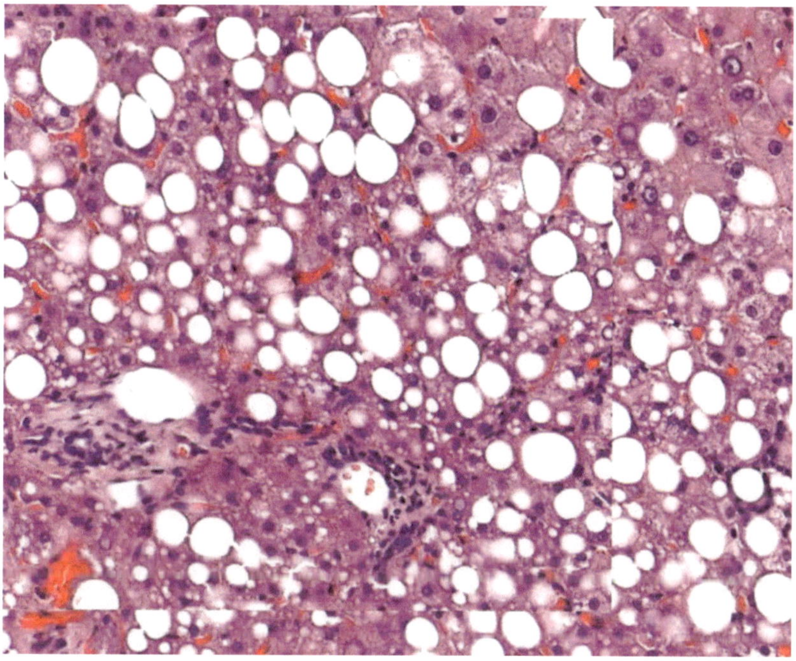

Fig. 7. In the liver multiple, large lipid vacuoles are seen representing a severe fatty degeneration (HE 400x).

Copper was demonstrated in 12, while nickel in 2 cases. None of the copper-positive patients suffered from Wilson disease. The amount of the metal granules was mild, and showed uneven distribution (Fig. 10.). In all but one specimens there were evidence of fatty degeneration, accumulation of connective tissue (septal fibrosis or cirrhosis), and inflammatory reaction. Presence of copper was observed in 1 case with normal liver. Histologically visible nickel was demonstrated just in 2 cases. One sample had a fatty change accompanied by infiltration of chronic inflammatory cells, the other specimen was taken from an alcoholic patients displaying fatty change and incomplete cirrhosis.

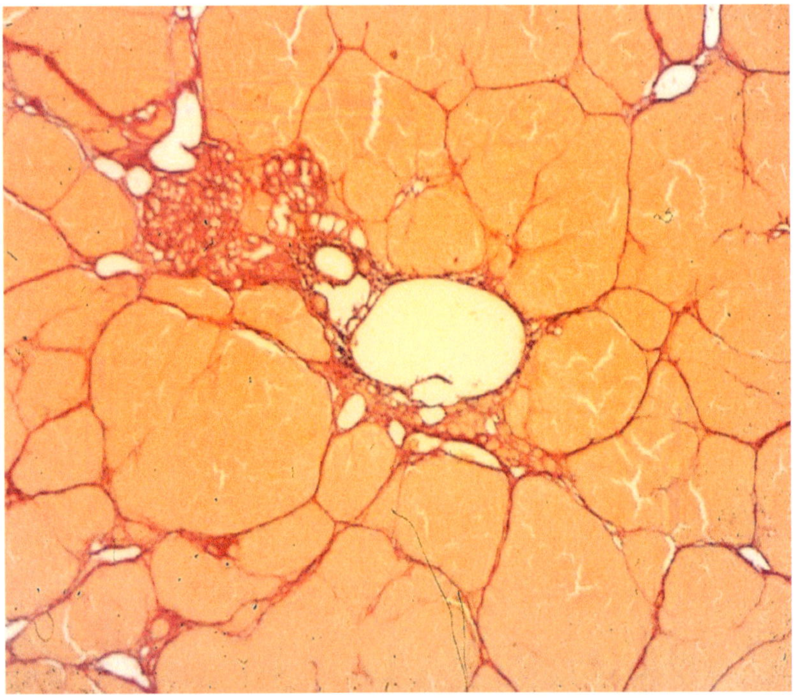

Fig. 8. The picrosirius red stain reveals a micronodular cirrhosis (200x).

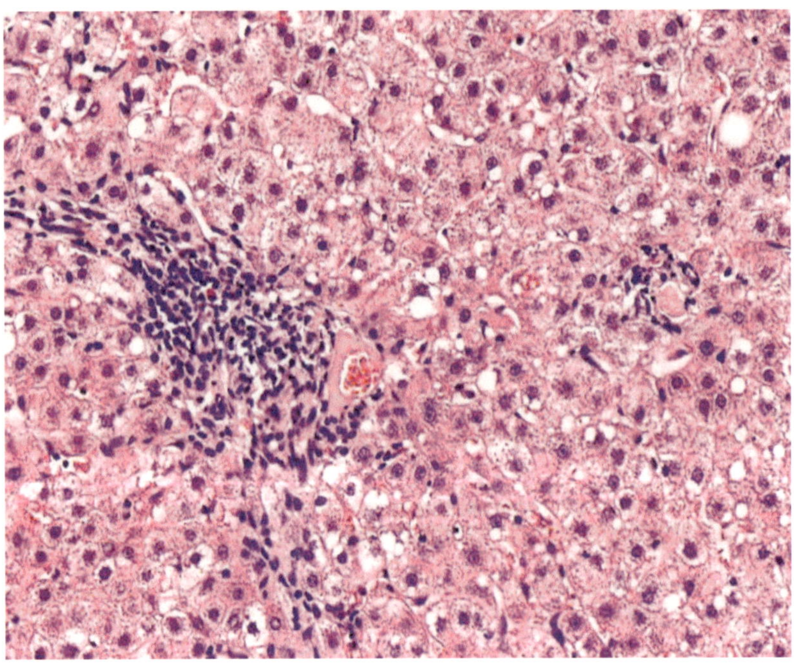

Fig. 9. The portal tract is loaded with moderate amount of chronic inflammatory cells. Moreover, focal, unicellular, intralobular necrosis is shown, surrounded by inflammatory cells (HE 300x).

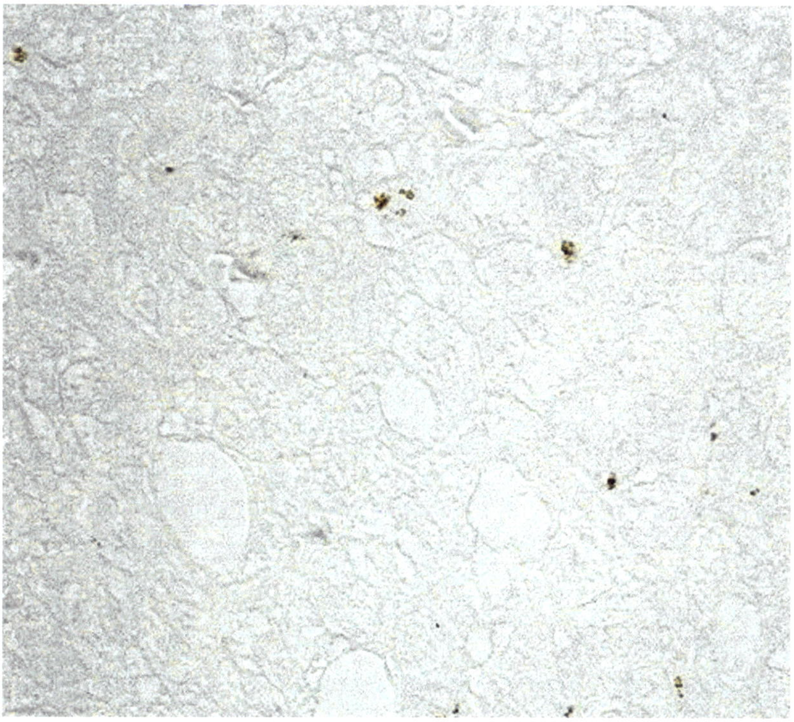

Fig. 10. Greenish-black copper-granules in the liver with fatty degeneration of intermediate degree. Rubeanic acid, 400x

Significant correlation was found between trace element determinations and the ultrasound and histopathological data in the case of Ni (Varga et al., 2005). This finding was confirmed in the present study with a larger sample size (Fig. 11.). In the normal and low attenuation (DI) type bright liver groups very low Ni concentrations were found, close to the detectability limit (Fig. 11.). On the contrary, in the high attenuation (DII) type bright liver group the Ni concentrations were substantially higher in all cases and some of them were extremely high, up to 700 µg/g (Fig. 11.). Decreased Fe concentration was also observed in the group of patients with steatosis. Distribution of elements within the liver was investigated taking biopsy samples from different localizations of a cadaveric liver. It is seen on table 3. in 3.2.4.2 , that the essential elements are uniformly distributed in the liver except the Cr. Ni showed surprisingly uneven distribution. The possible contamination with Ni can be excluded on the basis of our studies. Therefore the high Ni content of the liver can be taken as concomittant sign of fatty degeneration.

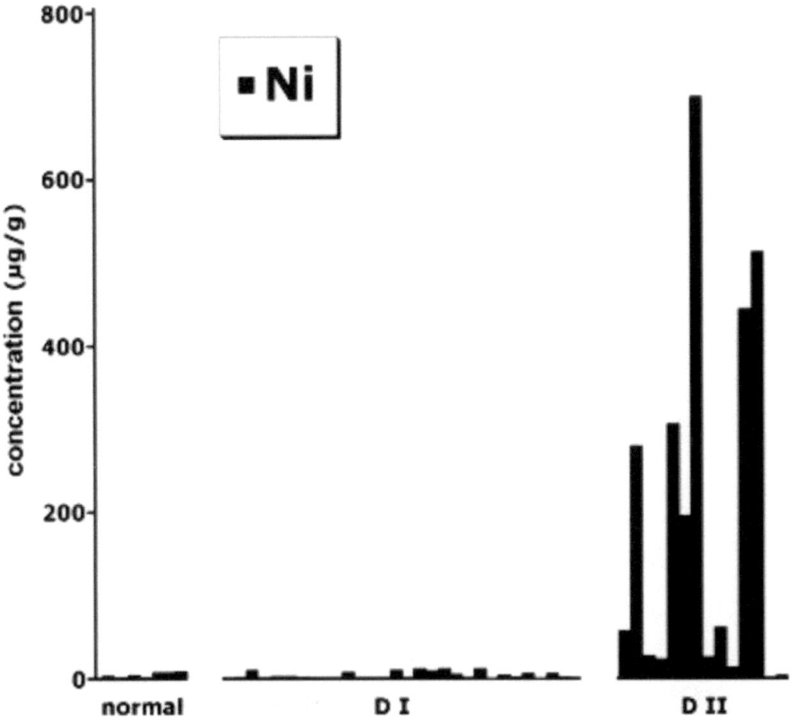


Fig. 11. Concentration of Ni in the three ultrasound based groups of patients. It is well seen, that the Ni content is much higher in the DII. type bright liver group, representing fatty liver, than in the normal, or DI type bright liver groups.

Three typical X-ray fluorescence spectra illustrate simultaneous analysis and distibution of maior, minor and trace elements obtained from liver biopsy samples. The only significant difference between the three ultrasonically determined groups was in the concentration of Ni and Fe as demonstrated on figures 12., 13. and 14. It is seen in figure 12., (normal ultrasonic pattern), that the Ni concentration is low, near to the quantification limit of the applied analytical method. On the 13. figure, originated from a liver biopsy sample of a patient with DI type bright liver the Ni concentration is in the normal range. On the contrary, on figure 14. the spectrum of a liver biopsy sample of a patient with fatty liver (ultrasonically DII type bright liver), high Ni concentration can be observed. Intense peak appearing at 2.7 keV energy is due to scattered radiation of the X-ray tube (Rh K-lines). As concerning the iron content, in the patient with liver steatosis (Fig. 14.), lower Fe concentration was found, than in the patients from the other groups (Figs. 12.,13.).

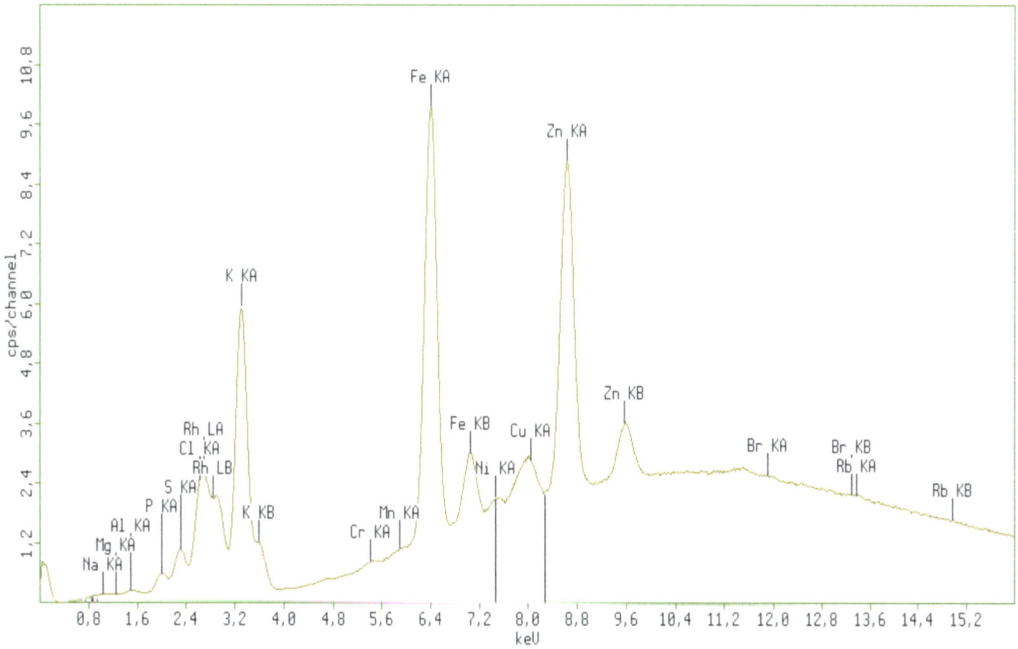


Fig. 12. TXRF spectrum of a liver biopsy sample of a patient from the normal group.

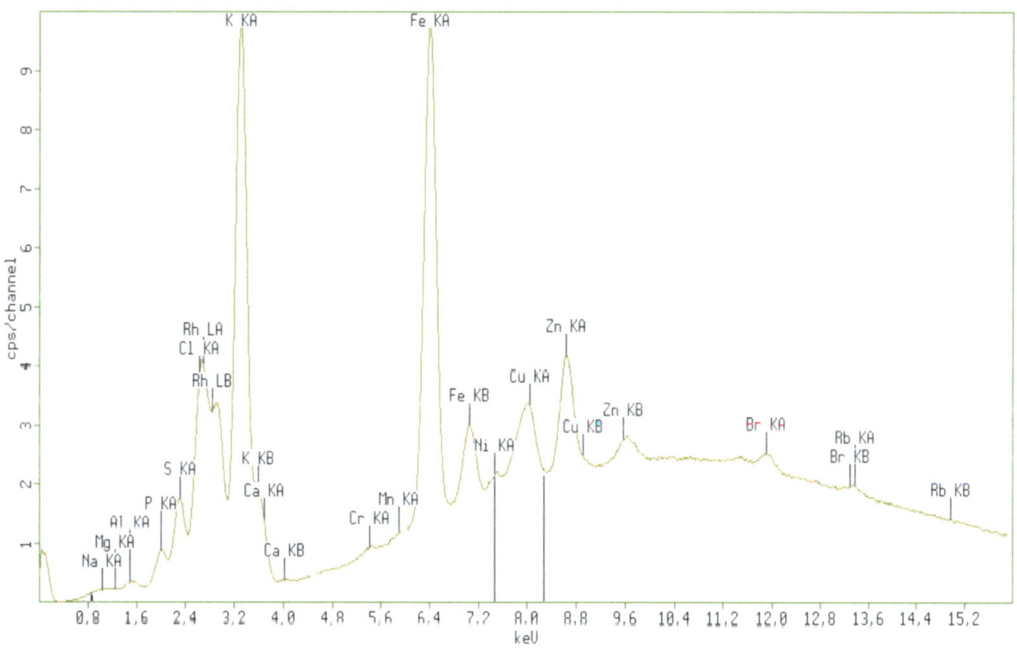


Fig. 13. TXRF spectrum of a liver biopsy sample of a patient from the DI type bright liver group.

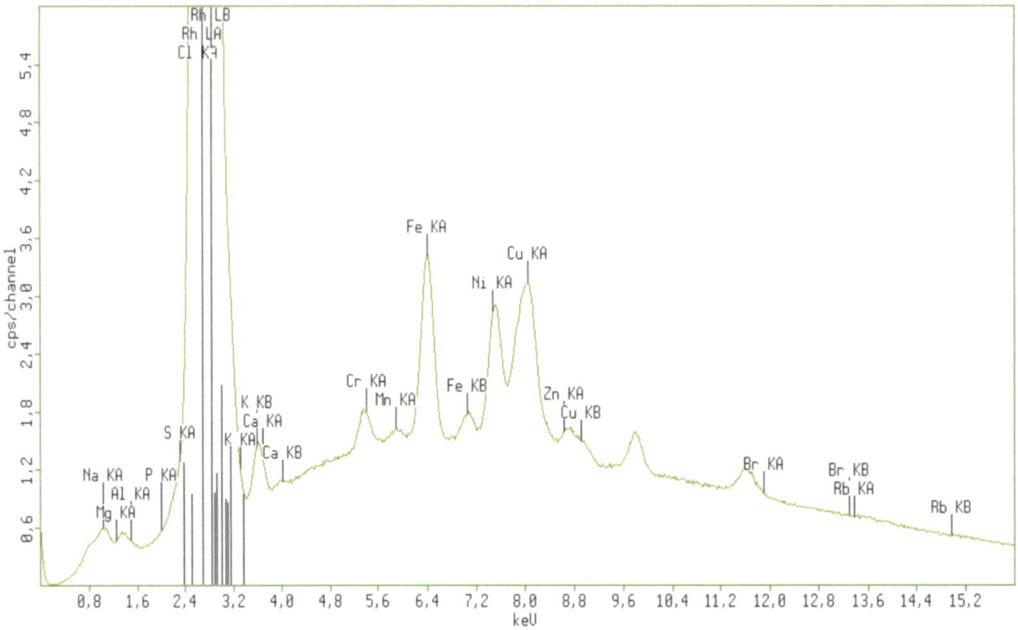


Fig. 14. TXRF spectrum of a liver biopsy sample of a patient from the DII type bright liver group (high Ni content).

## 5. Discussion

For the investigation of the pathological background of the different types of bright liver, quantitative measurement of the liver attenuation is necessary; a simple and reliable method was elaborated together with J.D. Satrapa (Satrapa, & Szebeni, 1996; Szebeni, & Satrapa, 1996). Evaluation of trace element analysis in subjects with normal ultrasound liver pattern and in patients with chronic diffuse liver diseases showing bright liver demonstrated, that the two types of ultrasound attenuation had different pathological background and also was not uniform from the point of view of trace element content. On the basis of attenuation measurements and semiquantitative histopathological analysis it was proved that low attenuation (DI) type bright livers show increase of connective tissue content while high attenuation (DII) type bright livers are associated with lipid deposition dominance (Szebeni, A. et al., 2006). It was also proved that some parameters, e.g. body mass index (BMI), subcutaneous fat thickness (SCF), could well be associated with the groups of liver ultrasound attenuation (Szebeni et al., 1999).

The different attenuation patterns reflect various histopathological alterations: fibrosis, fatty degeneration, chronic inflammation, alone, or in combination. DI pattern was mainly due to chronic, fibrotizing inflammation, while the severe fatty change was the major finding in DII cases.

Although trace metals are relatively frequently stored in the liver, the routine histological techniques rarely display their presence, therefore, if these metals do not reach the toxic levels, they may remain unidentified. Some technical notes also seem important, because it was found that reliable histological assessment for copper is only possible in formalin fixed liver tissue (Hoffmann et al., 2009), and not after alcohol fixation. The rubeanic acid stain is a very useful method for demonstration of copper in Wilson disease and in various liver diseases with cholestasis, but in our positive cases both possibilities could have been excluded. It has long been known that accumulation of intrahepatic copper is most frequently demonstrable in alcoholic cirrhosis, but it is not related to the concomitant cholestasis or to the activity of the process (Berresford et al., 1980). The cirrhotic process by itself, however, was not a decisive feature in our material, because in 10, histologically proven incomplete or complete cirrhosis no rubeanic acid positivity was observed. It is interesting that in most of the copper-containing liver specimens a fatty degeneration was seen. The relationship between the two condition is not clear, but it was published that in cultured rat hepatocytes Cu induced lipid peroxidation, while similar effect was not seen after Ni administration (Furono et al., 1996).

Nickel was histochemically identified just in 2 cases. In both cases fatty degeneration was seen. In the literature very few data are available about the non-toxicological appearance of this metal. Rezuke et al. have determined nickel concentrations in various human tissues from 10 postmortem specimens by using electrothermal atomic absorption spectrophotometry with Zeemann background correction (Rezuke et al., 1987). In their reference work they have found a relatively higher Ni-concentration in thyroid and adrenal gland as compared with other organs, and it was suggested that biliary excretion may be a significant route for the elimination of nickel in humans. It was found that in vitro Ni uptake by rat hepatocytes was partly through the Ca channel transport processes (Funakoshi, 1997). Exposure of HepG2 human hepatoma cells to nickel(2+) ions resulted in a stimulation of Ser/Thr Akt and this activation is most likely independent of oxidative processes, since no oxidation of cellular glutathion was detected (Eckers et al., 2009). The mitochondrium also seems to be the place of its effects, because there are data that Ni is a potent competitive inhibitor of calcium transport in mitochondria (Bragadin et al., 1997, Ligeti et al., 1981). So the hepatic fatty change and the presence of copper and nickel in these samples are not necessary independent findings.

Nowadays a lot of analytical laboratory use an inductively coupled plasma optical emission spectrometer (ICP-OES) or an inductively coupled plasma mass spectrometer (ICP-MS) for multielemental analysis of various samples. Generally analyses of various essential elements and potential toxic elements with relatively low concentration are required, for which an ICP-MS is needed due to much smaller detection limits of the elements.

To elaborate analytical methods for analysis of the examined elements with an inductively coupled plasma mass spectrometer the most important interfering effects (problems) were evaluated before analysis: 1) isobaric elemental, 2) isobaric molecular and 3) physical interferences (Montaser, 1998; *www.epa.gov)*. EPA 6020A describes the interferences in ICP-MS techniques (www.epa.gov):

- Isobaric elemental interferences:

  These types of interferences in ICP-MS are caused by isotopes of different elements forming atomic ions with the same nominal mass-to-charge ratio (m/z). An evaluation software must be used to correct for these interferences, however these types of interferences are not easily corrected.

- Isobaric molecular and doubly-charged ion interferences:

  These interferences are caused by ions consisting of more than one atom or charge, respectively. Most isobaric interferences that could affect ICP-MS determinations have been identified in different literature.

- Physical interferences:
  These are associated with the sample nebulization and transport processes as well as with ion-transmission efficiencies. Nebulization and transport processes can be affected if a matrix component causes a change in surface tension or viscosity. Changes in matrix composition can cause significant signal suppression or enhancement (Beauchemin et al., 1987). Dissolved solids can deposit on the nebulizer tip of a pneumatic nebulizer and on the interface skimmers (reducing the orifice size and the instrument performance). One or more suitable internal standards can be used to correct for physical interferences, if it is carefully matched to the analyte so that the two elements are similarly affected by matrix changes.
- Memory interferences:
  Sample deposition on the sampler and skimmer cones, spray chamber design, and the type of nebulizer affect the extent of observed memory interferences. The rinse period between samples must be long enough to eliminate significant memory interference.

The isobaric elemental, isobaric molecular and doubly-charged ion interferences caused by various ions consisting of one or more than one atom or charge. These types of possibly emerging interferences are listed in Table 4., which are described in the Plasmalab software (2007) made by Thermo Fisher for analysis of different samples and build an appropriate analytical method. Before analysis these interferences were evaluated and were taken into consideration for decrease or eliminate these interfering effects.

To eliminate the doubly-charged ion interferences, before analysis the tuning parameters were optimized considering the appropriate plasma temperature which ensures the minimum level of doubly-charged ions.

The interferences (Plasmalab, 2007) caused by various dimer, trimer or tetramer ions consisting of two, three or four elements were decreased by gas mixture using 7% hydrogen in helium (7% $H_2$ + 93% He) as collision cell technology (CCT) gas.

Collision/reaction cell technology has proved to be effective methods for decrease/eliminate the interferences caused by various dimer, trimer or tetramer ions and thus allow the determination of the major isotopes ($^{52}Cr$, $^{56}Fe$ and $^{80}Se$). This method needs a collision/reaction cell, which is composed of a multipole (quadrupole, hexapole or octopole) before the quadrupole analyzer. A collision/reaction gas is introduced into the cell where, by a number of different ion-molecule collision and reaction mechanisms, most of poly-atomic interfering ions were converted to harmless non-interfering species. The analyte ions continue the way into the quadrupole analyzer for normal mass separation and detection. Owing to the collision/reaction cell technology the most abundant and thus most sensitive isotope can be used for the analysis of a given element. Different collision and reaction gases or gas mixtures have been selected to apply in an ICP-MS. Generally a mixture of $H_2$ and He gases (7-8% $H_2$ in He), $NH_3$ (1% $NH_3$ in He) and $CH_4$ gases are widely applied in ICP-MS. Moreover $O_2$, $N_2O$ or other gases or mixtures can be used as collision/reaction gases also.

In the case of the analysis of the most abundant selenium isotope ($^{80}Se$) by ICP-MS the next possible mechanisms can be for reduction/elimination of polyatomic interferences.

- collisional dissociation:

$$\text{e.g. } ArAr^+ + He = Ar + Ar^+ + He$$

- chemical reaction:

$$\text{e.g. } ArAr^+ + H_2 = ArH + ArH^+$$

- charge transfer:

$$\text{e.g. } ArAr^{+} + H = ArAr + H^{+}$$

- collisional retardation/energy filtering:

$$\text{e.g. } ArAr^{+*} + He = ArAr^{+} + He^{*}$$

| Symbol | Abundance | Interferences |
|---|---|---|
| $^{25}$Mg | 10.11 | $^{40}$Ar+$^{15}$N, $^{16}$O+$^{39}$K, $^{14}$N+$^{41}$K, $^{1}$H+$^{54}$Fe, $^{1}$H+$^{54}$Cr, $^{15}$N+$^{40}$Ca, $^{36}$Ar+$^{19}$F, $^{12}$C+$^{43}$Ca, $^{109}$Ag$^{++}$, $^{110}$Pd$^{++}$, $^{110}$Cd$^{++}$ |
| $^{52}$Cr | 83.76 | $^{40}$Ar+$^{12}$C, $^{36}$Ar+$^{16}$O, $^{1}$H+$^{51}$V, $^{12}$C+$^{40}$Ca, $^{17}$OH+$^{35}$Cl, $^{13}$C+$^{39}$K, $^{16}$O+$^{36}$S, $^{103}$Rh$^{++}$, $^{104}$Ru$^{++}$, $^{104}$Pd$^{++}$ |
| $^{53}$Cr | 9.55 | $^{40}$Ar+$^{13}$C, $^{17}$OH+$^{36}$Ar, $^{14}$N+$^{39}$K, $^{1}$H+$^{52}$Cr, $^{16}$O+$^{37}$Cl, $^{12}$C+$^{41}$K, $^{13}$C+$^{40}$Ca, $^{18}$O+$^{35}$Cl, $^{17}$OH+$^{36}$S, $^{106}$Pd$^{++}$, $^{105}$Pd$^{++}$, $^{106}$Cd$^{++}$ |
| $^{55}$Mn | 100 | $^{40}$Ar+$^{15}$N, $^{16}$O+$^{39}$K, $^{14}$N+$^{41}$K, $^{1}$H+$^{54}$Fe, $^{1}$H+$^{54}$Cr, $^{15}$N+$^{40}$Ca, $^{36}$Ar+$^{19}$F, $^{12}$C+$^{43}$Ca, $^{109}$Ag$^{++}$, $^{110}$Pd$^{++}$, $^{110}$Cd$^{++}$ |
| $^{54}$Fe | 5.9 | $^{54}$Cr, $^{40}$Ar+$^{14}$N, $^{14}$N+$^{40}$Ca, $^{17}$OH+$^{37}$Cl, $^{1}$H+$^{53}$Cr, $^{12}$C+$^{42}$Ca, $^{15}$N+$^{39}$K, $^{19}$OH+$^{35}$Cl, $^{107}$Ag$^{++}$, $^{108}$Pd$^{++}$, $^{108}$Cd$^{++}$ |
| $^{56}$Fe | 91.52 | $^{40}$Ar+$^{16}$O, $^{1}$H+$^{55}$Mn, $^{16}$O+$^{40}$Ca, $^{17}$OH+$^{39}$K, $^{12}$C+$^{44}$Ca, $^{14}$N+$^{42}$Ca, $^{36}$Ar+$^{20}$Ne, $^{112}$Cd$^{++}$, $^{111}$Cd$^{++}$, $^{112}$Sn$^{++}$ |
| $^{58}$Ni | 67.76 | $^{58}$Fe, $^{40}$Ar+$^{18}$O, $^{12}$C+$^{46}$Ti, $^{17}$OH+$^{41}$K, $^{1}$H+$^{57}$Fe, $^{14}$N+$^{44}$Ca, $^{13}$C+$^{45}$Sc, $^{16}$O+$^{42}$Ca, $^{18}$O+$^{40}$Ca, $^{19}$OH+$^{39}$K, $^{115}$In$^{++}$, $^{116}$Sn$^{++}$, $^{116}$Cd$^{++}$, $^{115}$Sn$^{++}$ |
| $^{59}$Co | 100 | $^{19}$OH+$^{40}$Ar, $^{14}$N+$^{45}$Sc, $^{40}$Ar+$^{19}$F, $^{1}$H+$^{58}$Ni, $^{12}$C+$^{47}$Ti, $^{17}$OH+$^{42}$Ca, $^{36}$Ar+$^{23}$Na, $^{1}$H+$^{58}$Fe, $^{19}$OH+$^{40}$Ca, $^{16}$O+$^{43}$Ca, $^{118}$Sn$^{++}$, $^{117}$Sn$^{++}$ |
| $^{60}$Ni | 26.16 | $^{1}$H+$^{59}$Co, $^{40}$Ar+$^{20}$Ne, $^{12}$C+$^{48}$Ti, $^{14}$N+$^{46}$Ti, $^{16}$O+$^{44}$Ca, $^{15}$N+$^{45}$Sc, $^{36}$Ar+$^{24}$Mg, $^{12}$C+$^{48}$Ca, $^{17}$OH+$^{43}$Ca, $^{120}$Sn$^{++}$, $^{119}$Sn$^{++}$ |
| $^{65}$Cu | 30.91 | $^{14}$N+$^{51}$V, $^{17}$OH+$^{48}$Ti, $^{1}$H+$^{64}$Zn, $^{40}$Ar+$^{25}$Mg, $^{12}$C+$^{53}$Cr, $^{16}$O+$^{49}$Ti, $^{1}$H+$^{64}$Ni, $^{13}$C+$^{52}$Cr, $^{17}$OH+$^{48}$Ca, $^{130}$Te$^{++}$, $^{129}$Xe$^{++}$, $^{130}$Xe$^{++}$, $^{130}$Ba$^{++}$ |
| $^{64}$Zn | 48.89 | $^{64}$Ni, $^{12}$C+$^{52}$Cr, $^{40}$Ar+$^{24}$Mg, $^{16}$O+$^{48}$Ti, $^{1}$H+$^{63}$Cu, $^{17}$OH+$^{47}$Ti, $^{14}$N+$^{50}$Ti, $^{14}$N+$^{50}$Cr, $^{13}$C+$^{51}$V, $^{36}$Ar+$^{28}$Si, $^{14}$N+$^{50}$V, $^{19}$OH+$^{45}$Sc, $^{16}$O+$^{48}$Ca, $^{127}$I$^{++}$, $^{128}$Te$^{++}$, $^{128}$Xe$^{++}$ |
| $^{66}$Zn | 27.81 | $^{14}$N+$^{52}$Cr, $^{1}$H+$^{65}$Cu, $^{40}$Ar+$^{26}$Mg, $^{12}$C+$^{54}$Fe, $^{17}$OH+$^{49}$Ti, $^{16}$O+$^{50}$Ti, $^{16}$O+$^{50}$Cr, $^{12}$C+$^{54}$Cr, $^{15}$N+$^{51}$V, $^{16}$O+50V, $^{18}$O+$^{48}$Ti, $^{13}$C+$^{53}$Cr, $^{132}$Xe$^{++}$, $^{131}$Xe$^{++}$ |
| $^{75}$As | 100 | $^{40}$Ar+$^{35}$Cl, $^{16}$O+$^{59}$Co, $^{12}$C+$^{63}$Cu, $^{17}$OH+$^{58}$Ni, $^{1}$H+$^{74}$Ge, $^{14}$N+$^{61}$Ni, $^{1}$H+$^{74}$Se, $^{17}$OH+$^{58}$Fe, $^{36}$Ar+$^{39}$K, $^{19}$OH+$^{56}$Fe, $^{149}$Sm$^{++}$, $^{150}$Sm$^{++}$, $^{150}$Nd$^{++}$ |
| $^{78}$Se | 23.61 | $^{78}$Kr, $^{14}$N+$^{64}$Zn, $^{12}$C+$^{66}$Zn, $^{1}$H+$^{77}$Se, $^{16}$O+$^{62}$Ni, $^{17}$OH+$^{61}$Ni, $^{14}$N+$^{64}$Ni, $^{13}$C+$^{65}$Cu, $^{15}$N+$^{63}$Cu, $^{19}$OH+$^{59}$Co, $^{156}$Gd$^{++}$, $^{155}$Gd$^{++}$ |
| $^{80}$Se | 49.96 | $^{80}$Kr, $^{40}$Ar+$^{40}$Ar, $^{40}$Ar+$^{40}$Ca, $^{17}$OH+$^{63}$Cu, $^{1}$H+$^{79}$Br, $^{16}$O+$^{64}$Zn, $^{14}$N+$^{66}$Zn, $^{12}$C+$^{68}$Zn, $^{16}$O+$^{64}$Ni, $^{15}$N+$^{65}$Cu, $^{159}$Tb$^{++}$, $^{160}$Gd$^{++}$, $^{160}$Dy$^{++}$ |
| $^{82}$Se | 8.84 | $^{82}$Kr, $^{1}$H+$^{81}$Br, $^{17}$OH+$^{65}$Cu, $^{16}$O+$^{66}$Zn, $^{12}$C+$^{70}$Ge, $^{14}$N+$^{68}$Zn, $^{13}$C+$^{69}$Ga, $^{40}$Ar+$^{42}$Ca, $^{12}$C+$^{70}$Zn, $^{19}$OH+$^{63}$Cu, $^{164}$Dy$^{++}$, $^{163}$Dy$^{++}$, $^{164}$Er$^{++}$ |
| $^{111}$Cd | 12.86 | $^{12}$C+$^{99}$Tc, $^{40}$Ar+$^{71}$Ga, $^{17}$OH+$^{94}$Zr, $^{16}$O+$^{95}$Mo, $^{1}$H+$^{110}$Pd, $^{12}$C+$^{99}$Ru, $^{1}$H+$^{110}$Cd, $^{14}$N+$^{97}$Mo, $^{17}$OH+$^{94}$Mo, $^{36}$Ar+$^{75}$As, $^{13}$C+$^{98}$Mo, $^{18}$O+$^{93}$Nb |
| $^{114}$Cd | 28.81 | $^{114}$Sn, $^{40}$Ar+$^{74}$Ge, $^{12}$C+$^{102}$Ru, $^{16}$O+$^{98}$Mo, $^{14}$N+$^{100}$Ru, $^{1}$H+$^{113}$Cd, $^{14}$N+$^{100}$Mo, $^{17}$OH+$^{97}$Mo, $^{1}$H+$^{113}$In, $^{16}$O+$^{98}$Ru, $^{40}$Ar+$^{74}$Se, $^{12}$C+$^{102}$Pd, $^{15}$N+$^{99}$Tc, $^{13}$C+$^{101}$Ru |
| $^{208}$Pb | 52.38 | $^{16}$O+$^{192}$Os, $^{17}$OH+$^{191}$Ir, $^{14}$N+$^{194}$Pt, $^{40}$Ar+$^{168}$Er, $^{12}$C+$^{196}$Pt, $^{1}$H+$^{207}$Pb, $^{16}$O+$^{192}$Pt, $^{13}$C+$^{195}$Pt, $^{15}$N+$^{193}$Ir, $^{12}$C+$^{196}$Hg, $^{40}$Ar+$^{168}$Yb |

Table 4. The most important isobaric interference ions (Plasmalab, 2007)

Those inductively coupled plasma mass spectrometers which use CCT or reaction gases, have the best detection limits, for example the detection limit of selenium approximately 0.001 μg/l for $^{80}Se$ isotope. These best detection limits origin from using the collision and/or reaction gases to reduce the interfering effects on various element peak. CCT can eliminate approximately 99.99% of the $^{40}Ar^{40}Ar^{+}$ and $^{39}Ar^{39}Ar^{+}$ interferences on $^{80}Se$ and $^{78}Se$, respectively.
On the basis of the above we can conclude that a quadrupole inductively coupled plasma mass spectrometer which instrument applying a collision/reaction cell technique is the most appropriate to analyze ultra trace elements in routine analysis of human origin samples, which can decrease effectively the interference of polyadducts.
Sample contamination during autopsy was nominated the major source of uncertainty of trace element analysis of biological samples. Biopsies taken by the use of stainless steel needles were recommended to analyze only for non-steel metals (Versieck et al, 1973; Versieck et al, 1982). For urine and blood recommendations were outlined to eliminate possible contamination during sample collection (Cornelis et al., 1992). Burguera et al. (Burguera et al, 2005) reported that Mn contamination during Atomic Absorption Spectrometry (AAS) analysis of urine samples was avoided by using new plastic and glassware containers soaked for at least $4^h$ in 2 mol/l nitric acid. Christensen (Christensen, 1995) gave a detailed overview on contamination control in trace element analysis. The author concluded: Although it is impossible in most instances, the whole analytical procedure recommended to be carried out in clean room facilities. Blood samples were analyzed by Zeeman-ETAAS taken in a clean room. After puncture steel needle was withdrawn, venous blood was collected using a teflon catheter in 6 vials. Vial No. 5 was used for analysis in order to avoid contamination by steel-metals (Kristiansen et al., 1997). Oral mucosa biopsies were taken by $CO^2$-laser bistoury technique for minimizing the contamination during sample collection and 36 elements were determined by radiochemical neutron activation analysis (Foglio Bonda et al., 2001).
Multielement analysis of porcine liver and human cadaveric liver biopsy samples applying total reflection X-ray fluorescence spectrometry and inductively coupled plasma mass spectrometry are described with a special respect to Ni content. Porcine liver can be successfully applied to estimate the reproducibility of biopsy sampling and to investigate possible contamination by steel metals originating from the biopsy needles. Evidence of tissue contamination by steel-metals during hours of contact with the steel biopsy needle was shown. However, contamination was not measurable applying less than 6 min. contact as usual in the clinical practice.
The intra-individual variability of element concentrations was determined by the analysis of biopsies taken from a cadaveric human liver. Variability of Mn, Fe, Cu, Zn and Rb concentration was in the range of 9-18 %RSD. Pb, Ni and Cr found to be inhomogeneously distributed in the liver having variability of 28, 73 and 69 %RSD, respectively. It was beyond the scope of the present study to explore the causes of inhomogeneity. The result presented in this paper demonstrated that despite of its uneven distribution, Ni concentration in human liver biopsy samples seemed to be suitable for classification of patients.
Analizing trace elements by microanalitical methods in human liver biopsy samples, collected from 52 individuals in a previous work (Varga et al., 2005), a probable correlation between high nickel concentration and hepatic steatosis was found: accumulation of nickel was exclusively observed in cases of steatosis. Decreased Fe concentration was also observed in the group of patients with-steatosis. In the present study this finding could be

confirmed on a larger sample size, at 183 patients (Fig. 11.). Investigations of cadaver liver showed that Ni was the only element distributed unevenly within the cadaver liver. Nevertheless, absolute values of Ni concentrations were so much higher in every segment of fatty livers, than the very low levels in normal one and in other diffuse liver diseases, that despite of the inhomogeneous distribution this sign is considered characteristic to fatty liver. The cause of Ni enrichment is not known so far.

## 6. Conclusions

Histological staining methods were not enough sensitive for the demonstration of nickel in cases with chronic dissuse liver diseases.
TXRF and ICP-MS methods were successfully applied for element analysis of liver biopsy samples. The two methods gave essentially same results; yet, for certain elements ICP-MS was more sensitive.
It was proved that no contamination occurred at the sampling and preparation procedures.
It was demonstrated, that distribution of the examined trace elements - except Ni - was homogeneous, thus microquantities of liver material is informative.
In fatty degeneration of the liver, established by ultrasound and histology, the enrichment of Ni was found by TXRF and ICPMS methods, in some cases to extremely great extent. The Ni concentration was much higher than normal in every fatty liver cases, therefore, despite of the inhomogeneous distribution, this phenomenon can be interpreted as characteristic to fatty liver.

## 7. References

Amacher, D. (2011). Strategies for the early detection of drug-induced hepatic steatosis in preclinical drug safety evaluation studies. *Toxicology,* Vol. 279, No.1-3, (January, 2011), pp. (10-18), ISSN 0300-483

Beauchemin, D. Mclaren, J. & Herman, S. (1987). Study of the effects of concomitant elements in inductively coupled plasma mass spectrometry. *Spectrochimica Acta Part B: Atomic Spectroscopy,* Vol. 42, No. 3, (n.d.), pp. (467-490), ISSN 0584-8547

Berresford, P. Sunter, J. Harrison, V. & Lesna, M. (1980). Histological demonstration and frequency of intrahepatocytic copper in patients suffering from alcoholic liver disease. *Histopathology,* Vol. 4, No. 6, (November, 1980), pp. (637-643), ISSN 0309-0167

Boffetta, P. (1993). Carcinogenicity of trace elements with reference to evaluations made by International Agency for Research on Cancer. *Scandinavian Journal of Work Environment & Health,* Vol. 19. Suppl. 1. (n.d.), pp. (67-70), ISSN 0355-3140

Bragadin, M. & Viola, E. (1997). Ni++ as a competitive inhibitor of calcium transport in mitochondria. *Journal of Inorganic Biochemistry,* Vol. 66, No. 4, (n.d.), pp. (227-229), ISSN 0162-0134

Burguera, M. Burguera, J. Rivas, D. Rondon, P. Carrero, O. Alarcon, Y. de Pena, M. Brunetto, M. Gallignani, O. & Marquez, J. (2005). On-line electrochemical preconcentration and flame atomic absorption spectrometric determination of manganese in urine samples. *Talanta,* Vol. 68, No. 1, (December, 2005), pp. (219-225), ISSN 0039-9140

Christensen, J. (1995). Human exposure to toxic metals: factors influencing interpretation of biomonitoring results. *Science of the Total Environment,* Vol. 166, No. 1, (April, 21.), pp. (89-135), ISSN 0048-9697-

Copel, L. Sosna, J. Kruskal, J. & Kane, R. (2003). Ultrasound-guided percutaneous liver biopsy: indications, risks, and technique. *Surgical Technoigy. International,* Vol. 11, No. 12, (n.d.), pp. (154-160), ISSN 1090-3941

Cornelis, R. Heinzow, B. Herber, R. et al. (1995). Sample collection guidelines for trace elements in blood and urine. *Pure and Appied Chemistry,* Vol. 67, No. 8/9 (n.d.), pp. (1575-1608), ISSN 0033-4545

Eckers, A. Reimann, K. & Klotz, L. (2009). Nickel and copper ion-induced stress signaling in human hepatoma cells: analysis of phosphoinositide 3'-kinase/Akt signaling. *Biometals,* Vol. 22, No. 2, (April, 2009), pp. (307-316), ISSN 0966-0844

Foglio Bonda, P. Porrini, R. Rizzio, E. Pietra, R. Fortaner, S. Sabbioni, E. (2001). Trace metals in oral mucosa in relation to the lichen ruber planus pathology. A preliminary study carried out by neutron activation analysis. *Journal of Trace Elements in Medicine & Biology,* Vol. 15, No. 2/3, (n.d.), pp. (79-83), ISSN 0946- 672X

Funakoshi, T. Inoue, T. Shimada, H. & Kojima, S. (1997). The mechanisms of nickel uptake by rat primary hepatocyte cultures: role of calcium channels. *Toxicology,* Vol. 124, No. 1, (December, 1997), pp. (21-26), ISSN 0300-483X

Furono, K. Suetsuga, T. & Sugihara, N. (1996). Effects of metal ions on lipid peroxidation in cultured rat hepatocyte loaded with alpha-linolenic acid. *Journal of Toxicology and Environtal Health,* Vol. 48, No. 2, ( June, 1996), pp. (121-129), ISSN 1528-7394

Germani, G. Hytiroglou, P. Fotiadu, A. Burroughs, A. & Dhillon, A. (2011). Assessment of fibrosis and cirrhosis in liver biopsies: an update. *Seminars in Liver Disease,* Vol. 31, No. 2, (February 2011), pp. (82-90), ISSN 0272-8087

Hayes, R. (1997). The carcinogenicity of metals in humans. *Cancer Causes Control,* Vol. 8, No. 3, (May 1997), pp. (371-385), ISSN 0957-5243

Hoffmann, G. Ijzer, J. Brinkhof, B. Schotanus, B. van den Ingh, T. Penning, L. & Rothuizen, J. (2009). Comparison of different methods to obtain and store liver biopsies for molecular and histological research. *Comparative Hepatology,* Vol. 8, (July, 2009), p. 3, ISSN 1476-5926

Joseph, A. Dewbury, K. & Mc Guire, P. (1979). Ultrasound in the detection of chronic liver disease (the "bright liver"). *British Jounak of Radiology,* Vol. 52, No. 615, (March, 1979), pp. (184-188), ISSN 1748-880X

Karamashi, M. (2008). Performing percutaneous liver biopsy in parenchymal liver diseases. *British Journal of Nursing,* Vol. 17, No. 12, (June, 2008), pp. (746-752), ISSN 0966-0461.

Kovács, B. Prokisch, J. Széles, É. & Győri Z. (2006). Szelén- és arzéntartalom analízisének vizsgálata ICP-MS berendezés alkalmazásával. *Konferenciakiadvány. XV. Élelmiszer Minőségellenőrzési Tudományos Konferencia.* pp. (240-241), ISBN 963-229-636-2, Debrecen, March, 2006. (Hungarian).

Kristiansen, J. Christensen J. Iversen, B. Sabbioni, E. (1997). Toxic trace element reference levels in blood and urine: influence of gender and lifestyle factors. *Science of the Total Environment,* Vol. 204, No. 2, (September, 1997 ). pp. (47-160), ISSN 0048-9697

Labat, L. Dehon, B. & Lhermitte, M. (2003). Rapid and simple determination of selenium in blood serum by inductively coupled plasma-mass spectrometry (ICP-MS).

*Analytical and Bioanalytical Chemistry,* Vol. 376, No. 2, (May, 2003), pp. (270-273), ISSN 1618-2042

Lewindon, P. Stephen, R. Walsh, M. Greer, R. Williamson, R. Pereira, T. Frawley, K. Bell, S. Smith, J. & Ramm, G. (2011). Importance of hepatic fibrosis in cystic fibrosis and the predictive value of liver biopsy. *Toxicology,* Vol. 53, No. 1, (January, 2011), pp. (193-201), ISSN 1527-3350

Ligeti, E. Bodnar, J. Karoly, E. & Lindner, E. (1981). Ni2+, a new inhibitor of mitochondrial calcium transport. *Biochim Biophys Acta,* Vol. 656, No. 2, (December, 1981), pp. (177-182), ISSN 0006-3002

Lonardo, A. Bellini, M. Tartoni, P. Tondelli, E. (1997). The bright liver syndrome, Prevalence and determinants of a "bright" liver echopattern. *Italian Journal of Gastroenterology and Hepatology,* Vol. 29, No. 4, (August, 1979), pp. (351-356). ISSN 1125-8055

Marco, L. & Hernandez-Caraballo, E. (2004). Direct analysis of biological samples by total reflection X-ray fluorescence. *Spectrochimica Acta Part B,* Vol. 59, No. 8, (August, 2004), pp. (1077-1090), ISSN 0584-8547

Millos, J. Costas-Rodríguez, M. Lavilla, I. & Bendicho, C. (2008). Multielemental Determination in breast cancerous and non-cancerous biopsies by inductively coupled plasma-mass spectrometry following small volume microwave-assisted digestion. *Analytica Chimica Acta,* Vol. 622, No. 1-2, (August, 2008), pp. (77- 84), ISSN 0003-2670

Montaser, A. (1998). *Inductively Coupled Plasma Mass Spectrometry.* Wiley-VCH. ISBN 0-471-18620-1, New York

Navarro Silvera, S. & Rohan, T. (2007). Trace elements and cancer risk: a review of the epidemiologic evidence. *Cancer Causes Control,* Vol. 18, No. 1, (February 2007), pp. (7-27), ISSN 0957-5243

Nordberg, G. & Andersen, O. (1981). Metal Interactions in Carcinogenesis: Enhancement, Inhibition. *Environmental Health Perspectives,*Vol. 40, No. 8, (August, 1981), pp. (65-81), ISSN 0091-6765

Plasmalab software (2007). Thermo Fisher, Build Version: 2.5.1.289.

Quicke, D. & Brace, R. (1979). Differential and staining of cobalt-and nickel-filled neurones using rubeanic acid. *Journal of Micros*copy, Vol. 115, No. 2, (March, 1979), pp. (161 163), ISSN 0022-2720

Rezuke, W. Knight, J. & Sunderman, F. Jr. (1987). Reference values for nickel concentrations in human tissues and bile. *American Journal of Industrial Medicine,* Vol. 11, No. 4, pp. (419 426), ISSN 0271-3586

Satrapa, J. & Szebeni, A. (1996). New quantitative support for B-image and Color Doppler sonography. *European Journal of Ultrasound,* Vol. 4, No. 1, S. 58, ISSN 0929-8266.

Sky-Peck, H. (1986). Trace metals and neoplasia. *Clinical Physiology and Biochemistry,* Vol. 4, No. 1, pp. (99-111), ISSN 0252-1164

Sporea, I. Popescu, A. & Sirli, R. (2008). Why, who and how should perform liver biopsy in chronic liver diseases. *World Journal of Gastroenterology,* Vol. 14, No. 21, (June,2008), pp. (3396-3402), ISSN 1007-9327

Strauss, E. (2010). Usefulness of liver biopsy in chronic hepatitis C. *Annals of Hepatology,* Vol. 9, Suppl. 1. (received March, 20 2010, accepted April 20, 2010) pp. (39-42), ISSN 1665-2681

Szebeni, A. & Satrapa, J. (1996). New possibilities in ultrasonography of the liver. *38. Jahrestreffen der ungarischen Gesellschaft für Gastroenterologie, Z. Gastroenterol. XXXlV, 333*, ISSN 0044-2771, Balatonaliga, May, 1996.

Szebeni A. Satrapa, J. Tolvaj, Gy. Dávid, K. (1999). The role of ultrasound measurement of liver attenuation in patients with chronic diffuse liver diseases. In: *European Congress I.H.P.B.A. "Budapest 1999"*, Flautner L. Kupcsulik P. Rózsa I. pp. (264-271). Monduzzi Editore, Bologna, Italy, ISBN 88-323-0524-0, Budapest, Hungary, May, 1999.

Szebeni, A. Tolvaj, Gy. & Zalatnai A. (2006). Correlation of ultrasound attenuation and histopathological parameters of the liver in chronic diffuse liver diseases. *European Journal of Gastroenterolog & Hepatology*, Vol. 18, No. 1, (January, 2006), pp. (37-42), ISSN 0954-691X

Szendröi, M. Vajta, G. Kovács, L. Schaff, Zs. & Lapis, K. (1984). Polarization colours of collagen fibres: a sign of collagen production activity in fibrotic processes. *Acta Morphologica Hungarica*, Vol. 32, No. 1, (n.d.), pp. (47-55) , ISSN 0236-5391

Talwalkar, J. (2002). Motion - all patients with NASH need to have a liver biopsy: Arguments for the motion. *Canadian Journal of Gastroenterology*, Vol. 16, No.10, pp. (718-721), ISSN 0885-7900

Vacca, L. (1985). *Laboratory manual of histochemistry*, Raven Press, ISBN 0-89004-540-2, New York.

Varga, I. Szebeni, A. Szoboszlai, N. & Kovács, B. (2005). Determination of trace elements in human liver biopsy samples by ICP-MS and TXRF: hepatic steatosis and nickel accumulation. *Analytical and Bioanalytical Chemistry*, Vol. 383, No. 3, (October, 2005), pp. (476-482), ISSN 1618-2042

Versieck, J.,Speecke, A. Hoste J. Barbier, F. (1973). Trace element contamination in biopsies of the liver., *Clinical Chemistry*, Vol. 19, No. 5, (n.d.), pp. (472-475), ISSN 0009-9147

Versieck J. Barbier, F. Cornelis R. Hoste J. (1982). Sample contamination as a source of error in trace element analysis of biological samples. *Talanta*, Vol. 29, No. 11, (November, 1982), pp. (973-984), ISSN 0039-9140

Wingren, G. & Axelson, O. (1993). Epidemiologic studies of occupational cancer as related to complex mixtures of trace elements in the art glass industry. *Scandinavian Journal of Work Environment &Health*, Vol. 19, Suppl. 1, (n.d.) pp. (95-100), ISSN 0355-3140

www.epa.gov/sw-846/pdfs/6020.pdf: METHOD 6020A Inductively Coupled Plasma-Mass Spectrometry

# 7

# The Use of Flow Cytometric DNA Ploidy Analysis of Liver Biopsies in Liver Cirrhosis and Hepatocellular Carcinoma

Ashraf Tabll[1] and Hisham Ismail[2,3]
[1]*Microbial Biotechnology Dept., National Research Center, Giza,*
[2]*R&D Dept., Biotechnology Research Center, New Damietta,*
[3]*Biochemistry Division, Umm Al-Qura University, Aziziah, Makkah,*
[1,2]*Egypt*
[3]*Saudi Arabia*

## 1. Introduction

Hepatocellular carcinoma (HCC) is the fifth most common human cancer world-wide but the third most common cause of mortality and evidence has been accumulating in various countries that HCC is increasing (Andrisani et al., 2011; Parkin et al., 2000; Perkin, 2004). Major etiologic agents in HCC pathogenesis are chronic infection with hepatitis B virus or hepatitis C virus (Bruix et al., 2004; Poynard et al., 2003). Advanced liver fibrosis and HCC have been indicated to develop in about 30% of patients with chronic hepatitis B or C. Other causal factors of lower incidence include alcohol abuse, metabolic disorders, and environmental agents, e.g., exposure to aflatoxin B1 (Llovet et al., 2003). HCC typically develops in the cirrhotic liver in about 80% of cases and develops only in the non-cirrhotic liver in less than 20% of cases (Alkofer, 2011). When diagnosed at early stage, HCC remains eligible for potential curative options such as surgical resection, orthotopic liver transplantation or percutaneous destructions. The absence of advanced fibrosis or cirrhosis makes resection feasible more often. However, most of HCCs have widespread dissemination within the liver at diagnosis (intermediary stage) or show extrahepatic dissemination within the portal tract, lymph nodes or distant visceral metastasis (Llovet et al., 2008). As recommended by Llovet and Bruix (2008), new and efficacious therapies are needed, along with new diagnostic biomarkers for early detection of liver cancer.

Liver biopsy, since its initial introduction by Klatskin as a clinical tool 100 years ago, soon became the major diagnostic test for liver disease (Afdhal & Manning, 2008). Many studies have been performed to evaluate the use of readily available laboratory biomarkers to predict significant fibrosis or cirrhosis or HCC to substantially reduce the number of performed biopsies (Attallah et al., 2007; 2009a, Ismail, 2010; Pinzani, 2010). However, biomarkers alone are not sufficient to allow definitive decisions to be made for a given patient (Halfon et al., 2008). Reproducibility studies of noninvasive markers should be performed according to professional recommendations and respecting standards previously proposed by experts (Munteanu et al., 2008; Sanai FM, Jeeffe, 2011). However, histological examination of liver biopsy specimens is still the gold standard for evaluating the presence of liver fibrosis, pathogenesis of liver injury and assessment of anti-viral treatment. Besides establishing the diagnosis, the biopsy is often used to assess the severity of the disease in terms of both grade and stage (Patton et al., 2010).

The assessment of cellular kinetics of liver biopsies is of great importance for understanding the development of liver disease. Cellular DNA content can be measured by flow cytometry (FCM) with the aim of (1) revealing cell distribution within the major phases (G0/G1, S-phase and G2/M) of the cell cycle, (2) estimating the frequency of apoptotic cells with fractional DNA content, and/or (3) disclosing the DNA-ploidy of the measured cell population (Darzynkiewicz et al., 2010). On the other hand, Argyrophilic nucleolar organizer regions (AgNORs) proteins are a set of argyrophilic nucleolar proteins that accumulate in highly proliferating cells, whereas their expression is very low in nonproliferating cells (Fariña et al., 2011). The simple and universally applicable methods for staining fixed and non fixed liver cells will be described. Methods for staining of cell suspension from liver biopsies, and deconvolution of DNA-content-frequency histograms to estimate the percentage of cells in major phases of the cell cycle and frequency of apoptotic cells with fractional DNA content will be presented. In addition, the advantage and disadvantages of the DNA-FCM and AgNORs count in the assessment of cellular kinetics of liver biopsies in liver disease will be investigated.

## 2. Principles of flow cytometry

### 2.1 Basis of flow cytometry

Modern flow cytometers are able to analyze several thousand particles every second (analyzer flow cytometry) and can actively separate and isolate particles having specified properties; cell sorter flow cytometry (Darzynkiewicz et al., 2011). A flow cytometer is similar to a microscope, except that, instead of producing an image of the cell, flow cytometry offers "high-throughput" (for a large number of cells) automated quantification of set parameters . To analyze tissues, such as liver biopsies, a single-cell suspension must first be prepared using mechanical or enzymatic methods. The idea of flow cytoemtry is based on a beam of light (usually laser light) of a single wavelength is directed onto a hydrodynamically-focused stream of fluid (Cho et al., 2010).

A number of detectors are aimed at the point where the stream passes through the light beam: one in line with the light beam (Forward Scatter or FSC) and several perpendicular to it (Side Scatter (SSC) and one or more fluorescent detectors). Each suspended particle from 0.2 to 150 micrometers passing through the beam scatters the ray, and fluorescent chemicals (such as propidium iodide which used for binding to DNA) found in stained cells or attached to the particle (as conjugated fluoresce antibodies used for immunophenotyping) may be excited into emitting light at a longer wavelength than the light source (de Tute, 2011). This combination of scattered and fluorescent light is picked up by the detectors, and, by analyzing fluctuations in brightness at each detector. Forward scatter (FSC) correlates with the cell size and side scatter (SSC) depends on the inner complexity of the particle (i.e., shape of the nucleus, the amount and type of cytoplasmic granules or the membrane roughness) (Fig. 1).

Fluorescence-activated cell sorting (FACS) is a specialized type of flow cytometry. It provides a method for sorting a heterogeneous mixture of biological cells into two or more containers, one cell at a time, based upon the specific light scattering and fluorescent characteristics of each cell. It is a useful scientific instrument, as it provides fast, objective and quantitative recording of fluorescent signals from individual cells as well as physical separation of cells of particular interest. The cell sorted machines have ability to sort cells with highly sterility and purity more than 98%, so these cells can be use for tissue culture applications (Cho et al., 2010).

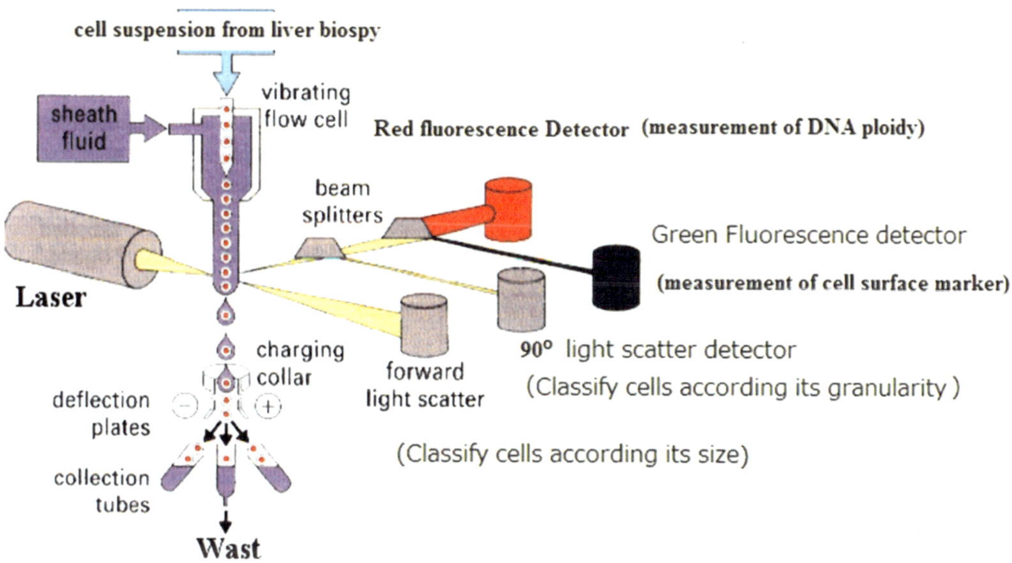


Fig. 1. Diagram of general components of flow cytometry.

## 2.2 DNA ploidy and cell cycle analysis

### 2.2.1 Cell cycle phases

The cell cycle is commonly divided into "phases" - interphase and mitosis. Interphase is further divided into three sub-phases, G1, S, and G2. In G1, cells integrate environmental and internal signals that are aimed at the "replicate"/"do not replicate" decision (Darzynkiewicz et al., 2010). The S phase is defined by the ability to synthesize genomic DNA. G2 was originally defined as the second gap between S and Mitosis, but is now known to function as a time of DNA damage repair, and likely, preparation for entering Mitosis (M phase). Mitosis has been traditionally sub-divided into stages defined by nuclear morphology - prophase, prometaphase, metaphase, anaphase A and B, and telophase. A final phase, division of the cytoplasm that overlaps telophase and is often lumped with mitosis, is cytokinesis (CK). The major cell cycle sub-phases, G1, S, G2+M can typically be identified by direct quantitative measurement of the DNA by flow cytometry based on staining of DNA with fluorescence dye such as propidium iodide (Fig. 2).

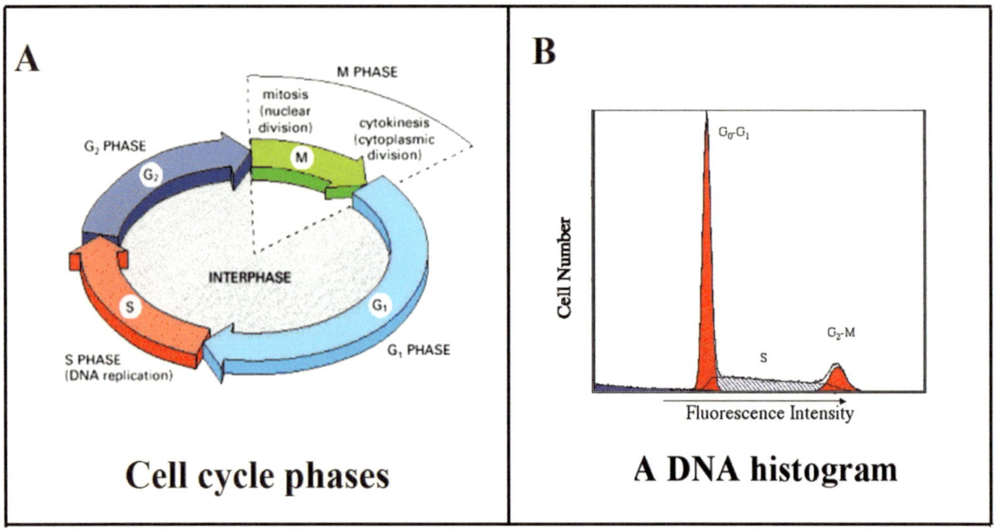


Fig. 2. The cell cycle phases (A) and diploid DNA histogram measured by flow cytometry (B).

### 2.2.2 DNA ploidy by flow cytometry

DNA content measurement by cytometry serves to estimate frequency of cells in particular phases ($G_{0/1}$ versus S versus $G_2M$) of the cell cycle as well as to assess DNA ploidy. In most situations DNA ploidy is being assessed in hematological or solid tumors; the evidence of aneuploidy by itself is a definitive marker of a presence of the tumor (Darzynkiewicz et al., 2010). Often is also considered to be a prognostic indicator of tumor progression and outcome of the treatment. To assess DNA ploidy of the tumor sample one has to compare DNA content of the $G_0/G_1$ cells population of the presumed tumor cells with that of normal (control) cells. Towards this end most frequently the peak value of the integrated fluorescence (peak channel) of $G_{0/1}$ population of normal cells is being considered to be DI = 1.0 and DNA ploidy of the tumor cells is expressed as a ratio of the peak value (channel) of fluorescence intensity of these cells with respect to that of the normal $G_{0/1}$ cells (Darzynkiewicz et al., 2011). It is also common to express DI of the tumor as a ratio of modal rather than the peak value of fluorescence intensity representing DNA content of $G_0/G_1$ population tumor cells to modal value of $G_{0/1}$ population of normal cells. Some authors still prefer to use the mean values of fluorescence intensity of $G_{0/1}$ population rather than the peak or modal values to obtain this ratio (Darzynkiewicz et al., 2010). In essence, when DNA measurement is done correctly and accurately, either of these approaches is expected to yield similar estimate of DI of aneuploid cells. From our experience, we can use normal lymphocytes, including lymphocytes from the same patient, as external standard control of DI = 1.0 (Fig. 3).

For comparison with the tumor it is necessary to use normal cells both as external and internal control standards. When used as external control they have to be subjected to identical processing and staining procedure and measured by cytometry under identical

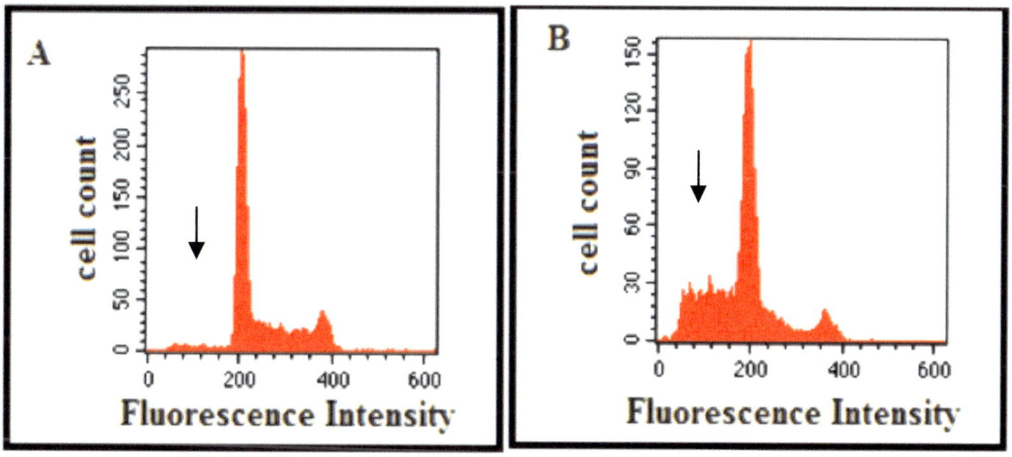


Fig. 3. Apoptotic cells (sub G0/G1 region) as measured by flow cytometry. Figure B shows high percentage of apoptotic cells (indicated by arrows) in comparison with low percentage shown in figure A.

laser and detector settings as tumor sample (Shankey and Rabinovitch, 2002). The external lymphocyte control cells should be measured prior to- and also after- measurement of tumor sample. This double- measurement of control cells allows one to detect the possible shift in fluorescence readout e.g., due to mis adjustment in instrument settings in the course of the sequential measurements. In addition to external control, normal cells should also be admixed (e.g., in 1:1 proportion) with the tumor sample cells and used then as internal control in another set of measurements (Darzynkiewicz et al., 2010). Often, normal stromal- or tumor infiltrating cells are already present in the tumor sample and they can be used as an internal control of DNA ploidy. In fact, when DNA ploidy is assessed based on measurement of nuclei isolated from paraffin blocks, the internal control provided by the presence of stromal and infiltrating normal cells that provide standard for DI = 1.0 is the only way to assess DNA ploidy of the tumor (Shankey et al.,1993). This is due to the fact that DNA stains ability after formaldehyde fixation and paraffin embedding is markedly altered making external standards useless (Darzynkiewicz et al., 2010). Two different types of reagents are necessary to ensure accuracy of DNA content analysis. Controls are used to assure proper instrument performance and to validate the DNA staining technique (Robinson et al., 2002). Fresh or fixed cells such as chicken erythrocytes (internal control or human lymphocytes (external control) have been used to determine staining consistency between samples, variations in DNA binding by different cell population can produce ambiguity in the correction definition of the diploid DNA content (Shankey et al., 1993, Darzynkiewicz et al., 2010) as shown in Fig. 4 & Fig. 5.

Fluorescent beads are useful controls to determine instrument performance and linearity because their fluorescence is consistent on a day-to day basis (Darzynkiewicz et al., 2010). These standards are used to define the amount of DNA related fluorescence that is equivalent to the amount that would be obtained from a diploid human cell.

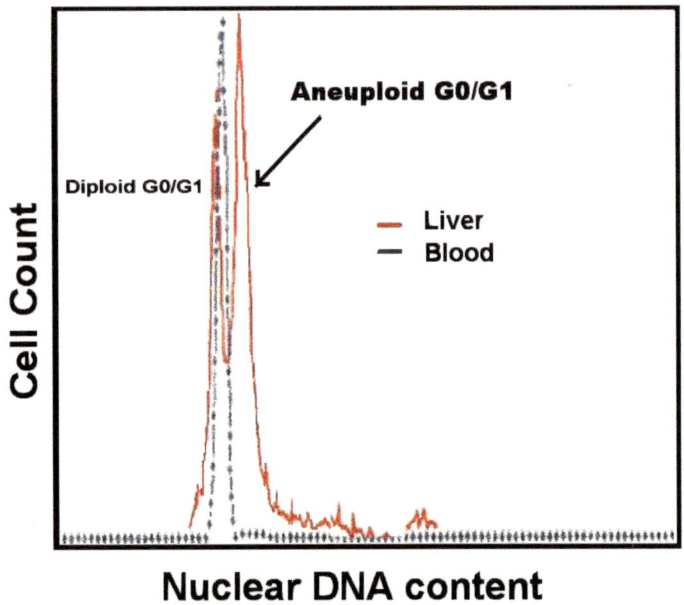


Fig. 4. Blood lymphocytes (blue) used as external control for DNA ploidy analysis by flow cytometry. DNA ploidy of liver biopsy from HCC patient (red).

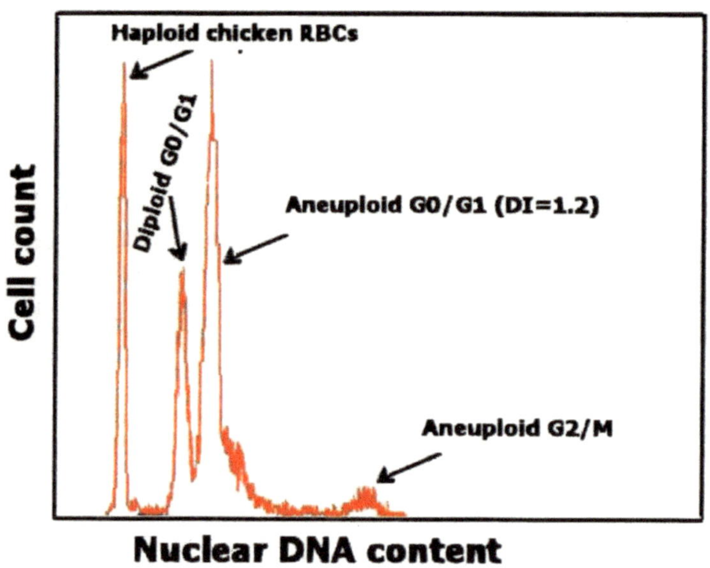


Fig. 5. Chicken red blood cells can be used as internal control during DNA ploidy analysis by flow cytoemtry.

### 2.2.3 Doublet discrimination

Because cells and especially fixated cells tend to stick together, cell aggregates have to be excluded from analysis through a process called doublet discrimination. This is important because a doublet of two cells in the $G_0/G_1$ phase has the same total amount of DNA and thus the same fluorescence intensity as a single cell in the $G_2/M$ phase (Wersto et al., 2001). $G_0/G_1$ doublets would therefore create false positive results for $G_2/M$ cells.

### 2.2.4 Analysis of cellular DNA content by flow cytometry

Flow cytometry analysis of ploidy and cell cycle analysis were one of the first applications of flow cytometry and this technique remains the only rapid and efficient means of making such measurements (López-Otero et al., 2010). As previously described, distribution of cells within the major phases of the cell cycle is based on differences in DNA content between the cells in pre replicative phase (G0/1) versus the cells that actually replicate DNA (S phase) versus the post replicative plus mitotic (G2 + M) phase cells (Darzynkiewicz et al., 2010). It is generally accepted that DNA content measured by cytometry (DNA ploidy) is defined as DNA index (DI) and for normal (non tumor, euploid) cells in G0/1 phase of the cell cycle DI = 1.0. Cells in G2/M phase of the cell cycle have DI = 2.0 and the S-phase normal cells are characterized by $1.0 < DI < 2.0$. Different histograms DNA ploidy measured using flow cytometry based on liver biopsied from HCC and liver cirrhosis with different DNA index are shown in Fig. 6. Analysis of DNA content reveals cell ploidy, provides information on cell position in the cell cycle and also allows one to estimate frequency of apoptotic cells that are characterized by fractional DNA content (Shankey et al., 1993, Darzynkiewicz et al., 2010). Such apoptotic cells can be identified as the cells with fractional DNA content ($DI < 1.0$). It is often being defined as "sub-G1" cell population.

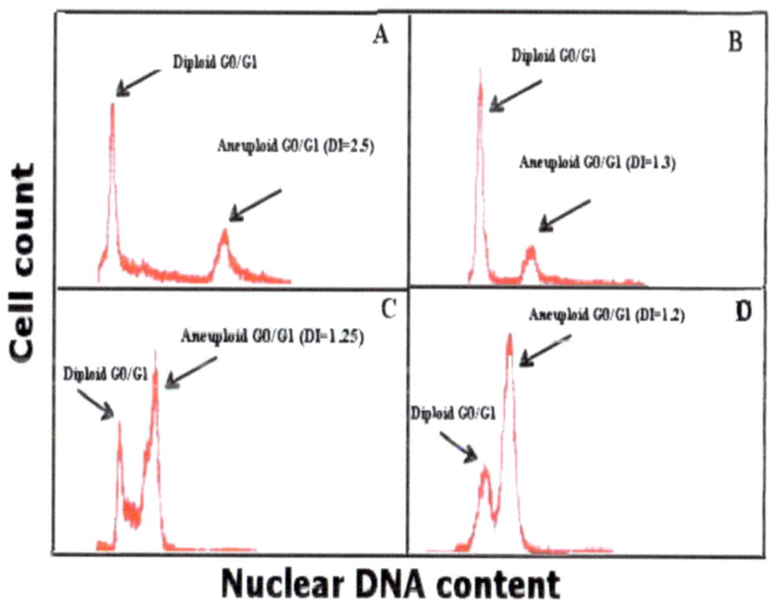


Fig. 6. Different ploidy histograms of liver biopsies from pateints with HCC. Figures A,C from tumor part and B,D from residual part (non tumor part) of HCC liver biospes.

## 3. Simple and universally applicable method for staining fixed and non fixed liver cells and analysis by flow cytoemtry

In cirrhotic patients with early HCC, a pre-operative liver biopsy should be performed because it has a low complication rate and it provides clinically useful information for the management of these patients (Colecchia et al., 2011). Knowledge of pre-operative tumor grade is crucial in the management of HCC because it can influence recurrence and survival after surgery. The accuracy of pre-operative needle biopsy in tumor grading has been assessed in only a few studies with conflicting results (D'Amico et al., 2009; Pawlik et al., 2007). Fine needle aspiration biopsy (FNA) is currently the preferred technique for diagnosing liver masses because of its safety and rapidity. The cytological diagnosis is usually taken as definitive, which makes it critical for patient management (Kocjan G 2010). However, in the literature it is reported that FNA of the liver has variable diagnostic sensitivity (60–100%), and that difficulties exist in diagnosing well-differentiated HCCs and in distinguishing primary from metastatic tumors (Kuo et al., 2004; Ligato et al., 2008). For this reason, additional studies that can be performed on cytological samples are desirable to aid diagnosis.

DNA analysis has diagnostic and/or prognostic significance in different human neoplasias, and can be performed on FNA samples. The following is the simple and universally applicable method for staining fixed and non fixed liver cells and analysis by flow cytoemtry. Single-cell suspensions can be prepared by mechanical dissociation of the fresh biopsy specimen in RPMI-1640 medium (Sigma Chemical Co., St. Louis, MO) or phosphate buffer saline (PBS) followed by filtration through a piece of fine nylon mesh (45 μm pore-size) and centrifugation to remove debris and cell clumps. Cells were permeabilized with Triton X-100 (Sigma) (0.1 % in di-ionized $H2O$ followed by staining using propidium iodide (Sigma) (50 μg/ ml in PBS) as a DNA specific fluorochrome. Core liver biopsy or cell suspension can be preserved in media (sterile DMEM media or phosphate buffer saline) in freezer - 20 $^0$C for more than one month. Also cells can fixed in absolute alcohol then be preserved at freezer - 20 $^0$C. Flow cytometric analysis can be performed with a any flow cytometer (such as Coulter EPICS profile II Coulter Corp., Hialeah, FL ), configured with a 488 nm argon ion laser. Peripheral blood lymphocytes were used as an external standard for tissue material. A total of 10000 events per sample were acquired. DNA aneuploidy was defined as any population with a distinct additional peak (s) or the presence of a tetraploid population greater than 15%. The coefficient of variation (CV) was defined as the standard deviation as a percentage of the mean DNA value of the diploid peak. Samples were excluded when CV exceeded 5%. Histograms showing only one G0/G1 peak was considered as diploid cells (normal) and those showing two distinct peaks were considered as aneuploid cells (Attallah et al., 2009b).

## 4. DNA-FCM in the assessment of cellular kinetics of liver biopsies in liver cirrhosis and HCC

It is scientifically and clinically important to better understand the intermediate events that predispose to neoplastic progression. Many neoplasms generate DNA-flow cytometry histograms which differ from the normal in having more than one peak with a different DNA content, the term aneuploid being used to describe these populations. Aneuploidy is believed to correlate with poor prognosis and early recurrence following surgery (Quinn and Wright 1990; Tripathi et al., 2008). According to the multi-step theory of neoplastic progression, cancer development is associated with the evolution of a clone of cells with an acquired genomic instability and abnormal proliferation, i.e. progression to malignancy is associated with the expansion of cells with altered DNA. In our previous study, (Attallah et al., 1999b), the cellular DNA content, known as ploidy state, of cells and expressed as DI revealed that normal liver showed a diploid pattern. Abnormal DNA content was observed in 78.6% of the tumor sites of HCC, (50% were aneuploid (1:15, DI, 1:8), 28.6% were tetraploid), in agreement with Chen et al. (1991). Mise et al. (1998) found that DNA aneuploidy was observed in 31 of 80 tumors (38.8%) while Kato et al. (1998) demonstrated that, aneuploidy was seen in 45% (9 of 20) of tumors. However, 21.4% of HCC patients were in a diploid state.

Ploidy study estimates quantitative changes in chromosome complement by measuring nuclear DNA content. At least two possibilities can be considered. One is that there may be a balanced translocations chromosomal rearrangement without change in chromosomal volume, point mutations or deletions (Hayashi et al., 1988; Hiddeman et al., 1984; Raiker, et al., 1989) which cannot be identified as abnormalities by flow cytometry measurement. The other possibility is the degree of quantitative change of chromosomes. It is difficult to identify a small change, such as a defect in the short arm of a chromosome (Hayashi et al., 1988) or an abnormal or small-sized chromosome (Maletz et al, 1986; Tripathi et al., 2008). Residual liver lesions of HCC had aneuploid cell populations in 43% of cases. Aneuploidy was found in 44.5% of the liver cirrhosis patients group. The high percentage of aneuploidy in residual liver lesions of the HCC group or the cirrhotic liver group did not agree with the data of Rua et al. (1996) which demonstrated that aneuploidy is found in only 11% of cirrhotic parts of peritumoral HCC. The discrepancy is not completely clear and may be due to the method used. In the study of Rua et al., parafin-embedded tissues were used while our samples were tested fresh. In addition, dysplasia was found in 66% of cirrhotic cases and this in agreement with Anthony et al., (1973) and Roncalliet al., (2010). Aneuploidy was found in 69% of dysplastic cases. The proliferative activity (S-phase and G2/M phases), measured by flow cytometry, revealed statistically a significant difference between the liver cirrhosis group and normal liver ($P < 0.05$) and this agrees with Rua et al. (1996), who suggested that S phase fraction of cirrhotic liver parenchyma may be employed as a new additional parameter in the prognostic evaluation of HCC patients. There may be a relationship between the development of carcinoma and an increased cell proliferation, presumably due to an increased rate of random mutations (Jain et al., 2010; Tarao et al., 1994a).

The survival of patients with HCC which developed in a cirrhotic liver with a diploid DNA content and a high S-phase fraction was significantly reduced (Rua et al., 1996). Tarao et al. (1994a) demonstrated that HCC developed within a 3-year period in 64.3% of the cirrhotic patients with high DNA synthesis activity and only in 14.3% of the cirrhotic patients with low DNA synthesis activity. Ballardini et al. (1994) found higher reactivity for proliferating cell nuclear antigen in the cirrhotic liver of patients who eventually developed HCC, and therefore they suggest a differentiated follow-up of these patients. In the present study, proliferation activity of diploid tumors and residual liver lesions showed an increase but was not statistically significant ($P < 0.06$, $P < 0.08$ respectively). Patients with cirrhosis and high cell proliferation rates are at increased risk of developing cancer as reported by Baker et al. (1995) and But et al., (2008). So, the presence of liver cell dysplasia (66%) and a high proliferation rate may explain the high percentage of aneuploidy in the cirrhotic patients group and in residual liver tissues of HCC. The increase of aneuploidy in liver cirrhosis patients and residual liver lesions of HCC demonstrated that liver cirrhosis is a premalignant lesion for HCC and that high proliferating activity and aneuploid cirrhotic patients must be followed up, as reported by Ballardini et al. (1994) and Roncalli et al., (2010). We can conclude that, DNA ploidy analysis of core liver biopsy specimens is useful in the investigation of the cell kinetics of liver cirrhosis and HCC. Dysplasia, cell proliferation and aneuploidy in liver cirrhosis may be an indication of a risk factor of liver cirrhosis for development of HCC. Also quantitative DNA content analysis using small needle liver biopsies is simple and technically convenient for flow cytometric ploidy analysis.

## 5. DNA ploidy and liver cell dysplasia in liver biopsies from patients with liver cirrhosis

There is controversy among pathologist when assessing the presence or absence of liver cell dysplasia in liver biopsies taken from cirrhotic patients (El-Sayed et al., 2004). Flow cytometry is a rapid cell proliferation (technique and can assess thousands of cells in a few minutes. Moreover, FCM can identify cases with high cell proliferation (high S phase and G2/M), which are very susceptible to different mutagenic agents or chemicals, which results in neoplastic transformation. FCM can therefore be considered as a better ancillary technique in the assessment of liver cell dysplasia because it is objective and not able to misinterpretation or inter-observer discordance (Attallah et al., 2009b). In our previous study (El-Sayed et al., 2004), liver cell dysplasia was found in 60 % of patients with liver cirrhosis, small cell dysplasia in 38 % and large cell dysplasia in 62 %. Our results are in agreement with finding of Roncalli et al (1989) and Lin et al., (1990). We used FCM to determine the DNA ploidy, cellular DNA content and proliferation index (PI). We found that 81.5 % of cases that were histopathologically shown to have liver cell dysplasia also had aneuploidy. In addition, aneuploidy was found in 11.1% of biopsies without liver cell dysplasia. This may be due to the higher sensitivity of FCM. These results confirm the aneuploidy nature of liver cell dysplasia (Anthony et al., 1973; Park and Roncalli et al., 1989; Roncalli et al., 2010).

The DNA content of liver cells expressed as DI was significantly higher ($P<0.0001$) in cases with liver cell dysplasia than cases without liver cell dysplasia, in accordance with the finding of other investigations (Henmi A, et al., 1985; Lee et al., 1997, Roncalli et al.,1989; van Dekken et al., 2005). Libbrecht et al., (2001) indicated that the presence of liver cell dysplasia in a needle liver biopsy of patients with the viral induced chronic liver disease is an independent risk factor for the development of HCC. At least two possibilities can be considered to explain the diploidy in liver cirrhosis biopsies with dysplasia. One is that there may be balanced translocations chromosomal rearrangements without change in chromosomal volume, point mutations, or deletions that con not be identified by FCM measurement (Fukushi et al., 2009; Hayashi et al., 1989; Tomioka, 2003). The other possibility may be due to the degree of quantitative change of chromosomes. It is difficult to identify a small change, such as a defect in the short arm of a chromosome. It is difficult to identify a small change, such as a defect short arm of a chromosome or an abnormal or small sized chromosome. Furthermore, the aneuploidy was found more commonly in large cell dysplasia (LCD) compared with small cell dysplasia (SCD), but no multiple aneuploid peaks (polypoidy) were found in either LCD or SCD. We showed that the cellular DNA contents were insignificant relation with activity of cirrhosis (El-Sayed et al., 2004), which is in agreement with Lin et al., (1990). Moreover, active cirrhosis was significantly (P<0.05) associated with a higher PI (S + G2M phases) than diploid cases with inactive cirrhosis and my due to liver response to cell injury (Pahlavan et al., 2006; Schaffner 1991). The value of detecting these cellular DNA changes in liver cirrhosis by FCM is of prognostic value in regards to early detection of preneoplastic changes in liver cirrhosis were found to be at increased risk of developing HCC (Clemente et al., 2007; Ruà et al., 1996; Tarao et al., 1994b). The presence of an aneuploid DNA pattern had been reported by Hoso and Nakanuma (1991), to a precancerous change in cases with atypical adenomatous hyperplasia, of the liver. Yet, the presence of liver cell dysplasia, although not specific as premalignant condition, could be considered as a serious hand mark in cases of liver cirrhosis. In our previous study, DNA aneuploidy was indentified in 46.7 % of patients with liver cirrhosis (El-Sayed et al., 2004). However, Thomas et al., (1992) reported a lower incidence (25 %) of DNA aneuploidy in patients with liver cirrhosis. This difference may be due to the use of archival material of paraffin embedded blocks. Also serum albumin levels was significantly lower (P<0.008) in patients with liver cell dysplasia than patients without dysplasia. Moreover, a significant negative correlation (P<0.05) was found between the serum albumin and the percentage of aneuploid cells. This may be a attributed to poor synthesis of albumin by these dysplastic hepatic cells as a result of change in the nuclear DNA contents of these aneuploid cells. So we can conclude that liver cell dysplasia is associated with aneuploidy, as measured by flow cytometry, may carry the risk for progression to HCC and liver cirrhotic patients with aneuploidy must be followed up.

## 6. Advantage and disadvantages of the DNA-FCM count in the assessment of cellular kinetics of liver biopsies in liver disease

Measurement of DNA content of individual cells by using flow cytometry offers a number of advantages over cytogenetic analysis (Nunez et al., 2004; Ritter et al., 1994). Unlike cytogenetic analysis, in which 20 to 40 cells are routinely analyzed, cytometric analysis can measure ten thousands of cells or nuclei. One of the most advantages of cytometric DNA content analysis is that it does not rely on metaphase cells, and cell in all phases of the cell cycle are generally included in the analysis. The critical limitation of cytometric analysis is the significantly lower resolution compared with karotyping. Flow cytometric DNA content analysis con not provide information on chromosome structure and is thus incapable of detecting balance chromosomal translocation (Dundar et al., 2010; Shankey et al., 1993). The limitation imposed on cytometric analysis even using high precision instruments and the most stiometric DNA binding fluorescence dye; DAPI (4, 6 diamidino 2-phenylindole), prevent cytometric from detecting chromosomal gains or losses involving more than about 5 % of the total DNA. In practical terms, this implies that the smallest change that can be detected theoretically is the gain or loss of equivalent of one large (e.g. A-group) chromosome (Shankey et al., 1993).

## 7. Nucleolar organizer regions

Nucleolar organizer regions (NORs) are situated within the nucleolus of a cell that are of central importance in the transcription of DNA to ribosomal RNA and hence in the ultimate assembly of proteins (Howat et al., 1989; Schwint et al., 1996; Uno et al., 1998). NORs are located, one each on the short arms of the five acrocentric chromosomes namely

13, 14, 15, 21, and 22 as secondary constrictions close to the centromere (Howell, 1982; Vuhahula et al., 1995). The number of NOR-bearing chromosomes are seen in the karyotype (Landini et al., 1990). NORs could be demonstrated in histological sections by means of the argyrophilia of their associated proteins using the structures and simple silver staining method and thus demonstrated as termed AgNORs (Crocker, 1995; Crocker & Skilbeck 1987; Trere`, 2000).

AgNOR proteins are a set of argyrophilic nucleolar proteins that accumulate in highly proliferating cells, whereas their expression is very low in nonproliferating cells. Some of these proteins remain associated with the NORs during mitosis. In situ, the expression of AgNOR proteins is measured globally by quantification of the level of silver staining using morphometry and image analysis (Sirri et al., 2000). The distribution of AgNORs and their quantities have been associated with proliferative activity and ploidy in different neoplastic and preneoplastic conditions. Several studies investigated the correlation of the number of detectable AgNORs with the degree of nucleolar dispersion or disaggregation, which is related directly to cell proliferation and the NOR-bearing chromosomes (Arora et al., 2002; Giri et al., 1989; Underwood & Giri, 1988).

### 7.1 Staining of nucleolar organizer regions

In our laboratories, liver biopsy samples were taken from the most representative area of the diseased tissue. The biopsy specimens were then fixed in 10% buffered formalin and subsequently processed to prepare paraffin blocks. Two separate sets of sections of 4 µm thickness were obtained from each block. One set stained by the hematoxylin and eosin (H&E) technique for routine histological evaluation and confirmation of diagnosis. Another set of sections were stained for localization and quantification of AgNORs according to the method described by Lindner et al., (1993). The sections were deparaffinized in xylene, and hydrated through 100% and 95% ethanol to water. Reduction of sections was done with 1% potassium iodide for 60 min. Silver staining solution was prepared by dissolving 2% gelatin in 1% formic acid at room temperature and filtered through syringe filter (Sigma Chemical Co., St. Louis, MO, USA). One part of the solution was mixed with two parts of 50% silver nitrate immediately before use. Staining was done in dark at room temperature for 30 min, then sections were immersed in 5% sodium thiosulphate for 5 min. Sections were washed in water, dehydrated in 95% and 100% ethanol, and mounted in permanent mounting media (Attallah et al., 2009b).

### 7.2 Counting of silver stained nucleolar organizer regions (AgNORs)

AgNORs appear as brown black dots inside the nucleus using silver stain. Counting of AgNORs was done without any knowledge of the histological or the clinical data. The slides were examined with an oil immersion objective at 1000 magnification. The examined fields were selected randomly. AgNORs were counted in 100 nuclei, which were randomly selected. The absolute number of AgNORs within each nucleus was counted and the mean number of AgNORs per nucleus (mAgNORs) was determined for each case (fig. 7). Background should be pale yellow and clear, the nucleus yellow and/or brown, and AgNOR sites intra-nucleolar black dots.

Most studies have shown that high AgNORs counts can reflect a tumor's degree of malignancy, differentiate among reactive, benign, and malignant conditions (Derenzini & Ploton 1991; Khan et al., 2006; Kummoona et al., 2008; Raikhlin et al., 2006). Crocher &

McGovern (1988) applied the AgNORs method to normal, cirrhotic, and carcinomatous livers and recognized a significant difference in their AgNORs scores. Study of Jain et al. (1998) indicated that both quantitative and qualitative analysis of AgNORs may be useful as an adjunct to routine hematoxylin and eosin stain to distinguish cirrhosis from HCC especially when the latter is well differentiated. Also, AgNORs count in the hyperplastic foci was significantly higher than that in the controls (Wakasa et al., 1998). Jagan et al. (2008) investigated the antiproliferative effect of gallic acid during diethylnitrosamine (DEN)-induced HCC in male Wistar albino rats. They used levels of AgNORs as a tumor marker, which can be an indicator of tumor response to therapy.

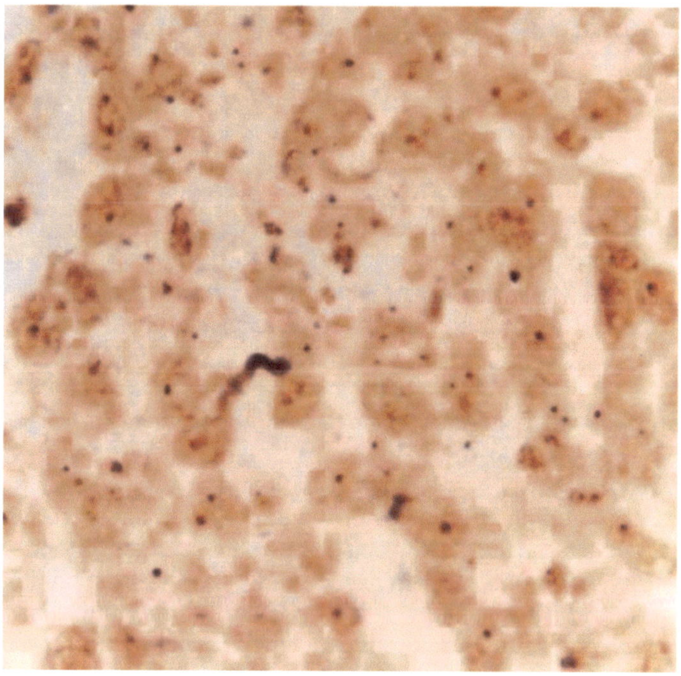

Fig. 7. The AgNORs staining in liver of patient with HCC. The findings were viewed following staining under the light microscope using 100X oil immersion lens and cedar wood oil. Nucleolar organizer regions appear as brown black dots inside the nucleus using silver stain (AgNORs count).

### 7.3 AgNOR count reflects DNA ploidy or proliferative activity

Several attempts have been made to determine whether mean AgNOR count reflects ploidy or proliferative activity. However, several studies have correlated the mean AgNOR count with Ki-67, bromodeoxyuridine (BrdU)-labeling indexes (Munakataet al., 1994; Trere et al., 1991), and proliferating cell nuclear antigen (PCNA) in mucosa-associated lymphoid tissues and gastrointestinal stromal tumors (Yu et al., 1992). Mikow et al. (1993) indicated that mean AgNOR reflects the proliferative activity rather than ploidy. Another study failed to show a relationship between AgNORs count and Ki-67 and BrdU-labeling indexes (Nyska, 1995), or between diploid and aneuploid tumors (Nagao et al., 1995). This is in a disagreement with a study of mean AgNOR in trophoblastic disease, which indicated that mean AgNOR is a reflection of ploidy and proliferative activities (Maier et al., 1990). However, in contrast to immunohistochemical methods merely determining the growth fraction of the cells by Ki-67 and proliferating cell nuclear antigen (PCNA) analysis AgNORs apparently reflect time-related proliferation rates and ploidy. Thus, AgNOR analysis may provide further insights concerning the biological behavior of the cell and is simple, inexpensive, and reliable method of evaluating the proliferative activity and ploidy of the cell (Meng et al., 1996).

Celikel (1995) found a correlation between mean AgNOR and ploidy and proliferation activity of urinary bladder tumor as measured by DNA flow cytometry. Also, Borzio et al. (1998) demonstrated that a high hepatocyte proliferation rate detected by AgNORs is a major risk factor for HCC development in the cirrhotic liver. Therefore, they indicated that the evaluation of the hepatocyte proliferation rate is very important to identify patients requiring stricter follow-up program for early diagnosis of HCC. High AgNOR count in cirrhotic liver as a marker of regenerative capacity has been associated with a significantly increased incidence in development of HCC in chronic liver disease (Derenzini et al., 1993). However, in liver cirrhosis, dysplasia had a significant relationship with ploidy and AgNORs. So, the incidence of high AgNORs count, dysplasia, and presence of aneuploidy by DNA flow cytometry suggest that liver cirrhosis may be considered as a more serious condition in the evolution of HCC.

Recently, we compared the results of DNA flow cytometry and AgNORs with the histopathological data. It was found that the lowest mean AgNOR count per nucleus was found in the normal liver (1.3± 0.9) and the highest count was (3.89± 0.827) in tumor lesion of HCC (Attallah et al., 2009b). A gradual increase in the AgNOR count per nucleus was noted as disease progressed from normal liver through liver cirrhosis to HCC tumor lesions. Analysis of AgNOR counts showed a significant difference between tumor and residual liver tissues of HCC or normal liver ($P < 0.001$) and this is in agreement with several studies (Shemizu et al., 1995; Siddiqui et al., 1999; Politi et al., 2004). However, Chen et al. (2003) revealed that AgNOR area and AgNOR area-count ratio are the most valuable features for differential diagnosis of normal, preneoplastic, and cancer cells. Spolidorio et al. (2002) found that the morphometric results were statistically different for normal mucosa, dysplasia, and microinvasive oral carcinoma and they concluded that an increase of NOR activity follows the disease progression and may reflect the degree of cellular proliferation and malignancy. Siddiqui et al. (1999) revealed a gradual increase in mean AgNOR counts from normal liver through cirrhosis to HCC. The difference in NOR counts was significant in these three groups. The hepatocellular carcinomas were graded according to the Edmondson-Steiner histological grading system. Grade I hepatocellular carcinomas show AgNOR counts ranging between 5 and 6/cell, a score that is much higher than in the normal liver, where it ranges between 1.2 and 2.0/cell. This technique can be used to assess the lesions where the distinction between normal liver and grade I HCC is difficult with the use of routine methods, on the light of the hypothesis of a relationship between the development of carcinoma and an increased cell proliferation, presumably by an increase of random mutations (Jain et al., 2010; Tarao et al., 1994a). So, quantification of AgNOR is considered to have putative relationship with ploidy in HCC. Our study presents complementary methods to histopathology, which are valuable to pathologists, when they have difficulty in diagnosis of early stages of HCC on the basis of liver biopsy. Finally, both AgNORs count and DNA ploidy analysis are useful and valuable indicators of cellular kinetics in HCC.

## 8. Conclusion remarks and future research

The assessment of cellular kinetics of liver biopsies is of great importance for understanding the development and diagnosis of liver disease. Flow cytometric analyses of ploidy and cell cycle were one of the first applications of flow cytometry and this technique remains the only rapid and efficient means of making such measurement particularly for core liver biopsies. AgNOR proteins are a set of argyrophilic nucleolar proteins that accumulate in highly proliferating cells, whereas their expression is very low in nonproliferating cells. The AgNOR tissue marker can be used as a routine complementary histopathologic study and DNA ploidy by flow cytometry, since the variations in its number and distribution indicate existence of cell alterations in a given lesion and the use of this technique is easy and inexpensive. Diagnosis of HCC using both DNA ploidy and mean AgNORs are useful in the detection of cellular and structural abnormalities. However, further research are required to confirm the relationship between viral infections such as HCV and cancer, cell proliferation and apoptosis based on liver biopsies from patients cirrhosis and HCC.
The detection of viral antigens based on specific monoclonal antibodies and/or the detection of viral hepatitis nucleic acids such as HCV RNA and HBV DNA in the liver biopsies and its relation to cell cycle analyses measured by flow cytometry will be the future research in this field.

## 9. Acknowledgment

This work was partially funded through the Science and Technology Development Fund (STDF), Egypt "Grant no. 894" to Dr. Ashraf Tabll.

## 10. References

Afdhal NH., & Manning D. (2008). Diagnosis of liver fibrosis in 2008 and beyond. *Gastroentérol Clin Bio* 32: 88-90.

Alkofer B., Lepennec V., & Chiche L. (2011). Hepatocellular cancer in the non-cirrhotic liver. *J Visc Sur,* 148, 3–11.

Andrisani OM., Studach L., & Merle L. (2011). Gene signatures in hepatocellular carcinoma (HCC). *Seminars Canc Biol,* 21: 4–9.

Anthony PP., Vogel CL., & Barker LF. (1973). Liver cell dysplasia: a premalignant condition. *J Clin Pathol,* 26(3), 217-23. PMID: 4700503

Arora B., Jain R., Kumar S., Rekhi B., Arora H., & Arora DR. (2002). Morphometric analysis of AgNORs in the lymph node lesions. *Adv Clin Path,* 6(2):95-99.

Attallah AM., Shiha G., Ismail H., Mansy SE., El-Sherbiny RE., & El-Dosoky I. (2009a). Expression of p53 protein in liver and sera of patients with liver fibrosis, cirrhosis or hepatocellular carcinoma associated with chronic HCV infection. *Clin Biochem,* 42: 455-461.

Attallah AM., Tabll AA., El-Nashar E., El-Bakry KA., El Sadany M., Ibrahim T., & El-Dosoky I. (2009b). AgNORs count and DNA ploidy in liver biopsies from patients with schistosomal liver cirrhosis and hepatocellular carcinoma. *Clin Biochem,* 42(16-17):1616-20.

Attallah AM., Tabll AA., Salem SF., El-Sadany M., Ibrahim TA., Osman S., & El-Dosoky I. (1999). DNA ploidy of liver biopsies from patients with liver cirrhosis and hepatocellular carcinoma: a flow cytometric analysis. *Cancer Lett,* 142(1):65-69. PMID: 10424782

Attallah AM., Zahran F., Ismail H., Omran M., El-Dosoky I., & Shiha G. (2007). Immunochemical identification and detection of serum fibronectin in liver fibrosis patients with chronic hepatitis C. *J Immunoassay Immunochem,* 28(4): 331-342.

Baker ME., Pelley R. (1995). Hepatic metastases: basic principles and implications for radiologists. *Radiology,* 197(2):329-37. PMID: 7480672

Ballardini G., Groff P., Zoli M., Bianchi G., Giostra F., Francesconi R., Lenzi M., Zauli D., Cassani F., & Bianchi F. (1994). Increased risk of hepatocellular carcinoma development in patients with cirrhosis and with high hepatocellular proliferation. *J Hepatol,* 20(2):218-22. PMID: 7911817

Barwick K., Rosai J., (1996). Liver. In: *Ackerman's Surgical Pathology,* 8th ed. J. Rosai, pp. 857, Mosby-Year Book, New York.

Borzio M., Trere D., Borzio F., Ferrari A., Bruno S., Roncalli M., Colloredo G., Leandro G., Oliveri F., & Derenzini M. (1998). Hepatocyte proliferation rate is a powerful parameter for predicting hepatocellular carcinoma development in liver cirrhosis. *Mol Pathol,* 51(2):96–101.

Bruix J., Boix L., Sala M., & Llovet JM. (2004). Focus on hepatocellular carcinoma. *Cancer Cell,* 5:215–9.

But DY., Lai CL., & Yuen MF. (2008). Natural history of hepatitis-related hepatocellular carcinoma. *World J Gastroenterol,* 14(11):1652-6. PMID:18350595

Celikel C. (1995). DNA Flow cytometric studies and AgNOR counts in patients with transitional cell carcinoma of bladder. *Eur Urol,* 28:152–157.

Chen M., Lee JC., Lo S., & Shen J. (2003). Argyrophilic nuclear organizer regions in nasopharyngeal carcinoma and paraneoplastic epithelia. *Head Neck,* 25(5):395–399.

Chen MF., Hwang TL., Tsao KC., Sun CF., & Chen TJ. (1991). Flow cytometric DNA analysis of hepatocellular carcinoma: preliminary report. *Surgery,* 109(4):455-8. PMID: 1706892.

Cho SH., Godin JM., Chen CH., Qiao W., Lee H., & Lo YH. (2010). Review Article: Recent advancements in optofluidic flow cytometer. *Biomicrofluidics,* 4(4):43001. PMID: 21267434.

Clemente C., Elba S., Buongiorno G., Guerra V., D'Attoma B., Orlando A., & Russo F. (2007). Manganese superoxide dismutase activity and incidence of hepatocellular carcinoma in patients with Child-Pugh class A liver cirrhosis: a 7-year follow-up study. *Liver Int,* 27(6):791-797. PMID: 17617122.

Colecchia A., Scaioli E., Montrone L., Vestito A., Di Biase AR., Pieri M., D'Errico-Grigioni A., Bacchi-Reggiani ML., Ravaioli M., Grazi GL., & Festi D. (2011). Pre-operative liver biopsy in cirrhotic patients with early hepatocellular carcinoma represents a safe and accurate diagnostic tool for tumour grading assessment. *J Hepatol,* 54(2):300–305. PMID: 21056498.

Crocker J., McGovern J. (1988). Nucleolar organizer region in normal, cirrhotic, and carcinomatous livers. *J Clin Pathol* 41:1044–1048.

Crocker J., Skilbeck N. (1987). Nucleolar organizer region associated proteins in cutaneous melanocytic lesions: a quantitative study. *J Clin Pathol,* 40: 885–889.

Crocker J. (1992). Nucleolar organizer regions (NORs) in neoplasms. In: *Oxford text book of pathology vol 1.* McGee JD, Issacson PG, et al, eds. pp. 586-590. Oxford university press; Oxford.

D'Amico F., Schwartz ME., Vitale A., Tabrizian P., Roayaie S., Thung S., Guido M., del Rio Martin J., Schiano T., & Cillo U. (2009). Predicting recurrence after liver transplantation in patients with hepatocellular carcinoma exceeding the up-to seven criteria. *Liver Transpl,* 15(10):1278–1287.

Darzynkiewicz Z., Halicka HD., & Zhao H. (2010). Analysis of cellular DNA content by flow and laser scanning cytometry. *Adv Exp Med Biol,* 676:137-147. PMID: 20687474.

Darzynkiewicz Z., Traganos F., Zhao H., Halicka HD., & Li J. (2011). Cytometry of DNA replication and RNA synthesis: Historical perspective and recent advances based on "click chemistry". *Cytometry A,* In press. PMID: 21425239.

de Tute RM. (2011). Flow cytometry and its use in the diagnosis and management of mature lymphoid malignancies. *Histopathology* 58(1):90-105. PMID: 21261686

Derenzini M., & Ploton D. (1991). Interphase nucleolar organizer region in cancer cells. *Int Rev Exp Pathol,* 32:149–152.

Derenzini M., Trerè D., Oliveri F., David E., Colombatto P., Bonino F., & Brunetto MR. (1993). Is high AgNOR quantity in hepatocytes associated with increased risk of hepatocellular carcinoma in chronic liver disease?. *J Clin Pathol* 46(8):727–729.

Dundar M., Kiraz A., Tasdemir S., Akalin H., Kurtoglu S., Hafo F., Cine N., & Savli H. (2010). Unbalanced 3;22 translocation with 22q11 and 3p deletion syndrome. *Am J Med Genet A,* 152A(11):2791-5. PMID: 20949503

El-Sayed SS., El-Sadany M., Tabll AA., Soltan A., El-Dosoky I., & Attallah AM. (2004). DNA ploidy and liver cell dysplasia in liver biopsies from patients with liver cirrhosis. *Can J Gastroenterol,* 18(2):87-91. PMID: 14997216.

Fariña RA., Becar M., Plaza C., Espinoza I., & Franco ME. (2011). Relation between single photon emission computed tomography, AgNOR count, and histomorphologic features in patients with active mandibular condylar hyperplasia. *J Oral Maxillofac Surg,* 69(2):356-361. PMID: 21122972

Fukushi D., Watanabe N., Kasai F., Haruta M., Kikuchi A., Kikuta A., Kato K., Nakadate H., Tsunematsu Y., & Kaneko Y. (2009). Centrosome amplification is correlated with ploidy divergence, but not with MYCN amplification, in neuroblastoma tumors. *Cancer Genet Cytogenet,* 188(1):32-41.

Giri D., Nottingham J., Lawry J., Dundas S., & Underwood J. (1989). Silver binding nucleolar organizer regions (AgNORs) in benign and malignant breast lesions: correlation with ploidy and growth phase by DNA flow cytometry. *J Pathol,* 157:307–313.

Halfon P., Munteanu M., & Poynard T. (2008). FibroTest-ActiTest as a non-invasive marker of liver fibrosis. *Gastroentérol Clin Bio,* 32:22-39.

Hayashi Y., Kanda N., Inaba T., Hanada R., Nagahara N., Muchi H., & Yamamoto K. (1989). Cytogenetic findings and prognosis in neuroblastoma with emphasis on marker chromosome 1. *Cancer,* 63(1):126-32. PMID: 2910410.

Henmi A., Uchida T., & Shikata T. (1985). Karyometric analysis of liver cell dysplasia and hepatocellular carcinoma. Evidence against precancerous nature of liver cell dysplasia. *Cancer,* 55(11):2594-9. PMID: 2986818

Hiddemann W., Schumann J., Andreef M., Barlogie B., Herman CJ., Leif RC., Mayall BH., Murphy RF., & Sandberg AA. (1984). Convention on nomenclature for DNA cytometry. Committee on Nomenclature, Society for Analytical Cytology. *Cancer Genet Cytogenet,* 13(2):181-3. PMID: 6478442

Hoso M., & Nakanuma Y. (1991). Cytophotometric DNA analysis of adenomatous hyperplasia in cirrhotic livers. *Virchows Arch A Pathol Anat Histopathol,* 418(5):401-404. PMID: 1852083

Howat AJ., Giri DD., Cotton DW., Slater DN. (1989). Nucleolar Organizer Regions in spitz nevi and malignant melanomas. *Cancer,* 63:474-478.

Howell, WM. (1982). Selective staining of nucleolus organizer regions (NORs). In: *The cell nucleus.* Busch, H., & Rothblum, L. (Eds.), pp. 89–143, Academic press, New York.

Ismail H., Al-Zahrany SA., Al-Ghamedy ZS., & Radway ON. (2010). Simple and rapid identification of liver status in HCV infection using blood biochemical markers. 2010. *Proceedings of the 25th annual meeting of the Saudi biological society,* King Faisal University, Al-Hasa, Saudi Arabia, May 2010.

Jagan S., Ramakrishnan G., Anandakumar P., Kamaraj S., & Devaki T. (2008). Antiproliferative potential of gallic acid against diethylnitrosamine-induced rat hepatocellular carcinoma. *Mol Cell Biochem,* 319(1-2):51–59.

Jain R., Malhotra V., Kumar N., & Sarin S. (1998). Nucleolar Organizer region in cirrhosis and hepatocellular carcinoma. *Trop Gastroenterol,* 19(3): 100–101.

Jain S., Singhal S., Lee P., & Xu R. (2010). Molecular genetics of hepatocellular neoplasia. *Am J Transl Res,* 2(1):105-18. PMID:20182587.

Kato A., Kubo K., Kurokawa F., Okita K., Oga A., & Murakami T. (1998). Numerical aberrations of chromosomes 16, 17, and 18 in hepatocellular carcinoma: a FISH and FCM analysis of 20 cases. *Dig Dis Sci,* 43(1):1-7. PMID: 9508509

Khan N., Sood P., Vasenwala SM., Afroz N., & Verma AK. (2006). Significance of AgNOR score in benign and malignant soft tissue tumours. *Indian J Pathol Microbiol,* 49(1):17–20.

Kocjan G. (2010). Fine needle aspiration cytology of the pancreas: a guide to the diagnostic approach. *Coll Antropol,* 34(2):749-56. PMID: 20698166.

Kummoona R., Jabbar A., & Kareem Al-Rahal D. (2008). Proliferative activity in oral carcinomas studied with Ag-NOR and electron microscopy. *Ultrastruct Pathol,* 32(4):139–146.

Kuo FY., Chen WJ., Lu SN., Wang JH., & Eng HL. (2004). Fine needle aspiration cytodiagnosis of liver tumors. *Acta Cytol* 48(2):142-8. PMID:15085744.

Landini G. (1990). Nucleolar organizing regions (NORs) in pleomorphic adenomas of the salivary glands. *J Oral Pathol Med,* 19:257-260.

Lee RG., Tsamandas AC., & Demetris AJ. (1997). Large cell change (liver cell dysplasia) and hepatocellular carcinoma in cirrhosis: matched case-control study, pathological analysis, and pathogenetic hypothesis. *Hepatology,* 26(6):1415-1422. PMID: 9397980.

Libbrecht L., Cassiman D., Verslype C., Maleux G., Van Hees D., Pirenne J., Nevens F., & Roskams T. (2006). Clinicopathological features of focal nodular hyperplasia-like nodules in 130 cirrhotic explant livers. *Am J Gastroenterol,* 101(10):2341-2346. PMID: 17032200.

Libbrecht L., Craninx M., Nevens F., Desmet V., & Roskams T. (2001). Predictive value of liver cell dysplasia for development of hepatocellular carcinoma in patients with non-cirrhotic and cirrhotic chronic viral hepatitis. *Histopathology,* 39(1):66-73. PMID: 11454046.

Ligato S., Mandich D., & Cartun RW. (2008). Utility of glypican-3 in differentiating hepatocellular carcinoma from other primary and metastatic lesions in FNA of the liver: an immunocytochemical study. *Mod Pathol*, 21(5):626-31. PMID:18264086

Lin HH., Shyu WC., Chen GL., Lin YH., Chen TJ., & Liaw YF. (1990). DNA measurements in chronic hepatitis, cirrhosis and hepatocellular carcinoma. *Liver*, 10(5):313-8. PMID: 2175006.

Lindner L. (1993). Improvements in the silver-staining technique for nucleolar organizer regions (AgNORs). *J Histochem Cytochem*, 41:439–445.

Llovet JM., & Bruix J. (2008). Molecular targeted therapies in hepatocellular carcinoma. *Hepatology*, 48:1312–1327.

Llovet JM., Burroughs A., & Bruix J. (2003). Hepatocellular carcinoma. *Lancet*, 362:1907–1917.

Llovet JM., Di Bisceglie AM., Bruix J., Kramer BS., Lencioni R., Zhu AX., Sherman M., Schwartz M., Lotze M., Talwalkar J., Gores GJ., & Panel of Experts in HCC-Design Clinical Trials. (2008). Design and endpoints of clinical trials in hepatocellular carcinoma. *J Natl Cancer Inst*, 100(10):698–711. PMID: 18477802.

López-Otero A., Ruiz-Delgado GJ., Hernández-Arizpe A., Ruiz-Argüelles A., & Ruiz-Argüelles GJ. (2010). The flow-cytometric DNA content of the plasma cells of patients with multiple myeloma is a prognostic factor: a single institution experience. *Hematology*, 15(6):378-381. PMID:21114899.

Maier U., Morimura M., & Ofner L. (1990). Argyrophilic nucleolar organizer regions (AgNORs) in human brain tumor: Relation with grade of malignancy and proliferative indices. *Acta Neuropathol*, 80:156–162.

Maletz N., McMorrow LE., Greco A., & Wolman SR. (1986). Ewing's sarcoma. Pathology, tissue culture, and cytogenetics. *Cancer*, 58(2):252-257. PMID: 3719518.

Meng F., Giwereman A., & Skakkebaek W. (1996). Investigation of carcinoma in situ cells of testis by quantification of argyrophilic nucleolar organizer region associated protein (AgNORs). *J Pathol*, 180:206–2013.

Mikow P., Kanavaros P., & Gorgoulis B. (1993). Nucleolar organizer region staining and proliferating cell nuclear antigen (PCNA) immunostaining in mucosa associated lymphoid tissue. *Pathol Res Pract*, 189:1004–1009.

Mise K., Tashiro S., Yogita S., Wada D., Harada M., Fukuda Y., Miyake H., Isikawa M., Izumi K., & Sano N. (1998). Assessment of the biological malignancy of hepatocellular carcinoma: relationship to clinicopathological factors and prognosis. *Clin Cancer Res*, 4(6):1475-1482. PMID: 9626465.

Munakata S., & Hendricks J. (1994). Multilabelling technique for simultaneous demonstration and quantitation of Ki-67 and nucleolar organizer regions (AgNORs) in paraffin embedded tissue. *J Histochem Cytochem*, 42: 789–793.

Munteanu M., Morra R., Imbert-Bismut F., Messous D., Thabut D., & Lebray P. (2008). Reproducibility of non-invasive fibrosis biomarkers, FibroMeter and FibroTest, could be improved by respecting the analytical standardizations. *Clin Biochem*, 41:1113–1114.

Nagao T., Ishida Y., Yamazaki K., & Kondo Y. (1995). Nucleolar organizer regions in hepatocellular carcinoma related to the cell cycle, cell proliferation and histologic grade. *Pathol Res Pract*, 191(10):967–972.

Nunez R., Garay N., Villafane C., Bruno A., & Lindgren V. (2004). Description of a flow cytometry approach based on SYBR-14 staining for the assessment of DNA content, cell cycle analysis, and sorting of living normal and neoplastic cells. *Exp Mol Pathol,* 76(1):29-36. PMID:14738866.

Nyska I. (1995). Assessment of nucleolar organizer regions by automated image analysis in benign and malignant colonic tumors. *J Comp Pathol,* 113:45–50.

Pahlavan PS., Feldmann RE., Jr, Zavos C., & Kountouras J. (2006). Prometheus' challenge: molecular, cellular and systemic aspects of liver regeneration. *J Surg Res,* 134(2):238-251. PMID: 16458925.

Park YN., & Roncalli M. (2006). Large liver cell dysplasia: a controversial entity. *J Hepatol,* 45(5):734-743. PMID: 16982109.

Parkin DM., Bray F., Ferlay J., & Pisani P. (2001). Estimating the world cancer burden: Globocan 2000. *Int J Cancer,* 94:153–156.

Parkin DM. (2004). International variation. *Oncogene,* 23:6329–6340.

Patton HM., Yates K., Unalp-Arida A., Behling CA., Huang TT., Rosenthal P., Sanyal AJ., Schwimmer JB., & Lavine JE. (2010). Association between metabolic syndrome and liver histology among children with nonalcoholic fatty liver disease. *Am J Gastroenterol,* 105(9):2093-2102. PMID: 20372110.

Pawlik TM., Gleisner AL., Anders AR., Assumpcao L., Maley W., & Choti MA. (2007). Preoperative assessment of hepatocellular carcinoma tumour grade using needle biopsy. Implications for transplant eligibility. *Ann Surg,* 245: 435–442.

Pinzani M. (2010). Non-invasive systems for staging compensated cirrhosis. *Arab J Gastroenterol,* 10: S32–S34.

Politi EN., Lazaris AC., Alexopoulou D., Lambropoulou S., Kavantzas N., & Koutselini H. (2004). Morphometric analysis of AgNORs in thin-layer, liquidbased liver specimens. *Anal Quant Cytol Histol,* 26(4):187–193.

Poynard T., Yuen MF., Ratziu V., & Lai CL. (2003). Viral hepatitis C. *Lancet,* 362:2095–2100.

Quinn CM., & Wright NA. (1990). The clinical assessment of proliferation and growth in human tumours: evaluation of methods and applications as prognostic variables. *J Pathol,* 160(2):93-102. PMID: 2181096.

Raiker A., Green W., Shabaik A., & Perlin E. (1989). Acute promyelocytic leukaemia following treatment of non-Hodgkin's lymphoma. *Cancer,* 63(7):1402-1406. PMID: 2646008.

Raikhlin NT., Bukaeva IA., Probatova NA., & Smirnov EA. (2006). Argyrophilic proteins in the regions of nucleolar organizers are markers of cell proliferation rate. *Arkh Patol,* 68(3):47–51.

Ritter MA., Albrechtson JL., Kim YJ., & Kinsella TJ. (1994). Tumor cell kinetics in mixed populations. *Cytometry,* 16(2):118-28. PMID:7924680.

Roncalli M., Borzio M., Brando B., Colloredo G., & Servida E. (1989). Abnormal DNA content in liver-cell dysplasia: a flow cytometric study. *Int J Cancer,* 44(2):204-207. PMID: 2759727.

Roncalli M., Park YN., & Di Tommaso L. (2010). Histopathological classification of hepatocellular carcinoma. *Dig Liver Dis,* 42(3):S228-34. PMID:20547308.

Ruà S., Comino A., Fruttero A., Torchio P., Bouzari H., Taraglio S., Torchio B., & Capussotti L. (1996). Flow cytometric DNA analysis of cirrhotic liver cells in patients with hepatocellular carcinoma can provide a new prognostic factor. *Cancer,* 78(6):1195-1202. PMID: 8826940.

Sanai FM., & Jeeffe EB. (2011). Liver biopsy for histological assessment: the case against. *Saudi J Gastroenterol,* 16(2):124-132.

Schaffner F. (1991). Structural and functional aspects of regeneration of human liver. *Dig Dis Sci,* 36(9):1282-1286. PMID: 1893815.

Schwint AE., Folco A., Morales A., Cabrini RL., & Itoiz ME. (1996). AgNOR mark epithelial foci undergoing malignant transformation in hamster cheek pouch carcinogenesis. *J Oral Pathol Med,* 25:20-24.

Shankey T., & Rabinovitch P. (2002). DNA content flow cytometry. In: *Manual clinical laboratory immunology, sixth edition.* Rose N, Hamilton R, Detrick B (ed), p171-184, ISBN 1-55581-215-5, ASM press Washinton D.C.

Shankey TV., Rabinovitch PS., Bagwell B., Bauer KD., Duque RE., Hedley DW., Mayall BH., Wheeless L., & Cox C. (1993). Guidelines for implementation of clinical DNA cytometry International Society for Analytical Cytology. *Cytometry,* 14(5):472-7. PMID: 8354117.

Shemizu K., Izumi R., Ii T., Muraoka K., Inoue T., Fukushima W., Sakamoto K., Tani T., Hashimoto T., Yagi M., Miyazaki I., & Monomura A. (1995). Prognostic significance of nuclear organizer region in hepatocellular carcinoma. *Hepatol,* 21:393–397.

Shimamoto T., Haruma K., Tanaka S., Todo H., Yoshihara M., Sumii K., & Kajiyama G. (1993). Usefulness of nucleolar organizer region staining in gastric myogenic tumors: correlation with ploidy by DNA flow cytometry. *Oncology,* 50(1):52-56. PMID: 8421598.

Siddiqui M., Soomro I., Kayani N., Muzaffar S., & Hasan S. (1999). Assessment of nucleolar organizer regions (NORs) in proliferative conditions of the liver. *Pathol Res Pract,* 195(6):421–426.

Sirri V., Roussel P., & Hernandez-Verdun D. (2000). The AgNOR proteins: qualitative and quantitative changes during the cell cycle. *Micron,* 31(2):121–126.

Spolidorio L., Neves K., Soares C., Spolidorio D., Basso M., Malavazzi I., & Almeida O. (2002). Evaluation of argyrophilic nucleolar organizer regions in oral tumor progression. *Micron,* 33(7- 8):605–608.

Tarao K., Hoshino H., Shimizu A., Ohkawa S., Nakamura Y., Harada M., Ito Y., Tamai S., Akaike M., & Sugimasa Y. (1994a). Role of increased DNA synthesis activity of hepatocytes in multicentric hepatocarcinogenesis in residual liver of hepatectomized cirrhotic patients with hepatocellular carcinoma. *Jpn J Cancer Res,* 85(10):1040-1044. PMID: 7961106.

Tarao K., Ohkawa S., Shimizu A., Harada M., Nakamura Y., Ito Y., Tamai S., Hoshino H., Inoue T., & Kanisawa M. (1994b). Significance of hepatocellular proliferation in the development of hepatocellular carcinoma from anti-hepatitis C virus-positive cirrhotic patients. *Cancer,* 73(4):1149-1154. PMID: 7508816.

Thomas RM., Berman JJ., Yetter RA., Moore GW., & Hutchins GM. (1992). Liver cell dysplasia: a DNA aneuploid lesion with distinct morphologic features. *Hum Pathol,* 23(5):496-503 PMID: 1314776.

Tomioka N., Kobayashi H., Kageyama H., Ohira M., Nakamura Y., Sasaki F., Todo S., Nakagawara A., & Kaneko Y. (2003). Chromosomes that show partial loss or gain in near-diploid tumors coincide with chromosomes that show whole loss or gain in near-triploid tumors: evidence suggesting the involvement of the same genes in the tumorigenesis of high- and low-risk neuroblastomas. *Genes Chromosomes Cancer*, 36(2):139-150. PMID: 12508242.

Trere D., Farabegoli F., & Derenzini M. (1991). AgNOR area in interphase nuclei of human tumor correlate with the proliferative activity evaluated by bromodeoxyuridine labeling and Ki-67. *J Pathol*, 165:53–59.

Trere` D. (2000). AgNOR staining and quantification. *Micron*, 31:127–131.

Tripathi P., Tripathi AK., Kumar A., Ahmad R., Balapure AK., Vishwakerma AL., & Singh RK. (2008). DNA aneuploidy study for early detection of chromosomal abnormality in patients with aplastic anemia: prognostic and therapeutic implications. *In Vivo*, 22(6):837-44.PMID:19181017.

Underwood J., & Giri D. (1988). Nucleolar organizer regions as diagnostic discriminate for malignancy. *J Pathol*, 156:95–96.

Uno T., Hashimoto S., Shimono M. (1998). A study of the proliferative activity of long junctional epithelium using AgNOR staining. *J Periodontal Res*, 33:298-309.

van Dekken H., Verhoef C., Wink J., van Marion R., Vissers KJ., Hop WC., de Man RA., Ijzermans JN., van Eijck CH., & Zondervan PE. (2005). Cell biological evaluation of liver cell carcinoma, dysplasia and adenoma by tissue micro-array analysis. *Acta Histochem*, 107(3):161-171. PMID: 16000213.

Vuhahula EA., Nikai H., Ogawa I., Miyauchi M., Takata T., & Ito H. (1995). Correlation between argyrophilic nucleolar organizer region (AgNOR) counts and histologic grades with respect to biologic behavior of salivary adenoid cystic carcinoma. *J Oral Pathol Med*, 24(10):437-442.

Wakasa K., Haba T., Sasaki M., Sakurai M., Ikebe T., Hirohashi K., & Kinoshita H. (1998). Heperplastic foci in chronic liver disease: their proliferative activity assessed by nucleolar organizing. *Pathol Interact*, 48(1):29–32.

Wersto RP., Chrest FJ., Leary JF., Morris C., Stetler-Stevenson MA., & Gabrielson E. (2001). Doublet discrimination in DNA cell-cycle analysis. *Cytometry*, 46(5):296-306. PMID: 11746105

Yu C., Fletcher C., & Goodlad G. (1992). Proliferating cell nuclear antigen (PCNA) immunostaining, nucleolar organizer region (AgNOR) staining and histological grading in gastrointestinal stromal tumors. *J Pathol*, 166:147–152.

8

# Electron Microscopy of Liver Biopsies

Theodore C. Iancu and Irena Manov
*The Rappaport Faculty of Medicine, Technion-Haifa*
*Israel*

## 1. Introduction

During the last years of the 20th century, diagnosis in liver pathology was enriched by additional methodologies including immunohistopathology and confocal microscopy. Nevertheless, it soon became obvious that ultrastructural examinations remain essential in both research and diagnosis. The present chapter focuses on the use of electron microscopy in diagnostic hepatology and research of unsolved mechanisms. Attention will be directed to the correct retrieval of specimens for electron-microscopic examination and their processing for obtaining maximal information. The revival of interest in both transmission (TEM) and scanning electron microscopy (SEM) follows continuous changes in the subjects under examination: new diseases or additional features of old diseases; new therapeutic agents and their potentially hepatotoxic effects; environmental factors affecting the liver; identification of viruses and/or other rare noxious agents; immune pathology including liver transplantation and rejection; the liver in systemic-genetic diseases; and ultrastructural pathology in both experimental animals and cell cultures. We herewith wish to provide the clinician (neonatologist, pediatrician, geneticist, and hepatologist-gastroenterologist) with information about the value of electron-microscopic examination *before* performing a liver biopsy and thus enabling him/her to preserve a minute sample for a valuable study.
In his limited size, the present chapter cannot be all-inclusive. Many areas, in which the contribution of electron-microscopy is limited to research investigations, have been left out. Similarly, areas in which histopathology and immune staining are major diagnostic tools, such as in hepatitis, were sidestepped.

## 2. Technical aspects

Whenever an electron microscopic examination is planned, *immediate fixation of the retrieved specimen is essential.* While most laboratories have their own preference, 2.5% buffered glutaraldehyde is universally accepted. Suggested primary fixative: 2.5% glutaraldehyde in 0.1M sodium Cacodylate buffer (Add 1ml of 25% glutaraldehyde stock to 9 ml of buffer). The specimen should not be larger than 1 mm in each direction to allow for good penetration of the fixative. It is advised to avoid the tip of the cylindrical needle biopsy specimen which may contain sub-capsular liver area and may not be diagnostic. After 2 hrs. (At room temperature or in the refrigerator) continue with the standard steps: osmium post-fixation, dehydration, infiltration, embedding. Do not

freeze at any stage! (For immune-electron microscopy, keep a separate deep-frozen specimen.)
*Toluidine blue staining of thick (semi-thin* 0.5 $\mu$m or 1.0 $\mu$m.*) sections for TEM,* used as guideline to the area of interest and further trimming: Reagents: 1% Toluidine Blue and 2% borate in distilled water. *Ultrathin sections,* 40-100 nm (regularly 60 nm for TEM) are spread mostly on 200 or 300 mesh copper grids and stained with uranyl acetate and lead citrate solutions. For iron-containing compounds, keep unstained sections or stained only 2 minutes with lead.
Table I summarizes findings in biopsies of most conditions encountered in clinical cases. The reader can find details in the many books and atlases on hand (Johannessen, 1978; Tanikawa et al., 1979; Ghadially, 1997)).

## 3. The liver biopsy – general features

Hepatocytes: The large, round nuclei usually show an even, round contour and contain 1-2 nucleoli, heterochromatin adjacent to their external border and distinct nuclear membranes and nuclear pores. Uneven, crenated nuclei can follow faulty fixation or other processing problems (Fig. 1). Chromatin margination and fragmentation can indicate apoptosis. In more advanced stages of damage, apoptotic and necrotic cells are seen (Figs. 2-6).

### 3.1 Damaged and dying liver cells

If the biopsy specimen has been retrieved and fixed correctly, it can be assumed that damaged liver cells indicate a pathological process. The sequences are: edema, swelling of mitochondria, cristolysis, flocculated matrix, nuclear chromatin clumping, margination and fragmentation, (apoptosis), RER denudation, dense deposits in mitochondria, peroxysomes and matrix, necrosis. (Figs. 1-6)

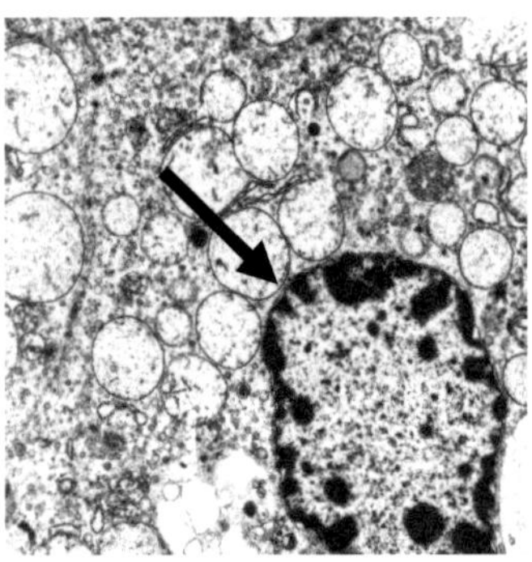

Fig. 1. Delayed fixation: cristolysis and "extracted" matrix of mitochondria; fragmented euchromatin (arrow). x 8,000

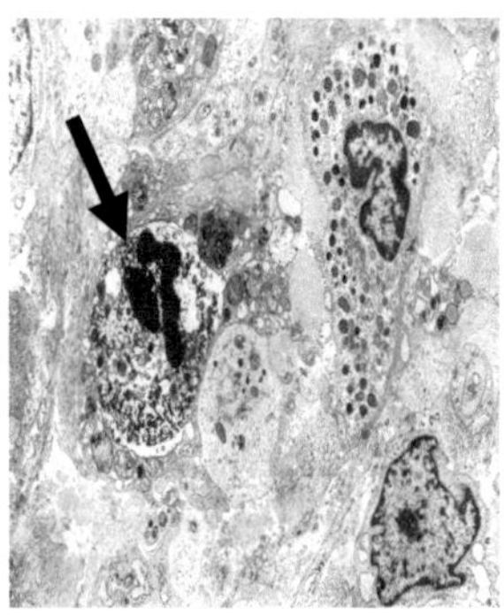

Fig. 2. Necrotic cells in periportal area. Residual necrotic nucleus (arrow). x 5,000

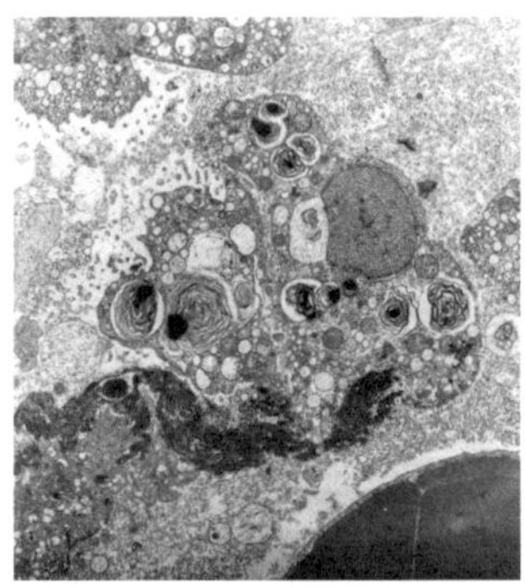

Fig. 3. Disintegrating cell in sinusoid: small nucleus, membraneous lysosomes and some collagen fibers (arrows). x 6,000

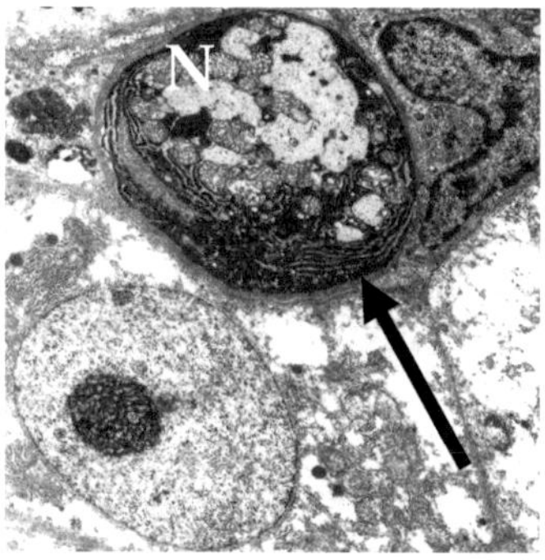


Fig. 4. Apoptotic body: parts of nucleus (N), RER (arrow) and remaining mitochondria in the center. x 6,000

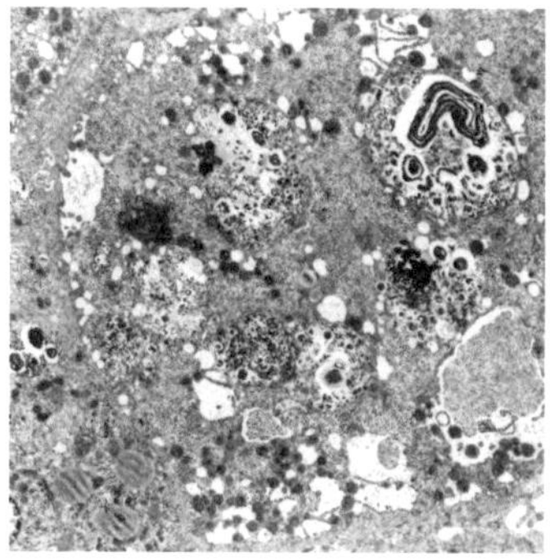

Fig. 5. Extreme biliary necrosis. x 4,000

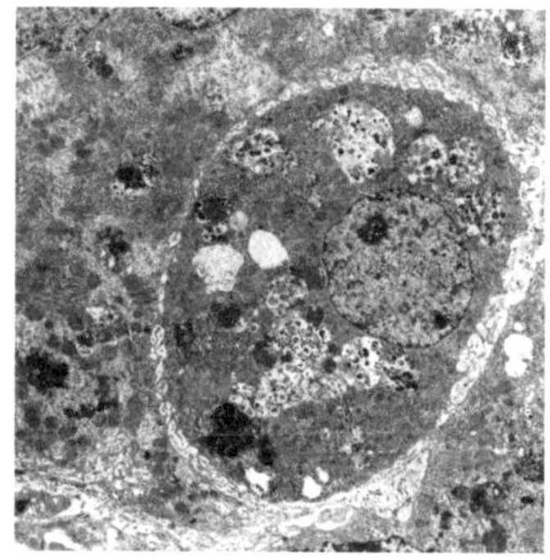

Fig. 6. Biliary necrosis in a detached hepatocyte in the sinusoid. x 5,000

## 4. Organelle pathology (1): Mitochondria

### 4.1 Shape and size

*Megamitochondria* (giant mitochondria, up to 10.0 μm long), existing in numerous metabolic abnormalities including drug reactions and fatty liver; they are frequently elongated along their longitudinal axis. They may contain crystals (Figs. 7, 8), (Sternlieb, 1979). *Amoeboid shape*, found in metabolic abnormalities and Reye syndrome (Partin et al., 1971); *Oncocytic transformation*: mitochondrial crowding similar to an oncocytoma (Tandler et al., 1970) is found generally in hepatocytes in mitochondrial DNA deficiency (Mandel et al., 2001).

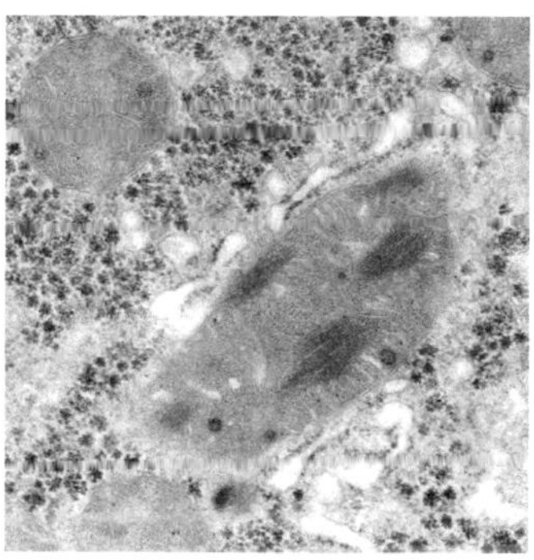

Fig. 7. Fatty liver - NAFLD. Megamitochondrion with longitudinal crystal formations. x 15,000

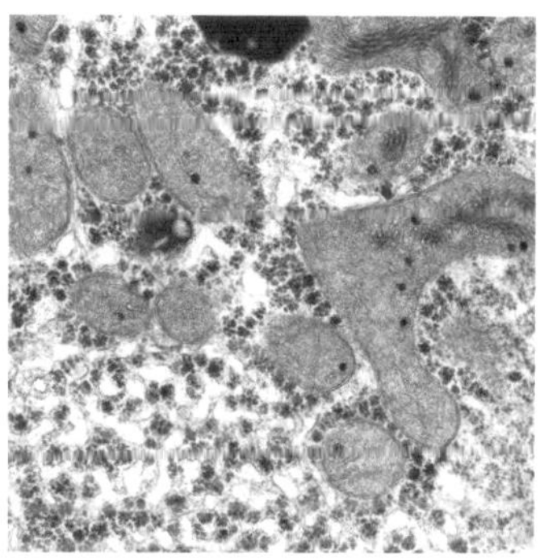

Fig. 8. Lactic acidosis. Angular mitochondrion with twisted and circular cristae. x 15,000

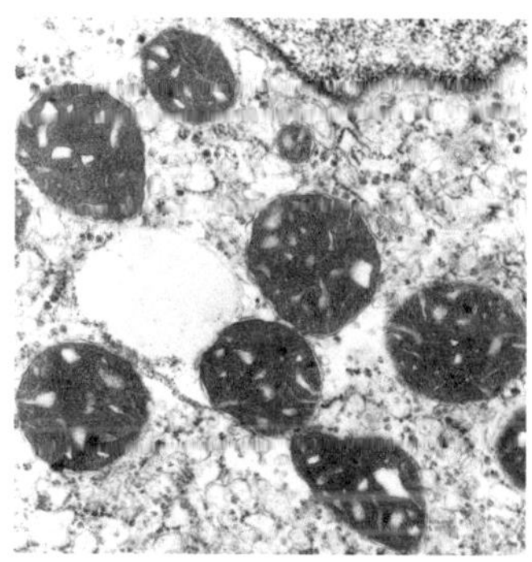

Fig. 9. "Condensed conformation" of mitochondria in "edge artifact". x 8,000

### 4.2 Content: matrix, cristae, crystals, granules, dense deposits

*Orthodox* vs. *Condensed* mitochondria. Surrounding conditions induce mitochondrial changes. Mitochondria with dilated cristae and condensed (opaque) matrix are labeled in *'condensed'* conformation, whereas the apparently 'normal' mitochondria are termed to be in *'orthodox'* conformation (Hackenbrock et al., 1971). Condensed mitochondria are seen at the periphery of a thin section, where *all* cellular components appear more diluted (Fig. 9). We have termed this finding as *edge artifact*. Condensed mitochondria may be seen in pathological conditions (*e.g.* Wilson disease) and thus have diagnostic significance. Therefore we suggest avoiding an *edge artifact* by assessing mitochondria also at safe distance away from the edge.

*Cristolysis* is a significant, non-specific, sign of mitochondrial injury, when only fragments of cristae remain visible, severed from inner mitochondrial membranes (see Reye syndrome).

*Circular or 'curled' cristae* are classically seen in cholestasis (Figs. 10, 11); (Phillips et al., 1987); occasionally the cristae are twisted (Figs. 8, 11, 12.). Other variations in amount, position and arrangement remain unexplained, such as: longitudinally stacked; transverse position, perpendicular to the outer membrane; or cartwheel arrangement (Menkes' kinky hair disease) (Ghadially, 1997).

*Autolytic changes*: specimens retrieved *post mortem* show 'extraction' of matrix and cristae, resulting in empty-looking organelles and nuclei, similar to that of defectively fixed specimens (Fig. 1). *Dense deposits in mitochondria* have been found in Wilson disease (Fig. 13); (Phillips et al., 1987) and in severe iron overload (Bessis & Weed, 1973).

*Matrical dense granules,* a common, normal feature of mitochondria, are known to contain calcium, but their precise role in mitochondrial function is unknown. However, their generalized absence is an indication of abnormality (drug toxicity, metabolic disturbance?). Large granules may show a hollow center (Fig. 11).

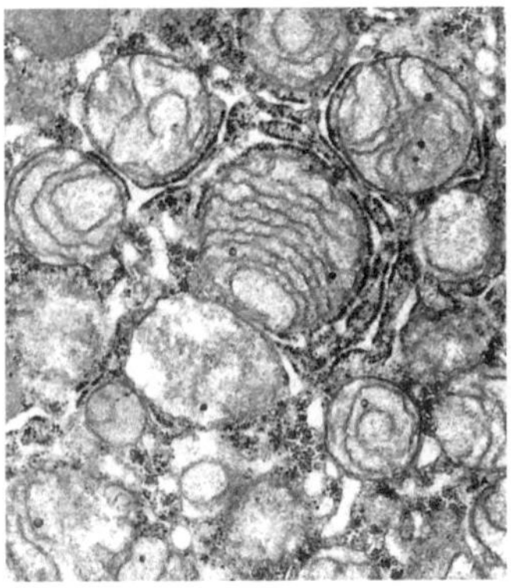

Fig. 10. Circular and stacked cristae in cholestasis. Neonatal hepatitis. x 10,000

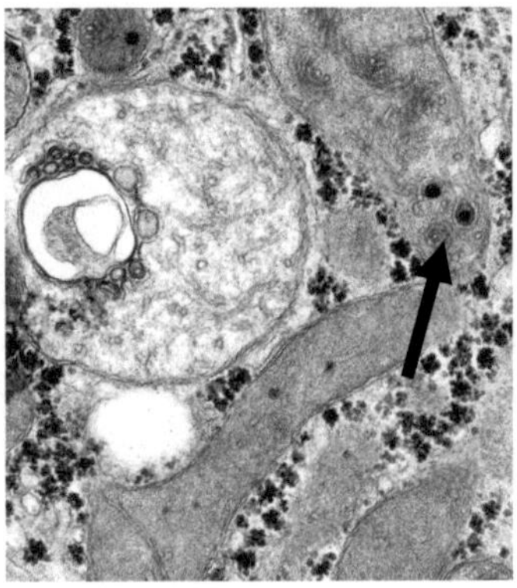

Fig. 11. Metabolic acidosis. Cristolysis and hollow granules (arrow), also in mitochondrion x 15,000

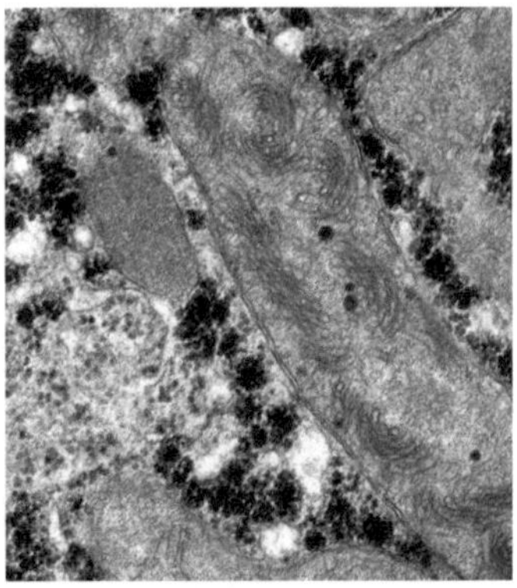

Fig. 12. Metabolic acidosis. Circular and twisted cristae in a mega-mitochondrion. x 20,000

*Intramitochondrial inclusions*: crystalline, paracrystalline, and filamentous. Crystalline inclusions, have been found in nuclei, cytoplasm and mitochondria (Ghadially, 1997) and show a highly ordered pattern of organization. Crystals with a less ordered arrangement have been named *crystalloid* or *paracrystalline.* The appearance of the crystals depends *'inter alia'* on the plane of sectioning in relationship to the plane of crystal lattice (Figs 7, 14, 15).

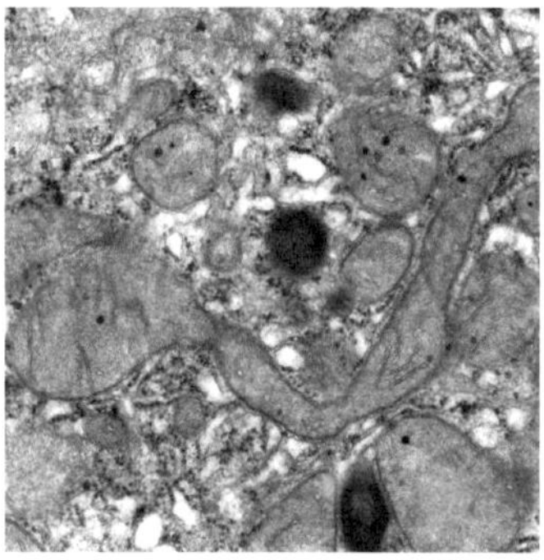

Fig. 13. Wilson disease. Elongated mitochondria and dense deposits. x 15,000.

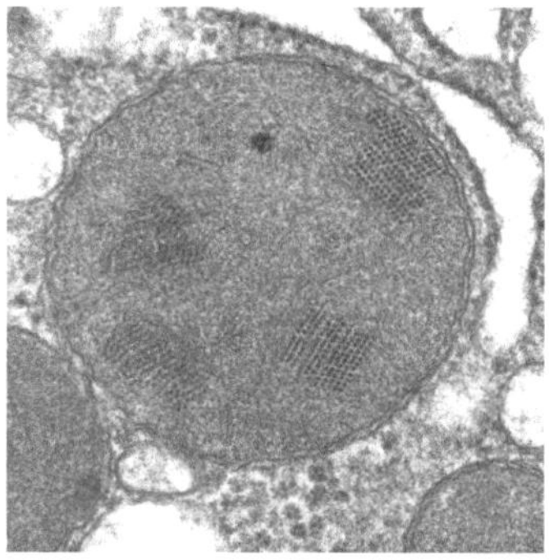

Fig. 14. Aspirin toxicity. Transverse section through paracrystalline formations. x 20,000.

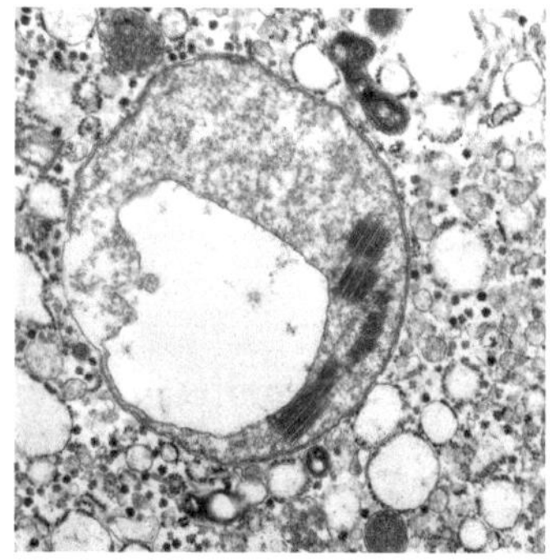

Fig. 15. Aspirin toxicity. Crystalline deposits in giant, abnormal mitochondrion. x 20,000

### 4.3 Organelle pathology (2): Peroxisomes

Peroxisomes (microbodies) are seen in hepatocytes as round, ellipsoid, slightly angular or elongated organelles. They contain a homogeneous, amorphous, finely granular or flocculent matrix, surrounded by a single tripartite membrane. Randomly distributed in the cytoplasm, they may form clusters. Their diameter is 0.25-1.34 μm and they may exhibit a peripheral terminal or marginal plate of about 0.4 μm long along their limit membrane (Fig. 16). They show variations in number, size, shape and matrix (Fig. 17). The major pathological finding is the absence of peroxisomes in the cerebrohepatorenal syndrome of Zellweger. Conditions with fewer peroxisomes (Table I) comprise *Infantile Refsum disease* (Fig. 18) whereas abundant organelles were reported in Reye syndrome, alcoholic liver disease, clofibrate and 6-mercaptopurine therapy and cholestatic jaundice of pregnancy (Sternlieb, 1979).

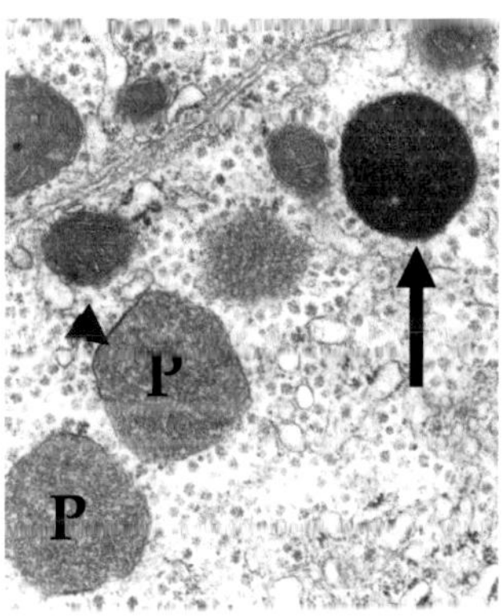


Fig. 16. Siderosome (arrow) *vs.* peroxysomes (P), one with a terminal plate (arrowhead) x 15,000

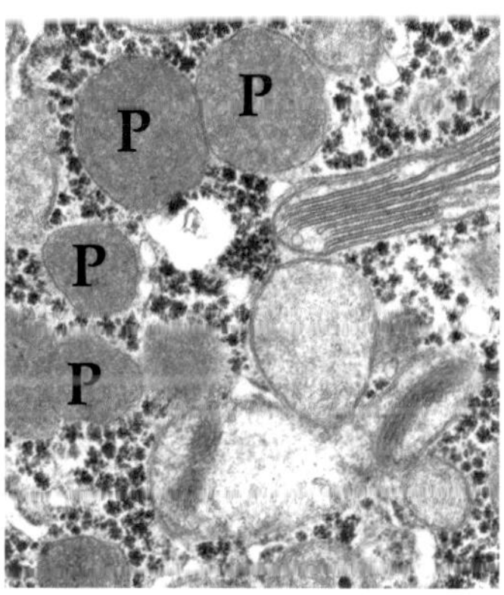


Fig 17 Metabolic acidosis. Longitudinal arrangement of cristae and multiple large peroxysomes (P). x 15,000

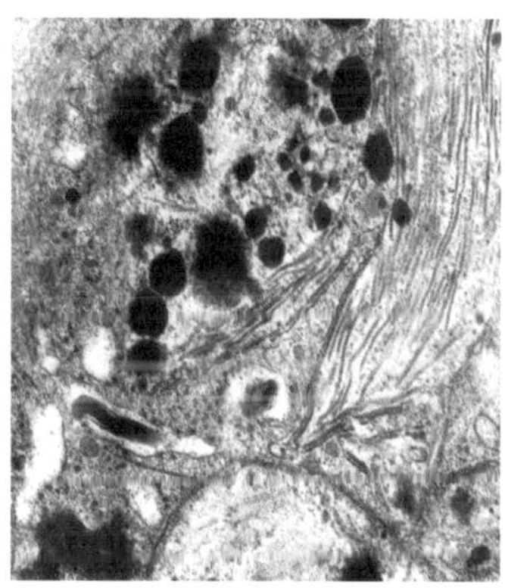

Fig. 18. Infantile Refsum disease, Zellweger variant, absent peroxisomes. Note trilaminar filaments and dense deposits. x 20,000

### 4.4 Organelle pathology (3): Lysosomes

These Golgi-derived organelles are of major importance in the interpretation of liver biopsies. Their role in autophagy (phagosomes; autophagosomes, autophagolysosomes) and apoptosis has been documented by numerous observations (Ghadially, 1997). In practice, some lysosomes are indicative, if no diagnostic, of *a group of conditions.* Within such a group, further differentiation requires additional (mainly genetic) information. For instance, among storage diseases, identifying a particular mucopolysaccharidosis can be difficult: the lysosomes are *similar,* apparently empty, round or oval single-membrane bound vacuoles (Figs. 19-21.) and may contain a small electron-dense 'nucleoid'. Such appearances have been designated as "the bull's eye" (Fig. 19).

In some cases, the lysosome content discloses the origin of the partially degraded component secluded by autophagy: Glycogen storage disease type II (GSD II, acid maltase or lysosomal alpha-glucosidase deficiency) is typically diagnostic by the presence of modified glycogen molecules (Fig. 22), (McAdams et al., 1974). Siderosomes contain ferritin and/or hemosiderin (Iancu, 1992) and aurosomes and platinosomes the respective metals (Ghadially, 1997); lipolysosomes contain fat droplets (Hayashi & Sternlieb, 1975); Experiments with Thorotrast and carbon particles have demonstrated the phagocytic capacities of lysosomes (Ghadially, 1997).

## 5. Inborn lysosomal and metabolic diseases

### 5.1 Lysosomal diseases

The established criteria for this group of conditions have been postulated by Hers (Hers, 1963) as follows: "genetic deficiency of one of the acid hydrolases that is normally localized within the lysosome; consequent accumulation of undigested material within single-membrane-bound organelles that are altered lysosomes". The classical example of lysosomal storage disease, GSD II is due to lysosomal alpha-glucosidase deficiency, an enzyme encoded in humans by the *GAA* gene.

Lysosomal storage disorders have been listed in numerous publications and recently by Pastores (Pastores, 2010). This classification, as well as the present Table I, is based on the relevant substrate involved. We have selected previously unpublished electron micrographs to exemplify diagnostic features.

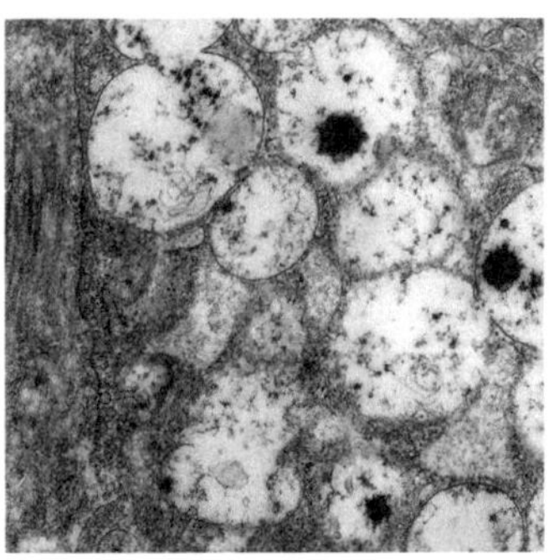

Fig. 19. "Bull's eye" appearance of nucleoid-containing lysosomes in mucopolyscaccharidoses. (Hurler). x 15,000

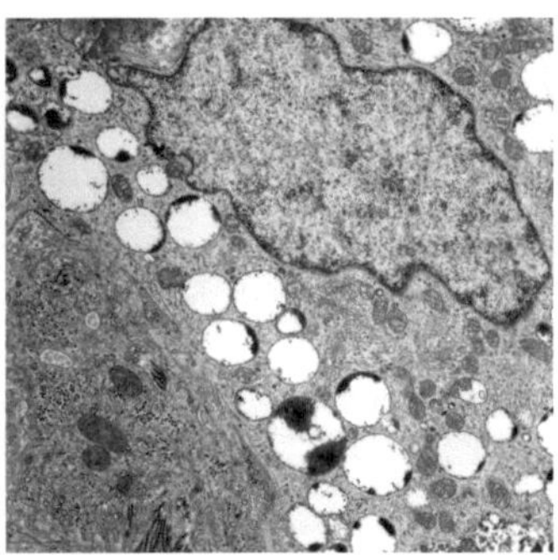

Fig. 20. Sinusoidal cell: Mucopolysaccharidosis (Hunter). Note typical lysosomes. x 6,000

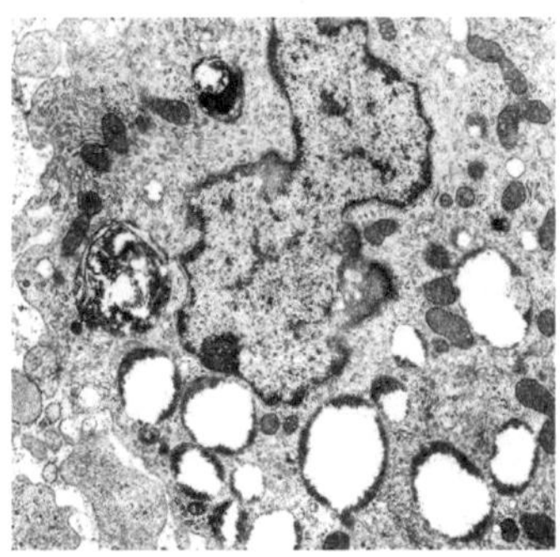

Fig. 21. Mucopoly-saccharidosis. "Empty looking" lysosomes and degraded phagolysosomes. (Morquio). x 6,000

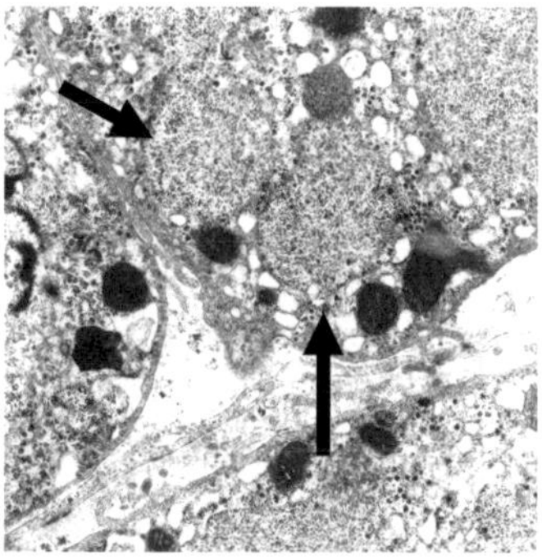

Fig. 22. Acid maltase deficiency (Pompe). Monoparticulate glycogen in membrane-limited bodies (arrows). x 10,000

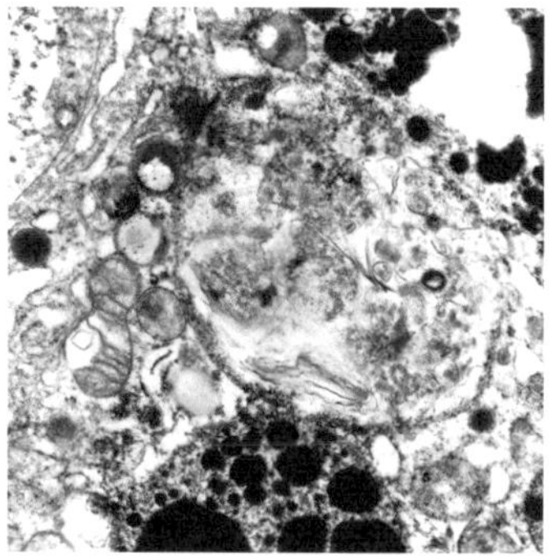

Fig. 23. GM1 Gangliosidosis (Landing). Filaments in a large lysosome; dense deposits, possibly related to TPN. x 10,000

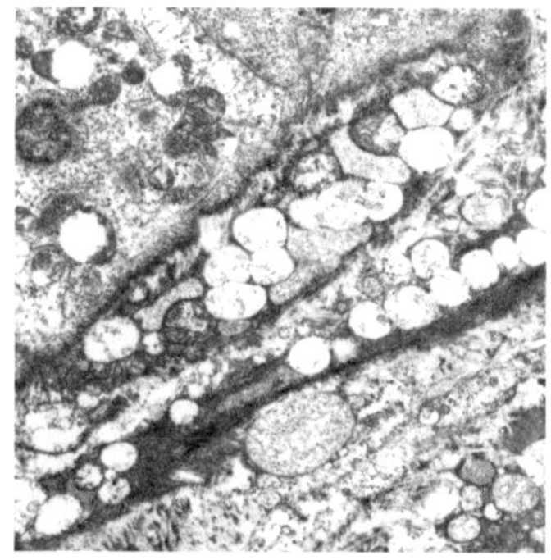

Fig. 24. Sialidosis: numerous single-membrane limited lysosomes in a sinusoid. x 5,000

### 5.1.1 Mucopolysaccharidoses (MPS)

This group includes diseases with intralysosomal storage and urinary excretion of partially degraded mucopolysaccharides. By TEM, single-membrane-bound bodies show scarce flocculent and particulate precipitate lying in a lucent matrix in many tissues (Tondeur and Neufeld, 1975). They are found in various diseases of the group (see Table 1), with only minor differences (Figs. 19-21). Of interest is the presence of a "nucleoid", remnant after extraction by processing of lysosomal content (Fig. 19). The appearance of several other conditions with empty-looking lysosomes and occasional electron-dense deposits may generate diagnostic difficulties, *e.g.* gangliosidosis (Fig. 23) sialidosis (Fig. 24), fucosidosis, mannosidosis.

### 5.1.2 Gaucher disease (GD)

The most prevalent lysosomal storage disease, GD is due to a deficiency of glucocerebrosidase leading to accumulation of glucosylceramide in "Gaucher cells", in the liver and other organs. These cells can be found in other conditions (*pseudo*-Gaucher cells) but characteristically in the three forms of GD: Type I-chronic non-neuropathic, (90% in Ashkenazi Jews); Type II (acute neuropathic); and Type III (subacute neuropathic). Bone marrow or liver biopsy examinations for diagnosis have been replaced by glucocerebrosidase determination in leukocytes or cultured fibroblasts, or by mutation analysis. Liver biopsy is reserved for *hydrops fetalis* in congenital GD or unclear cases of hepatosplenomegaly. The pale-staining cytoplasm of the large, multinucleated Gaucher cells, show by TEM large lysosomes containing long tubules, some twisted and intermingled (Fig. 25). (Chakrapani & Green, 2004)

### 5.1.3 Niemann–Pick Disease (NPD) including type A (NPA), B (NPB) and C (NPC)

NPDs of various types can begin as fetal disease or neonatal jaundice. Some types and mutants can show relatively late-onset hepatosplenomegaly. The histopathological characteristic of this group of storage diseases is the presence of "foamy cells" storing sphyngomyelin. While diagnosis of NPA and NPB is by sphingomyelinase assays and mutation analysis, NPC1 need be diagnosed by mutational analysis at the level of cDNA and/or assaying cultured fibroblasts for cholesterol esterification and staining for unesterified cholesterol with filipin (Meiner et al., 2001). The advantage of TEM over these methods is that it can provide a more rapid diagnostic confirmation by identifying suspicious cells, usually liver or amniotic cells (Fig. 26), (Spiegel et al., 2009).

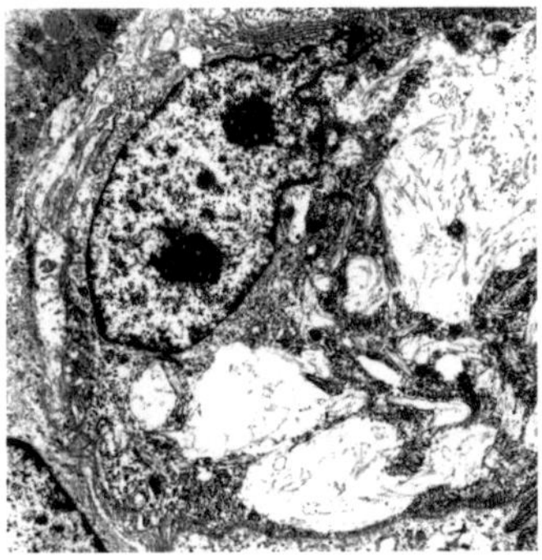

Fig. 25. Part of Gaucher cell showing typical fibrils. x 10,000

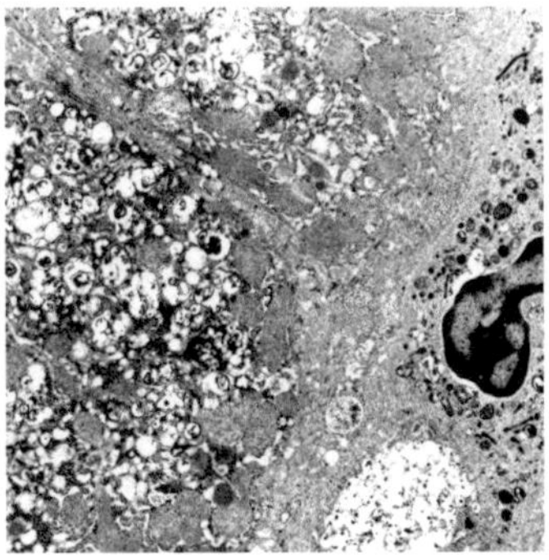

Fig. 26. Niemann-Pick C: membranous whorls fill hepatocytes. x 4,000

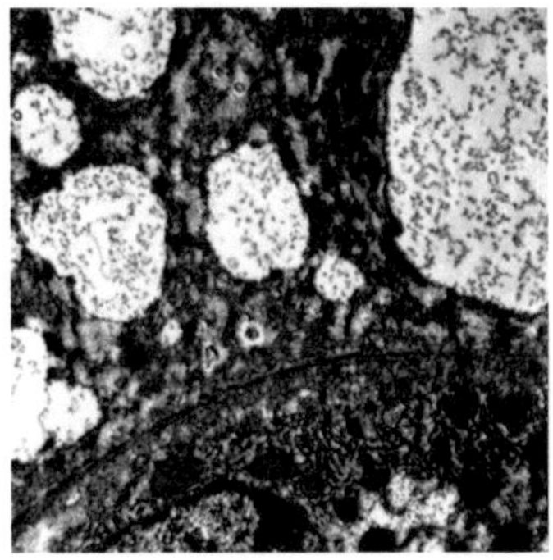

Fig. 27. "Fructose holes" in hereditary fructose intolerance. x 6,000

### 5.2 Cholestasis

Cholestasis, appearing in conditions in which the bile flow is blocked, is still differentiated as extra-hepatic- and intra-hepatic. There are only few differential features revealed by electron microscopy.

Pre-and post-natal bile-production and secretion may be hindered by morphological and functional abnormalities. Neonatologists are more troubled by jaundice associated to *direct-binding (conjugated) bilirubin* frequently indicating the possibility of structural abnormalities, such as *biliary atresia*. Liver biopsy is usually required to confirm this life-saving surgical correction. Other conditions associated with conjugated bilirubin are listed in Table 1 and several reviews (Balistreri, 2002); Suchy, 2004). Meanwhile, new clinical, morphological and genetic characteristics continue to emerge (Bull et al., 1997; Bezerra & Balistreri, 1999; Davit-Spraul et al., 2009). Other conditions, in which basic conditions are associated with cholestasis, are listed for differential diagnosis (Roberts, 2004 a).

#### 5.2.1 Ultrastructural features of cholestasis

Hepatocytic mitochondria show circular, concentric or curled cristae (Fig. 10, 28). With continuing cholestasis, bile-containing bodies are seen as clusters, mostly around bile canaliculi. In their outer limit, a membranous structure is occasionally identified. The bile-containing bodies, considered lysosomes, are electron-opaque organelles, usually 0.5-2.0 (0.1-10.0) μm diameter (Fig. 29). Bile canaliculi display distension and damaged microvilli (Fig. 30). In time, spicular conglomerates become visible (Fig. 31). Myelin-like membranes are noticeable in long-standing cholestasis (Fig. 32).

Bile leakage into the cytosol (amorphous, without limit membrane) appears after prolonged, severe cholestasis. Cells other than hepatocytes (Kupffer cells, sinusoidal lining cells, stellate cells, bile duct epithelia) exhibit variable degrees of cholestasis, mainly as bile-containing lysosomes. *Focal biliary cytoplasmic necrosis* is the extreme form of bile-induced hepatocytic damage, other than biliary cirrhosis (Fig. 33).

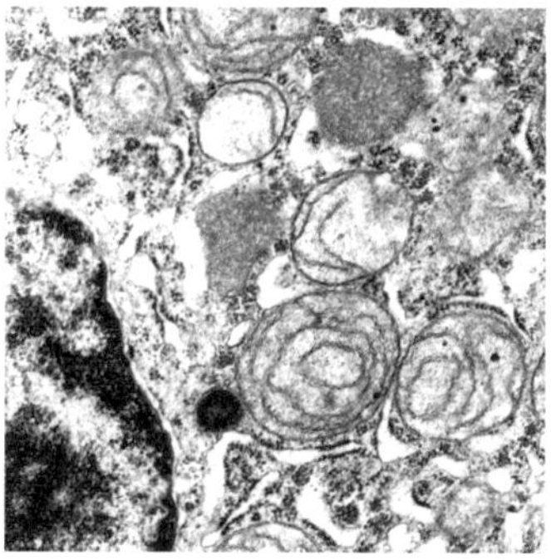

Fig. 28. Hepatocyte. Circular and curled cristae in cholestasis. Peroxysomes (P). x 8,000

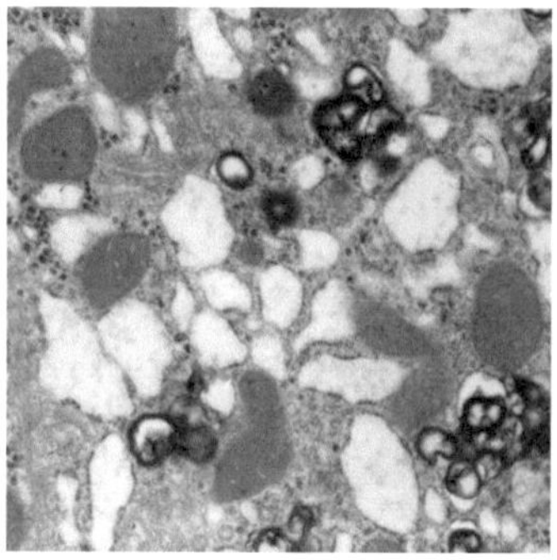

Fig. 29. Bile-containing lysosomes in the pericanalicular area. Note dilated RER. x 4,000

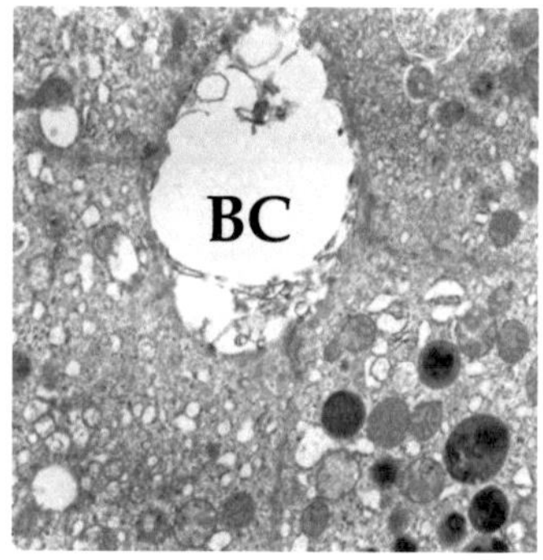


Fig. 30. Distension of canaliculus (BC) and loss of microvilli in cholestasis. x 4,000

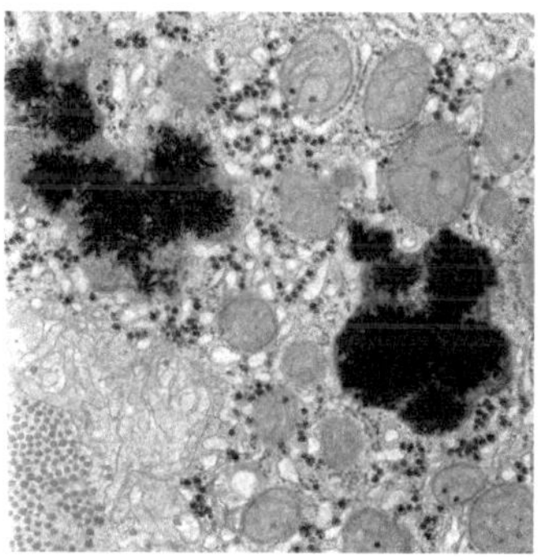

Fig. 31. Severe cholestasis: spicular bile x 10,000

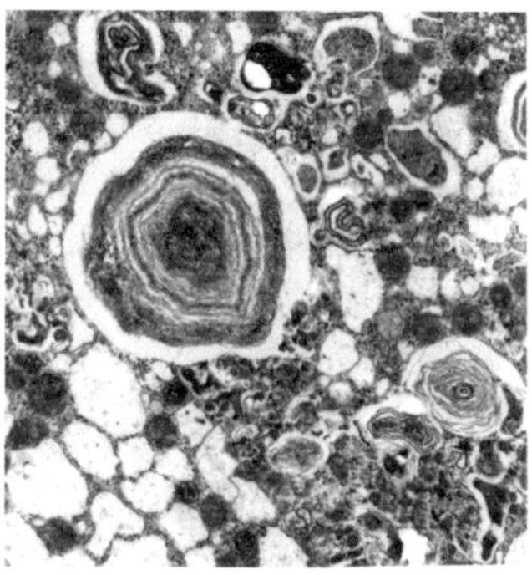

Fig 32. Myelin-like lysosomes in a degraded hepatocyte. x 8,000

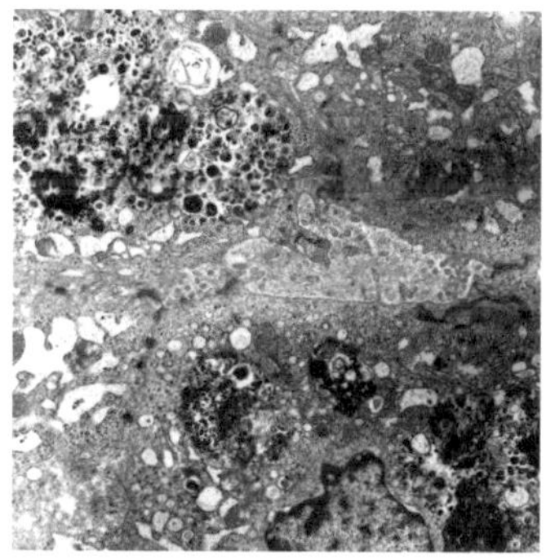

Fig. 33. Focal biliary cytoplasmic necrosis, near bile canaliculi. x 4,000

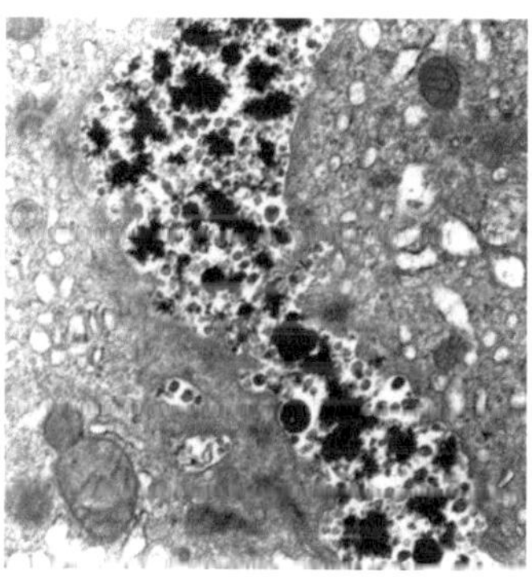

Fig. 34. Cholestatic jaundice. "Byler-like" bile in PFIC-1. x 6,000

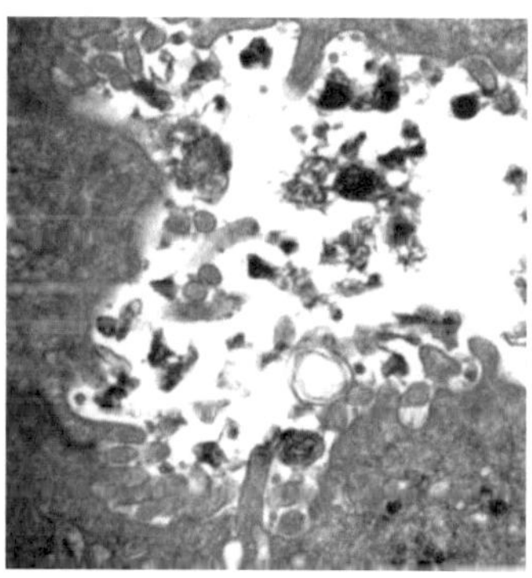

Fig. 35. PFIC-1. "Byler-like" bile. Distended canaliculus, injured microvilli. X 4,000

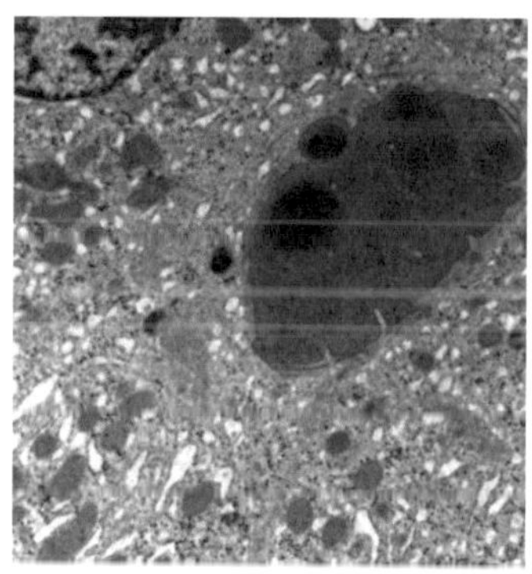

Fig. 36. Bile plug in biliary atresia. x 4,000

### 5.2.2 PFIC-1, PFIC-2 and PFIC-3

PFIC-1 (former Byler disease) is caused by a mutation in the *ATP8B1* gene on chromosome 18q21-22. Byler-like bile, seen in PFIC-1, is formed of coarse granular bile in distended canaliculi with damaged/absent microvilli (Figs. 34-35). In contrast, the bile in PFIC-2 is not granular but filamentous, important for differential diagnosis. Bile plugs are typically seen in severe obstructive cholangiopathies including biliary atresia (Fig. 36).
PFIC-2 is caused by a mutation in the *ABCB11* gene on chromosome 2q24 that encodes the bile salt export pump (BSEP). BSEP is the major canalicular bile acid pump, and thus the loss of BSEP function results in severe hepatocellular cholestasis. Both PFIC-1 and PFIC-2 are characterized by low gamma-glutamyl peptidase (GGT) levels. Although genetically distinct, PFIC1 and PFIC2 are both caused by the absence of a gene product required for canalicular export and bile formation. Clinically and histologically there are few differences between these conditions, which may both advance to cirrhosis. An important contribution of electron microscopy to the otherwise ample description of histopathological features of PFIC, is the finding of the coarsely granular *"Byler bile"* in dilated canaliculi that lack microvilli and are cuffed by a thick layer of microfilaments. "Byler bile", is apparently related to the defect in canalicular bile acid transport with primary retention of hydrophobic bile salts. Weber suggested the microfilament collar was a feature of cholestasis in another ethnic group (Weber et al., 1981). Bull and co-authors reported that "Byler bile" was found only in children who were homozygous for the microsatellite haplotype at 18q21-q22 (PFIC 1)(Bull et al., 1997). It should be noted that Byler bile can be seen occasionally in cholestatic conditions other than PFIC 1 or PFIC 2, such as Familial Progressive benign cholestasis (Phillips et al., 1987).
The absence of bile salts in the bile ducts in PFIC1 and PFIC2 and their presence in the bile ducts in PFIC3 accounts for the difference in biochemical tests. In PFIC3, as in most cholestatic diseases, exposure of duct cell membranes to bile salts results in solubilization of GGT, absorption of the enzyme into the circulation, and elevated serum GGT levels. In contrast, in PFIC1 and PFIC2 there are low levels of bile salts, the GGT is never solubilized, and the serum GGT is normal. Rather than defective bile acid export, patients with PFIC3 have deficient hepatocellular phospholipid export. The lack of phospholipids produces destabilized micelles and promotes lithogenic bile with crystallized cholesterol which could produce small bile duct obstruction (Davit-Spraul et al., 2009). The histological and ultrastructural features are similar to other forms of PFIC, except for the absence of Byler bile. In PFIC-3 the bile is amorphous or filamentous. The patients become symptomatic at various ages, from 1 month to 20 years, and progression to cirrhosis can be rapid (first decade).
Recently (Verhulst et al.), 2010), reported on the critical role of ATP8B1 (deficient in PFIC-1) in apical membrane organization, potentially relevant for development of cholestasis and extrahepatic manifestations associated with ATB8B1 deficiency (such as disorganized apical actin cytoskeleton and defective microvilli formation)

### 5.2.3 Crigler-Najjar

This syndrome is divided into two types: type I and type II, with the latter sometimes called Arias syndrome. These two types, along with *Gilbert's syndrome, Dubin-Johnson syndrome,* and *Rotor syndrome,* make up the five known *hereditary defects in bilirubin metabolism.* Unlike Gilbert's syndrome, only a few hundred cases of Crigler-Najjar syndrome are known to exist (Kelly, 2004).

### 5.2.4 Dubin-Johnson syndrome

Originally termed canalicular multiple organic anion transporter (cMOAT) defect, it is also known as *multidrug resistance protein 2 (MRP2)* and is a member of the *ABC transporter superfamily*. The gene that encodes the transporter is *ABCC2* is found on chromosome 10. Rare cases of neonatal hepatitis have been reported; in older children, histology and TEM show typical melanin-containing pigment predominantly in the centrilobular area, around bile canaliculi (Fig. 37).

### 5.2.5 Alagille syndrome (Arteriohepatic dysplasia)

Described in 1975, the syndrome comprises infantile cholestasis, hepatic ductular hypoplasia, typical facies, peripheral pulmonic stenosis, vertebral anomalies and physical and mental retardation. The persistence of cholestasis is not associated to extra-hepatic obstruction but paucity of intralobular bile ducts is frequent. Valencia-Mayoral et al. have found ultrastructural changes suggesting a block in the Golgi apparatus or in the pericanalicular cytoplasm (Valencia-Mayoral et al., 1984). These TEM findings in Alagille syndrome appear to be distinctive when compared to other cholestatic syndromes.

### 5.2.6 Alpha-1-antitrypsyn deficiency (A1AT)

This disorder is a relatively common autosomal co-dominant condition causing chronic lung and liver disease. $\alpha_1$-antitrypsin is a protease inhibitor belonging to the *serpin superfamily*. It is generally known as serum trypsin inhibitor. A point-mutation induces aggregation-prone properties to a secretory protein so that the retained mutant protein is not secreted into blood or body fluids. Accumulation of the mutant A1AT in the RER of hepatocytes, typically seen with the TEM (Fig. 38) causes liver inflammation and carcinogenesis by a gain-of-toxic function mechanism. Studies performed over the last years have shown the importance of autophagy in disposal of mutant, a phenomenon also demonstrated by TEM. In infancy, A1AT is an important cause of cholestatic jaundice, with giant cell hepatitis, mimicking biliary atresia and Alagille syndrome (Mowat, 1994)

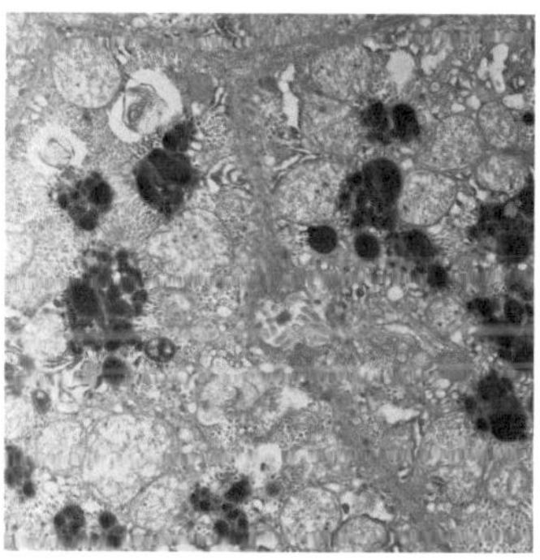

Fig. 37. Dubin-Johnson syndrome. Electron-dense accumulations adjacent to bile canaliculus. x 5,000

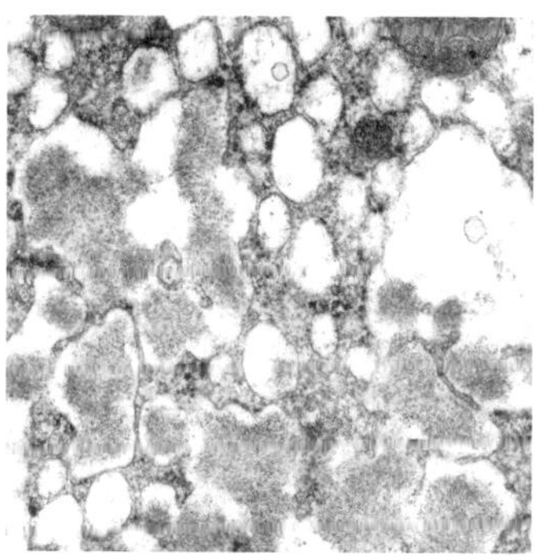

Fig. 38. Alpha-1-antitrypsin deficiency: amorphous accumulations in RER. x 6,000

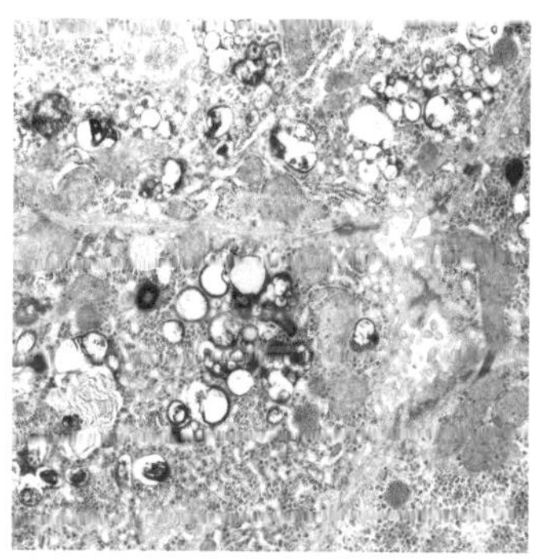

Fig. 39. Congenital disorder of glycosylation (CDG). Pericanalicular clusters of single-membrane-bound bodies. x 5,000

### 5.3 Congenital disorders of glycosylation (CDG)

This new group of genetic diseases characterized by defective glycoprotein biosynthesis exemplifies the value of electron microscopic diagnosis by liver biopsy (Iancu et al., 2007) The patients can present either with a neurological form (psychomotor retardation, cerebellar hypoplasia and retinitis pigmentosa, or with a multivisceral form with neurological and extra-neurological manifestation including liver, cardiac, renal or gastrointestinal involvement). A form with liver involvement and/or cardiomyopathy, enteropathy and hypoglycemia has also been reported. Elevated transaminases may focus attention to the liver. The biopsy shows increased cellularity, distorted bile ducts and small- and medium size lipid droplet steatosis. TEM shows, in addition, the presence of numerous myelinosomes. These organelles are mainly empty whorls measuring 0.02-0.1 µm and forming conglomerates ("grape-like") close to bile canaliculi (Fig. 39). Isoelectric focusing of transferrin provides an easy method of identification of CDG's.

### 5.4 Galactosemia, fructose intolerance, tyrosinemia

These inherited metabolic disorders are included here because of their common presentation with jaundice and elevated transaminases, as evidence of liver involvement. Although TEM results are not always specific, if a biopsy is performed, the findings can be supportive for life-saving diagnosis (Phillips et al., 1987; Mowat, 1994).
*Galactosemia:* enlarged hepatocytes, dilated RER, fatty liver, focal cytoplasmic degeneration, biliary necrosis;
*Hereditary fructose intolerance:* punched-out cytoplasmic lysis - "fructose holes" (Fig. 27).
*Tyrosinemia:* Increased lipid, dilated RER, pleomorphic mitochondria and focal necrosis.

### 5.5 Siderosis

Inorganic iron is revealed by TEM in *unstained* or slightly stained sections. The compounds are electron-dense due to the presence of *ferritin* and/or *hemosiderin* (Iancu, 1983; Iancu, 1992) and (rarely) *iron-containing micelles* (Fig. 40), (Bessis & Weed, 1973; Iancu, 1983; Iancu, 1992). The octahedral storage molecule ferritin (Holoferritin = ferritin core (Fe hydroxyphosphate) + apoferritin protein coat) becomes visible by TEM when the core contains more than about 1,500 inorganic iron molecules, up to a maximum of 4,500 molecules (*iron-rich ferritin).* Ferritin molecules (cores) can be seen randomly dispersed within the cell sap of hepatocytes, sinusoidal and Kupffer cells (Fig. 41, 42) in amounts depending on the origin of overload (absorptional or transfusional). The accumulation of iron is easier detectable in *lysosomes.* Iron-containing lysosomes are termed *siderosomes.* They contain electron-dense iron in 3 forms: a) ferritin molecules (mostly iron-rich variety), frequently associated with pseudo-membranous layers and forming arrays or hexagonal crystals; b) coalesced ferritin particles (after degradation of their apoferritin coat) forming 'clumps' of hemosiderin with extreme electron-density; c) siderosomes in which smaller particles can be resolved, apparently an intermediate stage between a) and b). Yet, a strict electron-microscopic definition of these compounds emphasizes that *hemosiderin* is formed when the coat of apoferritin is smaller than 0.25 nm and thus the distance between two ferritin molecules is reduced to less than 0.5 nm (Fischbach et al., 1971)
The TEM study of liver siderosis reveals: presence of ferritin and/or hemosiderin within various cells; relationship with additional conditions (e.g. cirrhosis, hepatitis, and carcinoma); quantification of the iron-containing compound by mass spectrometry or other analytical methods; and assessment of putative effect of a chelating agent. TEM confirmed that iron

overload from excessive absorption (hemochromatosis HFE) produces parenchymal overload with an initial mild reticuloendothelial (RES) overload, while transfusional iron is located mostly in the RES, followed by re-distribution of excess iron among both compartments.

### 5.5.1 Genetic hemochromatosis (HFE) "classical" hemochromatosis, type 1

Hemochromatosis HFE is most often caused by a mutation in the gene HFE on chromosome 6p21.3. Four types were identified (Muir et al., 1984), with differences between the degrees of liver iron loading. Children as young as 4 years had juvenile forms. The various stages of overload were followed by TEM (Iancu et al., 1997).

### 5.5.2 Other iron-loading conditions

In homozygous β-thalassemia, excess iron originates from hemolysis, increased absorption and frequent blood transfusions. In the liver, "foreign "transfused iron is channeled to the (RES), whereas iron from excessive absorption reaches parenchymal cells. The end-result is severe overload possibly followed by cirrhosis and/or hepatocellular carcinoma. In aplastic anemia and dialysis, iron derives from transfusions, with predominant initial RES overload, followed by redistribution towards hepatocytes and aggravation of liver siderosis as seen at the ultrastructural level. (Iancu, 1989; Iancu, 2011).

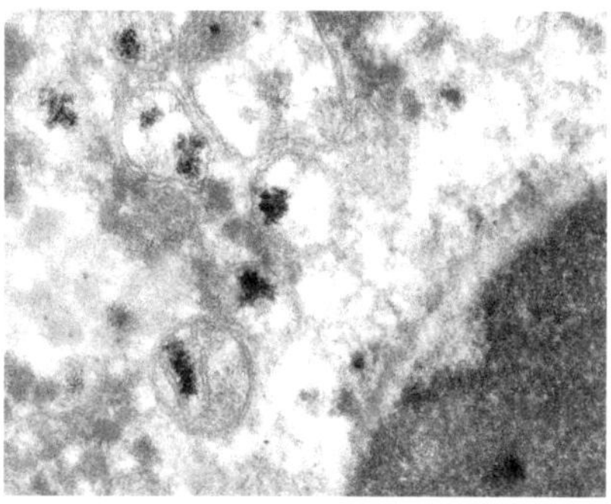

Fig. 40. Homozygous beta-thalassemia: Electron-dense iron micelles within mitochondria. x 20,000, unstained

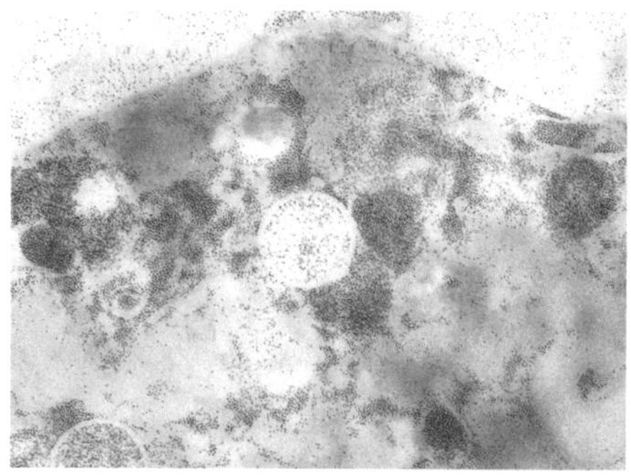

Fig. 41. Genetic hemochromatosis HFE. Ferritin cores in a Kupffer cell, dispersed and/or aggregated. x 20,000, unstained

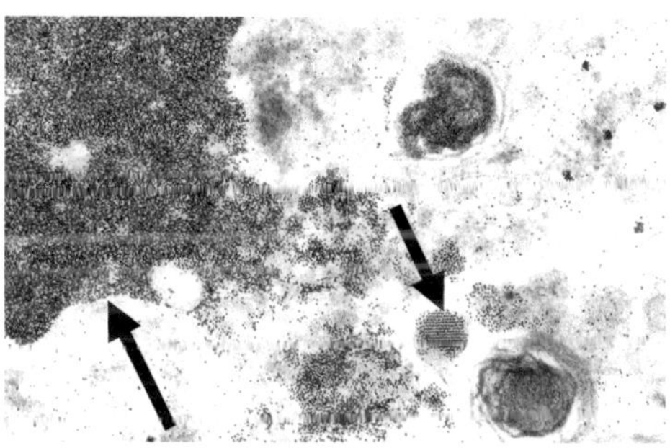

Fig. 42. Hepatocyte from β-thalassemia major. Ferritin dispersed or coalesced in crystals (curved arrow). In hemosiderin, (arrows) ferritin particles cannot be resolved anymore. x 20,000, unstained

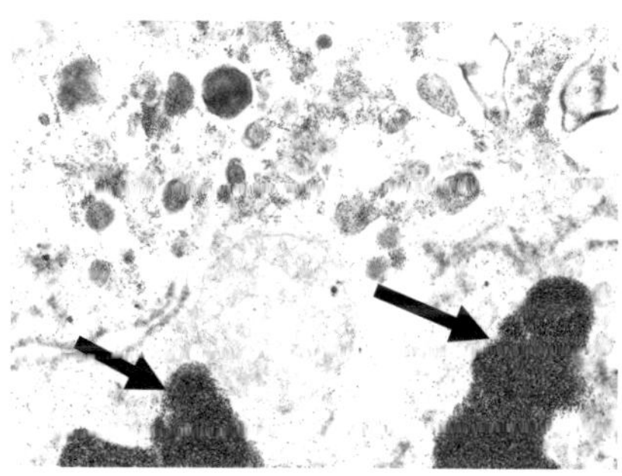

Fig. 43. Neonatal hemochromatosis, similar to genetic hemochromatosis: note ferritin of variable electron-density ("iron-rich" *vs.* "iron-poor") and hemosiderin "clumps" (arrows). x 20,000, unstained.

### 5.5.3 Neonatal hemochromatosis (NH)

In the neonatal period, the liver normally contains relatively large amounts of ferritin and hemosiderin, which diminish during the first year of life.

Neonatal hemochromatosis is a severe, frequently fatal condition. It has been found in fetuses and newly born infants presenting with rapidly progressing liver failure. The pattern of liver siderosis is similar to that of hereditary hemochromatosis (HFE) but the pace of pathological changes is fulminant: there is a striking difference between the iron-loaded hepatocytes and the sinusoidal cells which show only minor iron deposition. Perls' stain reveals siderosis in extra-hepatic locations (pancreas, thyroid, heart). Until recently, the cause and mechanism of this condition were unknown. Presently, NH is considered an alloimmune disease in which maternal antibodies damage the hepatocytes, especially post-partum. The siderosis is seen as secondary to the damaged liver cells and not the primary metabolic abnormality (Knisely & Vergani, ; Whitington, 2007). Because of the life-endangering condition of these infants, liver biopsy is rarely performed. TEM reveals iron mainly in hepatocytes, stored similarly to other parenchymal loading disorders (Fig. 43).

The role of iron in the brain and in Parkinson and Alzheimer diseases is under continuous study. Iron-induced lipid peroxidation and the formation of toxic free radicals appear to contribute to the development of the latter conditions (Zhu et al., 2007). Ongoing experimental work is focused on the effect of new chelating agents, capable to pass the blood-brain-barrier (Gal et al., 2006) and reduce the damaging effects of iron. Using cultured hepatoma-derived Hep3B cells loaded with inorganic iron, we could demonstrate the effect of a new bimodal chelator M30 capable of reducing ferritin in these cells, as seen by immunofluorescence (personal communications, Y Bashenko, 2009-2011).

### 5.5.4 Wilson disease (WD)

In this copper metabolism abnormality, there are numerous ultrastructural changes in liver cells as the liver lesions change in time, from chronic hepatitis to acute liver failure or cirrhosis. Alterations involve nuclei, mitochondria, peroxisomes, RER, fatty changes with lipolysosomes and neocholangioles with copper deposits (Figs. 44-47) (Sternlieb, 1979) Phillips et al., 1987).

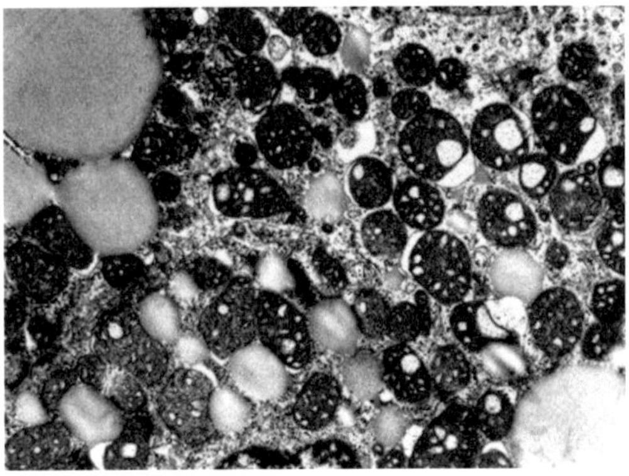

Fig. 44. Punched-out mitochondria and fat droplets in WD. x 6,000

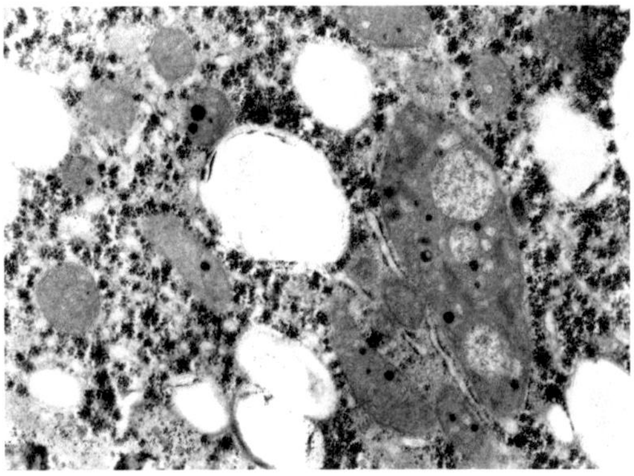

Fig. 45. Giant mitochondrion with punched-out areas and fat droplets. x 10,000

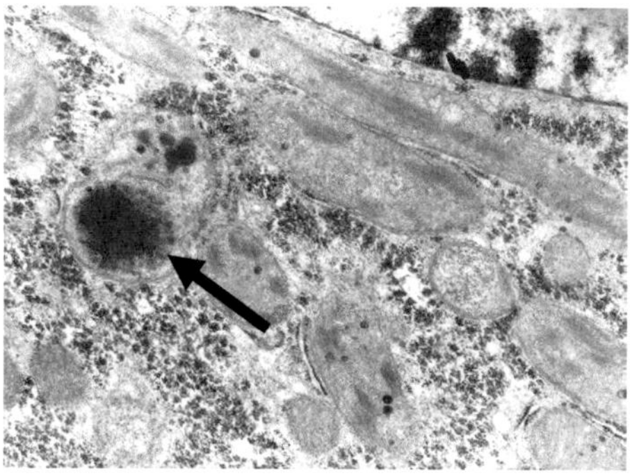

Fig. 46. WD: Mitochondria with crystalline deposits and dense deposits (arrow) x 8,000

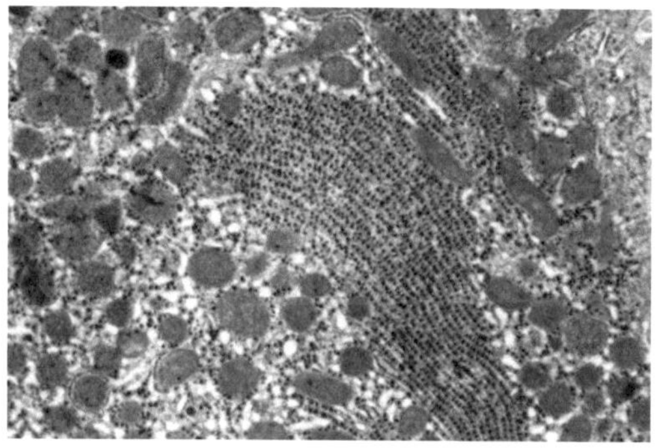

Fig. 47. Glycogen body (RER) frequently seen in WD. x 6,000

### 5.6 Reye syndrome

Around 1970, TEM had a major diagnostic role showing changes considered typical for Reye syndrome: generalized steatosis, glycogen depletion, increased frequency of peroxisomes and "amoeboid", occasionally giant mitochondria; their matrix was described as "flocculent" and frequently contained crystalline inclusions and lacked dense matrical granules (Figs. 48-49). Towards 1980, possibly following the reduced aspirin consumption, the frequency of Reye syndrome decreased dramatically. However, sporadic cases still occurred without a clear relationship to aspirin ingestion. The ultrastructural findings were similar to those described in Reye syndrome, and were therefore named "Reye-like" (Phillips et al., 1987). In the UK, over 10% of reported cases with an initial diagnosis of Reye's syndrome have later been revised to an *Inborn Metabolic Disorder (IMD)* which may mimic Reye's syndrome. IMD includes defects in fat oxidation, amino acid metabolism, carbohydrate metabolism and disorders of ammonia detoxification. The relationship with aspirin ingestion was not firmly established, as Reye syndrome appeared in areas where aspirin was never used (Australia) and continued to appear after aspirin was discontinued (France).

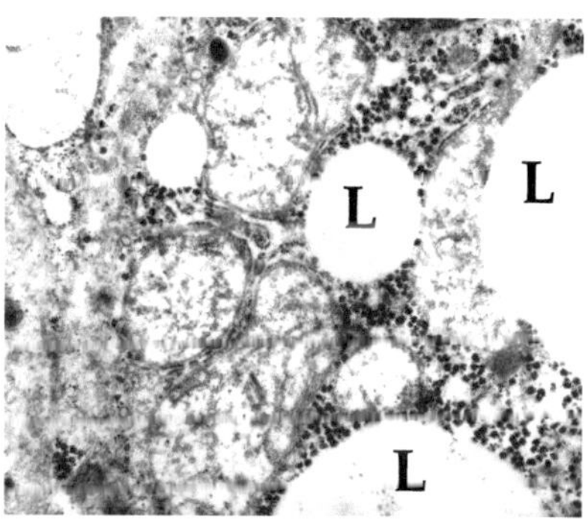


Fig. 48. Reye syndrome. Cristolysis and generalized lipid deposition (L) x 20,000

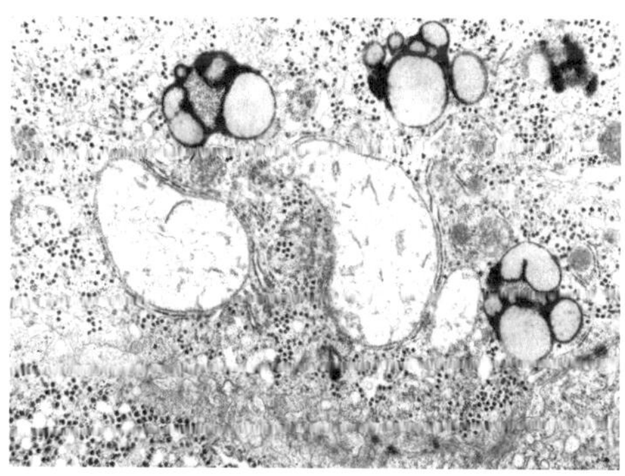

Fig. 49. Reye syndrome. Expanded mitochondria, cristolysis, lipofuscin and absent matrical granules. x 10,000

## 5.7 Steatosis

This group includes presently: 1. Alcoholic liver disease; 2. NAFLD (non-alcoholic fatty liver disease) which encompasses most forms of fatty liver, including "simple steatosis", without inflammation, seen in an important percent of adult population (Fig. 50), and 3. NASH, (non-alcoholic steatohepatitis) which by definition involves inflammation and/or fibrosis (Roberts, 2004 b) and may progress to cirrhosis more frequently than simple steatosis.

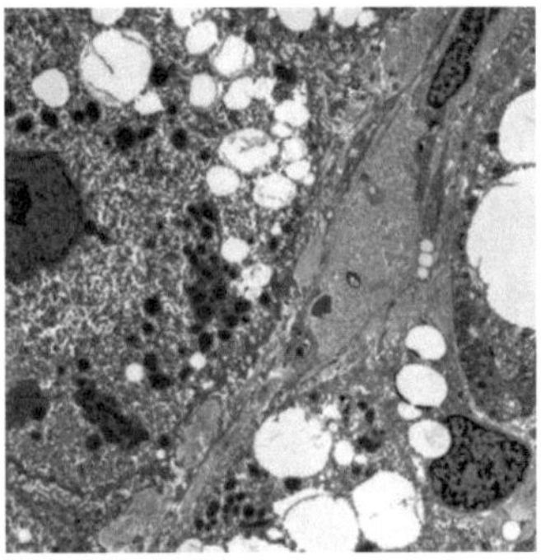

Fig. 50. Fatty liver - NAFLD: Large droplets present in hepatocytes and sinusoidal cells x 4,000

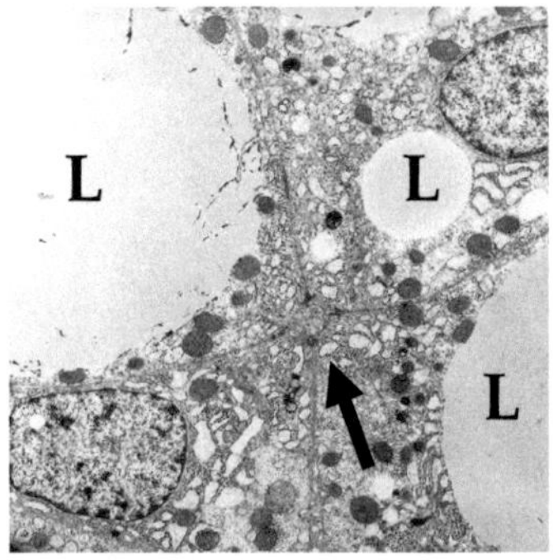


Fig. 51. Total parenteral nutrition. Lipid droplets (L) strangle a minute bile canaliculus (arrow). x 6,000

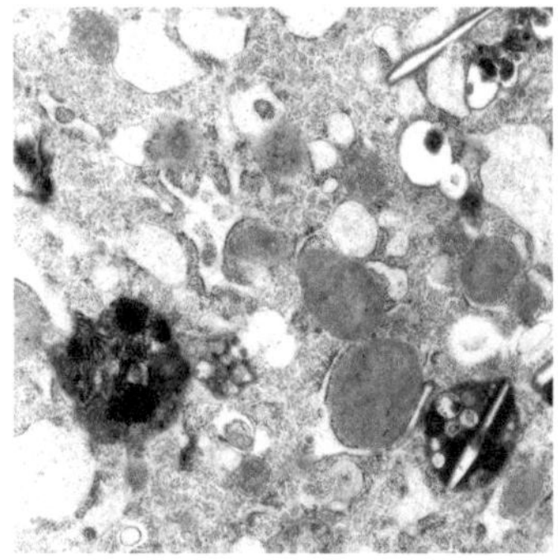

Fig. 52. Total parenteral nutrition. Spicular cholesterol within dense bodies. Abnormal mitochondria. x 8,000

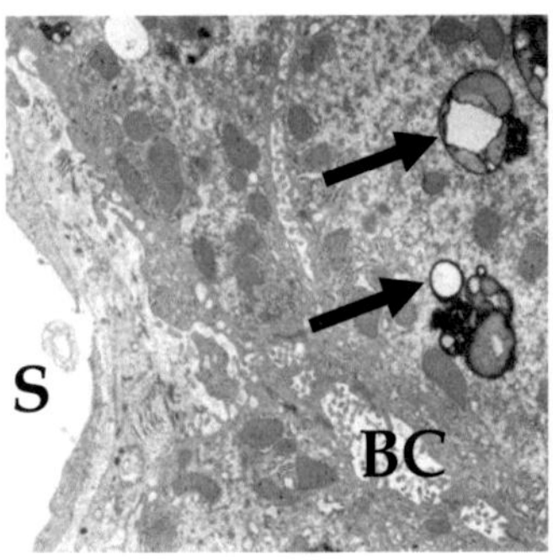


Fig. 53. NAFLD. Lipofuscin- lipolysosomes (arrows) near the sinusoid (S) and bile canaliculus (BC). x 4,000

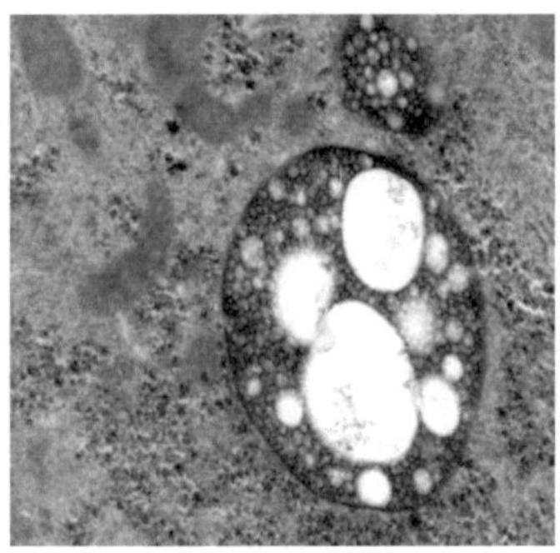

Fig. 54. Hepatocyte. Typical lipolysosomes, Wilson disease. x 6,000

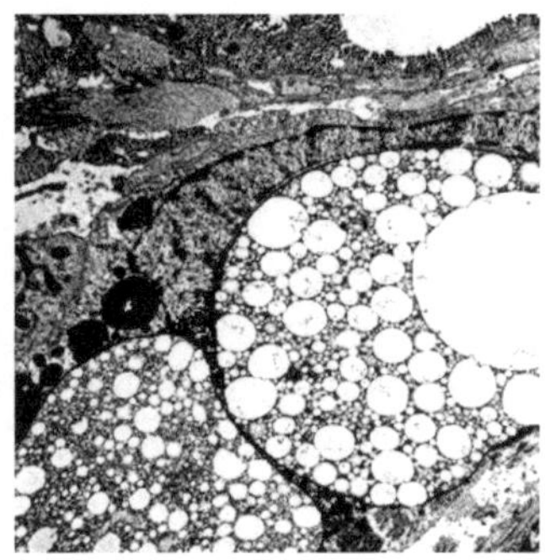

Fig. 55. Compound lipolysosome. Note extreme size compared to adjacent nuclei; x 6,000

For electron-microscopic characterization of liver steatosis, the classical terms "large droplet"(macrovesicular) and "small droplet"(microvesicular) are still used. Macrovesicular steatosis is mostly seen in nutritional abnormalities including: kwashiorkor, obesity, prolonged parenteral nutrition (Figs. 51-52), diabetes mellitus, glycogenoses, Wilson disease, hyperlipidemias, A-(or hypo) betalipoproteinemia, familial lipoprotein deficiency, total lipodystrophy (Sherlock & Doodley, 1993). Microvesicular steatosis is frequently found in mitochondrial dysfunctions, urea cycle enzyme defects, lysosomal storage diseases, Reye- and Reye-like syndromes, lipodystrophies and certain drug toxicities such as salicylates and valproate).

Fat droplets of various sizes can be seen mostly, but not only, in hepatocytes. The ubiquitous triglyceride droplets have a round contour, are only slightly electron dense and usually have no surrounding limit membrane. Even in cells apparently completely filled-up with fat droplets, the changes in other organelles are rare, with the exception of crystal formation in mitochondria, seen more frequently. Occasionally, a fat droplet can be seen in the nucleus as well.

### 5.7.1 Atypical lipid-containing organelles

Membrane-bound lipid droplets (lipolysosomes) are frequently seen in hepatocytes in association with triglyceride-containing droplets.
We distinguish between several types of lipid-containing, membrane-bound bodies:

1. *Lipolysosomes* as described by Hayashi and Sternlieb, and Kanai et al.(Hayashi & Sternlieb, 1975; Hayashi et al., 1983; Kanai et al., 1994). Electron-lucent droplets, usually up to 10 μm in diameter, with uniform content and surrounded by a trilaminar membrane. Of special interest are vesicles (attachments) to the outer leaflet of the surrounding membrane and associated lipofuscin (Figs. 53).
2. *Multivesicular bodies,* described by Phillips et al. (1987) as lipolysosomes, containing numerous smaller droplets with lipidic aspect (Fig. 54). Such lipolysosomes have been observed frequently in Wilson disease and in patients with NAFLD. They are frequently seen in hepatocytes showing increased amounts of typical lipofuscin
3. *Giant lipolysosomes* (Fig. 55) which we suggest to name "compound lipolysosomes", observed in cases of extreme overweight (Haimi et al., 2011). They appear to be formed by the fusion of numerous lipolysosomes of usual size, through a process similar to the formation of "compound siderosomes" describe in iron overload (Roy & Ghadially, 1967).

## 6. Infections and infestations (See Table 1)

Negative staining is required for identification of some viral particles while others display characteristic features in cytosol or nucleus in various liver cells. In acute hepatitis, remnants of *apoptotic* hepatocytes form eosinophilic *acidophilic bodies (Fig. 56).* They are then expelled from the cell aggregate and later phagocytized by macrophages. Other cells undergo necrosis without an identifiable apoptotic stage (Fig. 57).

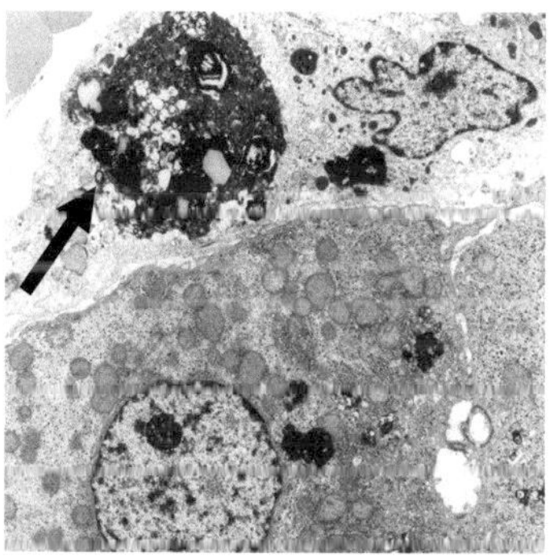

Fig. 56. Acidophilic body (arrow) in the sinusoid. Fat droplets, disintegrated nucleus and phagolysosomes are still recognizable. x 5,000

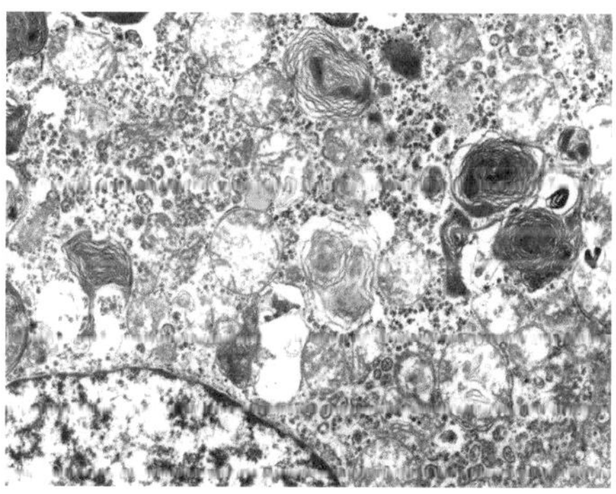

Fig. 57. Acute hepatitis: Membranous phagolysosomes in a necrotic hepatocyte. x 6,000

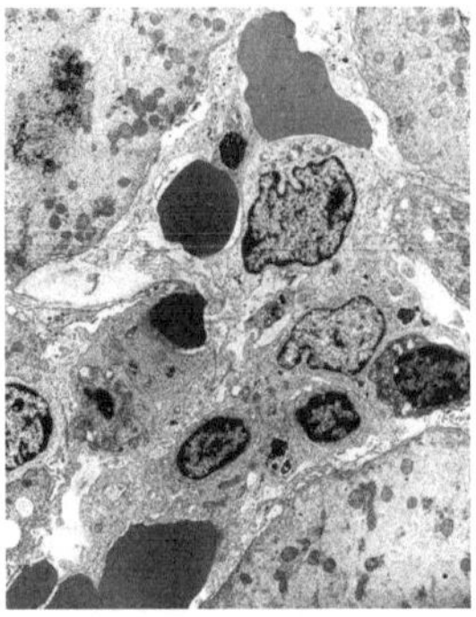

Fig. 58. Acute hepatitis. Mononuclear cells in sinusoid. x 4,000

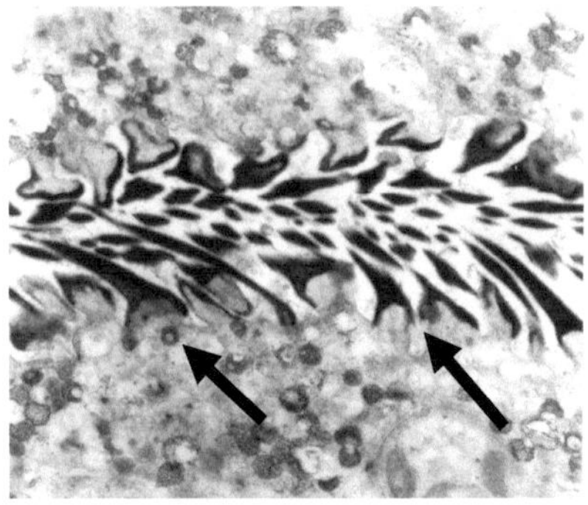

Fig. 59. Echinoccocus granulosum: hooklets (arrows) in the liver biopsy retrieved at surgery. x 10,000

The presence of inflammatory reactions, mostly of viral origin, is visualized by TEM initially by the presence of mononuclear cells in sinusoids (Fig. 58). Focal cytoplasmic degeneration precedes changes recognizable by light microscopy, to be followed by apoptosis and eventually necrosis. The identification of various hepatitis etiological agents is beyond the routine liver biopsy examination. The occasional encounter with parasites (Fig. 59) has an investigational character,

## 7. Drug hepatotoxicity

With the exponential increase in the number of drugs (medication) there is a parallel increase in the number of side- and toxic effects reported by patients. Many of these are related to liver function and metabolism and to the major de-toxifying role of this organ. In drug-induced damage, autophagosomes are frequently seen (Fig. 60) occasionally containing mitochondria (Fig. 61). In this review we will exemplify only a few of these toxic changes as seen by electron microscopy: non-specific effects, from mild and reversible to severe and life-endangering are listed in Table 1. In addition, there are some specific features which enable diagnosis of the offending compound: amiodarone, NSAIDs, aspirin, corticosteroids.

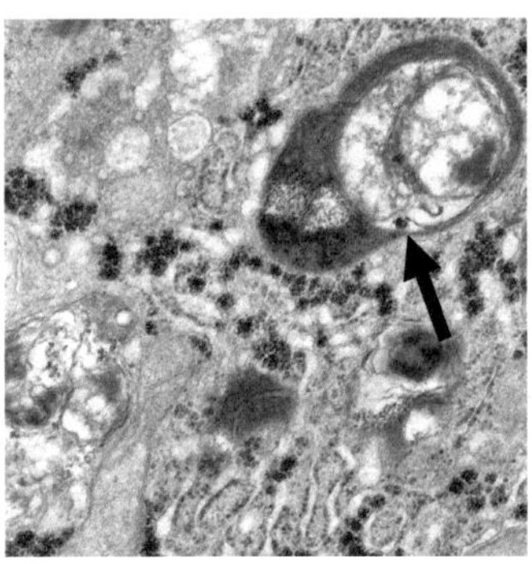

Fig. 60. Drug toxicity. Autophagosomes (arrows) contain fat and multiple membranes. x 15,000

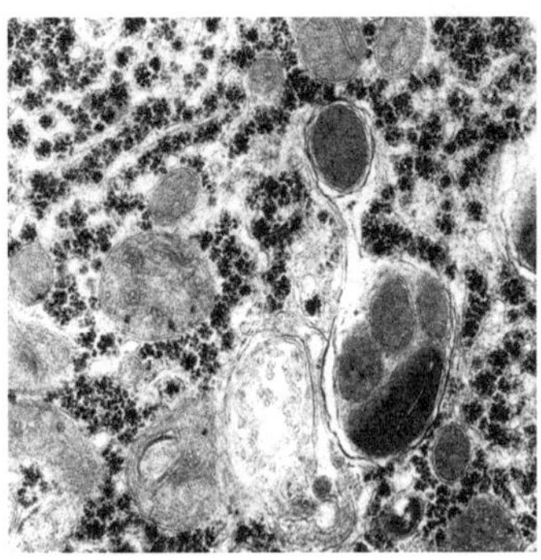

Fig. 61. Valproate toxicity. Mitochondria secluded in autophagolysosome. x 15,000

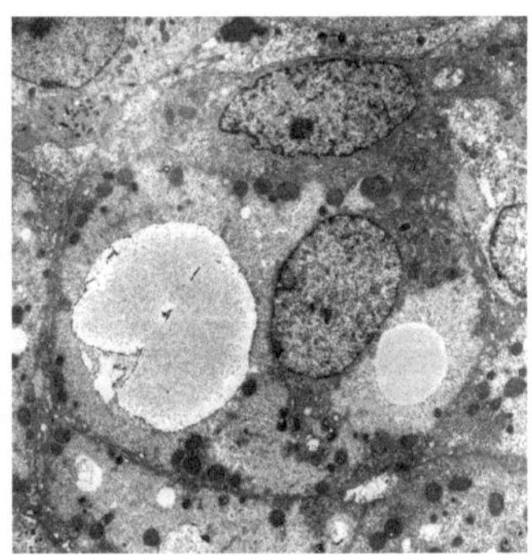

Fig. 62. Corticosteroid effect. Lipid and excessive glycogen in a bi-nucleated hepatocyte. x 6,000

| Condition | EM findings |
|---|---|
| **Artefacts** | |
| Delayed fixation<br>Inadequate fixation | Mitochondrial matrix with dense deposits<br>'Ballooned' mitochondria, 'Extraction' of nuclei<br>Myelin-like whorls in mitochondria |
| **Infections/ infestations** | |
| Hepatitis, herpes-varicella group virus | viral particles |
| Hepatitis, acute (HBV) | viral particles (HBsAg)<br>Nuclear Dane particles (HBcAg) |
| Infectious mononucleosis | Ebstein-Barr virus |
| Cytomegalovirus infection | Electron-dense particles in hepatocytes (no virus) |
| Kala-Azar | Leishmania bodies in Kupffer cells |
| Malaria | Schizonts in Kupffer cells |
| Ecchinococosis | Fragments in tissue |
| | |
| **Bilirubin retention syndromes** | |
| **Unconjugated hyperbilirubinemia - Inherited disorders (Constitutional, non-hemolytic)** | |
| Crigler-Najjar syndromes, type 1 & 2 | Intracanalicular bile thrombi, increased intercellular space. |
| Gilbert's disease | Flattening of hepatocyte microvilli, reduced RER, proliferated SER. |
| **Conjugated hyperbilirubinemia** | |
| Cholangiopathies - Cholestasis (most etiologies) | Curled cristae in mitochondria; dense deposits in cell sap; amorphous and/or filamentous bile cytolysosomes mostly around bile canaliculi; focal biliary necrosis; dilated & distorted bile canaliculi with abnormal microvilli and bile plugs. Pericanalicular cytoplasm may show microfilaments. |
| Biliary atresia - Biliary duct obstruction | Extensive cytoplasmic cholestasis, cytoplasmic biliary necrosis; pericanalicular filamentous cuff. |
| Cystic fibrosis | Cholestasis in infancy; aggregates of osmiophilic material in lumen; collagen; steatosis; ductule dilatation; many stellate cells. |
| Alagille | Numerous bile-containing cytolysosomes and vesicles in Golgi; canaliculi can be empty. |
| PFIC 1 (ATP8B1) | Severe cholestasis (hepatocytes, sinusoidal cells, bile ducts, granular Byler bile). |

| | |
|---|---|
| PFIC 2 (ABCB11) | As in PFIC-1 but amorphous and filamentous bile in canaliculi. |
| PFIC 3 (ABCB4) | As in PFIC 1 & PFIC 2 but amorphous and filamentous bile in canaliculi. |
| Dubin-Johnson syndrome | Lipofuscin-like pigment, abnormal bile canaliculi. |
| Rotor syndrome | Megamitochondria, reduced microvilli in bile canaliculi. |
| | |
| **Carbohydrate metabolism** | |
| Glycogen Storage Diseases (GSD) Type I,(I-a) III, VI, VIII, IX, X, XI | Accumulation of cytosolic glycogen in hepatocytes; displacement of organelles; frayed α-glycogen in types VI, VIII, IX, X. |
| Type IIa, b, c | Abnormal glycogen-containing lysosomes: glycogenosomes. |
| Type IV (amilopectinosis) | Abnormal structural glycogen, collagen deposition and cirrhosis. |
| Diabetes mellitus | As for GSD I and III; micro- and macrovesicular steatosis. Hyperglycogenation of nuclei. Lipolysosomes, lipofuscin; mitochondrial crystalline inclusions. |
| Hereditary fructose intolerance | Concentric membranous arrays in hepatocytes; Areas of cytoplasmic damage: 'Fructose holes': abundant glycogen, prominent lipid droplets, large autophagic glycogen-containing vacuoles, myelin figures, focal cytoplasmic degradation. |
| Galactosemia | Hepatocytes: rosette or pseudoglandular formation; multinuclear hepatocytes. Cholestasis; large lipid droplets; distended RER |
| | |
| **Disorders of glycoprotein metabolism** | |
| **Mucopolysaccharidoses** : Hurler, Hunter, Sanfilippo, Scheie, Morquio, Maroteaux-Lamy | Abnormal lysosomes in hepatocytes, RER, sinusoidal cells and vascular epithelia; empty-looking vacuoles, occasional 'bull's eye' appearance. |
| **Glycoproteinoses** | |
| Fucosidosis | Lysosomes with variable membranous content. |
| Sialidosis (Mucolipidosis I) | Fine reticular-granular content of lysosomes (hepatocytes and sinusoidal cells). |
| Mannosidosis | Fine reticular-granular content of lysosomes. Electron-opaque globules in Kupffer cells. |

| | |
|---|---|
| Salla disease | "Empty lysosomes ": parenchymal & sinusoidal cells. |
| Glutamyl ribose 5-phosphate glycoproteinosis | Vacuoles with floccular material in Kupffer cells. |
| | |
| **Mucolipidoses** | |
| Mucolipidosis II (I-cell disease) | Cytoplasmic membrane- bound vacuoles containing fibrillose-granular material. |
| Mucolipidosis III (Pseudo-Hurler) | Vacuoles in cultured fibroblasts. |
| Mucolipidosis IV | Hepatocytes: lamellar inclusions; Kupffer cells: fibrogranular material in lysosomes. |
| Alpha-1-AT deficiency | Amorphous accumulations in hepatocytic RER. |
| | |
| **Disorders of lipid metabolism** | |
| **Sphingolipidoses - Gangliosidoses** | |
| GM1 (generalized gangliosidosis) Landing) | Membranous cytoplasmic bodies. Lipid-laden histiocytes (liver). |
| GM2 (Tay-Sachs, Sandhoff disease) | Membranous cytoplasmic bodies. |
| Glycosphingolipid lipidosis (Fabry disease) | Lysosomal concentric arrays disease. |
| Lactosyl ceramidosis | Lysosomal lamellae. |
| Sulphatidosis (metachromatic leukodystrophy) | Hepatocytic lamellar inclusions "Herring bone" |
| Glucocerebrosidosis (Gaucher disease) | Gaucher cells. |
| Ceramidosis (Farber disease) | Hepatocytic vacuoles and dense bodies; curved tubular structures in Kupffer cells. |
| **Sphingomyelinosis (Niemann-Pick disease)** | |
| (All types) | Lysosomal concentric membranes in hepatocytes and sinusoidal cells. |
| Abetalipoproteinemia | Macrovesicular liver steatosis.<br>Deficient trans-Golgi vacuole formation |
| Familial lipoprotein deficiency | Lipolysosomes in foam cells of RES. |
| Acid lipase deficiency & Wolman disease | Foamy histiocytes containing acicular crystal lipid droplets in hepatocytes and histiocytes. |
| Cholesteryl ester storage disease | Cholesteryl ester crystals in Kupffer cells. |
| Ceroid lipofuscinosis | Lipofuscin and tubular structures in lysosomes. |
| Chanarin Dorfman disease | Ichthyosis, fatty liver, cirrhosis. |
| Steroid therapy, prolonged | Macrovesicular liver steatosis. |
| Total lipodystrophy & Parenteral nutrition | Macrovesicular steatosis, lipid lakes, cholestasis |
| **Disorders of protein metabolism** | |
| Tyrosinemia | Cholestasis, steatosis, abnormal MV, collagen in space of Disse. |

| | |
|---|---|
| Aspartylglucoaminuria | Large lysosomes in hepatocytes &Kupffer cells. Membranous structures in mitochondria. |
| Carbamyl phosphate synthetase deficiency | Concentric RER, small mitochondria with high matrix density. |
| Lysinuric protein intolerance with deficient transport of basic amino acids | Increased SER; large vesicles filled with fibrogranular material. |
| Carnitine palmoyl transferase deficiency | Large-droplet fatty liver. |
| Hyperornithinemia | Megamitochondria, abnormal shapes and membranes. |
| Cystinosis | Crystals in Kupffer cell lysosomes. |
| Homocystinuria | Mitochondria abnormal shapes, SER. proliferation, peribiliary lysosomes. |
| | |
| **Metals** | |
| **Iron** | |
| Primary and secondary hemochromatosis | Ferritin in cytosol and lysosomes (siderosomes) Hemosiderin only in lysosomes (most cell lines) |
| Transfusional siderosis | RES hemosiderin loading, less in parenchyma. |
| Neonatal hemochromatosis<br><br>Aceruloplasminemia | Heavy parenchymal siderosis, less in RES (distribution similar to hemochromatosis)<br>Brain and systemic siderosis, including liver |
| Association with lipofuscin | Ferritin and hemosiderin in compound lysosomes with lipofuscin. |
| **Copper** | |
| Wilson disease | Abnormal mitochondria, abnormal peroxisomes, lipolysosomes, fatty liver, electron-dense deposits. |
| Menkes' kinky hair syndrome | Cartwheel-like cristae in mitochondria. |
| | |
| **Peroxisomal disorders** | |
| Zellweger syndrome | Absent peroxisomes. |
| Hepatic acatalasia syndrome | Absent peroxisomes. |
| Neonatal adrenoleukodystrophy | Few, small, peroxisomes. |
| Primary hyperoxaluria Type I | Few, small, peroxisomes |
| Infantile Refsum's disease | Few, small peroxisomes; angulated lysosomes. |
| | |
| **Drug Toxicity** - general features | Mitochondrial changes(absent dense matrical granules, paracrystalline formation); RER dilatation, SER proliferation; increased. frequency of lysosomes (autophagolysosomes); apoptosis, focal necrosis, lipofuscinosis. |

| | |
|---|---|
| Corticosteroid therapy, high dosage, short term | Glycogen accumulation in hepatocytes. |
| | |
| **Miscellaneous** | |
| Kwashiorkor, protein-calorie malnutrition | Large droplet fatty liver, abnormal mitochondria. |
| Chediak-Higashi disease | Abnormal inclusions in Kupffer cells and hepatocytes. |
| Erythrohepatic-protoporphyria | Amorphous or needle-like pigment in hepatocytes and Kupffer cells. |
| Erythroblastosis fetalis | Erythroblasts and reticulocytes in liver parenchyma. |
| GVH disease | Immune cell infiltrate. |
| Langerhans Cell Histiocytosis | Birbeck granules. |
| Parenteral nutrition | Mitochondrial changes, vesiculated SER, cholestasis, lipofuscin, in hepatocytes and Kupffer cells. |
| Reye syndrome & Reye-like syndrome | Microvesicular fatty liver, abnormal mitochondria, many peroxisomes. |

Table 1. Electron Microscopic findings in different conditions

### 7.1 Corticosteroid effect

Fatty liver has been reported among the side-effects of prolonged large-dose steroid therapy (Sherlock & Doodley, 1993). Three patients aged 8, 10 and 12 year respectively, treated with medium-high doses of corticosteroids presented with hepatomegaly and elevated transaminases of unknown origin. Liver biopsy performed to elucidate these findings, revealed (by TEM) excessive glycogen in hepatocytes, to the extent of justifying hepatomegaly. The increased amount of hepatocytic glycogen displaced mitochondria and other components towards the nucleus and plasma membrane (Fig. 62). The pattern was similar to that of glycogen storage diseases observed in type III and IX. Lipid droplets were scarce. After the steroid therapy was discontinued, the liver size returned to normal (Iancu et al., 1986).

### 7.2 Amiodarone

Changes similar to alcoholic liver injury are commonly found. Steatosis, is the most frequent histopathological feature. Ballooning of hepatocytes, Mallory bodies, and fibrosis are common. Other changes include nuclear unrest, acidophilic bodies, foam cells, hyperglycogenated nuclei, and portal inflammation. Characteristic lamellar lysosomal inclusion bodies representing phospholipidosis should be better designed as "myelinosomes"(Fig. 63), (Ghadially, 1997). The cytotoxic pseudoalcoholic changes could be an independent phenomenon in susceptible patients unable to metabolize the drug. The true incidence of hepatic injury from amiodarone remains to be determined from prospective evaluations of pretreatment and follow-up liver biopsies (Lewis et al., 1990).

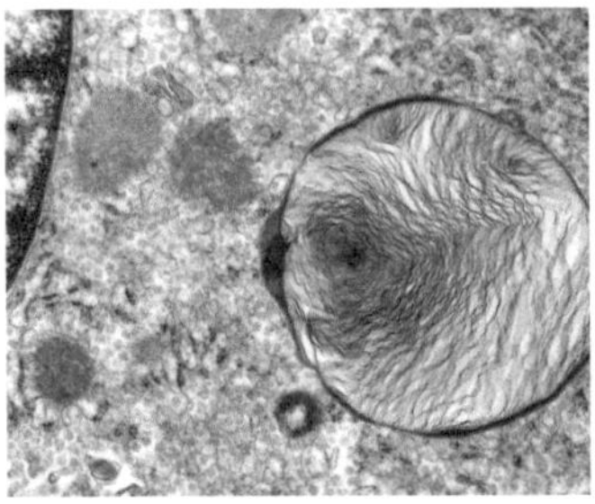

Fig. 63. Amiodarone toxicity: lamellar phosphorlipidosis in a lysosome x 10,000

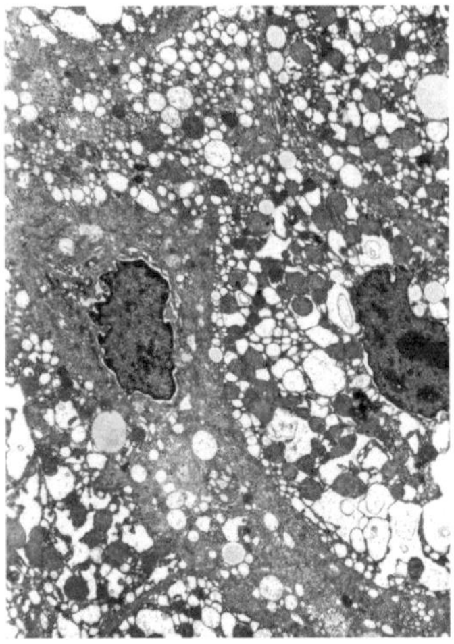

Fig. 64. Aspirin toxicity: dilated RER; steatosis, shrunken nuclei. x 4,000

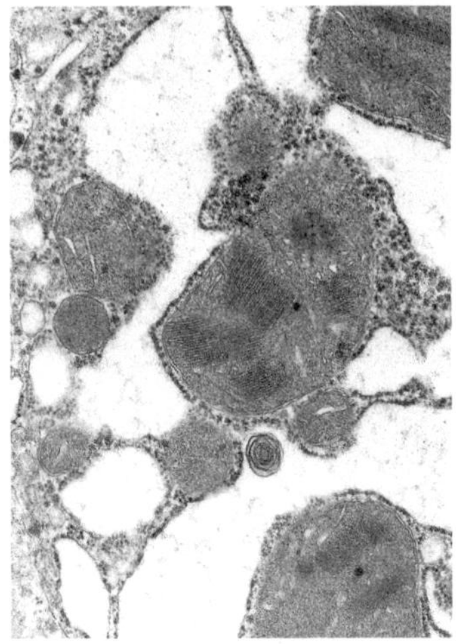

Fig. 65. Aspirin toxicity: dilatation of RER; crystalline deposits. x 10,000

### 7.3 Acetylsalicylic acid (Aspirin)

In addition to its suspected relationship to Reye syndrome, aspirin, in large doses, has been found to increase the level of transaminases, a reversible reaction. TEM of a liver biopsy of a patient disclosed hepatotoxicity: dilatation of RER, mitochondrial changes (megamitochondria, crystalline formation), nuclear changes and lipofuscinosis (Figs. 64-65), (Iancu & Elian, 1976).

### 7.4 Acetaminophen (Paracetamol)

Frequently used as a suicidal drug, paracetamol can precipitate fatal liver failure when dosage is beyond 8–10g. TEM of experimental animals and cultured hepatoma-derived cells (HepG2 and Hep3B) disclosed the different stages of dose-related toxicity. Of note, the anti-oxidant *N*-acetylcysteine did not protect cultured cells against acetaminophen-induced apoptosis (Manov et al., 2002; Manov et al., 2004). Various aspects of ultrastructural damage induced by non-steroidal anti-inflammatory drugs (NSAIDs) are described in detail in a review of hepatotoxicity of anti-inflammatory and analgesic drugs (Manov et al., 2006).

## 8. Conclusions

Transmission electron microscopy of liver biopsies provides:

1. **Typical diagnostic findings** for a relatively small, but important, number of pathological conditions.
2. **Supportive information** for a larger group of suspected conditions which require further confirmation.
3. **Important exclusion** of conditions which were considered in differential diagnosis.

Furthermore, it remains an essential research tool in all areas of bio-pathology.

## 9. Acknowledgments

The electron-microscopic work was supported by The Milman Fund for Pediatric Research and the Dan David Foundation (Grant 03-06, 2010) and by a joint grant to Dr. I. Manov from The Center of Absorption in Science of the Ministry of Immigrant Absorption and the Committee for Planning and Budgeting of the Council for Higher Education, in the framework of the Kamea Program.

The following colleagues submitted liver specimens for examination: D. Berkowitz, H. Bitterman, J. Bujanover, D. Bransky, E. Broide, I. Dalal, M. Haimi, C. Hartman A. Lerner, A. Levine, H. Mandel, A. On, A. Pecht, S. Peleg, H. Shamali, R. Shaoul, R. Shamir, R. Shapiro, R. Spiegel, R. Regev, M. Wilschanski, N. Zelnick, E. Zuckerman.

## 10. References

Balistreri, W. F. (2002). Intrahepatic cholestasis. *J Pediatr Gastroenterol Nutr*, Vol. 35 Suppl 1, No. S17-23

Bessis, M. & Weed, R. I. (1973). *Living blood cells and their ultrastructure. Translated [and edited] by Robert I. Weed,* Springer-Verlag, New York,

Bezerra, J. A. & Balistreri, W. F. (1999). Intrahepatic cholestasis: order out of chaos. *Gastroenterology*, Vol. 117, No. 6, 1496-8

Bull, L. N.; Carlton, V. E.; Stricker, N. L.; Baharloo, S.; DeYoung, J. A.; Freimer, N. B.; Magid, M. S.; Kahn, E.; Markowitz, J.; DiCarlo, F. J.; McLoughlin, L.; Boyle, J. T.; Dahms, B. B.; Faught, P. R.; Fitzgerald, J. F.; Piccoli, D. A.; Witzleben, C. L.; O'Connell, N. C.; Setchell, K. D.; Agostini, R. M., Jr.; Kocoshis, S. A.; Reyes, J. & Knisely, A. S. (1997). Genetic and morphological findings in progressive familial intrahepatic cholestasis (Byler disease [PFIC-1] and Byler syndrome): evidence for heterogeneity. *Hepatology*, Vol. 26, No. 1, 155-64

Davit-Spraul, A.; Gonzales, E.; Baussan, C. & Jacquemin, E. (2009). Progressive familial intrahepatic cholestasis. *Orphanet J Rare Dis*, Vol. 4, No. 1

Fischbach, F. A.; Gregory, D. W.; Harrison, P. M.; Hoy, T. G. & Williams, J. M. (1971). On the structure of hemosiderin and its relationship to ferritin. *J Ultrastruct Res*, Vol. 37, No. 5, 495-503

Gal, S.; Fridkin, M.; Amit, T.; Zheng, H. & Youdim, M. B. (2006). M30, a novel multifunctional neuroprotective drug with potent iron chelating and brain selective monoamine oxidase-ab inhibitory activity for Parkinson's disease. *J Neural Transm Suppl*, Vol. No. 70, 447-56

Ghadially, F. N. (1997). *Ultrastructural pathology of the cell and matrix,* Butterworth-Heinemann, Boston

Hackenbrock, C. R.; Rehn, T. G.; Weinbach, E. C. & Lemasters, J. J. (1971). Oxidative phosphorylation and ultrastructural transformation in mitochondria in the intact ascites tumor cell. *J Cell Biol*, Vol. 51, No. 1, 123-37

Hayashi, H., Sameshima, Y., Lee, M., Hotta, Y. & Kosaka, T. (1983). Lipolysosomes in human hepatocytes: their increase in number associated with serum level of cholesterol in chronic liver diseases. *Hepatology*, Vol. 3, No. 2, 221-5

Hayashi, H. & Sternlieb, I. (1975). Lipolysosomes in human hepatocytes. Ultrastructural and cytochemical studies of patients with Wilson's disease. *Lab Invest*, Vol. 33, No. 1, 1-7

Hers, H. G. (1963). alpha-Glucosidase deficiency in generalized glycogenstorage disease (Pompe's disease). *Biochem J*, Vol. 86, No. 11-6

Iancu, T. & Elian, E. (1976). Ultrastructural changes in aspirin hepatotoxicity. *Am J Clin Pathol*, Vol. 66, No. 3, 570-5

Iancu, T. C. (1983). Iron overload. *Mol Aspects Med*, Vol. 6, No. 1, 1-100

Iancu, T. C. (1989). Ultrastructural pathology of iron overload. *Baillieres Clin Haematol*, Vol. 2, No. 2, 475-95

Iancu, T. C. (1992). Ferritin and hemosiderin in pathological tissues. *Electron Microsc Rev*, Vol. 5, No. 2, 209-29

Iancu, T. C. (2011). Ultrastructural aspects of iron storage, transport and metabolism. *Journal of neural transmission (Vienna, Austria : 1996)*, Vol. No.

Iancu, T. C.; Deugnier, Y.; Halliday, J. W.; Powell, L. W. & Brissot, P. (1997). Ultrastructural sequences during liver iron overload in genetic hemochromatosis. *J Hepatol*, Vol. 27, No. 4, 628-38

Iancu, T. C.; Mahajnah, M.; Manov, I.; Cherurg, S.; Knopf, C. & Mandel, H. (2007). The liver in congenital disorders of glycosylation: ultrastructural features. *Ultrastruct Pathol*, Vol. 31, No. 3, 189-97

Iancu, T. C.; Shiloh, H. & Dembo, L. (1986). Hepatomegaly following short-term high-dose steroid therapy. *J Pediatr Gastroenterol Nutr*, Vol. 5, No. 1, 41-6

Johannessen, J. V. (1978). *Electron microscopy in human medicine,* McGraw-Hill International Book Co., New York

Kanai, M.; Watari, N.; Soji, T. & Sugawara, E. (1994). Formation and accumulation of lipolysosomes in developing chick hepatocytes. *Cell Tissue Res*, Vol. 275, No. 1, 125-32

Knisely, A. S. & Vergani, D. "Neonatal hemochromatosis": a re-vision. *Hepatology*, Vol. 51, No. 6, 1888-90

Lewis, J. H.; Mullick, F.; Ishak, K. G.; Ranard, R. C.; Ragsdale, B.; Perse, R. M.; Rusnock, E. J.; Wolke, A.; Benjamin, S. B.; Seeff, L. B. & et al. (1990). Histopathologic analysis of suspected amiodarone hepatotoxicity. *Hum Pathol*, Vol. 21, No. 1, 59-67

Mandel, H.; Hartman, C.; Berkowitz, D.; Elpeleg, O. N.; Manov, I. & Iancu, T. C. (2001). The hepatic mitochondrial DNA depletion syndrome: ultrastructural changes in liver biopsies. *Hepatology*, Vol. 34, No. 4 Pt 1, 776-84

Manov, I.; Hirsh, M. & Iancu, T. C. (2002). Acetaminophen hepatotoxicity and mechanisms of its protection by N-acetylcysteine: a study of Hep3B cells. *Exp Toxicol Pathol*, Vol. 53, No. 6, 489-500

Manov, I.; Hirsh, M. & Iancu, T. C. (2004). N-acetylcysteine does not protect HepG2 cells against acetaminophen-induced apoptosis. *Basic Clin Pharmacol Toxicol*, Vol. 94, No. 5, 213-25

Manov, I.; Motanis, H.; Frumin, I. & Iancu, T. C. (2006). Hepatotoxicity of anti-inflammatory and analgesic drugs: ultrastructural aspects. *Acta Pharmacologica Sinica*, Vol. 27, No. 259-272

McAdams, A. J.; Hug, G. & Bove, K. E. (1974). Glycogen storage disease, types I to X: criteria for morphologic diagnosis. *Hum Pathol*, Vol. 5, No. 4, 463-87

Meiner, V.; Shpitzen, S.; Mandel, H.; Klar, A.; Ben-Neriah, Z.; Zlotogora, J.; Sagi, M.; Lossos, A.; Bargal, R.; Sury, V.; Carmi, R.; Leitersdorf, E. & Zeigler, M. (2001). Clinical-biochemical correlation in molecularly characterized patients with Niemann-Pick type C. *Genet Med*, Vol. 3, No. 5, 343-8

Mowat, A. P. (1994). *Liver disorders in childhood*, Butterworth-Heinemann, Oxford

Muir, W. A.; McLaren, G. D.; Braun, W. & Askari, A. (1984). Evidence for heterogeneity in hereditary hemochromatosis. Evaluation of 174 persons in nine families. *Am J Med*, Vol. 76, No. 5, 806-14

Partin, J. C.; Schubert, W. K. & Partin, J. S. (1971). Mitochondrial ultrastructure in Reye's syndrome (encephalopathy and fatty degeneration of the viscera). *N Engl J Med*, Vol. 285, No. 24, 1339-43

Pastores, G. M. (2010). *Lysosomal storage disorders : principles and practice*, World Scientific, Singapore

Spiegel, R.; Raas-Rothschild, A.; Reish, O.; Regev, M.; Meiner, V.; Bargal, R.; Sury, V.; Meir, K.; Nadjari, M.; Hermann, G.; Iancu, T. C.; Shalev, S. A. & Zeigler, M. (2009). The clinical spectrum of fetal Niemann-Pick type C. *Am J Med Genet A*, Vol. 149A, No. 3, 446-50

Sternlieb, I. (1979). Electron Microscopy of Mitochondria and Peroxysomes of Human Hepatocytes, In: *Progress in Liver Diseases*, P. Hans and S. Fenton, (Ed.), 81-104, Grune & Stratton, New York

Tandler, B.; Hutter, R. V. & Erlandson, R. A. (1970). Ultrastructure of oncocytoma of the parotid gland. *Lab Invest*, Vol. 23, No. 6, 567-80

Tanikawa, K.; Eguchi, T. & Ikejiri, N. (1979). *Ultrastructural aspects of the liver and its disorders*, Igaku-Shoin, Tokyo ; New York

Valencia-Mayoral, P.; Weber, J.; Cutz, E.; Edwards, V. D. & Phillips, M. J. (1984). Possible defect in the bile secretory apparatus in arteriohepatic dysplasia (Alagille's syndrome): a review with observations on the ultrastructure of liver. *Hepatology*, Vol. 4, No. 4, 691-8

Verhulst, P. M.; van der Velden, L. M.; Oorschot, V.; van Faassen, E. E.; Klumperman, J.; Houwen, R. H.; Pomorski, T. G.; Holthuis, J. C. & Klomp, L. W. A flippase-independent function of ATP8B1, the protein affected in familial intrahepatic cholestasis type 1, is required for apical protein expression and microvillus formation in polarized epithelial cells. *Hepatology*, Vol. 51, No. 6, 2049-60

Weber, A. M.; Tuchweber, B.; Yousef, I.; Brochu, P.; Turgeon, C.; Gabbiani, G.; Morin, C. L. & Roy, C. C. (1981). Severe familial cholestasis in North American Indian children: a clinical model of microfilament dysfunction? *Gastroenterology*, Vol. 81, No. 4, 653-62

Whitington, P. F. (2007). Neonatal hemochromatosis: a congenital alloimmune hepatitis. *Semin Liver Dis*, Vol. 27, No. 3, 243-50

Zhu, W.; Xie, W.; Pan, T.; Xu, P.; Fridkin, M.; Zheng, H.; Jankovic, J.; Youdim, M. B. & Le, W. (2007). Prevention and restoration of lactacystin-induced nigrostriatal dopamine neuron degeneration by novel brain-permeable iron chelators. *Faseb J*, Vol. 21, No. 14, 3835-44

9

# Quantitative Morphometric Analysis of Liver Biopsy: Problems and Perspectives

Tokin Ivan B.[1], Tokin Ivan I.[2] and Filimonova Galina F.[1]
[1]*St.-Petersburg State University,*
[2]*St.-Petersburg State Medical Academy,*
*Russia*

## 1. Introduction

The liver biopsy has long been the gold standard for the evaluation of the state of liver diseases in patients, especially in chronic hepatitis. Hepatic fibrosis plays the most important role in the evolutionary process from chronic hepatitis to cirrhosis. Therefore, accurate assessment of the degree of hepatic fibrosis in chronic viral hepatitis is important to understand not only the clinical condition and prognosis of patients, but also the natural history of hepatitis. Information on a stage of chronic viral hepatitis C is essential to make prognosis and decide antiviral treatment. Semi quantitative scoring systems have been used in most studies that have relied upon liver biopsy to evaluate changes in fibrosis (Knodell et al., 1981, Desmet et al., 1994, Chevallier et al., 1994, French METAVIR, 1994, Ishak et al. 1995). Comparative characteristic of different scoring systems is presented by Brunt (2000) and Goodman (2007). However, these methods cannot completely avoid the observer's bias. Recent studies have reported that the estimation of fibrosis by semi quantitative scoring system is not always accurate and high rate of inter- and intraobsrever discrepancies takes place (Scheurer, 2003). The alternative to semi quantitative fibrosis scores is direct measurement of the amount of fibrosis, or necroinflammatory lesions, or portal zones in the biopsy by computer-assisted morphometric image analysis (O'Brien et al., 2000), or stereological morphometric analysis (Filimonova et al., 2010). Cell population analysis gives additional information about structure of parenchyma elements (liver plates and sinusoids).

## 2. Patients and methods

### 2.1 Patients

The different groups of patients with chronic viral hepatitis C (HCV) and chronic viral hepatitis B (HBV) were investigated. The patients with weak, moderate and expressed degree of fibrosis according to Ishak (Ishak et al., 1995) and METAVIR group classification (French METAVIR, 1994) participated. The diagnosis of chronic HCV or chronic HBV was established after careful examination of patients: the anamneses of diseases and life, laboratory analyses, virological and morphological studies. Serum level of ALT was expressed. The upper limit of normal (ULN) was 41 U/L for men and 31 U/L for women. The classification of chronic liver diseases, accepted by the International Congress of Gastroenterology (Los Angeles, 1994), was used during the formulation of the diagnosis.

## 2.2 Histological evaluation

All liver biopsies were performed according to the routine medical follow up program, using the standard Menghini procedure (Menghini, 1970, Mengini et al., 1975). Samples were formalin-fixed and paraffin-embedded. Serial paraffin sections were cut at 5 mcm. Criteria for adequacy of the biopsy specimens included a core length of 10 mm and at least 5-6 portal tracts. Hematoxylin-eosin stain was used. Each biopsy for necro-inflammatory activity and fibrosis was assessed by two hepatologists. For each biopsy specimen, a numerical score was established, both for the grading of necroinflammatory activity and to determine the stage of fibrosis. Knodel Histology Activity Index (HAI) was used to grade histopathological lesions (Knodell et al., 1981). HAI was graded according to 3 components: periportal inflammation with or without bridging necrosis (scale, 0-10), intralobular degeneration and focal necrosis (scale, 0-4), and portal inflammation (scale, 0-4). In accordance with the previously cited studies, the intensity of HAI was scaled as follows: A0 denoted no histological activity; A1, minimal activity (scale units, 1-3); A2, mild activity (scale units, 4-8); moderate activity (scale units, 9-12); and A4, severe activity (scale units, > 12). METAVIR group scoring system was used for detecting the stage of fibrosis (French METAVIR, 1994). Fibrosis was staged on a scale from F0 to F4, as follows: F0 = no fibrosis, F1 = portal fibrosis without septa, F2 = few septa, F3 = numerous septa without cirrhosis, and F4 = cirrhosis. None of the included patients showed any signs of cirrhosis.

## 2.3 Computer digital analysis

Fibrosis ratio for each liver biopsy specimen was calculated using an image analysis system consisting of a microscope (Leica DM 2500) with attached digital camera (Leica DFC 320 R2) and a computer. Serial pictures of biopsy slices of patients with HBV were photographed by light microscope and saved electronically. The further process was performed with the computer program Adobe Photoshop CS 4. Image was converted into a binary image. The two-dimensional patterns were measured by direct pixel counting on the binary images under a simultaneous visual control of light microscopy. The total area of serial sections was the sum of the area of all microscopic fields including parenchyma and non-parenchymal areas. Fibrosis in the space of Disse was not calculated. We considered that non-parenchymal elements included the sum of portal areas and intralobular infiltrates and necroses.

## 2.4 Stereometric analysis

The stereometric analysis is based on the determination methods of the specific volumes of different structure (Hamilton and Allen, 1995). Samples of biopsy from the patients with HBV were investigated. The calculation was carried out using the standard graticule (400 squares). Morphometry was applicated on counting the points or intersections in the field of microscope at the magnification of x400. The field of vision of microscope at the magnification of x400 as a standard unit was accepted. In each field of sight a quantity of intersections of non-parenchymal liver structure - portal tracts, with nearby piecemeal and bridging necroses, venous vessels and intralobular necroses - were calculated. Other liver structures were studied together with parenchyma (liver plates and sinusoids). The measurement of portions (percentage) of portal areas, foci of intralobular necroses and vessels was estimated. The total area of the sections was the sum of the area of all microscopic fields including parenchyma and non-parenchymal elements. Fibrosis in the space of Disse was not evaluated.

### 2.5 Cell population analysis

The comparative investigation was performed at the samples of biopsy from the patients with both chronic hepatitis, HCV and HBV. Proportion between the portion of the area occupated with liver plates and intralobular sinusoids was detected by stereometric morphometric analysis. The number of lytic necroses of hepatocytes, binucleate hepatocytes and polymorphous hepatocytes with large nuclei was calculated in composition of liver plates. The number of Kupffer cells and endoteliocytes was determined in composition of sinusoids. Calculation was performed in the standard field of vision of microscope at the magnification x400 in region of middle zone of liver lobule. Twenty standard fields of vision were investigated for each biopsy.

### 2.6 Statistical analysis

Variables, differing significantly according to the quantity of non-parencymal elements in the estimation group were identified by univariate analysis. Therefore, all variates were included in a multivariate forward stepwise regression analysis to determine the morphometric data. Pearson and Spearman correlation coefficients were used to evaluate whether changes in morphometric data were correlated with ALT. Student and Satterwhite criterions, Pearson and Spearman correlation coefficients were used to evaluate the structure of population. Statistical analysis was performed by tabulated processor Microsoft Excel 2003 and STATISTIKA 9.0.

## 3. Results

### 3.1 Quantitative image analysis for evaluation of pathological changes in liver structure

A biopsy is an important key factor for the prediction and tactics of treatment of patients with chronic viral hepatitis (Friedman, 2003, Friedman et al., 2007). Numerical fibrosis scoring systems (Knodell et al., 1981, French METAVIR, 1994, Ishak et al., 1995, Brunt, 2000) are usually used to assess the degree of activity and fibrosis stage. These systems are semi quantitative: the assessment of inflammatory, degenerative and fibrotic changes is determined in scale units. Many investigators recognize that there may be purely subjective error in numeral fibrosis scoring. Thus, the variability of fibrosis staged is estimated at 20% (Friedman, 2003). It is believed that the more indicators are presented in a given system, the more misunderstandings can occur.

Consequently, the assessment activity and the stage of process were usually performed by two independent experts. However, correct assessment of the degree of liver damage at the time of initial biopsy is extremely important for a treating physician. Thus, it effects the choice of treatment (antiviral or symptomatic treatment) and the ability to forecast progression of fibrosis.

Recently the computer morphometry has been used to assess the stage of fibrosis (Manabe et al., 1993; Chevallier et al., 1994; Kage et al., 1997; Pilette et al., 1998; Duchatelle et al., 1998; Masserolli et al., 2000; O'Brien et al., 2000). Chevallier et al. (1994) compared the computerized fibrosis ratio with a detailed subjective scoring system. That incorporated evaluation of central veins, pericellular fibrosis, portal tracts, and the number and width of septa in patients with chronic liver diseases. Duchatelle et al. (1998) used computerized image analysis to measure liver fibrosis in groups of patients with chronic hepatitis C treated with interferon alfa. Significant correlation was observed between evaluations of fibrosis degree using two methods: a semi quantitative method with a staging scoring system and a computed image system (Kage et al., 1997).

Pilette et al. (1998) compared fibrosis ratios and subjective scores (METAVIR) in series of patients with chronic liver disease in a study of the validity of serum markers of fibrosis. The area of fibrosis, as determined by image analysis and the semi quantitative score was well correlated. However, for serum markers the correlation was higher with the area of fibrosis than with the semi quantitative score. Authors supposed that such characteristics as reproducibility, rapidity, simplicity, adaptability, and exhaustiveness also favored image analysis.

O'Brien et al. (2000) found an overall statistically significant correlation between fibrosis ratio and ordinal score, but subset analysis showed that this correlation was restricted to biopsy specimens with high scores (3-6, early bridging fibrosis to established cirrhosis). The fibrosis ratio was the total area of fibrosis divided by the total area of the section. Authors found that the fibrosis ratio of liver biopsy specimens calculated by digital image analysis was not always reflecting fibrosis in chronic hepatitis as indicated by subjective scoring classifications. This applied particularly to livers that were normal or in early fibrosis (stage 0-2).

Masserolli et al. (2000) described the design and validation of an original image analysis-based application, FibroQuant, for automatically and rapidly quantifying perisinusoidal, perivenular and portalperiportal and septal fibrosis in liver histological specimens. Sometime morphometric image analysis was used for evaluation of fibrosis progression (Goodman et al., 2007, 2009). Morphometry demonstrated complex, non-linear changes in fibrosis over time in heterogenous cohort of patients with interferon-refractory chronic hepatitis C (Goodman et al., 2009).

The purpose of this study was to explore the possibilities of using computer morphometry for quantitative assessment of histological parameters biopsies of patients with chronic hepatitis B. The group of patients with minimal, mild, moderate and severe activity, but without cirrhosis was studied. Two major indicators were selected for evaluation: the portal area or its fragments and intralobular infiltrates.

According to portal areas we calculated next variants:

- portal area without changes;
- expansion of portal area without damages of limiting plate;
- portal area with damage of limiting plate and development of short septa;
- portal area with damage of limiting plate and development of piecemeal necroses;
- portal area with marked bridging necroses;
- portal area with extensive fibrosis changes;
- portal area with extensive lymphoid infiltration;
- occasional fibrosis septa.

Intralobular infiltrates were divided into 2 groups:

- lymphohistiocyte infiltrates;
- lymphohistiocyte infiltrates with damaged hepatocytes.

So, our calculation included the evaluation of not only fibrosis changes, but also inflammatory area in portal and intralobular zones.

Different morphological pictures of samples of biopsy from patients with chronic viral hepatitis B are presented at Figures 1 - 4.

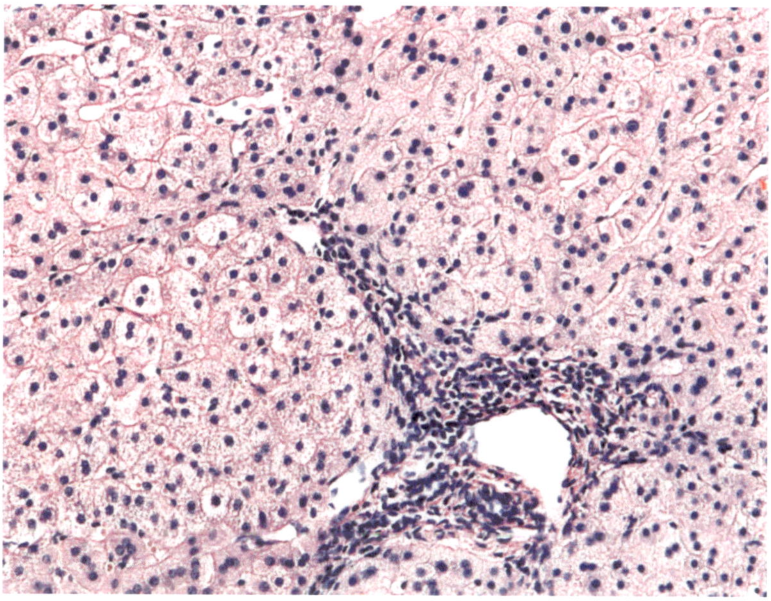

Fig. 1. Section of the liver biopsy specimen of patient with chronic hepatitis B. Portal area with damage of limiting plate and development of short septa. Hematoxylin-eosin. Obj.x20

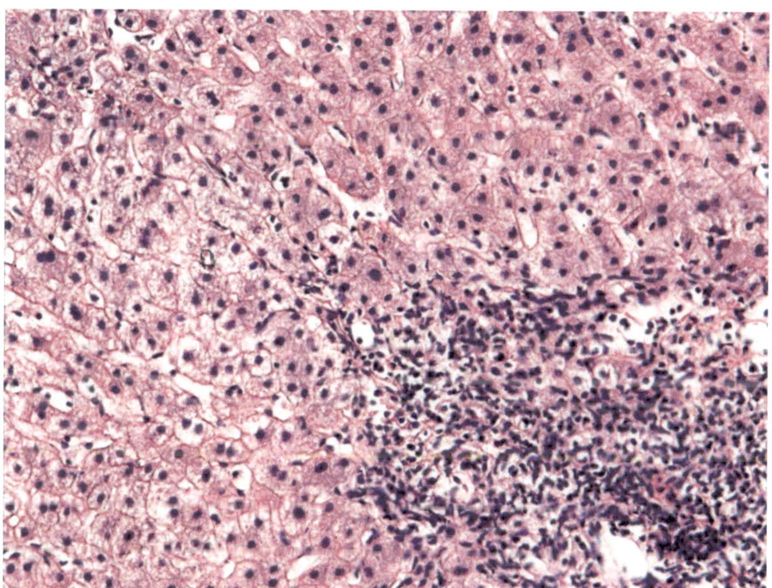

Fig. 2. Section of the liver biopsy specimen of patient with chronic hepatitis B. Portal tract with damage of limiting plate and development of piecemeal necroses (interface hepatitis). Hematoxylin-eosin. Obj.x20

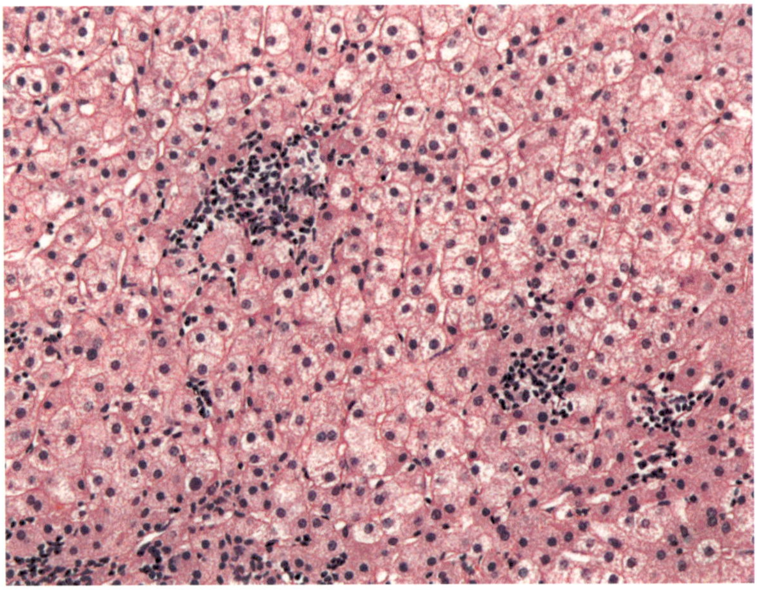

Fig. 3. Section of the liver biopsy specimen of a patient with chronic hepatitis B. Focal intralobular necroses in the middle zone of liver lobule. Hematoxylin-eosin. Obj.x20

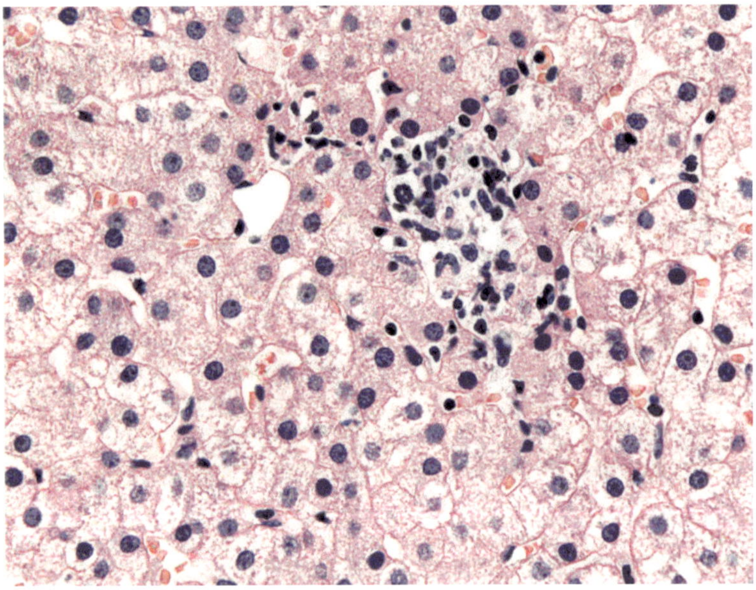

Fig. 4. Section of the liver biopsy specimen of a patient with chronic hepatitis B. Intralobular necrosis of hepatocytes with participation of lymphoid infiltration. Hematoxylin-eosin. Obj.x40

The special panoramic application of biopsy samples was performed by Photoshop CS4 program for computer analysis (Figure 5). This program allows you to connect serial micrographs of biopsy and get a computer image of the whole biopsy.

The program gives the possibility to unite serial micrographs of the single biopsy sections and create computer image of the total biopsy. The pixel count performs on the total square of the biopsy after the computer montage of individual micrographs. The squares of portal zones and intralobular infiltrates in pixels were determined separately, after that the special parts (percentage) of these components were counted. Further, after identification the areas of portal zones and intralobular infiltrates are calculated in pixels and transformed into percentage. The data obtained are summarized in Table 1.

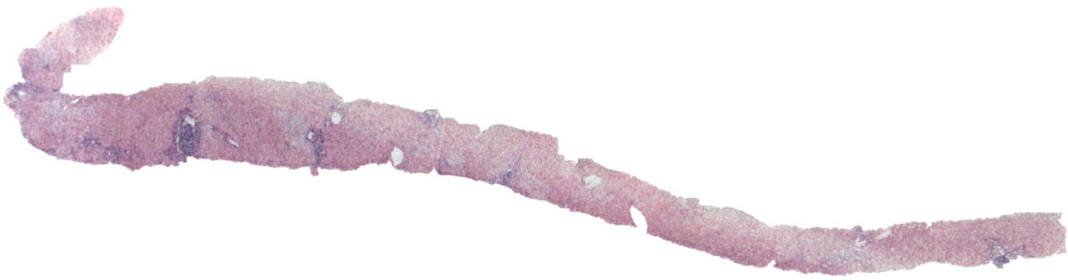

Fig. 5. General picture of liver biopsy composed by computer microscopy (Obj.x20) using Adobe Photoshop CS4. This picture contains 142 standard computer microphotographs of biopsy. Total area of biopsy is 327342640 in pixels

| Biopsy number | Total area of biopsy (in pixels) | Total area of parenchyma, % | Total area of non-parenchymal elements, % | Total area of portal zones and septa, % | Total area of intralobular necroses, % |
|---|---|---|---|---|---|
| 1 | 126077500 | 99.05 | 0.95 | 0.65 | 0.3 |
| 2 | 151379671 | 98.50 | 1.50 | 1.32 | 0.18 |
| 3 | 63388283 | 98.35 | 1.65 | 1.22 | 0.43 |
| 4 | 80293713 | 98.24 | 1.76 | 1.59 | 0.17 |
| 5 | 88550390 | 97.65 | 2.35 | 2.20 | 0.15 |
| 6 | 127210818 | 97.63 | 2.37 | 2.13 | 0.24 |
| 7 | 257720901 | 97.50 | 2.50 | 2.14 | 0.36 |
| 8 | 99280000 | 97.05 | 2.95 | 2.77 | 0.18 |
| 9 | 62243476 | 95.81 | 4.19 | 3.03 | 1.16 |
| 10 | 96036721 | 95.13 | 4.87 | 4.45 | 0.42 |
| 11 | 327342640 | 88.85 | 11.15 | 9.75 | 1.40 |

Table 1. Computer morphometric analysis of the total area of parenchymal and non-parenchymal elements of liver biopsy in percents and total area of biopsy in chronic hepatitis B. The samples of biopsies are arranged in sequence of increasing of non-parenchymal elements independently from biopsy sizes

This study focuses on the consideration of parameters of liver non-parenchymal elements, which includes all types of portal zones (Figures 1 and 2) and different variants of intralobular infiltrates and necroses (Figures 3 and 4). Liver plates and sinusoids were attributed to the hepatic parenchyma. As can be seen from the Table 1, the total area of the samples of biopsies is variable. Thus, the maximum biopsy size in pixels was 327324640, whereas the minimum - only 6224347 pixels. It is already possible to determine the suitability of a biopsy for further work at this stage. The absolute value of the area of any structures (in pixels) depends on the size of biopsy. Therefore, we have calculated the percentage of these structures.

Computer morphometric analysis discovered that the portions of the area of non-parenchymal elements of different biopsies of patients with HBV strongly varied from 0.95% to 11.5%. The area portions of the portal zones varied from 0.65% to 9.75%. Both indexes increased in biopsies of given group unidirectional and linearly. Intralobular necroses presented in all biopsies. Their specific parts varied from 0.15 % to 1.40 %. At the same time the percentage part of intralobular necroses did not depend on the indexes of percentage parts of portal zones. We supposed that separate quantitative evaluation of portal zones and intralobular necroses could be useful to indicate the severity and the progression of chronic hepatitis.

### 3.2 Histological evaluation of liver biopsies by stereometric analysis

The application of computer morphometry is not always possible, because it demands the complex expensive equipment (microscope, digital video camera and computer).

Nevertheless, the quantitative value of fibrosis development in liver is possible without using such complex equipment. In this case, usual light microscope may be effectively used for stereometric analysis (Filimonova et al., 2010).

We used this method for quantitative study of liver biopsies of patients with chronic viral hepatitis B. Information about the special group of patients selected for stereometric analysis is given in the Table 2.

| | |
|---|---|
| Age (years) | 20 ±1,3 |
| Sex | male |
| Duration of hospitalization (days) | 13,5±2,6 |
| Duration of infection (years) | 9,5±2,5 |
| Initial ALT | 371,5±277 |
| Initial bilirubin | 30,7±14,2 |
| Drug user | 1 person (10%) |

Table 2. Characteristics of patients with chronic hepatitis B

The morphological investigation of liver biopsies of the patients of this group found the presence of some essential changes, such as moderate fibrosis, expansion of a part of portal zones, increasing of the numbers of the cells with vacuolated nuclei, the appearance of the intralobular infiltrates, dilatation of portal veins, pronounced polymorphism of the hepatocytes and its nuclei.

Morphometric analysis was used to study three indexes: determination of the area of portal zones, focal infiltrates, terminal hepatic venules and sublobular veins. At first we determined for each case the portion of selected indexes (in points of intersections), and then calculated the corresponding parts (in percentage) of the parenchyma, portal zones, focal infiltrates and vessels taken over the standard unit of microscopic fields (Table 3).

The sum of the area of portal zones, focal infiltrates and vessels was referred to non-parenchymal elements. The results of analysis are placed in the Tables in the sequence of increasing part of the non-parenchymal elements in the biopsy.

The amount of the fields of view of biopsies of patients with HBV varied from 141 to 350 i.e. was 228.3±23.55 on the average. The sum amount of intersections by morphometric analysis varied from 43710 to 108500 number of points i.e. was 70773±7301.51 on the average.
The part of the non-parenchymal elements in liver biopsies of patients with chronic HBV varied from 2.39% to 12.46% (Table 3), but was essentially lower than in liver biopsies of patients with chronic HCV (Filimonova et al., 2010). The specific part of non-parenchymal elements did not exceed 4.62% in total, these indexes were essentially higher only from biopsies of two patients (8.41% и 12.46%, respectively).

| Biopsy number | ALT | Total area of morphometry (points of intersections) | Parenchymal elements, % | Non-parenchymal elements, % | Portal zones, % | Focal intralobular infiltrates, % | Hepatic veins, % |
|---|---|---|---|---|---|---|---|
| 1 | 45 | 90520 | 97,61 | 2,39 | 1,39 | 0,25 | 0,75 |
| 2 | 16 | 92380 | 97,24 | 2,76 | 1,25 | 0,19 | 1,33 |
| 3 | 89 | 56420 | 97,22 | 2,78 | 1,09 | 0,66 | 1,04 |
| 4 | 71 | 108500 | 97,18 | 2,82 | 1,54 | 0,99 | 0,30 |
| 5 | 29 | 66960 | 97,14 | 2,86 | 1,64 | 0,13 | 1,10 |
| 6 | 15 | 43710 | 96,76 | 3,24 | 2,33 | 0,13 | 0,78 |
| 7 | 414 | 49290 | 9568 | 4,32 | 2,87 | 0,07 | 1,38 |
| 8 | 41 | 89590 | 95,38 | 4,62 | 2,79 | 0,08 | 1,75 |
| 9 | - | 43710 | 91,59 | 8,41 | 7,59 | 0,24 | 0,58 |
| 10 | 2842 | 66650 | 87,54 | 12,46 | 10,98 | 1,05 | 0,43 |

Table 3. Quantitative characteristic of liver biopsies of the patients with chronic hepatitis B according to morphometric analysis

The mean value of the non-parenchymal elements in liver biopsies of the patients of this group was 4.66%; the correlation of the portion of the non-parenchymal elements with the level of the ALT was less obvious than in chronic HCV (Filimonova et al., 2010). The high level of the ALT (2842 U/L) was observed only by maximal increasing of the specific part of the non-parenchymal elements (up to 12.46%).

| Biopsy number | Total area of portal zones (points of intersections) | Area of portal zones, % | Number of portal zones in biopsy | Maximal area of portal zone (points of intersections) | Maximal area of portal zone at single microscopic fields, % |
|---|---|---|---|---|---|
| 1 | 1262 | 1,39 | 16 | 236 | 76,13 |
| 2 | 1152 | 1,25 | 32 | 83 | 26,78 |
| 3 | 616 | 1,09 | 17 | 71 | 22,90 |
| 4 | 1674 | 1,54 | 48 | 110 | 35,48 |
| 5 | 1098 | 1,64 | 20 | 212 | 68,39 |
| 6 | 1017 | 2,33 | 30 | 99 | 31,94 |
| 7 | 1415 | 2,87 | 20 | 376 | 121,29 |
| 8 | 2497 | 2,79 | 39 | 335 | 108,06 |
| 9 | 3316 | 7,59 | 21 | 439 | 141,61 |
| 10 | 7319 | 10,98 | 42 | 532 | 171,61 |

Table 4. Quantitative characteristic of portal zones of liver biopsies of the patients with chronic hepatitis B according to morphometric analysis

The specific part of the portal zones (Table 4) of the liver of the most patients varies from 1.09% to 2.87%, these indexes were essentially higher only from biopsies of two patients (7.59% и 10.98%, respectively). The mean value of specific part of the portal zones varies from 33.9 points to 78.8 points in general, i.e. it occupies from 11% to 25% of the standard sight of view. Maximal areas of portal zones varied from 22.9% till 171, 61% (or from 71 till 532 points respectively) at single microscopic field (Table 4). The portal tracts of two patients with expressed activity of the process of the disease were increased to 157.9 and 174.26 points; it was corresponded with the 51% and 56% of the square of the standard field of the microscope view. The focal interlobular infiltrates were observed in liver of all the patients (Tables 3 and 5).

| Biopsy number | Small focal infiltrates | Large focal infiltrates | Total number of infiltrates |
|---|---|---|---|
| 1 | 6 | 6 | 12 |
| 2 | 5 | 5 | 10 |
| 3 | 6 | 15 | 21 |
| 4 | 15 | 24 | 39 |
| 5 | 5 | 4 | 9 |
| 6 | 9 | 4 | 13 |
| 7 | 1 | 3 | 4 |
| 8 | 2 | 2 | 4 |
| 9 | 3 | 9 | 12 |
| 10 | 6 | 24 | 30 |

Table 5. The number of focal infiltrates at one standard square unit (100 fields of sight under the magnification ×400) in liver biopsies of patients with chronic hepatitis B

The specific part of focal infiltrates varied from 0.07% to 1.05%. Large focal infiltrates predominated in liver of approximately the half of the patients (Table 5). It is characteristic that the specific part of focal infiltrates did not depend on the specific part of non-parenchymal elements and did not correlate with ALT level. The amount of focal necroses (15.4±3.6) in liver of these patients in 100 standard fields of the microscope view was two times less than in liver of patients with hepatitis C (29.6±5.2) (Filimonova et al., 2010).

The specific square of hepatic veins varied from 0.30% to 1.75% and did not depend on the specific part of non-parenchymal elements (Table 3). The mean specific square of vessels varied from 16.05 to 56.67 points. The growth of the venules from the portal tracts occurred often in liver of the majority of patients with chronic HBV.

On the whole the inflammation-necrotic changes in liver of the given selected group of the patients were manifested weakly; fibrosis indexes did not exceed F0 and F1, both in the METAVIR system and Ishak system. Bridging and piecemeal necroses presented in liver of only two patients (№ 7 and № 10), both of them had the high ALT index and strongly enlarged the specific part of non-parenchymal elements.

So the morphometric calculation of the non-parenchymal elements in liver biopsies of patients with HBV allows giving the complex evaluation of the replacement level of functional parenchyma by necro-inflammatory and fibrosis structures.

Stereological quantitative morphometry allows to getting more correct evaluation of some morphological parameters of pathologically changed liver in patients with chronic viral hepatitis. It is very important for establishment of either positive of negative dynamic changes in liver, especially during estimation of efficiency of antiviral treatment. We supposed that the stereological morphometry is a suitable tool for quantitative evaluation of liver biopsies in therapeutics trials.

### 3.3 Cell population structure of liver biopsies from the patients with both chronic hepatitis, HCV and HBV

Only sufficiently large biopsies with 5-6 portal zones can be suitable for quantitative evaluation of parenchymal elements of liver by methods of stereological or computer morphometry. Nevertheless, biopsies used have frequently small sizes or consist of fine fragments without portal zones in clinical practice. Quantitative analysis of parenchyma elements (liver plates and sinusoids cells) is advisable in these cases.

In our investigation the cell population analysis of liver biopsies from the patients with both chronic hepatitis, HCV and HBV included the comparative evaluation of the specific part of non-parenchymal elements, analysis of the liver plates and sinusoids areas, cell population of liver plates and sinusoids.

#### 3.3.1 Comparative analysis of the specific part of non-parenchymal elements

The specific part of non-parenchymal elements in liver biopsies of patients with HCV (Table 6) strongly varies: from 2.16% to11.93% (mean value is 6.9 ± 0.8%).

| Biopsy number | Non-parenchymal elements, % | Liver plates, % | Sinusoids, % | Lytic necroses of hepatocytes | Binucleate hepatocytes | Polymorphous hepatocytes | Endotheliocytes | Kupffer cells |
|---|---|---|---|---|---|---|---|---|
| 1 | 2,16 | 96,77 | 3,23 | 2,70 | 0,90 | 0,40 | 5,80 | 11,10 |
| 2 | 2,46 | 92,68 | 7,32 | 1,60 | 2,40 | 0,90 | 7,30 | 6,90 |
| 3 | 3,6 | 94,23 | 5,77 | 3,80 | 2,70 | 0,60 | 8,00 | 9,10 |
| 4 | 4,3 | 95,10 | 4,90 | 3,50 | 1,00 | 1,30 | 7,20 | 5,30 |
| 5 | 4,63 | 94,90 | 5,10 | 4,60 | 1,50 | 0,80 | 10,20 | 10,90 |
| 6 | 4,7 | 93,74 | 6,26 | 2,80 | 0,30 | 0,00 | 8,90 | 6,90 |
| 7 | 5,06 | 95,42 | 4,58 | 5,70 | 1,30 | 0,10 | 12,00 | 6,90 |
| 8 | 5,18 | 93,32 | 6,68 | 2,60 | 0,30 | 0,10 | 7,60 | 10,70 |
| 9 | 6,64 | 93,55 | 6,45 | 5,20 | 0,30 | 0,50 | 7,70 | 9,80 |
| 10 | 9,46 | 94,68 | 5,32 | 4,40 | 1,70 | 0,80 | 12,80 | 15,80 |
| 11 | 9,68 | 94,35 | 5,65 | 5,70 | 0,50 | 0,70 | 9,90 | 8,80 |
| 12 | 10,56 | 92,16 | 7,84 | 4,60 | 1,10 | 0,90 | 11,30 | 12,00 |
| 13 | 10,89 | 94,94 | 5,06 | 5,50 | 1,30 | 0,00 | 7,20 | 7,00 |
| 14 | 11,76 | 93,00 | 7,00 | 3,80 | 2,70 | 1,90 | 9,70 | 14,00 |
| 15 | 11,93 | 92,87 | 7,13 | 3,10 | 0,90 | 0,60 | 10,40 | 9,20 |

Table 6. Cell population structure of liver plates and sinusoids in patients with chronic hepatitis C

The piecemeal and bridging necroses are presented, as a rule, in liver biopsies of the patients with high index of non-parenchymal elements. The piecemeal necroses are described in 11 cases from 15, bridging necroses in 7 cases from 15. Such distribution shows that during the ordinary course of the disease the piecemeal necroses arise from the beginning, the bridging necroses are discovered later.

The specific part of non-parenchymal elements changes from 2.39% to 8.41% (mean value is 3.8 ± 0.9) in liver biopsies of patients with HBV (Table 7). The piecemeal necroses were observed only in one biopsy, the bridging necroses in two biopsies.

The data regarding the specific parts of non-parenchymal elements shows that liver damages of patients with HCV are more significant in comparison with the analogical indexes of patients with HBV.

| Biopsy number | Non- paren-chymal elements, % | Liver plates, % | Sinusoids, % | Lytic necroses of hepatocytes | Binucleate hepatocytes | Poly-morphous hepato-cytes | Endothelio-cytes | Kupffer cells |
|---|---|---|---|---|---|---|---|---|
| 1 | 2,39 | 91,65 | 8,35 | 6,75 | 1,00 | 1,00 | 6,25 | 7,15 |
| 2 | 2,76 | 91,81 | 8,19 | 5,35 | 3,85 | 2,15 | 5,50 | 8,40 |
| 3 | 2,78 | 93,29 | 6,71 | 2,05 | 1,80 | 1,15 | 8,05 | 8,45 |
| 4 | 2,82 | 93,65 | 6,35 | 3,70 | 0,85 | 0,90 | 6,90 | 6,10 |
| 5 | 2,86 | 85,77 | 14,23 | 1,30 | 4,10 | 2,35 | 7,35 | 6,15 |
| 6 | 3,24 | 91,16 | 8,84 | 5,70 | 1,20 | 1,20 | 5,10 | 5,15 |
| 7 | 4,32 | 93,87 | 6,13 | 4,91 | 1,36 | 0,91 | 8,64 | 5,73 |
| 8 | 4,62 | 91,39 | 8,61 | 3,20 | 1,95 | 1,60 | 8,30 | 6,50 |
| 9 | 8,41 | 86,26 | 13,74 | 3,55 | 4,90 | 1,70 | 8,45 | 8,40 |

Table 7. Cell population structure of liver plates and sinusoids in patients with chronic hepatitis B

### 3.3.2 Analysis of the liver plates and sinusoids

Morphometric investigation shows that the specific parts of liver plates of patients with HCV slightly vary from 92.16% to 96.77% (mean value is 94.1±0.31). The specific parts of sinusoids vary from 3.23% to 7.84% (mean value is 5.9±0.4). Such variations are more significant in livers of patients with HBV. The specific parts of liver plates in this case vary from 85.77% to 93.87% (mean value is 90.98±0.32), the specific parts of sinusoids vary from 6.13% to 14.23% (mean value is 9.02±0.32). Morphological and morphometric studies show (Figures 6 and 7; Tables 6 and 7) that the sinusoids of liver biopsies of patients with HCV are significantly narrowed than such of patients with HBV. Respectively the conditions of intralobular blood circulation are significantly differ under various types of hepatitis.

Thus, the connection between the disease severity and specific parts of liver plates and sinusoids are not established.

### 3.3.3 Cell population of liver plates

In liver biopsies of patients with chronic HCV (Table 6) the amount of lost hepatocytes (lytic necroses) in liver plates varies from 1.6% to 5.7% in standard field of vision (mean value is

3.97±04). The number of binucleate hepatocytes varies from 0.3 to 2.7 (mean value is 1.26±0.2). The number of polymorphous hepatocytes in standard field of vision varies from 0.0 to 1.9 (mean value 0.64±0.1).

In liver biopsies of patients with HBV (Table 7) the amount of lost cells varies from 1.3 to 6.75 (mean value is 4.06±0.59). The number of binucleate hepatocytes varies from 0.85 to 4.9 (mean value is 2.33±0.5). The number of polymorphous hepatocytes at standard field of vision varies from 0.9 to 2.35 (mean value is 1.44±0.3).

Thus, the amount of single lytic necroses of hepatocytes does not differ in liver biopsies of patients with HBV and with HCV. At that time the number of binucleate hepatocytes and polymorphous hepatocytes is certainly higher in liver biopsies of patients with HBV. This situation may be connected with the different level of processes of regeneration.

### 3.3.4 Cell population of liver sinusoids

The amount of endotheliocytes in sinusoids of liver biopsies of patients with HCV (Table 6) strongly varies: from 5.8 to 12.8 cells in standard field of sight (mean value is 9.0±0.5). The amount of Kupffer cells is also significantly differing from 5.3 to 15.8 in the field of sight (main value is 9.6±0.7). Nevertheless, the precise linear dependence between the both of indexes is not revealing.

The amount of endotheliocytes in sinusoids of liver biopsies of patients with HBV (Table 7) weakly varies from 5.1 to 8.64 cells in standard field of sight (mean value is 7.17±0.13). The amount of Kupffer cells changes from 5.15 to 8.45 in the field of sight (mean value is 6.89±0.31).

Thus, the amount of endotheliocytes and Kupffer cells is essentially more in liver biopsies of patients with HCV. This circumstance is probably connected with the peculiarities of virus influence on the vessel component of liver parenchyma.

The cell population structure of liver biopsies of patients with HBV and HCV changes unequally. So, the using of Student and Satterwhite criteria allows discovering the statistically significant distinctions between mean values of all the indexes with the exception of the amount of lost hepatocytes in liver plates.

The coefficients of correlation between the indexes of specific parts of liver plates and the number of binucleate cells, between the indexes of specific parts of liver plates and the number of polymorphous cells are statistically significant for the cluster of liver biopsies of patients with HBV.

The statistically significant coefficients of correlation Pearson does not detected for the cluster of liver biopsies of patients with HCV.

The strong linear dependence between the indexes of specific parts of liver plates and the number of binucleate cells and the number of polymorphous cells was revealed in liver biopsies of patients with HBV.

The using of Spearmen coefficients of correlation allowed establishing the connection between the number of cells in sinusoids and the specific part of non-parenchymal elements in liver biopsies of patients with HBV. This circumstance could be used for indirect characteristics of the development of fibrotic changes in liver.

In total, the quantitative analysis of cell population structure in liver biopsies in the course of chronic hepatitis, especially in the case of defective biopsies, could be used for diagnostic and prognoses by expert evaluation.

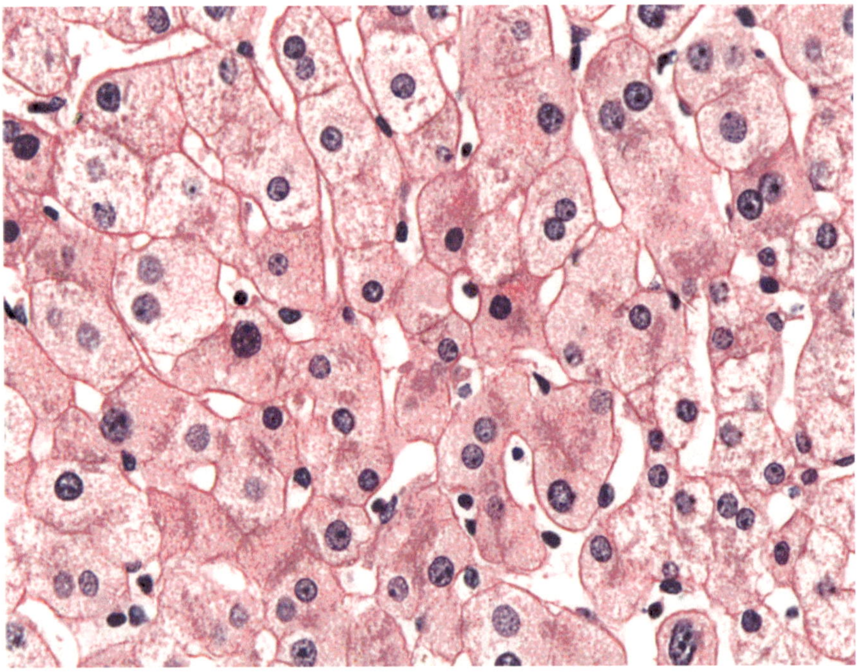

Fig. 6. The fragment of parenchyma with polymorphous hepatocytes and distorted sinusoids in liver of a patient with chronic hepatitis B. Hematoxylin-eosin. Obj.x40

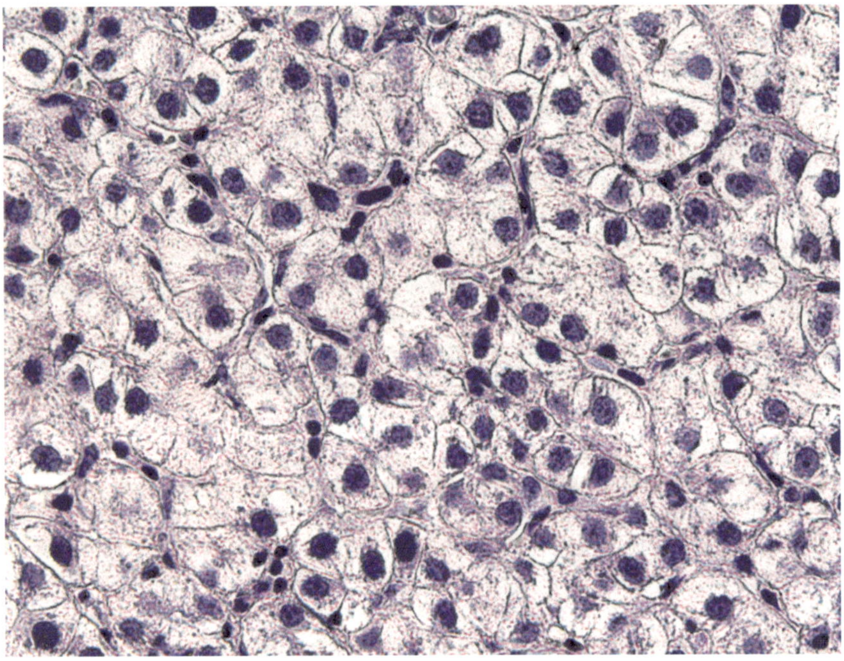

Fig. 7. The fragment of parenchyma with unimorphous hepatocytes and narrow sinusoids in liver of a patient with chronic hepatitis C. Alcian blue. Obj.x 40

## 4. Conclusion

Evaluation of fibrosis in liver biopsy remains as a point for the diagnosis, monitoring of disease prognosis, and response to treatment. Quantitative stereological and computer morphometric analysis as well as cell population analysis was used for more correct evaluation of dynamic of liver damages in patients with chronic hepatitis B and chronic hepatitis C.

Stereometric analysis of quantitative morphological changes in liver biopsies using conventional light microscopy yields good results. Especially effective is the application of quantitative analysis of elements in liver parenchyma (ratio between liver plates and sinusoids, counting the number of hepatocytes and sinusoidal cells in a standard field of view) for the analysis of non-standard biopsies (small size, fragmentation). These data are essential for predicting disease and an overall assessment of the liver in each case. However stereometric analysis is time consuming and requires special skills in work.

Colorimetric detection of zones of differential staining of collagen (Manabe et al., 1993; Duchatelle et al., 1998) or immunohistochemical markers of fibrogenesis (Kweon et al., 2001) with subsequent determination of the area of fibrosis in the percentage of the total field is commonly used in computer morphometry.

In our investigation the total registration of non-parenchymal elements in liver biopsies of patients with chronic viral hepatitis carried out using a special program that allowed quantifying the presence of fibrotic, inflammatory and necrotic changes in the liver.

It is particularly important to evaluate separately the number and the area of focal necroses, which characterize the activity of intralobular hepatocyte death. We believe that the increase of the area of non-parenchymal elements of liver demonstrates a degree of replacement of functioning parenchyma by inflammatory infiltrates, necroses and scars. Our studies show the advisability of separate accounting bridging necroses and septa, as this may serve as a prognostic sign of distortion of the architectonics of liver lobules, usually preceded by cirrhosis. In some biopsies we observed the early development of septa without noticeable changes in portal tracts. Computer and stereological morphometry can also registrate the degree of expansion of portal tracts.

Our research suggests that four percents or more increasing of the portion of portal zones area and increasing of specific parts of intralobular focal infiltrates are unfavorable factors for development of chronic liver diseases.

Thus, computer morphometry is a modern and reliable method for quantifying inflammatory, necrotic and fibrotic changes in liver biopsies of chronic diseases. At the same time this method requires the creation of a single algorithm to study the reproducibility and easy comparison of results obtained in different laboratories.

Some of the perspectives and problems of computer analysis of liver biopsies are summarized below.

Perspectives:

1. Computer microscopy and morphometry are ideal for digital archiving of samples of biopsies for comparison with repeated biopsies.
2. Quantitative information about the parameters of the biopsy improves the accuracy in diagnosing of disease and allows to optimize the treatment tactics and to adjust quickly the course of treatment.
3. Digital image of a biopsy can be sent by e-mail and be immediately consulted. It is also gives the possibility of participation of a large number of specialists for analysis of digital images biopsy in complicated cases, thus avoiding medical errors.

4. Quantitative analysis of digital images of biopsies is indispensable to study the effectiveness of testing new drugs developed by pharmaceutical companies. The effect can be calculated as a percentage.
5. Quantitative indicators of morphological parameters of biopsies may serve as a basis for developing mathematical models of the dynamics of chronic liver disease.

Problems:

1. It is necessary to work out some common standards of the quantitative computer evaluations of biopsy morphological changes, including the development of fibrosis. That will make possible the correct comparison of the results in different studies.
2. Comprehensive assessment and computer analysis of biopsies require the participation of medical specialists having the practice with chronic viral hepatitis patients and combining the ability to analyze the morphological changes in the liver with high skills as computer users.
3. A digital image of microscopic slides has a large amount of files (up to 2 - 3 gigabytes per biopsy), so high-power computers are necessary for the digital processing of biopsies.

## 5. References

Brunt, E. (2000). Grading and Staging the Histopathological Lesions of Chronic Hepatitis: The Knodell Histology Activity Index and Beyond. *Hepatology*. Vol.31, No.1, (January 2000), pp. 241-246, ISSN 0270-9139

Chevallier, M.; Guerrer, S.; Chossegros, P.; Gerard, F. & Grimaud, J. (1994). A Histological Semiquantitative Scoring System for Evaluation of Hepatic Fibrosis in Needle Liver Biopsy Specimens: Comparison with Morphometric Studies. *Hepatology*. Vol.20, No.2, (August 1994), pp. 349-355, ISSN 0270-9139

Desmet, V.; Gerber, M.; Hoofnagle, J.; Manns, M. & Sheuerr, P. (1994). Classification of Chronic Hepatitis: Diagnosis, Grading and Staging. *Hepatology*. Vol.19, No.6, (June 1994), pp. 1513-1520, ISSN 0270-9139

Duchatelle, V.; Marcellin, P.; Giostra, E.; Bregeaud, I.; Pouteau, M.; Boyer, N.; Auperin, A.; Guerret, S.; Erlinger, S.; Henin, D. & Degott, C. (1998). Changes in Liver Fibrosis at the End of Alpha Interferon Therapy and 6 to 18 Months later in Patients with Chronic Hepatitis C: Quantitative Assessment by a Morphometric Method. *Journal of Hepatology*. Vol.29, No.1, (July 1998), pp. 20-28, ISSN 0168-8278

Filimonova, G.; Tokin, I.I.; Tokin, I.B. & Hussar, P. (2010). An Assessment of Morphometric Analysis in Liver Biopsy Specimens of Patients with Chronic Hepatitis C. *Papers on Anthropology*. Tartu, Estonia. Vol. XIX, pp. 69-80, ISSN 1406-0140

French METAVIR Cooperative Study Group (1994). Intraobserver and Interobserver Variations in Liver Biopsy Interpretation in Patients with Chronic Hepatitis C. *Hepatology*. Vol.20, No.1, (July 1994), pp. 15-20, ISSN 0270-9139

Friedman, S. (2003). Liver Fibrosis – from Bench to Bedside. *Journal of Hepatology*. Vol. 38, Supplement 1, pp. S38 – S53, ISSN 0168-8278

Friedman, S.; Rockey, D. & Bissel D. (2007). Hepatic Fibrosis 2006: Report of the Third AASLD Single Topic Conference. *Hepatology*. Vol.45, No.1, (January 2007), pp. 242-249, ISSN 0270-9139

Goodman, Z. (2007). Grading and Staging System for Inflammation and Fibrosis in Chronic Liver Diseases. *Journal of Hepatology*. Vol.47, No.4, (August 2007), pp. 598-607, ISSN 0168-8278

Goodman, Z.; Becker, R.; Pockros, P. & Afdhal,N. (2007). Progression of Fibrosis in Advanced Chronic Hepatitis C: Evaluation by Morphometric Image Analysis. *Hepatology*. Vol.45, No.3, (September 2007), pp. 886-894, ISSN 0270-9139

Goodman, Z.; Stoddard, A.; Bonkovsky, H.; Fontana, R.; Ghany, M.; Morgan, T.; Wright, E.; Brunt, E.; Kleiner, D.; Shiffmann, M.; Everson, G.; Lindsay, K.; Dienstag, J.; Morishimo, C. & the HALT-C Trial Group. (2009). Fibrosis Progression in Chronic Hepatitis C: Morphometric Image Analysis in the HALT-C Trial. *Hepatology*. Vol.50, No.6, (December 2009), pp. 1738-1749, ISSN 0270-9139

Hamilton, P. & Allen, D. (1995). Morphometry in Histopathology. *Journal of Pathology*. Vol.175, No.4, (April 1995), pp. 369-379, ISSN 0022-3417

Ishak, K.; Baptista, A.; Bianchi, L.; Callea, F.; De Groote, J.; Gudat, F.; Denk, H.; Desmet, V.; Korb, G.; MacSween, R.; Phillips, M.; Portmann, B.; Poulsen, H.; Sheuer, P.; Schmid, M. & Thaler, H. (1995). Histological Grading and Staging of Chronic Hepatitis. *Journal of Hepatology*. Vol.22, No.6, (June 1995), pp. 696-699, ISSN 0168-8278

Kage, M.; Shimamatu, K.; Nakashima, E.; Kojiro, M.; Inoue, O. & Yano M. (1997). Long-Term Evolution of Fibrosis from Chronic Hepatitis to Cirrhosis in Patients with Hepatitis C: Morphometric Analysis of Repeated Biopsies. *Hepatology*. Vol.25, No.4, (April 1997), pp.1028-1031, ISSN 0270-9139

Knodell, R.; Ishak, K.; Bkack, W.; Chen, T.; Craig, R.; Kaplowitz, N.; Kiernan, T. & Wollman, J. (1981). Formulation and Application of a Numerical Scoring System for Assessing Histological Activity in Asymptomatic Chronic Active Hepatitis. *Hepatology*. Vol.1, No.5, (September/October 1981), pp. 431-435. ISSN 0270-9139

Kweon, Y.; Goodman, Z.; Dienstag, J.; Schiff, E.; Brown, N,; Burkhandt, E.; Schoonhoven, R.; Brenner, D. & Fried, M. (2001). Decreasing Fibrogenesis: An Immunohistochemical Study of Paired Liver Biopsies Following Lamivudin Therapy for Chronic Hepatitis B. *Journal of Hepatology*. Vol.35, No.6, (December 2001), pp. 749-755, ISSN 0168-8278

Manabe, N.; Chevallier, M., Chossegross, P., Causse, X.; Guerret, S. & Trepo Grimaud J. (1993). Interferon-alpha 2b Therapy Reduces Liver Fibrosis in Chronic A, Non-B hepatitis: A Quantitative Histological Evaluation. *Hepatology*. Vol.18, No.6 (December 1993), pp. 1344-1349, ISSN 0270-9139

Masserolli, M.; Caballero, T.; O'Valle, F.; Del Moral, R.M.G; Perez-Milena, A. & DelMoral R.G. (2000). Automatic Quantification of Liver Fibrosis: Design and Validation of a New Image Analysis Method: Comparison with Semi-quantitative Indexes of Fibrosis. *Journal of Hepatology*. Vol.32. No.3, (March 2000), pp.453-464, ISSN 0168-8278

Menghini, G. (1958). One-second Needle Biopsy of the Liver. *Gastroenterology*. Vol. 35, No.2, (August 1958), pp.190-199

Menghini, G.; Lauro, G. & Caraseni, M. (1975). Some Innovations in the Technic of the One second Needle Biopsy of the Liver. *American Journal of Gastroenterology*. Vol.64, No.3, (September 1975), pp.175-180, ISSN 0002-9270

O'Brien, M.; Keating, N.; Elderiny, S.; Cerda, C.; Keaveny, A.; Afdhal, N. & Nunes D. (2000). An Assessment of Digital Image Analysis to Measure Fibrosis in Liver Biopsy

Specimens of Patients with Chronic Hepatitis C. *American Journal of Clinical Pathology*. Vol.114, No.5, (November 2000), pp.712-718, ISSN 0002-9173

Pilettte, C.; Rousselet, M.; Chappard, D.; Oberti, F.; Riffet, H.; Maiga, M.; Gallois, Y. & Cales, P. (1998). Histopathological Evaluationof Liver Fibrosis: Quantitative Analysis vs Semi-quantitative Scores. Comparison with Serum Markers. *Journal of Hepatology*, Vol.28, No.3, (October 1997), pp. 439-446, ISSN 0168-8278

Poynard,T.; Mathurin, P.; Ching-Lung Lai; Quyader, D.; Poupon, R.; Tainturier, M.-H.; Myers, R.; Muntenau, M.; Ratziu, V.; Manns, M.; Arndt, V.; Capron, F.; Chedid, A. & Bedossa, P. for the PANFIBROSIS Group. (2003). A Comparison of Fibrosis Progression in Chronic Liver Diseases. *Journal of Hepatology*. Vol.38, No.3, (September 2003), pp. 257-265, ISSN 0168-8278

Scheuer, P.J. (2003) Assessment of Liver Biopsies in Chronic Hepatitis: How is it Best Done? *Journal of Hepatology*. Vol.38, No.2, (February 2003), pp.240-242, ISSN 0168-8278

# 10

# Ishak *versus* METAVIR: Terminology, Convertibility and Correlation with Laboratory Changes in Chronic Hepatitis C

Gamal Shiha and Khaled Zalata
*Internal medicine department & pathology department, Mansoura faculty of medicine Egypt*

## 1. Introduction

Ishak (modified Knodell score) and METAVIR scores are the most widely accepted scoring systems for assessment of fibrosis and necroinflammation in dealing with chronic hepatitis C. In METAVIR, only interface hepatitis and lobular necrosis determine the grade of activity, while in Ishak, portal infiltrate and confluent necrosis are included with the two previous parameters. Confluent necrosis is very rare in chronic hepatitis C, that in most patients the actual score limit is 12 instead of 18 (Ishak score), that mostly underscore the actual necroinflammation. Also, portal inflammatory infiltrate may reflect immunological response rather than necroinflammation. This may explain the discrepancy between enzyme elevation and necroinflammatory score as determined by Ishak score (modified HAI) in assessment of chronic hepatitis C biopsy specimens. On the other hand, no study has clearly tested such discrepancy in applying METAVIR.

Some of the terminologies applied in METAVIR are in need of revision or declaration. For example; the term "septa" is used to mean actual fibrous bridges, while in Ishak score both terms; septa and bridges; are applied by different meaning. Ishak et al, 1995, in their system, applied both terminologies (septa & bridges), however in completely different meaning. Septa, means expansion of portal tract edges without formation of bridges or actual connection between portal areas or portal area and central vein **(1)**. On the other hand, the term bridge was applied to actual fibrous connection between two portal areas or portal area and central vein. Because of this confusion, some studies comparing both scoring systems have committed some mistakes.

Some studies have compared both Ishak and METAVIR systems, but they included small number of patients or included hepatitis B and hepatitis C. Therefore, the objectives of this chapter are:

- Revision of histological grading and staging in chronic hepatitis C.
- Clarification of the METAVIR terminology for future applications.
- Establishing an Ishak to METAVIR fibrosis score conversion table.

## 2. Histological grading and staging in chronic hepatitis C

The new approach to classify chronic hepatitis C involves three separate considerations. The first is a comment on etiology. Frequently, this cannot be determined on the basis of histological appearance alone, and the diagnosis is made on the basis of other laboratory investigations. The second assessment relates to the severity and distribution of necroinflammatory activity (histological "grade"). Thirdly, an attempt should be made to assess the degree of fibrosis (histological "stage") **(2)**.

## 3. Patterns of necroinflammatory activity

Inflammatory activity in the liver can be divided into two main components. The first involves portal tracts (portal hepatitis) with variable extension into the adjacent periportal regions (periportal hepatitis). The second involves liver parenchyma (lobular hepatitis). These different patterns of inflammation are probably related to the different pathways whereby circulating inflammatory cells can gain access to the liver **(3)**.

### 3.1 Portal / periportal hepatitis

Inflammatory cells migrating across the endothelium of portal vessels pass into portal connective tissue which is rich in antigen presenting dendritic cells. A predominantly portal inflammatory infiltrate is one of the characteristic histological features of chronic hepatitis. However it should kept in mind that portal hepatitis by itself does not necessarily indicate a diagnosis of chronic hepatitis. Mild portal inflammatory changes, indistinguishable from low-grade chronic viral hepatitis, can be seen in a variety of conditions including systemic illness, nearby space-occupying lesion and even in some livers, which otherwise would be considered as normal. Furthermore, a predominantly portal inflammatory infiltrate is sometimes present in cases of acute viral hepatitis, without any implication of chronicity **(4)**. Considerable attention has focused on the extension of portal inflammatory cells into the adjacent liver parenchyma associated with destruction of the limiting plate and damage to periportal hepatocytes (interface hepatitis) **(5)**.

### 3.2 Lobular hepatitis

Inflammatory cells migrating across the endothelium of hepatic sinusoids can gain direct access to the liver parenchyma causing lobular inflammation. Typically this presents as "spotty" inflammation dispersed randomly throughout the liver parenchyma. In some cases inflammatory changes are more pronounced in perivenular (acinar zone 3) region and are associated with areas of confluent necrosis. When areas of zone 3 necrosis link vascular structures, in particular portal tracts to hepatic venules, the term "bridging necrosis" is used. Rarely in severe cases, there may be complete destruction of hepatocytes in one or more acini (panacinar necrosis or multiacinar necrosis) **(6)**.

### 3.3 Functional significance of necroinflammatory activity

The main purpose in identifying different patterns of necroinflammatory activity is that these may have different functional and prognostic significance in terms of progression to fibrosis and ultimately cirrhosis.

Interface hepatitis has long been considered as an important lesion in the evolution of chronic hepatitis to cirrhosis. In the original classification proposed by De Groote et al, 1968 **(7)**, chronic persistent hepatitis (portal inflammation without piecemeal necrosis) was thought to have a favorable prognosis, whereas chronic active hepatitis (portal inflammation with piecemeal necrosis) was regarded as having substantial risk for progression to cirrhosis. Interface hepatitis with associated periportal liver cell loss and collapse of the reticulin framework can readily be visualized as a mechanism for the development of periportal fibrosis **(2)**.

There have been few attempts to validate this lesion as a prognostic feature in serial biopsies. One study showed that the presence of interface hepatitis in initial biopsies from patients with chronic hepatitis correlate with subsequent development of cirrhosis **(8)**. Two other studies have demonstrated an association between the severities of necroinflammatory activity (including interface hepatitis as a major component) in an initial biopsy and the development of fibrosis or cirrhosis in follow up biopsies **(9)**.

Bursts of lobular inflammatory activity are thought to be particularly important in pathogenesis of chronic hepatitis C infection, where progression to cirrhosis is common despite the lack of interface activity **(10)**. For these reasons it has been suggested that the pattern and severity of lobular inflammation should be taken in account in assessing the outcome in cases of chronic hepatitis **(11)**.

### 3.4 Assessment of hepatic fibrosis

In the majority of cases fibrosis begins as expansion of portal tracts occurring in association of interface hepatitis. As fibrosis progresses, there is formation of septa with the development of portal-portal linkage. Eventually hepatocyte nodules are completely surrounded by fibrous tissue. Development of established cirrhosis usually takes several years. However, in some situations (e.g. viral hepatitis recurring following liver transplantation) cirrhosis can develop much more quickly. Parenchymal fibrosis can also occur in presence of lobular inflammation, particularly in areas of bridging necrosis **(12)**. This may be responsible of for formation of portal-central septa, which have been regarded as more significant in the development of cirrhosis than portal-portal linkages **(13)**.

## 4. Historical perspectives: The terminology of chronic hepatitis

The work of the two decades preceding the Knodell HAI provided the foundation for our current understanding of the histopathology of chronic hepatitis. Early descriptions and classifications focused on differentiating acute and chronic hepatitis and on lesions that predicted disease progression. The first histological classification, which was published by De Groote in 1968 **(7)**, codified the terminology, ***chronic persistent*** and ***chronic aggressive*** hepatitis. Both conditions involved portal inflammation, but were distinguished by the severity of piecemeal necrosis, inflammation, and structural remodeling of the liver. Inflammatory activity was graded as moderate or severe, but exact criteria were not given. The classification system also incorporated the concept that chronic persistent hepatitis had a generally good prognosis whereas chronic aggressive hepatitis could evolve to cirrhosis **(7)**.

Popper and Schaffner (1971) **(14)** affirmed the value of liver biopsy for diagnosis and prognosis and recommended use of "topographic" descriptors for hepatitis, that is, ***chronic lobular, chronic portal***, or ***chronic periportal hepatitis***. The last of these, synonymous with chronic aggressive hepatitis, was believed to progress, whereas chronic portal hepatitis, synonymous with chronic persistent hepatitis, was considered a non-progressive process. ***Chronic lobular hepatitis*** was a term for histological findings similar to those of acute hepatitis, but with a clinical duration of more than 3 months. It was thought to be non-progressive except when seen in combination with chronic periportal hepatitis.

The explosion of scientific information on viral and non-viral hepatitis in the last decades of the 20th century led pathologists to question the conventional nomenclature of chronic persistent and chronic active (aggressive) hepatitis because of a growing understanding that etiology may be more significant than morphological classification in predicting the natural history of liver disease. This shift in thinking was driven largely by the apparent dissociation between the mild histology of non A-non B hepatitis (hepatitis C) and its progressive clinical course. It was found that, in many cases, the lesions of this form of viral hepatitis fell between those described as chronic persistent and chronic active hepatitis and could not be clearly categorized **(15)**.

The lack of severe piecemeal necrosis and confluent lobular necrosis resulted in the diagnosis of chronic persistent hepatitis, implying a benign course. At the same time, the lobular component was being recognized as more significant than portal lesions with respect to disease progression. Also, confluent necrosis, which when present in severe autoimmune hepatitis and hepatitis B confers an ominous prognosis, is uncommon in hepatitis C, and yet progression to fibrosis or cirrhosis occurs in all 3 diseases **(2)**.

## 5. Scoring systems currently in use

For a system to be effective in every day diagnostic practice, it must be simple to understand, simple to apply, communicate effectively to the treating clinician, and clinically relevant **(16)**. The system that is most appropriate for clinical practice may not be the most informative for investigative work **(17)**.

## 6. Histological grading and staging of chronic hepatitis (1) (Table 1)

This scheme represents an extension of the original Knodell system, with a number of minor modifications. Firstly, a continuous scale is used for scoring each of the features assessed. Secondly, necroinflammatory activity and fibrosis are considered as separate categories. Thirdly, confluent necrosis is separated from periportal hepatitis and is included as a separate category of necroinflammatory activity. The term interface hepatitis was used in place of "piecemeal necrosis," to reflect the growing evidence that apoptosis, not necrosis, occurs at the limiting plate.

*The first category* (piecemeal necrosis) scores are defined as follows: 0, no piecemeal necrosis; 1, focal piecemeal necrosis in few portal areas; 2, focal piecemeal necrosis in most portal areas; 3, continuous piecemeal necrosis around <50% of tracts or septa; 4, continuous piecemeal necrosis around >50% of tracts or septa.

*The second category* (Confluent Necrosis) scores are defined as follows: 0, no confluent necrosis; 1, focal confluent necrosis; 2, zone 3 necrosis in some areas; 3, zone 3 necrosis in most areas; 4, zone 3 necrosis and occasional portal-central (P-C) bridging; 5, zone 3 necrosis and multiple (P-C) bridging; 6, panacinar or multiacinar necrosis.

*The third category* (focal lytic necrosis, apoptosis, and focal inflammation) scores are defined as follows: 0, No focal necrosis; 1, one focus or less per 10x objective; 2, two to four foci per 10x objective; 3, five to ten foci per 10x objective; 4, more than ten foci per 10x objective.

*The fourth category* (portal inflammation) scores are defined as follows: 0, no portal inflammation; 1, mild in some or all portal areas; 2, moderate in some or all portal areas; 3, moderate to marked, all portal areas; 4, marked in all portal areas. By combining scores for each of the four individual necroinflammatory categories, histological grading scores ranging from 0-18 can now be achieved. The overall activity scores are defined as follows: 1-3, minimal; 4-8, mild; 9-12, moderate; 13-18, severe **(1)**.

| Modified HAI Grading: Necroinflammatory Scores | | | | | | | |
|---|---|---|---|---|---|---|---|
| **Periportal or Periseptal Interface Hepatitis (piecemeal necrosis) (A)** | **Score** | **Confluent Necrosis (B)** | **Score** | **Focal (spotty) Lytic Necrosis, Apoptosis, and Focal Inflammation* (C)** | **Score** | **Portal Inflammation (D)** | **Score** |
| Absent | 0 | Absent | 0 | Absent | 0 | None | 0 |
| Mild (focal, few portal areas) | 1 | Focal confluent necrosis | 1 | One focus or less per 10x objective | 1 | Mild, some or all portal areas | 1 |
| Mild/moderate (focal, most portal areas) | 2 | Zone 3 necrosis in some areas | 2 | Two to four foci per 10x objective | 2 | Moderate, some or all portal areas | 2 |
| Moderate (continuous around <50% of tracts or septa) | 3 | Zone 3 necrosis in most areas | 3 | Five to ten foci per 10x objective | 3 | Moderate/marked, all portal areas | 3 |
| Severe (continuous around >50% of tracts or septa) | 4 | Zone 3 necrosis + occasional portal-central (P-C) bridging | 4 | More than ten foci per 10x objective | 4 | Marked, all portal areas | 4 |
| | | Zone 3 necrosis + multiple P-C bridging | 5 | | | | |
| | | Panacinar or multiacinar necrosis | 6 | | | | |
| *Does not include diffuse sinusoidal infiltration by inflammatory cells. | | | | | | | |

| Modified Staging: architectural changes, fibrosis and cirrhosis | |
|---|---|
| **Change** | **Score** |
| No fibrosis | 0 |
| Fibrous expansion of some portal areas, with or without short fibrous septa | 1 |
| Fibrous expansion of most portal areas, with or without short fibrous septa | 2 |
| Fibrous expansion of most portal areas with occasional portal to portal (P-P) bridging | 3 |
| Fibrous expansion of portal areas with marked bridging [portal to portal (P-P) as well as portal to central (P-C)] | 4 |
| Marked bridging (P-P and/or P-C) with occasional nodules (incomplete cirrhosis) | 5 |
| Cirrhosis, probable or definite | 6 |

**Additional features that should be noted but not scored**: bile-duct inflammation and damage; lymphoid follicles; steatosis, mild, moderate, or marked; hepatocellular dysplasia, large- or small-cell; adenomatous hyperplasia; iron or copper overload; intracellular inclusions (e.g. PAS-positive globules, Mallory bodies); and immunohistochemical findings. Information on viral antigens, lymphocyte subsets, or other features, when available, should be recorded and may be semi-quantitatively expressed.
Modified and reprinted **(1)**.

Table 1. Ishak Modified HAI (1995) (1).

The fibrosis scores are defined as follows: 0, no fibrosis; 1, fibrous expansion of some portal areas, with or without short fibrous septa; 2, fibrous expansion of most portal areas, with or without short fibrous septa; 3, fibrous expansion of most portal areas with occasional portal to portal bridging; 4, fibrous expansion of most portal areas with marked bridging (portal to

portal as well as portal to central); 5, marked bridging with occasional nodules (incomplete cirrhosis); 6, cirrhosis, probable or definite **(1)**.
Difficulties with the Ishak system have been noted. Use of the X10 objective for the evaluation of necroinflammatory foci raises concerns of reproducibility, because the size of the field may vary among microscopes. In addition, definitions of a "focus" of lymphocytic aggregates, apoptotic hepatocytes, or confluent necrosis may vary among pathologists **(18)**.

## 7. Algorithm for the grading of activity in chronic hepatitis (METAVIR system) (Table 2)

The French METAVIR Cooperative Study Group stated that another possible approach for grading the necroinflammatory activity is to consider that periportal and intra-lobular necroinflammatory lesions are related to the same pathologic mechanism and that they must be globally assessed. A panel decided to define activity according to its potential predictive value for the occurrence of liver fibrosis. They chose to include in algorithm only two features (piecemeal necrosis and lobular necrosis) **(19)**.
Portal inflammation was excluded from the algorithm, because this feature is a prerequisite for the definition of chronic hepatitis even without activity. Furthermore they observed a strong correlation with piecemeal necrosis, making these two features redundant criteria.
Piecemeal necrosis was chosen as the first decision criterion because of its proven potential value in other types of chronic hepatitis. It was then suspected that another feature, lobular necrosis, was of major importance in the prediction of liver fibrosis. It is believed that aggravation of chronic hepatitis C occurs through a burst of lobular necrosis, a lesion that is frequently present in chronic hepatitis C. The two lesions were therefore combined to propose a simple algorithm that defined activity.
In several existing classifications, the degree of piecemeal and lobular necrosis was independently assessed and their scores then added, thus giving each of these two lesions the same weight in the definition of activity. The METAVIR system included both piecemeal necrosis and lobular necrosis in the definition of activity, but with different values. The rationale for overweighting the piecemeal necrosis item by comparison with lobular necrosis is that piecemeal necrosis is the major discriminating factor used to grade activity, as shown by stepwise discriminate analysis.
*The first criterion* (piecemeal necrosis) scores are defined as follows: 0, absent; 1, focal alteration of the periportal plate in some portal tracts; 2, diffuse alteration of the periportal plate in some portal tracts or focal lesion around all portal tracts; 3, diffuse alteration of the periportal plate in all portal tracts.
*The second criterion* (focal lobular necrosis) scores are defined as follows: 0, less than one necroinflammatory foci per lobule; 1, at least one necroinflammatory foci per lobule; 2, several necroinflammatory foci per lobule or confluent or bridging necrosis. The overall activity scores are defined as follows: 0, No activity; 1, mild; 2, moderate; 3, severe **(20)**.
The fibrosis scores are defined as follows: F0, no fibrosis; F1, portal fibrosis without septa; F2, portal fibrosis with rare septa; F3 numerous septa without cirrhosis; F4, cirrhosis **(19)**.
The METAVIR system has the advantage of simplicity, reproducibility and application to a large number of biopsies **(20)**. This score is composed of a two-letter and two-number coding system: A= histological activity and F= fibrosis (Table 2).

## Algorithm for evaluation of histological activity

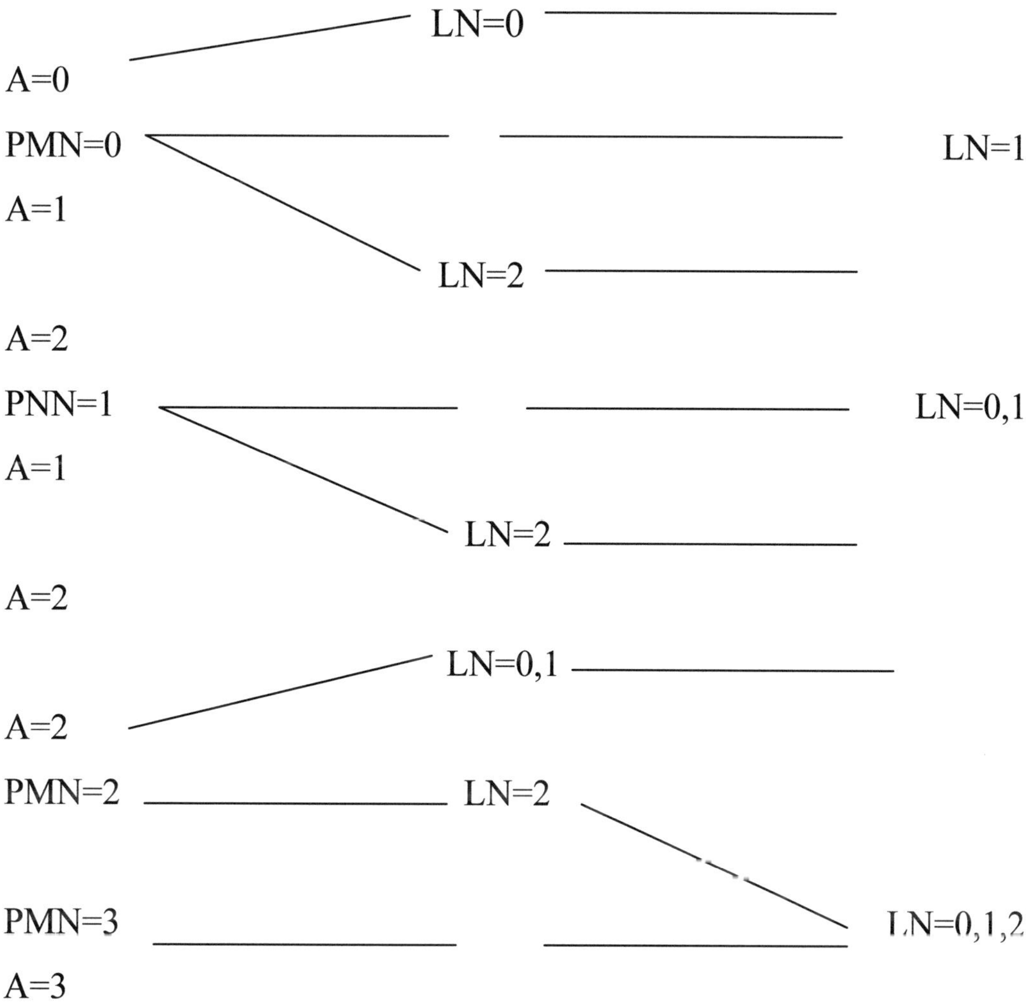


PMN, piecemeal necrosis; 0, none; 1, mild; 2, moderate; 3, severe; LN, lobular necrosis; 0, no or mild; 1, moderate; 2, severe; A, histological activity; 0, none; 1, mild; 2, moderate; 3, severe.

| Fibrosis Scoring | |
|---|---|
| **Score** | **Description** |
| 0 | No fibrosis |
| 1 | Stellate enlargement of portal tract but without septa formation |
| 2 | Enlargement of portal tract with rare septa formation |
| 3 | Numerous septa formation |
| 4 | Cirrhosis |

Modified and reprinted **(20)**.

Table 2. The METAVIR System.

## 8. Problems with histological scoring

There are a number of problems which apply to all the scoring systems currently in use.

- Lack of scientific validation:

A fundamental problem with histological "scoring" is that the numbers which are generated do not represent measurement of continuous variable. Instead, they simply represent different categories of severity. This contrasts with biochemical measurements, for example, serum transaminases, for which a true numerical progression can be more readily justified **(21)**.

- Observer variation:

There are problems in obtaining reproducible results, even when scoring system is applied by experts in the field of liver pathology. In general, better reproducibility has been obtained for scoring fibrosis than for scoring inflammatory activity. This is probably due to imprecise terminology which is used in individual histological features. Terms such as "occasional", "some", or "mild', "moderate and "severe" are used without defining precisely what these mean **(22)**.

- Sampling Variation:

Much of the knowledge regarding this problem has come from the examination of hepatectomy specimens obtained at liver transplantation. Sampling variation exist, both for the grade of necroinflammatory activity and for the stage of fibrosis. For example, small areas of multiacinar necrosis can often be found in a liver which otherwise show a relatively inactive cirrhosis. These areas are typically subcapsular in location but may be also present elsewhere. If a needle biopsy is taken from one of these areas, a "falsely high" inflammatory score may be obtained. Chronic viral hepatitis may affect the liver uniformly, but considerable variation in the severity of fibrosis can be seen when whole liver are available for examination **(2)**.

- Etiological considerations:

The scoring systems currently in common use incorporate histological features which may be seen in all types of chronic hepatitis. However, different types of chronic hepatitis have marked differences in natural history and response to therapy. These differences in behavior may be reflected by different patterns of histological damage. For example, ballooning, rosetting, and giant cell transformation may be regarded as signs of severe damage in cases of autoimmune hepatitis, even in the absence of conspicuous inflammatory activity. Direct cytopathic damage (e.g. ballooning or fatty change) may be important in the pathogenesis of fibrosis in chronic hepatitis C infection **(2)**.

## 9. Terminology in METAVIR

Terminology in METAVIR as regard fibrosis stage assessment is not clear and confusing; with narrow range (F0-F4). F3 indicates numerous septa, however, in practical application early (developing) cirrhosis is included too, irrespective of being not described in the score details. On the other hand, Ishak fibrosis score is wider (0-6), more sensitive, as well clearly separate incomplete (developing, early) cirrhosis from established cirrhosis **(1,20,23)**.

Rozario and Ramakrishna, 2003**(24)** have built their analysis, tables and comparison on the inaccurate idea that F2 of METAVIR (rare septa) is equal to stage 2 of Ishak. However, the correct is that, F1 stage of METAVIR is equal to stages 1&2 of Ishak, and F2 of METAVIR is equal to stage 3 of Ishak (occasional bridging fibrosis). This resulted in a defect that may affect the idea and the conclusion (4).

Applying semi-quantitative terminology reflecting grades of necroinflammatory injury as recorded by Ishak may underestimate the severity of these changes. In Ishak scoring, 6 points out of the 18 are related to confluent necrosis, which is a rare event in chronic hepatitis C.

Elzbieta and Marek, 2005 **(25)** reported that, the comparison of three histological scoring systems used to evaluate chronic hepatitis (Batts and Ludwig, Ishak *et al.* and METAVIR scoring systems) revealed a high coefficient of positive correlation between the respective scales. Thus, the systems seem comparable in the estimation of the inflammation grade and stage of fibrosis. Table 2 may be advised for converting fibrosis score from Ishak to METAVIR.

Goodman in his review 2007**(26)**, considered Ishak stage 5 (incomplete cirrhosis) to be included in METAVIR F4 stage, that is different from the opinion of Bedossa and others of METAVIR group. This is a pitfall that may affect the results of some research studies.

## 10. Current applications of Ishak and METAVIR scoring systems

In assessment of regression of fibrosis after autoimmune hepatitis treatment, Abdalla et al, 2009 have reported higher sensitivity of Ishak compared with METAVIR in detection of fibrosis regression **(27)**. They also found statistically higher sensitivity for quantitative assessment of fibrosis by analysis of digitalized pictures of sirus red. Czaja and Carpente 2004, reported a sensitivity of Ishak in assessment of fibrosis regression **(28)**. Esmat et al, 2007 (applying Ishak fibrosis score) have demonstrated a correlation between fibrosis score and hyaluronic acid level **(29)**. Tsochatzis1 et al 2011, in their meta-analysis of diagnostic accuracy of elastography for the diagnosis of severity of fibrosis in chronic liver disease, the different stages of fibrosis (scoring systems) were converted to comparable stages in METAVIR **(30)**. Goodman 2007, suggested application of METAVIR in routine work, and Ishak score in clinical trials, because of higher sensitivity in fibrosis assessment **(28)**. Lefkowitch 2007 and Guido et al, 2011, suggested application of any of the scoring systems, that is not home made, and the clinicians with whom they work prefer **(31,32)**.

Although liver biopsy has long been regarded as a gold standard procedure, it has obvious limitations. It represents an approximation of liver fibrosis for the whole liver and is, therefore, not the gold standard for fibrosis assessment. Nevertheless, it is the best procedure currently available **(33)**. Germani et al 2010 recommend liver pathologists to perform computer-assisted digital analysis of Sirius red-stained histological sections in addition to the scoring system established to describe the stage of the liver disease **(34)**.

## 11. Conclusions

*Regarding fibrosis:*

- Ishak and METAVIR are nearly identical; however, Ishak is of a wider scale.
- The term "Septa" in METAVIR is equal to "bridging fibrosis" in Ishak.
- F3 stage in METAVIR score includes incomplete (developing) cirrhosis.

*Regarding necroinflammatory injury*

- METAVIR is more sensitive to severe activity and more reproducible. However, without numerical scoring that let it less effective for monitoring minor changes.
- Ishak modified HAI has a wider scale. However, 6 points of it (confluent necrosis) are nearly out of the chronic hepatitis C scope. This minimizes the actual scoring to 12 points instead of 18 in practical application.

- The proposed table is advised for unidirectional converting fibrosis scores from Ishak to METAVIR.
- METAVIR F3 stage may better be subdivided into F3a: Marked bridging fibrosis and F3b: incomplete (early cirrhosis) (developing cirrhosis).

More work is needed in:

- Assessing the validity of the current scoring systems in post-liver transplant patients with recurrent HCV especially those with a back ground of graft pathologies such as rejection and those with associated HBV or cytomegalovirus and HIV infections.
- Convertibility of the results of these scoring systems and image pattern of contrast enhanced ultrasound of the liver.

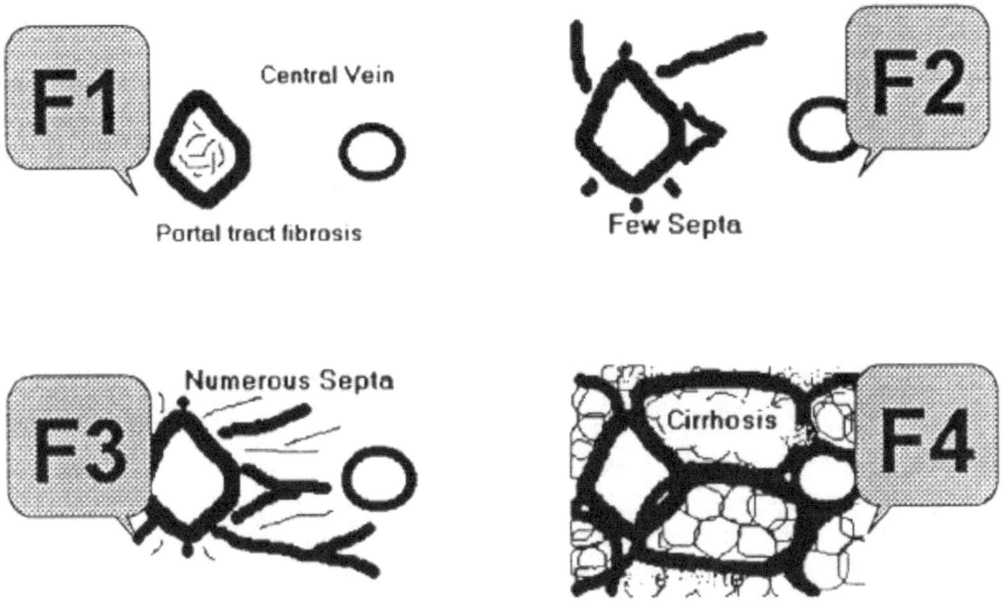


Modified and reprinted **(19)**.

| **Ishak, 1995.**<br>**Fibrosis: 0-6** | METAVIR Score.<br>Fibrosis: F 0-4 |
|---|---|
| 0 | 0 |
| 1-2 | 1 |
| 3 | 2 |
| 4-5 | 3 |
| 6 | 4 |

Fig. 1. **The METAVIR Fibrosis staging system.** F0 is normal liver (no fibrosis). F1 = portal fibrosis. F2 = few septa. F3 = many septa. F4 = cirrhosis.

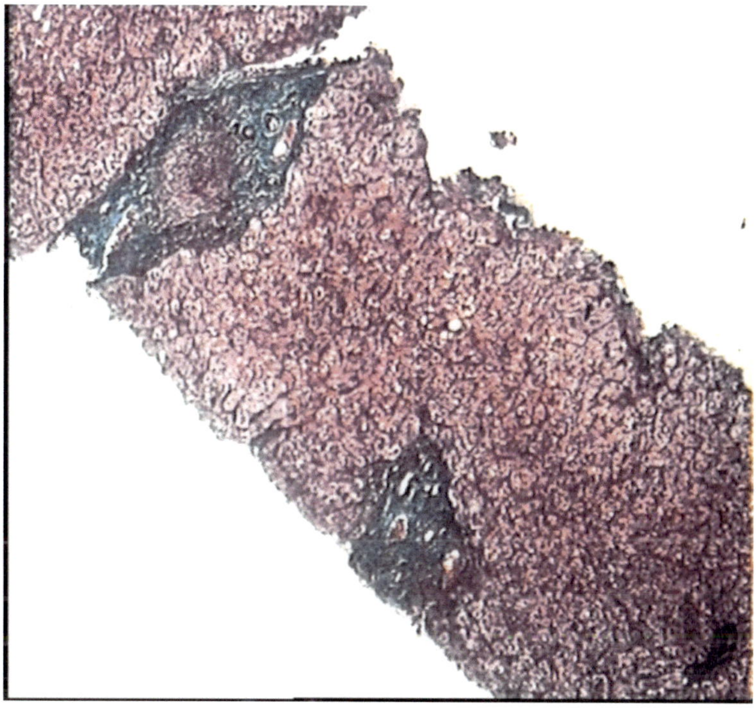

Fig. 2. Portal tract expansion by fibrosis, Masson trichrom stain.

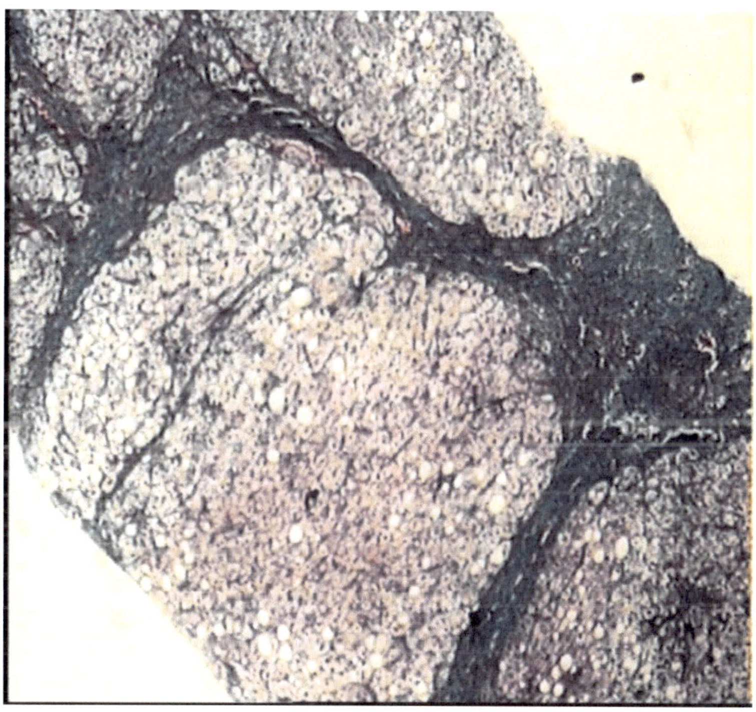

Fig. 3. Bridging fibrosis , Masson trichrom stain.

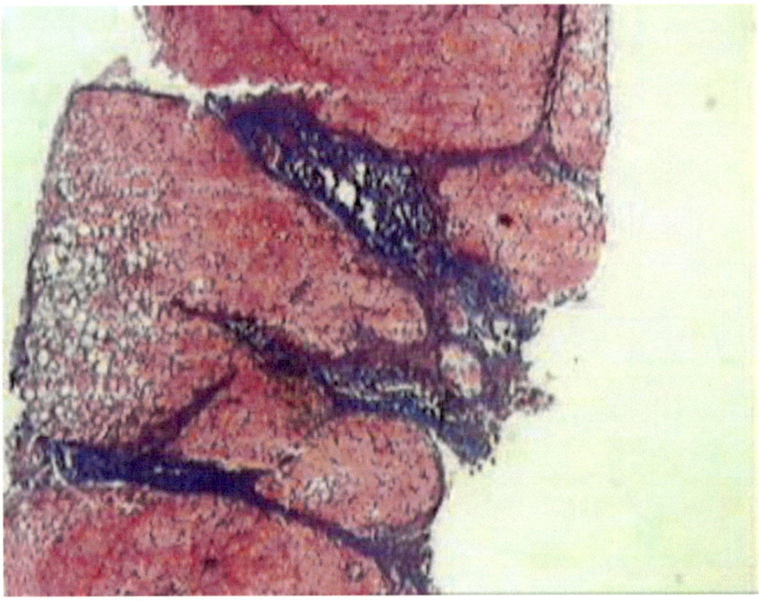

Fig. 4. Multiple portal-portal bridges, , Masson trichrom stain.

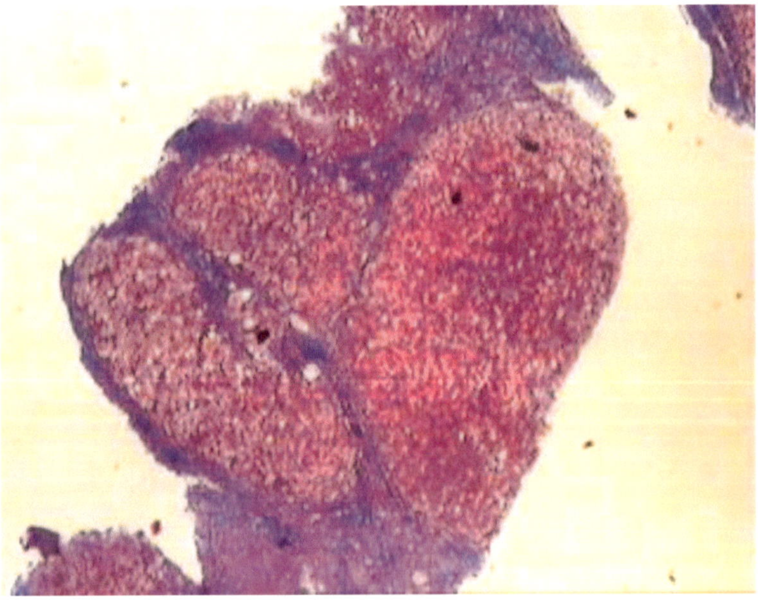

Fig. 5. Regenerating nodules rimmed by fibrosis, Masson trichrom stain.

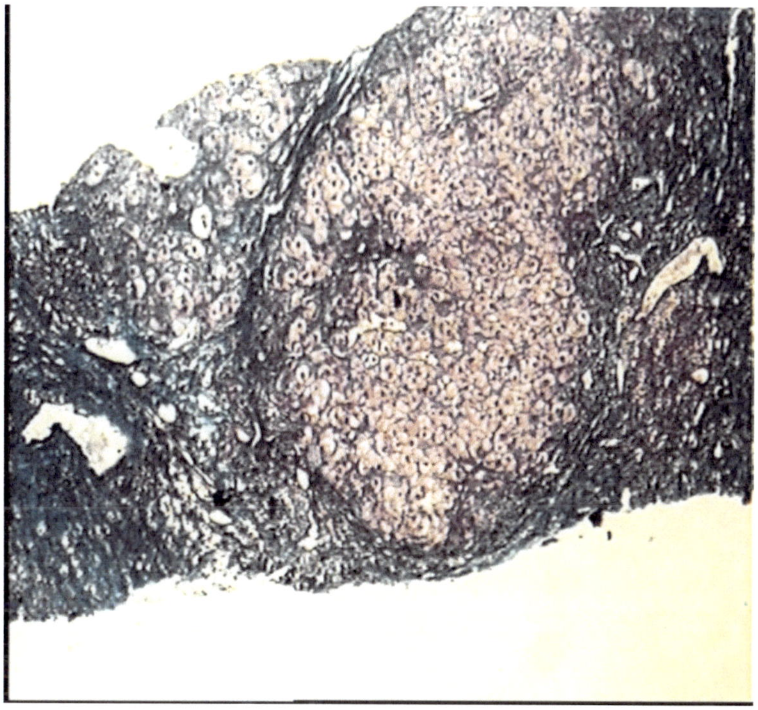

Fig. 6. Regenerating nodules rimmed by dense fibrosis, Masson trichrom stain.

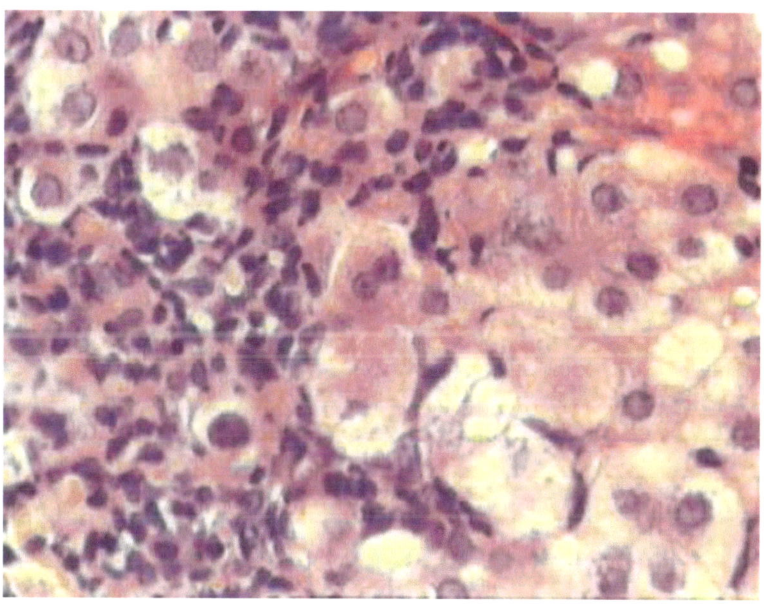

Fig. 7. Interface hepatitis, H&E stain.

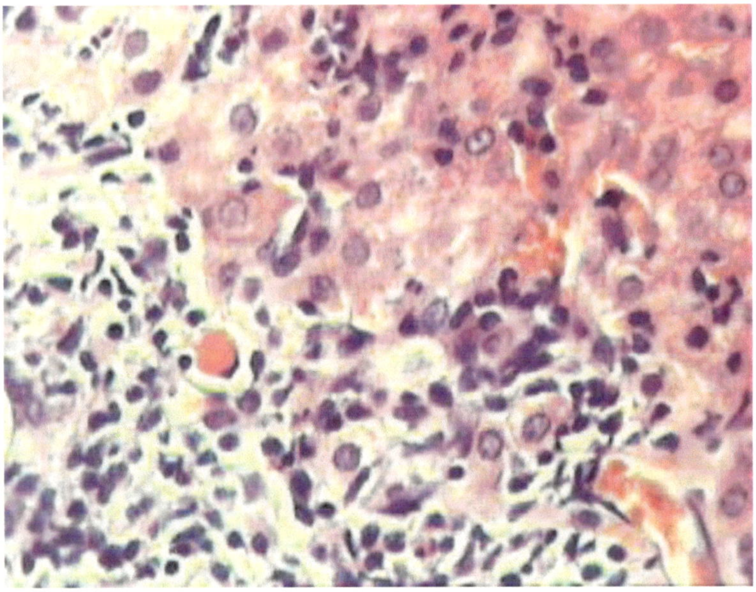

Fig. 8. Evident interface hepatitis with apoptosis, H&E stain.

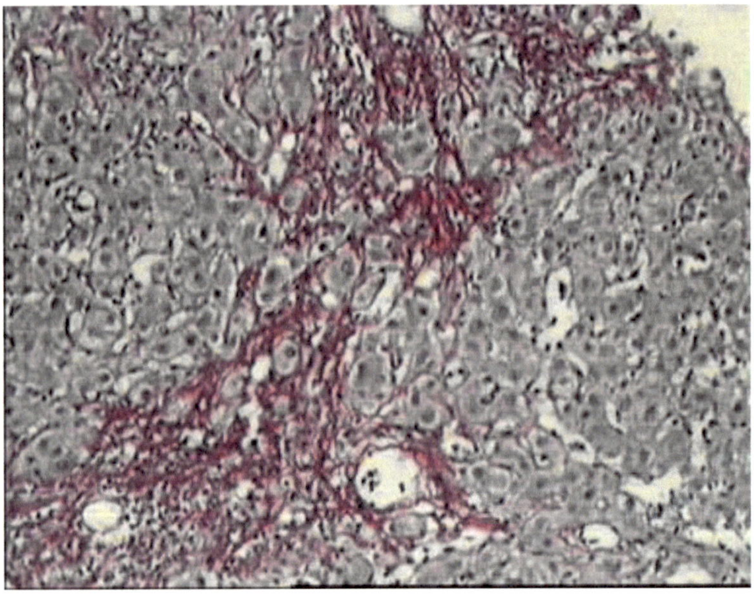

Fig. 9. Confluent necrosis, reticulin collapse , sirus red stain.

## 12. References

[1] Ishak K, Baptista A, Bianchi L, et al. Histologic grading and staging of chronic hepatitis. J Hepatol 1995;24:289-293.

[2] Hübscher S. Histological grading and staging in chronic hepatitis: clinical applications and problems. J Hepatol 1998;29:1015-1022.

[3] Salmi M, Adams D, Jalkanen S. Cell adhesion and migration. IV Lymphocyte trafficking in the intestine and liver. Am J Physiol 1998;274:1-6.

[4] Kay FW, O'Dowd J, Thomas R, et al. Mild abnormalities in liver histology associated with chronic hepatitis: distinction from normal liver histology. J Clin Pathol 1997;50:929-931.

[5] Galle P. Apoptosis in liver disease. J Heptol 1997;27:405-412.

[6] MacSween R, Desmit V, Roskams T, et al. Developmental anatomy and normal structure in: MacSween R, Burt A, Portman B, Ishak K, Scheuer P, and Anthony P (eds): Pathology of the liver. 4th edition (2002), Churchill, Livingston, PP: 1-66.

[7] De Groote J, Desmet VJ, Gedigk P, et al. A classification of chronic hepatitis. Lancet 1968;2:626-628.

[8] Mattson L, Weiland O, Glaumann H. Application of numerical scoring system for assessment of histological outcome in patient with chronic post transfusion non-A, non-B hepatitis with or without antibody to hepatitis C. Liver 1990;10:257-263.

[9] Poynard T, Bedossa P, Opolon P. Natural history of liver fibrosis progression in patients with chronic hepatitis C. Lancet 1997;349:825-832.

[10] Lefkwitch J, Schiff E, Davis G, et al. Pathological diagnosis of chronic hepatitis C: a multicenter comparative study with chronic hepatitis B. Gastroenterology 1993;104:595-603.

[11] Popper H. Changing concepts of the evolution of chronic hepatitis and the role of piecemeal necrosis. Hepatology 1983;5:758-762.

[12] Cooksley W, Bradbear R, Robinson W, et al. The prognosis of chronic active hepatitis without cirrhosis in relation to bridging necrosis. Hepatology 1986;6:345-348.

[13] Desmet V, Gerber M, Hoofnagle J, et al. Classification of chronic hepatitis: diagnosis, grading and staging. Hepatology 1994;19:1513-1520.

[14] Popper H, Schaffner F. The vocabulary of chronic hepatitis. N Engl J Med 1971;284:1154-1156.

[15] Scheuer P. Chronic hepatitis: what is activity and how should it be assessed? Histopathology 1997;30:103-105.

[16] Okafor O, Ojo S. A comparative analysis of six current histological classification schemes and scoring systems used in chronic hepatitis reporting. Rev Esp Pathol 2004;37:269-277.

[17] Brunt E. Grading and staging the histopathological lesions of chronic hepatitis: the Knodell histology activity index and beyond. Hepatology 2000;31:241-246.

[18] Westin J, Lagging LM, Wejstal R, et al. Interobserver study of liver histopathology using the Ishak score in patients with chronic hepatitis C virus infection. Liver 1999;19:183-187.

[19] Poynard T Ratziu V, Benmanov Y, et al. Fibrosis in patients with chronic hepatitis C: detection and significance. Semin Liv Dis 2000;20:47 55.

[20] Bedossa P, Poynard T and the French METAVIR Cooperative Study Group. An algorithm for grading activity in chronic hepatitis C. Hepatology 1996;24:289-293.

[21] Scheuer P. Classification of chronic viral hepatitis: a need for reassessment. J Hepatol 1991;13:372-374.

[22] Golden R, Golden J, Burt A, et al. Intra-observer and inter-observer variation in the histopathological assessment of chronic viral hepatitis. J Hepatol 1996;25:649-654.
[23] Bedossa P, Callard P, Degott C, et al. Intraobserver and interobserver variations in liver biopsy interpretation in patients with chronic hepatitis C. Hepatology 1994;20:15-20.
[24] Rozario and Ramakrishna. Histopathological study of chronic hepatitis B and C: a comparison of two scoring systems. J Hepatol 2003;38:223-229.
[25] Maria Elzbieta SL, Marek LD. Histological outcome of chronic hepatitis B in children treated with interferon alpha. World J Gastroenterol 2005;11:7179-7182.
[26] Goodman ZD. Grading and staging systems for inflammation and fibrosis in chronic liver diseases. J Hepatol 2007;47:598-607.
[27] Abdalla AF, Zalata KR, Ismail AF, et al. Regression of fibrosis in pediatric autoimmune hepatitis: morphometric assessment of fibrosis versus semiquantiatative methods. Fibrogenesis Tissue Repair 2009;2:2.
[28] Czaja AJ, Carpenter HA. Autoimmune hepatitis with incidental histologic features of bile duct injury. Hepatology 2001;34:659-665.
[29] Esmat G, Metwally M, Zalata KR, et al., Evaluation of serum biomarkers of fibrosis and injury in Egyptian patients with chronic hepatitis C. J Hepatol 2007;46:620-627.
[30] Tsochatzis EA, Gurusamy KS, Ntaoula S. Elastography for the diagnosis of severity of fibrosis in chronic liver disease: A meta-analysis of diagnostic accuracy. J Hepatol 201;54:650-659.
[31] Lefkowitch JH. Liver biopsy assessment in chronic hepatitis. Arch Med Res 2007;38:634-643.
[32] Guido M, Mangia A, Faa G. Chronic viral hepatitis: the histology report. Dig Liver Dis 2011;43(Suppl 4):S331-343.
[33] Bedossa P. Liver biopsy. Gastroenterol Clin Biol 2008;32(6 Suppl 1):4-7.
[34] Germani G, Burroughs AK, Dhillon AP. The relationship between liver disease stage and liver fibrosis: a tangled web. Histopathology Histopathology 2010;57:773-784.

# 11

# Transgastric Liver Biopsy Using the NOTES Technique: An Animal Study

Nobumi Tagaya and Masatoshi Oya
*First Department of Surgery,
Dokkyo Medical University Koshigaya Hospital,
Koshigaya, Saitama,
Japan*

## 1. Introduction

Liver biopsy (LB) is an important procedure in the diagnosis and treatment of liver diseases. At present, there are two minimally invasive techniques for liver tissue sampling: image-guided percutaneous liver biopsy (PLB) and transjugular liver biopsy (TJLB) [1-4]. Both techniques have several disadvantages, such as the risk of bleeding and subcapsular hematoma in the former, and the small sample size, longer procedure time and the need for considerable interventional skill in the latter. Recently, innovative intra-abdominal procedures that require no incision of the anterior abdominal wall have become possible by accessing the peritoneal cavity through natural orifices [5,6]. Natural orifice translumenal endoscopic surgery (NOTES) for access to the peritoneal cavity was first reported by Kalloo et al. [7]. To develop a new strategy for minimally invasive LB in humans, we have investigated a novel procedure for transgastric liver biopsy (TGLB) using the NOTES technique in experimental animals.

## 2. Materials and methods

The aim of this study was to determine the technical feasibility of peroral TGLB using a flexible endoscope. This experimental study was approved by the animal care institutional review board at the Dokkyo Medical University. The utility of transgastric peritoneoscopy was evaluated in three 15-kg farm pigs and five 8-kg dogs.

Under general anesthesia with an endotracheal intubation, a forward-viewing, double-channel endoscope (GIF-2T-240, Olympus, Tokyo) was advanced into the esophagus and stomach. Puncture of the gastric wall was performed with a 3-mm cutting-wire needle knife (KD-10Q-1, Olympus). The puncture site was enlarged to 8mm with a balloon dilator (CRE W.G. esophageal balloon 5839, Boston Scientific) and the endoscope was advanced into the peritoneal cavity. The peritoneal cavity was inflated with air through the endoscope. The liver was easily visualized by retroflexion of the endoscope (Fig.1).

LB was performed using routine biopsy forceps (FB-230K, Olympus) from the edge of the liver (Fig.2) and hemostasis of biopsy sites was achieved using electrocautery with the biopsy forceps (Fig.3). A gastric orifice was closed by endoscopic clips (HX-610-135, HX-610-090L, Olympus). The animals were sacrificed and necropsy was performed.

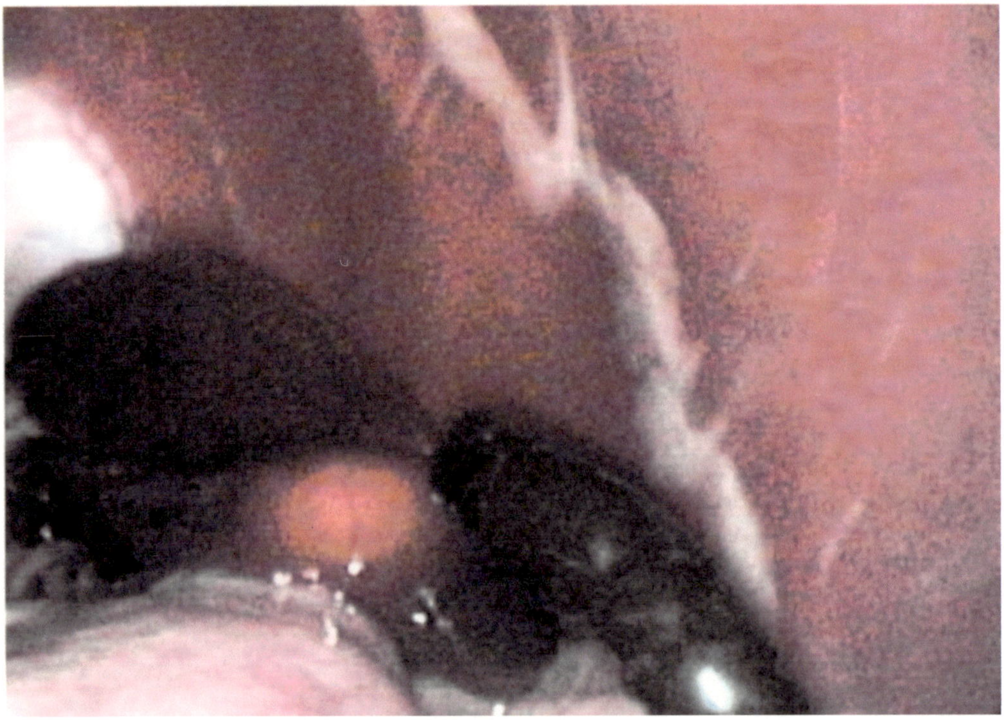

Fig. 1. Retroflexion of the endoscope easily visualized the liver

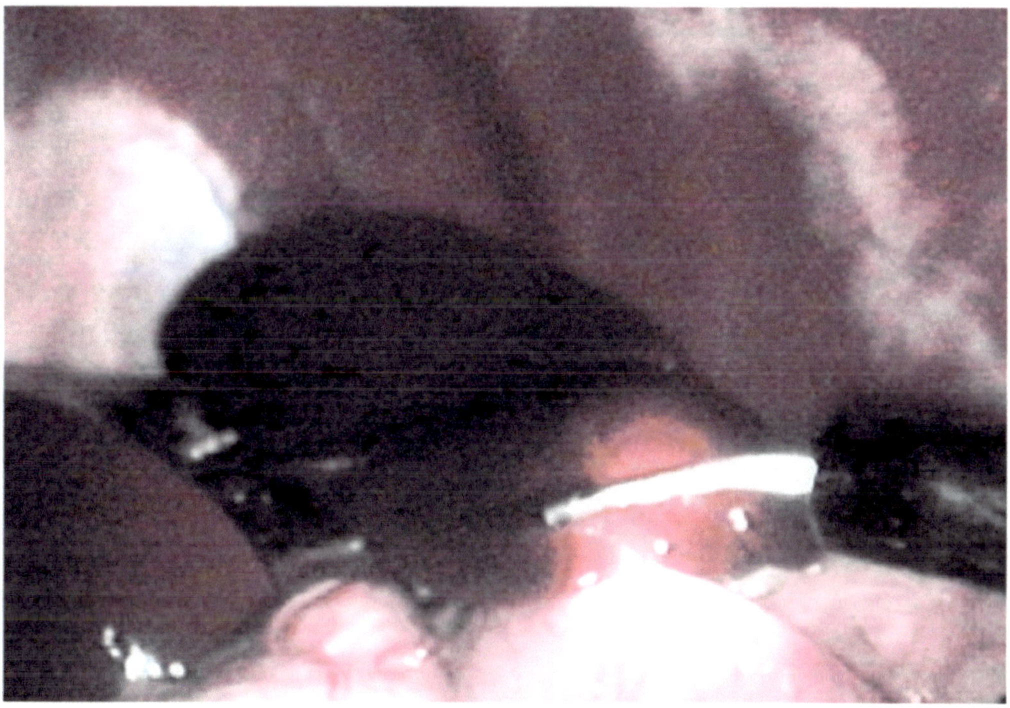

Fig. 2. Liver biopsy was performed using routine biopsy forceps from the edge of the liver.

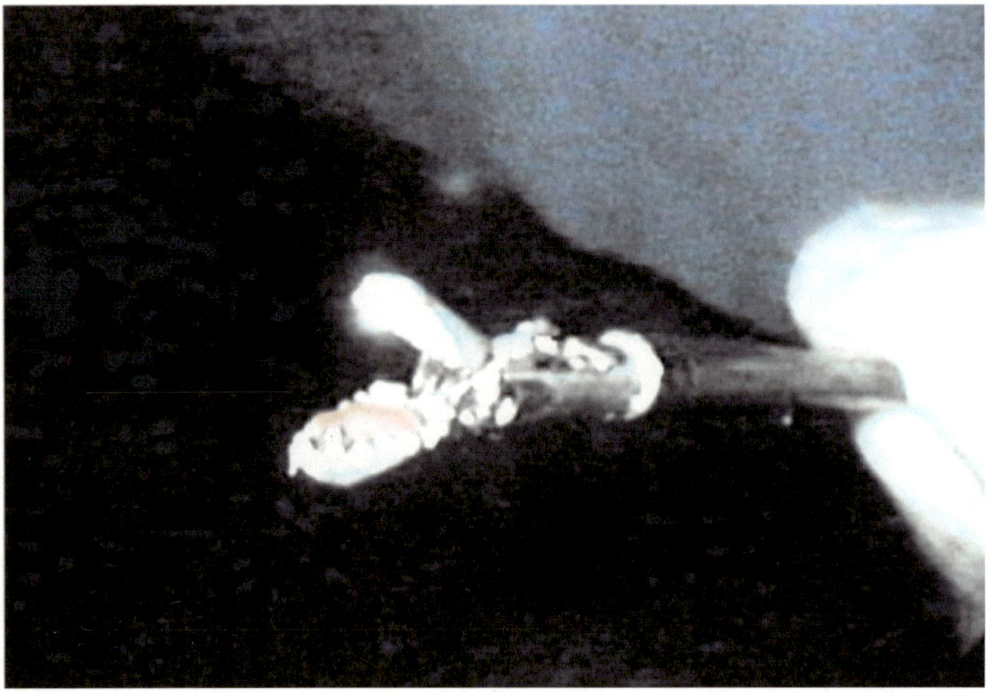

Fig. 3. An adequate sample was retrieved by biopsy forceps.

## 3. Results

None of the eight animals developed complications, including adjacent organ injury or bleeding, during incision of the gastric wall, entry into the peritoneal cavity, and the closure of the gastric wall. Visualization of the intraperitoneal organs through the endoscope using standard endoscopic techniques had no problems. Peritoneoscopy revealed a good operative view of abdominal cavity in all possible directions. LB was successfully performed without any trouble bleedings and yielded adequate samples for histopathologic examination in all cases. Minor bleeding occurred in three cases and was stopped by an endoscopic electrocoagulation (Fig 4).

Necropsy revealed no particular damages to other intraperitoneal organs related with this transgastric procedure. The acute experiments demonstrated the technical feasibility of this approach.

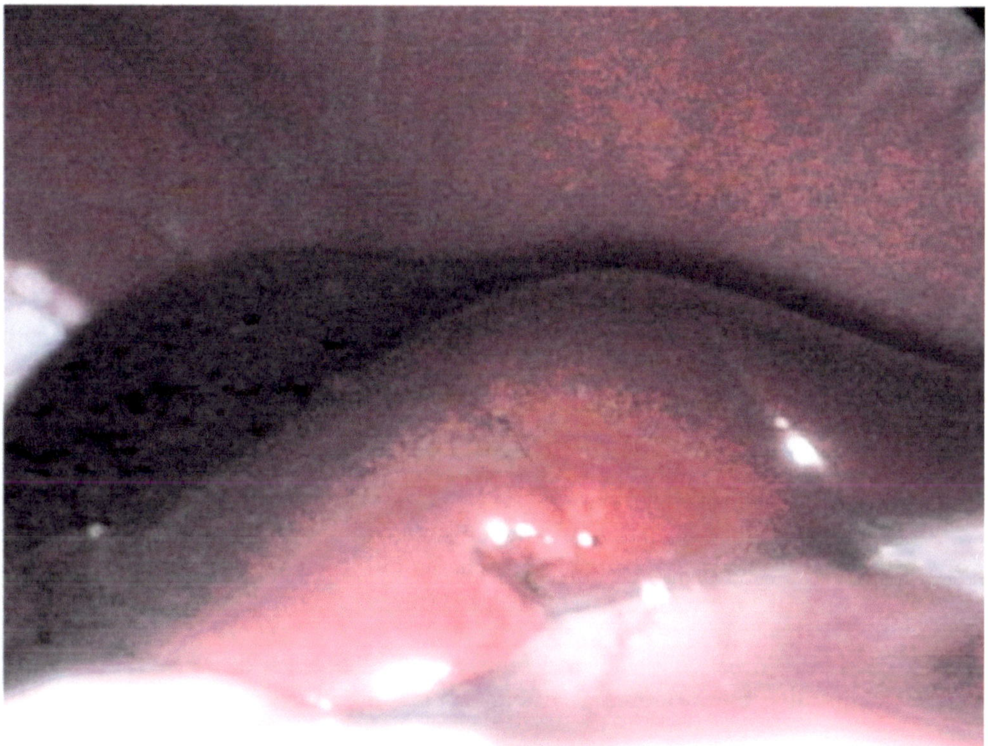

Fig. 4. Hemostasis was confirmed at the site of liver biopsy.

## 4. Discussion

In general, LB is a necessary procedure to evaluate the chronic liver disease, and a standard one to diagnose liver tumors pathologically. In performing LB, there are two procedures consisting of percutaneous and transjugular routes. However, those procedures revealed several disadvantages including post procedural hemorrhage, small sample size for diagnosis, the differences of the severity of fibrosis in the sites of LB, and so on [2]. We have to resolve or minimize those issues in this era. Recently, endoscopic approach in LB became attractive with minimally invasiveness to human bodies and no skin damage. We introduced TGLB by NOTES [5-7] as an endoscopic approach, and reported the evaluation of TGLB in diagnostic and therapeutic aspects for liver diseases.
The method of PLB is divided into blind, ultrasound (US) or computed tomographic guidance. Those results greatly depend on the skills of the gastroenterologist, hepatologist or radiologist as an operator and the technical possibilities including the quality of the ultrasonography itself. However, the most careful event is complications after PLB. Piccinino et al. [8] reported that 61% of the complications appeared in the first 2 hours after the biopsy, 82% in the first 10 hours, and 96% in the first 24 hours. We should have the strict observation for the first 24 hours after PLB. Several large studies showed that the rate of major complication after PLB ranged from 0.09% to 2.3%, severe complications appeared in 0.57%, and mortality ranged from 0.03% to 0.11% [9-11]. And the complications of blind PLB

are significant high rates compared with those of US-guided one [12-14], PLB under US guidance is recommended as a reasonable and cost-efficient procedure [1, 13, 15]. In fact, morbidity and mortality rates are not high. Furthermore, regarding bleeding after PLB, Alotaibi et al. [4] described that the positive color Doppler sign in US indicated bleeding along a biopsy tract and US-guided compression was effective in achieving appropriate hemostasis, and tract-plugging means that the biopsy tract is filled with Gelfoam or other thrombotic agents, it is an important procedure to decrease the risk of bleeding and subcapusular hematoma in PLB [2]. Nevertheless, in patients with ascites, abnormal coagulation profiles, another procedure is considered because of the high risk due to bleeding complications.

The TJLB via the internal jugular vein approach using the method described by McAfee et al. [16] is thought to be a safer biopsy option in patients with ascites, coagulopathy, thrombocytopenia or medical conditions with bleeding disorders such as hemophilia being considered as contraindications for PLB [17,18] because the patients will "bleed" back into the vein rather than into the abdomen. However, TJLB is a limited technique as a result of small sample size and caliber, longer procedure time, and the need for a skilled interventional radiologist [18]. Furthermore, it is also not without complications, which arise when the liver capsule or capsular veins are perforated, and does not prevent this risk, and it actually seems to increase risk in ascitic patients [3]. Therefore, the TJLB still needs a further study to evaluate indication, technique and complications.

The attractive points of LB by NOTES technique consist of no skin damage in the outside of the body and the direct observation of biopsy site in the inside of the body against PLB or TJLB. In clinically, the introduction of NOTES is required to resolve the identification of safe access to the peritoneal cavity, the complete closure of access route, the prevention of infection, the intra-abdominal orientation, the development of a multitasking platform, the management for the accidental complications, the outlining physiologic unanticipated events and the training of NOTES as White paper from American Society for Gastrointestinal Endoscopy and Society of American Gastrointestinal and Endoscopic Surgeons declared, [5,6]. In particular, infection or bacterial contamination in the abdomen due to the open of the digestive tract is a great concern in NOTES. However, transgastric peritoneoscopy being developed by Kalloo et al. [7, 19] showed no association with serious infection or other complications in the peritoneal cavity during their long-term survival experiments. Furthermore, Hazey et al. [20] reported that although contamination in the abdomen was documented, no clinically significant episode of the peritoneal cavity was observed without abscess formation or infectious complications during laparoscopic Roux-en-Y gastric bypass. From those findings, although the peroral TGLB required to add the artificial injury for normal organs, it will become one of alternatives to another LB methods.

In fact, there are several successful experimental reports of liver biopsy using a pig model [19, 21-23]. Mintz et al. [22] reported that LB can be performed safely and obtained from the edge of the liver using routine endoscopic punch biopsy forceps, and adequate hemostasis also obtained by an electrocautery. This report was similar to our procedure and results. In clinical, Hazey et al. [20] reported that LB was uneventfully performed from the transgastric access route in a patient who underwent a diagnostic laparoscopic evaluation of pancreatic mass. Steele et al. [24] also reported that LB from segments II, III, or IVb under flexible transgastric peritoneoscopy during Roux-en-Y gastric bypass for morbid obesity was

performed in 3 patients with only minor bleeding from the liver biopsy sites. Exploration of the peritoneal cavity with a flexible endoscope and a LB took 2.1 min to 6.0 with a mean of 4.1 min. The postoperative period in all patients was uneventful without any local or systemic complications. Above those findings revealed that LB could be a feasible and safe procedure without any critical complications even in humans.
In conclusion, this approach to peritoneal cavity is technically feasible and has the potential to be an alternative to routine LB. Transgastric endoscopic approach has a wide range of diagnostic and therapeutic interventions.

## 5. References

[1] Lindor KD et al. (1996). The role of ultrasonography and automatic-needle biopsy in outpatient precutaneous liver biopsy. Hepatology, 23, pp.1079-1983
[2] Sporea I et al. (2008). Why, who and how should perform liver biopsy in chronic liver disease. World J Gastroenterol, 14, pp.3396-3402.
[3] Hardman RL et al. (2010). Single-institution results of image-guided nonplugged percutaneous versus transjugular liver biopsy. Cardiovasc Intervent Radiol, [DOI 10.1007/s00270-010-9924-9].
[4] Alotaibi M et al. (2010). The positive color Doppler sign post biopsy: effectiveness of US-directed compression in achieving hemostasis. Pediatr Radiol, [DOI 10.1007/s00247-010-1848-7]
[5] ASGE & SAGES. (2006). ASGE/SAGES working group on natural orifice translumenal endoscopic surgery: White paper October 2005. Gastrointest Endosc, 63, pp.199-203.
[6] Rattner D & Kalloo A: ASGE/SAGES Working Group. (2006). ASGE/SAGES working group on natural orifice translumennal endosopic surgery. October 2005. Surg Endosc, 20, pp.329-33.
[7] Kalloo AN et al. (2000). Flexible transgastric peritoneoscopy: a novel approach to diagnostic and therapeutic interventions in the peritoneal cavity [abstract]. Gastroenterology, 118, pp.A1039.
[8] Piccinino F et al. (1986). Complications following percutaneous liver biopsy. A multicentre retrospective study on 68,276 biopsies. J Hepatol, 2, pp.165-173.
[9] Poynard T et al. (2000). Appropriateness of liver biopsy. Can J Gastroenterol, 14, pp.543–548.
[10] McGill DB et al. (1990). A 21-year experience with major hemorrhage after percutaneous liver biopsy. Gastroenterology, 99, pp.1396–1400.
[11] Cadranel JF et al. (2000). Practices of liver biopsy in France: results of a prospective nationwide survey. For the Group of Epidemiology of the French Association for the Study of the Liver (AFEF). Hepatology, 32, pp.477-481.
[12] Pasha T et al. (1998). Cost-effectiveness of ultrasound-guided liver biopsy. Hepatology, 27, pp.1220-1226.
[13] Younossi ZM et al. (1998). Ultrasound-guided liver biopsy for parenchymal liver disease: an economic analysis. Dig Dis Sci, 43, pp.46-50.
[14] Farrell RJ et al. (1999). Guided versus blind liver biopsy for chronic hepatitis C; clinical benefits and costs. J Hepatol, 30, pp.580-587.

[15] Adam T & Lewis JH. (2002). Percutaneous liver biopsy. Clin Perspectives Gastroenterol: 117-121.

[16] McAfee JH et al. (1992). Transjugular liver biopsy. Hepatology, 15, pp.726-732.

[17] Bravo AA et al. (2001). Liver biopsy. N Engl J Med, 344, pp.495-500.

[18] Rockey D et al. (2009). Americal Association for the study of Liver Diseases. Liver biopsy. Hepatology, 49, pp.1017-1044.

[19] Kalloo AN et al. (2004). Flexible transgastric peritoneoscopy: a novel approach to diagnostic and therapeutic interventions in the peritoneal cavity. Gatroitest Endosc, 60, pp.114-117.

[20] Hazey JW et al. (2008). Natural-orifice transgastric endoscopic peritoneoscopy in humans: Initial clinical trial. Surg Endosc, 22, pp.16-20.

[21] Lima E et al. (2006). Transvesical endoscopic peritoneoscopy: a novel 5 mm port for intra-abdominal scarless surgery. J Urol, 176, pp.802-805.

[22] Mintz Y et al. (2007). NOTES: The hybrid technique. J Laparoendosc Adv Surg Tech, 17, pp.402-406.

[23] Mintz Y et al. (2008). NOTES: A review of the technical problems encountered and their solutions. J Laparoendosc Adv Surg Tech,18, pp.583-587.

[24] Steele K et al. (2008). Flexible transgastric peritoneoscopy and liver biopsy: a feasibility study in human beings (with video). Gastrointest Endosc, 68, pp.61-66.

# Part 2

# Non-Invasive Alternatives to Liver Biopsy

# 12

# Noninvasive Alternatives to Liver Biopsy

Ludmila Viksna[1] et al.*
[1]*Riga Stradins University,*
*Latvia*

## 1. Introduction

During the past 60 years the role and importance of liver biopsy have changed. In 1950s the introduction of liver puncture biopsy was absolute innovation, e.g. in Latvia, and had an invaluable significance. The possibility to compare and/or oppose alterations of liver structure and liver function was achieved and it caused the information explosion. The spectrum of morphological research included investigations of liver tissue damage on different levels that explained the mechanisms of biochemically detected cytolysis and cholestasis syndrome, fibrosis and liver cirrhosis development. Relatively, in least degree the morphological phenomena of apoptosis and its role in acute and chronic liver diseases were examined.

Frequently conventional liver function tests are limited to quantifying hepatic function. Despite major progress in the diagnostics and therapy of liver diseases of different etiologies, the assessment of liver function continues to present a major clinical problem. Most of liver function tests are not sufficiently specific and do not accurately predict liver failure and outcome of it.

Liver biopsy is an essential part of the diagnostics and follow-up of many liver diseases giving clinically important information as well as scientific data. At present, it is the most specific test to assess the nature and severity of liver damage (Bravo et al., 2001). However, the role of liver biopsy in the evolution of medical science is dynamic. It became possible with the development of methods able to bring sufficient amount of liver tissue as well as to ensure the safety of the procedure itself. The methods used to obtain liver tissue include transcutaneous needle biopsy and transvenous approach via jugular or femoral vein. Occasionally, liver can be biopsied during laparoscopy or open abdominal surgery. Aseptics and antiseptics are of importance. There is an obvious necessity to ensure the monitoring of the patient and control of possible albeit rare complications. It seems reasonable to expect further developments in the field of liver morphology that might include both in-depth studies of tissue (Dioguardi et al., 2008) as well as elaboration of novel, completely different diagnostic methods.

The indications for liver biopsy include 1) the grading and staging of chronic viral hepatitis, alcohol-related liver damage, non-alcoholic steatohepatitis and autoimmune hepatitis; 2)

---

* Valentina Sondore[2], Jāzeps Keiss[2], Agita Jeruma[2], Pēteris Prieditis[1], Ilze Strumfa[1],
Arturs Sochnevs[1] and Baiba Rozentale[2].
*1 Riga Stradins University, Latvia,*
*2 State agency „Infectology Center of Latvia", Latvia.*

evaluation of hemochromatosis and Wilson's disease; 3) diagnostics of biliary diseases; 4) evaluation of patient with abnormal biochemical liver tests; 5) evaluation of medication toxicity; 6) diagnosis of focal liver lesion; 7) evaluation of liver transplant; 8) evaluation of patient with fever of unknown origin (Bravo et al., 2001). Liver biopsy ensure accurate diagnosis in 90% of patients with abnormal biochemical liver tests (Hultcrantz&Gabrielsson, 1993) and is informative in transplant patients revealing rejection, recurrence of primary disease, drug toxicity and other causes of liver damage (Brown et al., 2000).

The general limitations of liver biopsy represent the risk of complications (Poynard et al., 2004), sampling error (Poynard et al., 2004; Skripenova et al., 2007) and inter- and intra-observer variability (Poynard et al., 2004). However, the risk of serious complications is low (Shiha et al., 2009) - 3 per 1000 (Poynard et al., 2004), and the general risk of complications is estimated as 1% (Standish et al., 2006). The described risk of mortality has been between 0.1% - 0.01% (Standish et al., 2006). The variability can be reduced by scoring systems, and sampling error can be partially limited by keeping the standards. Namely, liver biopsy can be considered representative if it contains at least 11 portal fields or measures at least 1 cm (Skripenova et al., 2007). If the tissue fragment is markedly less than 1 cm, immediate rebiopsy can be performed.

Liver biopsy allows to perform visual examination of tissue structure. To ensure this, the logistics is mostly routine, not placing high requirements. The biopsied tissues are fixed in formalin and embedded in the paraplast. The paraffin blocks and stained sections can be archived thus providing several benefits. The biopsy can be re-evaluated and/or sent for second opinion. The second opinion can be obtained faster by application of full slide scanning and exchange of electronic files. The tissues can be later subjected to any novel examination methods in accordance with the development of medical science and practice. Scientific studies can also benefit from those materials, especially in large medical centres. The turnover time for liver biopsy is reasonable - 24 hours for routine logistics or 4 hours using fast processing.

The informativity of biopsy is highly dependent on the applied protocol of visualisation methods. The routine protocol could include haematoxylin-eozin (Gamble&Wilson, 2002), PAS (Totty, 2002), Masson's trichrome (Jones, 2002) and Perls' stain (Churukian, 2002) although modifications can definitely exist. Reticulin stain (Jones, 2002) can be advised. Stains for Wilson's disease can be applied to selected cases (Churukian, 2002). Immunohistochemistry for cytokeratins 7 and / or 19 helps to highlight bile ducts and is very useful in the assessment of general morphology, bile duct damage, ductopenia, ductular reaction. Viral antigens should be sought for (Desmet&Rosai, 2004). The differential diagnostics of focal lesions involves the need to differentiate between benign and malignant lesion, primary and metastatic malignancy including the complex question of identifying the origin of cancer of unknown primary. Thus, wide spectrum immunohistochemistry and search for chromosomal translocations are the requirements for diagnostics.

Further, we will describe in short the informativity of biopsy in different clinical situations, with the emphasis on the limitations.

The application of serologic and virologic examination has mostly replaced the use of biopsy for the diagnostics of acute viral hepatitis. If biopsy is performed, the type and degree of hepatocellular damage, the inflammatory acivity and presence or absence of regeneration can be assessed (Desmet&Rosai, 2004). Predominance of lobular parenchymal lesions is characteristic. The alternative diagnoses or combined liver lesion can be revealed in biopsy. It can be clinically reasonable to perform liver biopsy in order to differentiate between acute and chronic hepatitis. If marked fibrosis is present the morphological diagnosis is straightforward. However, this situation can also represent one of the limits of morphological diagnosis as the portal infiltrate in acute hepatitis may be marked and cause some degree of damage to limiting plate thus resembling chronic active hepatitis. In turn, some cases of chronic hepatitis show only mild changes. In case of severe acute hepatitis, the biopsy might reveal bridging or submassive necrosis. However, the condition of the patient can preclude the biopsy in such situations. The representativity of biopsy can be the limiting factor in the evaluation of submassive liver necrosis due to focality of lesions.

In case of chronic hepatitis, semiquantitative scoring systems provide useful prognostic information, improve the consistency of reporting the disease activity and stage and ensure acceptable intra- and interobserver variability. The examples of such systems include the Histological Activity (HAI) index or Knodell index (Knodell et al., 1981), the Scheuer scoring system (Scheuer, 1991), the modified HAI by Ishak (Ishak et al., 1995) and METAVIR system (Bedossa&Poynard, 1996). The extent of liver fibrosis can be evaluated directly in the biopsy. This assessment is highly accurate in cirrhosis, bridging fibrosis and portal fibrosis and yields clinically unexpected data only occasionally. Liver biopsy is the procedure of choice to assess the amount of fibrosis in the tissue (Shiha et al., 2009). The biopsy allows assessing even slight tissue damage. Even mild hepatitis can progress as reflected by increasing level of fibrosis in repeated liver biopsies (Ryder et al., 2004). Liver steatosis is frequently found in chronic hepatitis patients and can contribute to the elevation of transaminases level in blood. The degree and type of liver steatosis can be assessed separately from the necroinflammatory activity. Biopsy can also reveal combined liver damage. The limitations of biopsy in the diagnostics of chronic viral hepatitis are represented by the lack of specific morphologic changes, particularly regarding chronic viral hepatitis C. Thus, the biopsy must be used in conjunction with serologic and virologic data.

Liver biopsy can be used for the diagnosis of steatosis and steatohepatitis. Quantitative evaluation is possible for steatosis and fibrosis. Although fat stains can be used high quality routine histological slides stained with haematoxylin and eozin and PAS usually ensure the diagnosis. The limitations are caused by inability to distinguish between non-alcoholic steatohepatitis and alcohol – related hepatitis in abstaining patient.

Liver biopsy is considered important in establishing the diagnosis of autoimmune hepatitis (Oo et al., 2010). The information about features typical for autoimmune hepatitis is helpful as reflected by inclusion of these data in the diagnostic criteria. The absence of biliary abnormalities or steatosis is also of importance helping to exclude alternative diagnoses. The effect of immunosuppresion can be predicted (Feld, 2005) and monitored by biopsy (Oo et al, 2010). Biopsy is recommended before treatment withdrawal (Carpenter&Czaja, 2002; Montano-Loza et al, 2007; Czaja&Carpenter, 2003). Due to lack of specifity and possibility of plasma cell paucity in autoimmune hepatitis, the serologic data must be evaluated together with the biopsy.

Examination of liver biopsy for biliary diseases represents a complex problem. The most common questions target primary sclerosing cholangitis and primary biliary cirrhosis. Primary sclerosing cholangitis is a chronic cholestatic liver disease that typically affects young and middle-aged men, frequently suffering from inflammatory bowel disease (Silveira&Lindor, 2008a, 2008b). Although the disease is rare, it is among frequent indications for liver transplantation in Europe and USA, and is dangerous for the increased risk of cholangiocarcinoma. The evaluation of liver biopsy for primary sclerosing cholangitis can both bring information and face problems. Primary sclerosing cholangitis is characterised by loss of medium and large-sized bile ducts. The fibro-obliterative lesions and lack of bile duct in the portal area adjacent to large artery and vein are characteristic. However, ducts of such size are not typically captured in a percutaneous liver biopsy. The concentric periductal fibrosis is characteristic but present in less than 15% of patients. However, the evaluation of autoantibodies is also not very helpful thus increasing the role of biopsy.

The primary biliary cirrhosis (Hohenester et al., 2009; Kumagi&Heathcote, 2008) is an immune-mediated chronic progressive inflammatory liver disease characterised by the destruction of small portal bile ducts leading to progressive cholestasis, fibrosis and cirrhosis. Serum antimitochondrial autoantibodies are highly characteristic. Histologically, biliary duct damage and ductopenia are typical. Biopsy is not mandatory, but can be helpful in revealing typical picture, excluding other causes of liver damage and providing stage information.

Hereditary haemochromatosis, a group of inherited disorders that result in progressive iron overload, occurs mostly due to mutations in the *HFE* gene (Clark et al., 2010). The tests are available to reveal the two clinically relevant mutations C282Y and H63D. However, the penetrance of the disease seems to be low: 28.4% for males and 1.2 % in females homozygous for C282Y (Clark et al., 2010). Liver biopsy can determine the severity of liver disease; reveal other causes and *HFE*-mutation negative hemochromatosis.

In case of Wilson's disease, liver biopsy can be implemented in the primary diagnostic work-up. As clinically the course of fibrosis has been found difficult to follow, repeated biopsies are advocated for monitoring (Yokoyama et al., 2010).

In addition, liver biopsy is valuable in the evaluation of focal liver damage including the important and complex question of tumour diagnostics and differential diagnostics. Liver cell tumours and tumour-like lesions represent a wide diagnostic area, including focal nodular hyperplasia, liver cell adenoma, hepatocellular carcinoma, hepatoblastoma, bile duct tumours, epithelioid hemangioendothelioma and other lesions. In the diagnostics of hepatocellular carcinoma, the sensitivity and specifity of liver biopsy is 96% and 95%, correspondingly (Bialecki&Bisceglie, 2005). In contrast, the application of other methods can result in false-positive diagnosis with the rate as high as 33% (Hayashi et al., 2004). In case of malignancy, metastasis should always be considered. The implementation of immunohistochemistry has resulted in higher diagnostic yield of liver biopsy for neoplastic lesions. The identification of the primary origin of metastatic tumours can be reached in a fraction of cases. Inflammatory focal lesions as echinococcosis or liver abscess can be diagnosed reliably.

As shown, liver biopsy is used and should be used as a part of the complex examination for the analysis of the etiology, activity and extent of diffuse and focal liver damage as well as assessment of the treatment results.

Liver biopsy is an invasive method, there are potential adverse effects and complications. Certain precautions and means minimize the risks of adverse events. Biopsy conducted by a trained physician, use of only a limited number of passes and ultrasound quidance can significantly decrease the risk of complications, thereby enhancing the safety of biopsy (Bedossa&Carrat, 2009).

The main drawbacks (Bedossa, 2009; Reddy&Schiff, 2002; Rousselet et al., 2005; Colli&Fraqeulli, 2009) of liver biopsy as a diagnostic procedure lie in sampling and observation errors. Observer variation is a potential limitation of biopsy that is related to the discordance between pathologists in biopsy interpreation.

The main alternatives to liver biopsy that have been developed in the past 10 years are based on two very different concepts: serum markers and liver stiffness (Manning&Afdhal, 2008). These are noninvasive procedures.

Biochemical marker combinations are being developed as alternatives to liver biopsy in patients with liver diseases, especially with chronic liver diseases. Noninvasive tests are being developed to replace liver biopsy, and thus avoid the risk of biopsy-related adverse events. Noninvasive tests also have the potential to avoid limitations of liver biopsy including the risk of sampling errors and inter- and intra-pathologist variability.

Although clinicians already use liver biopsy substitutes - surrogate markers in their practices, offers are waiting for more valid tests (Mehta et al., 2009), especially for staging fibrosis and apoptosis identification and confirmation.

Fibrosis is not an autonomous feature, but rather a tissue lesion resulting from other pathologic mechanisms such as inflammatory, degenerative or dystrophic processes leading to other pathologic mechanisms such as hepatocellular carcinoma and portal hypertension.

The physiological process of apoptosis (programmed cell death) can be transformed into a pathological process, which can stimulate hepatic fibrosis, e.g. in hepatitis C, or can contribute to treatment failure (Schinoni et al., 2006). Over the last years, the importance of apoptosis for the pathogenesis of various diseases has been extensively investigated. Apoptosis is a greek term that means „the fall of the old leaves of the autumn trees". This term describes the process by which undesirable, damaged old cells are eliminated from multicellular organisms.

Apoptosis differs from cellular necrosis, because it is actively controlled, and the membrane integrity is maintained, avoiding extravasation of intracellular material and an inflammatory response. In order to discover the probable mechanisms by which hepatitis viruses and other agents perpetuate in the liver, apoptosis in liver disorders should be investigated. Apoptosis is the first step in hepatic lesions, and fibrosis is the final response of hepatic stellate cells to this process. There may be a direct relationship between these two processes.

Apoptosis and cell necrosis can be differentiated by morphology. However, liver diseases are often accompanied by a combination of both processes, so that there is mostly no clear borderline. Apoptosis assessment is still not frequent in liver biopsy. At the same time several apoptosis biochemical markers in blood are available at present (cytochrome C, cytokeratin-18 neoepitopes etc.), but are not widely used in the practice.

Fibrosis is a consequence of the necroinflammatory process. The process of fibrogenesis results in an increase in the extracellular matrix of: 1) collagen, 2) glycoproteins and 3) proteoglycans (e.g. hyaluronic acid).

Fibrotic status is usually assessed by liver biopsy, which has numerous disadvantages (Bottero et al., 2009), therefore prompting the development of several noninvasive methods for assessing fibrosis. However, the etiology of liver disease and the existence of co-morbidities impact the performance of non-invasive markers and cut-off values (Bottero et al., 2009).

Liver biopsy is currently the gold standard for assessment of liver fibrosis, yet it faces competition from non-invasive markers, which are easier to use, more acceptable to patient

and repeatable over time. Besides, biopsy sample is usually too small to diagnose the disease accurately and diagnostic opinions often differ among pathologists (Rousselet et al., 2005). As a result, a morphological examination does not always provide an accurate diagnosis. Recently, blood hyaluronic acid has been available for the assessment of liver fibrosis as a rapid and less invasive method.
The specific course of disease might be explained also by the diverse immunogenetic backgrounds of the individual patient. The host ability to react to viral antigens has often been associated with the human leukocyte antigen (HLA), mainly HLA class II antigens. Many studies suggest that the cellular immune response, e.g. to HCV, particularly the T helper (Th) lymphocyte response, plays a crucial role. The cell-receptors recognize only peptides bound to HLA class II molecules. Polymorphisms due to amino acid substitutions at specific positions may intervene within the HLA class II molecule and interact with both the peptide and T-cell-receptor; therefore, the HLA type characterizing each individual may influence the subject's immune response to particular pathogens. Certain HLA alleles have been shown to influence the outcome of other chronic viral infections, and a few recent studies have examined class II HLA alleles in the context of HCV clearance. The present study, which considers the relationship between HCV and HLA class II antigens from the locus DRB1* of view, aimed to investigate whether diferences of HLA class II antigens exist among HCV - infected patients with respect to healthy controls. The possibility that these antigens are associated with resistance or susceptibility to chronic HCV infection was also considered. The HLA class III human leukocyte antigens (DRB1*) are central to the host immune response and thus are ideal candidate genes to investigate for associations with HCV outcomes. During the study we investigated whether human leukocyte antigen (HLA-DRB1) alleles were associated with the response to PEG-interferon+Ribavirin (combined therapy) and Realdiron therapy in patients with chronic hepatitis C.
Our aim was to identify the new non-invasive methods to be used for the assessment of liver function in acute and chronic liver diseases and to evaluate the clinical diagnostic and prognostic accuracy of these methods, including immunogenetic methods, to cover advantages and disadvantages of noninvasive alternatives to liver biopsy, and to share experience and impressions accumulated in area of hepatology.

## 2. Materials and methods

During the process of apoptosis the sequential activation of caspases (they all are proteases that cleave proteins at aspartic acid residue) creates an expanding cascade of proteolytic activity which leads to digestion of structural proteins in cytoplasm and generates, e.g. apoptotic cytokeratin 18 (CK-18) neoepitopes.
To define the role of apoptosis in the development of acute and chronic HBV and HCV infection, the quantitative detection of serum CK-18 neoepitope was performed by using noninvasive method for caspase-generated CK-18 fragments determination (M30-Apoptosense®, ELISA kit, PEVIVA, Sweden) in 11 patients with acute hepatitis B, 14 - with acute hepatitis C, 132 - with chronic hepatitis C and, for comparison, in 23 patients with acute alcoholic hepatitis, all treated in the Infectology Center of Latvia.
The mitochondrial pathway involvement in the process of apoptosis was evaluated by determination of serum cytochrome C according to „Human cytochrome C ELISA", Bender MedSystems (Austria) in 129 patients with chronic hepatitis C, in 12 patients with acute hepatitis B and in 29 patients with acute alcoholic hepatitis.

Serum hyaluronic acid (HA) as a potential marker of fibrosis evolution was measured by ELISA (Corgenix Inc., Colorado, USA) according to description of manufacturer in 16 patients with acute hepatitis B, 9 – with acute hepatitis C, 22 – with acute alcoholic hepatitis and 132 patients with chronic hepatitis C.
The study was conducted in compliance with the Declaration of Helsinki and in accordance with Good Clinical Practice guidelines and local regulations and was approved at the Ethics Committee of Riga Stradins University (Riga, Latvia).
Diagnosis was based on modern immunochemical hepatitis marker assays and clinical, biochemical and morphological findings. Results were expressed as means±SE. For the comparison of two groups the unpaired Student's t-test was used; $p \geq 0.05\%$ was considered significant.
168 patients were enrolled in immunogenomic study and divided into four groups. Group A included 59 patients with HCV infection, treated with PEG-interferon + Ribavirin. Group B consisted of 45 patients with HCV infection and the same treatment regimen, but ineffective. Group C consisted of 30 patients with HCV infection (effective Realdiron therapy). Group D included 34 patients with HCV infection treated with Realdiron (non-responders). In group E, 100 healthy donors were included as the control group.
HLA typing low-resolution for HLA- DRB1* was performed by polymerase chain reaction (PCR) with amplification using sequence-specific primers (SSP). PCR products were separated on 3% agarose, the amplified bands were visualized, and the DRB1 type was deduced.
The distribution of HLA-DRB1* genes in all five groups (A, B, C, D and E controls) was compared using the chi-squared test with Yates' correction or Fisher's Exact. Odd ratios (OR) were calculated according to the Woolf's formula. All reported p-values were compared to a level of significance set to 0.05.

## 3. Results and discussion

Performed studies showed very high serum level of CK-18 neoepitope in patients with acute hepatitis B (1362.3±108.9 U/L), that is higher than in patients with alcoholic hepatitis (1003.9±104.3 U/L; $0.02<p<0.05$). CK-18 neoepitope concentration in acute hepatitis C (712.2±124.4 U/L) and chronic hepatitis C (232.3±15.8 U/L; $0.001<p<0.01$) was significantly lower (Table 1). Besides, about 1/3 of chronic hepatitis C patients had normal serum ALT activity, but elevated serum CK-18 neoepitope concentration.
Normally, cytochrome C is not detectable in serum, but 47.45% of patients with chronic hepatitis C had the increased level (0.29 ±0.05 ng/ml) of this apoptosis indicator (Table 1). Serum concentration of cytochrome C was even higher in acute hepatitides of viral and toxic etiologies.

| Patients | Cytokeratin-18 U/L (mean±SE) | Cytochrome C ng/ml (mean±SE) |
|---|---|---|
| **Acute hepatitis B** | 1362.3±108.9 (n=11) | 1.52±1.14 (n=14) |
| **Acute hepatitis C** | 712.2±124.4 (n=14) | 3.15±1.84 (n=3) |
| **Chronic hepatitis C** | 232.3±15.8 (n=132) | 0.29±0.05 (n=129) |
| **Acute alcoholic hepatitis** | 1003.9±104.3 (n=23) | 0.59±0.19 (n=58) |

Reference intervals for: Cytokeratin-18 – 47.1-103.9 U/l, Cytochrome C -0

Table 1. Level of apoptosis markers in serum from patients with acute and chronic liver diseases.

Very high serum concentration of HA was found in patients with acute alcoholic hepatitis (1015.50±58.83 ng/ml). Serum HA level was significantly higher in acute hepatitis B (228.13±51.71 ng/ml) than in acute hepatitis C (58.33±27.22 ng/ml, p<0.001). The level of serum HA in patients with chronic hepatitis was 103.82±15.47 ng/ml (Table 2).

| **Patient group** | **Number of patients** | **Hyaluronic acid ng/ml (mean±SE)** |
|---|---|---|
| **Acute hepatitis B** | 16 | 228.13±1.71 |
| **Acute hepatitis C** | 9 | 58.33±27.22 |
| **Chronic hepatitis C** | 132 | 103.82±15.47 |
| **Acute alcoholic hepatitis** | 22 | 1015.50±58.83 |

Reference interval: 0-75 ng/ml

Table 2. Serum hyaluronic acid in patients with acute and chronic liver diseases.

In the present study we identified HLA-DRB1 alleles associated with the risk of HCV infection or protection in comparison with healthy subjects. Some differences in the strength of those markers are presented in Table 3.

HLA DRB1*07 (OR=7.0, p<0.0001), HLA-DRB1*03 (OR=1.95, p<0.035) and HLA-DRB1*05 (OR=1.66, p<0.026) alleles were observed with the highest frequency, but DRB1*06, (OR=0.56, p<0.034) and DRB1*15 alleles (OR=0.59, p<0.020) - with the lowest frequency among patients with HCV infection.

Table 4 shows the association of different alleles of HLA class II genes with HCV infection and therapy. One hundred four patients received PEG-interferon + Ribavirin therapy. Fifty nine patients were characterized as responders, and the remaining 45 as non-responders.

| **Alleles DRB1*** | **HCV (n=336)** | **Controls (n=200)** | **Odds Ratio** | ***(p)*** |
|---|---|---|---|---|
| *01 | 48 | 31 | 0.91 | <0.701** |
| *15 | 49 | 45 | **0.59** | **<0.020** |
| *03 | 43 | 14 | **1.95** | **<0.035** |
| *04 | 39 | 23 | 1.01 | <0.970** |
| *05 | 83 | 33 | **1.66** | **<0.026** |
| *06 | 29 | 28 | 0.56 | <0.034 |
| *07 | 42 | 4 | **7.0** | **<0.000** |
| *08 | 3 | 14 | **0.12** | **<0.000** |
| *09 | 0 | 2 | - | - |
| *10 | 0 | 5 | - | - |

**Cornfield not accurate. Extract limits preferred.
Bold-face type highlihts statistically significant associations for patient's vs controls.
p-probability (l-p) *100%, OR – odds ratio
n=number of haplotypes (eg, 336 alleles from 168 individuals). Nature of valve lesions was not reported on 2 patients.

Table 3. The frequency of identified DRB1* alleles in HCV patients and control subjects.

| DRB1* alleles | *01 | *15 | *03 | *04 | *05 | *06 | *07 |
|---|---|---|---|---|---|---|---|
| Patients in total n=168 (general group) | 0.18 | **0.59/ (0.020)** | **1.95/ (0.035)** | | **1.66/ (0.026** | **0.56/ (0.034)** | **7.0/ (0.000)** |
| Effective PEG INF+Ribavirin therapy (group A) n=59 | 0.14 | 0.14 | 0.13 | **1.79/ 0.014** | 0.21 | **4.29/ (0.003)** | 0.03 |
| Noneffective PEG INF+Ribavirin therapy (group B) n=45 | 0.16 | 0.16 | 0.12 | 0.08 | **0.62/ 0.013** | 0.06 | **0.18/ 0.005** |
| Effective Realdiron therapy (group C) n=30 | **2.58/ 0.071** | 0.13 | 0.13 | 0.08 | 0.22 | 0.07 | 0.13 |
| Noneffective Realdiron therapy (group D) n=34 | 0.09 | 0.16 | 0.13 | **0.53/ 0.065** | 0.77 | 0.74 | 1.15 |
| Control subjects (group E) n=100 | 0.16 | 0.23 | 0.07 | 0.12 | 0.17 | 0.15 | 0.02 |

Bold-face type highlights statistically significant associations for patient's vs controls.
gf (gene frequency), p (probability), OR (odds ratio) and value are reported only for significant associations (p<0.05). n=number of haplotypes (eg, 336 alleles from 168 individuals).

Table 4. Association of different alleles of HLA class II genes with HCV infection and therapy.

Sixty four patients received Realdiron therapy. Thirty patients were characterized as responders, and the remaining 34 as non-responders. All individuals in the study were genotyped for HLA class II DRB1*alleles.

HLA-DRB1*06(OR=4.29, p<0.003)and HLA-DRB1*04 (OR=1.79, p<0.014) Major Histocompatibility class II alleles were significantly associated with the effective response to PEG interferon + Ribavirin therapy in patients. Our results therefore provide evidence that the presence of HLA DRB1*06 and HLA-DRB1*04 is an important additional factor for predicting a long-term response to PEG-interferon + Ribavirin therapy in patients with chronic hepatitis C.

The results of class II HLA distribution in patients with HCV are presented in Table 4.

HLA-DRB1*01 was detected among patients of group C and D and it was significantly associated (OR=2.58, p<0.071)with the effective response to Realdiron therapy in chronic hepatitis C patients. HLA-DRB1*04 (OR=0.53, p<0.065) was found as an indicator of non-responders to Realdiron therapy in group D. In both groups - C and D, the frequency of the remaining HLA antigens was of minor importance.

Liver biopsy is not always possible or reproducible, it cannot be performed frequently and is a costly invasive procedure with a certain, although low, risk of serious complications. Histological examination of the liver does not provide information about the dynamics of hepatic fibrogenesis, liver biopsy provides only static information about fibrotic process. Non-invasive markers that reflect fibroproliferative activity in the liver and the treatment response would be preferable. Serum hyaluronic acid has been identified as a potential marker of fibrosis evolution.

The clinical benefit of the existing markers may be limited by the etiology or stage of disease. Hyaluronate can be used as a specific marker to detect liver fibrosis (Afdhal&Nunes, 2004) and has been found to correlate with severity of the disease (Lackner C. et al., 2005). Findings of Kawamoto et al. (2006) suggest that hyaluronate can be used to assess severe liver fibrosis or cirrhosis, but it would be difficult to assess liver fibrosis at its early stage.

According to Suzuki et al. (2005), hyaluronic acid has been reported to have a high diagnostic performance in assessing the severity of hepatic fibrosis in patients with alcoholic liver disease.

In the context of above mentioned our findings don't contradict with conclusions of those investigators, particularly, in case of acute alcoholic hepatitis, when level of hyaluronic acid in blood serum is very high (see Table 2).

Performed parallel histological investigations of liver biopsies from patients with chronic hepatitis C illustrated the heterogeneity of hepatic fibrosis degree. Serum HA levels didn't significantly correlate with the degree of hepatic fibrosis found in these patients. HA could be a marker of hepatic fibrosis progression. In chronic liver diseases, serial HA levels have been advocated as the means to monitor disease progression and to limit the need for follow-up liver biopsy.

The results of performed investigation on main apoptosis markers (cytokeratin-18 neoepitope, cytochrome C) demonstrated very significant involvement of apoptosis (including mitochondrial way) in pathogenesis of acute hepatitis, independently of etiology. This presumption was confirmed by high level of apoptosis markers in serum (see Table 1). The delineation of the signalling patways that mediate apoptosis has changed the paradigms of understanding of many liver diseases (Schattenberg et al., 2006). Apoptosis is the normal physiological response to many chemical, physical and biological stimuli. Mitochondria and cell surface receptors mediate the two main pathways of apoptosis (Reed, 2000). Hypoxia has been shown to promote apoptosis (Holmgren L. et al., 1995). As apoptosis is closely involved in the process of liver disease progression, the treatment of ischemic injury remains one of the most challenging areas of hepatology today.

Apoptosis defines a type of cell death distinct from the more conventional necrotic death on the basis of characteristic morphological features. Although these descriptions and distinctions are useful, there is a great deal of overlap between apoptosis and necrosis in morphological features and biochemical events. Indeed, apoptosis is frequently followed by secondary necrosis of cells, especially, if there is failure of clearance or ingestion of apoptotic bodies (Bennett, 2002).

One of the aims of our study was to confirm the influence of HLA class II genes on the progression of HCV infection and to assess a possible relationship between these genes and different therapies. For this purpose we used the PCR-SSP test which permits the routine determination of the distribution of HLA class II genes. We confirmed that the frequency of HLA-DRB1*06 (4.29/0.003)and *04(1.79,0.014) was significantly higher in patients from group A than in patients from group B. In general group HLA-DRB1*07 and HLA-DRB1*05 alleles were observed.HLA-DRB1*07 was found as an indicator of non-responders to PEG-interferon + Ribavirin therapy (group B).

In all HCV patient groups, a correlation was found between certain HLA genes and the extent of liver damage. Among the host-related factors which have an important role in determining the outcome of HCV infection, certain HLA class II genes appear crucial for resolution or progression of hepatitis C.

Accumulation evidence regarding the limitations of biopsy have led some to suggest that non-invasive markers should replace biopsy as the initial method for disease staging. But further research is needed to evaluate the long-term effectiveness of the these strategies before a global recommendation can be made (Mehta et al., 2009). It is widely appreciated that substantial error has been observed when biopsy specimens have been compared to the full liver (Colloredo et al., 2003).

There are several advantages in using non-invasive markers: they can be used to accurately define an appropriate time for treatment initiation, they can help monitoring and assess the therapeutic efficacy of antiviral treatment in case of liver fibrosis and cirrhosis, etc., they are crucial to evaluate the performance of non-invasive markers used for diagnosis of liver fibrosis and apoptosis in HAV, HBV, HCV, HIV-infected patients.

A number of radiological methods are used in diagnosis of various chronic liver diseases. The first of them most often is ultrasonography (US). Signs of liver cirrhosis in B-mode image are well known. They are the irregularity and nodularity of liver surface, coarse nodularity of parenchyma structure, *lobus caudatus* hypertrophy, as well as symptoms of portal hypertension such as splenomegaly, ascites and portocaval shunts. The specificity of the method in detection of cirrhosis is in the range from 80% to 100%, sensitivity - from 43% to 88% (Needleman et al, 1986; Giorgio et al., 1986; Di Lelio et al., 1989; Gaiani et al., 1997; Colli et al., 2003; Vigano M. et al., 2005). Irregularity and nodularity of the liver surface caused by altering foci of regeneration nodules and necrosis (Poff et al., 2008) can be better assessed using high-frequency linear probe (Colli et al., 2003.; Nishiura et al., 2005). Nodularity of the structure is a prognostic sign of increased risk of developing hepatocellular carcinoma. This symptom is more common in liver cirrhosis of HDV hepatitis origin (51%), less common in other causes of diseases (9%) (Caturelli et al., 2003). A significant sign of liver cirrhosis is splenomegaly. The spleen size which overexceeds 15 cm is a symptom with 98% specificity and 57% sensitivity (O'Donohue et al., 2004). By combining sonographic symptoms of B-mode imaging in a common system several researchers have gained increment of specificity of the method (Nishiura et al., 2005). Liver cirrhosis is characterized by changes in liver size and its proportion: atrophy of the right lobe and the medial segment of the left lobe as well as hypertrophy of *lobus caudatus* and the lateral segment of the left lobe (Giorgio et al., 1986; Lafortune et al., 1998). In total, the diagnostic accuracy of US in detection of liver cirrhosis is high enough, while its applicability in precirrhotic stages of the disease is limited.

As chronic liver disease progresses, numerous processes occur in the structure altering liver blood flow. Under normal conditions liver receives 70-75% of blood through the portal vein, 25-30% through the hepatic artery, leaving a very small fraction for such tiny blood vessels as aberrant gastric veins, particularly the right (Matsui et al., 1995) which occurs in about 6-14 % of patients, *a.phrenica dx*, parabiliary veins (Couinaud, 1988), gallblader vein, which sometimes is drained directly to the liver. As a result of cirrhotic and fibrotic processes presinusoidal and sinusoidal occlusion develops there which increases resistance for the blood flow through the liver. A portal hypertension develops, if the pressure gradient overexceeds 10 mm $H_2O$ (Zwiebel&Pellerito, 2005). Due to the increased resistance as the portal blood flow diminishes, there is a compensatory increment of the flow in the hepatic artery (Burton-Opitz, 1911; Kock et al., 1972). As a result of the increment of the pressure in the portal vein, its size and pulsations are altered, blood flow slows down and later changes its direction from hepatopetal to hepatofugal. Increase in pressure in the portal vein is compensated through portocaval anastomoses. The hepatic artery itself does not have such a mechanism. It is compensated through very tiny (under normal conditions) anastomoses between portal and arterial system, which are located in the liver sinusoides, *vasa vasorum* of the portal vein and peribiliary vascular plexes. If transhepatic resistance overexceeds resistance of portosystemic collaterals, a shunting of arterial flow to the portal system starts to occur (Sacerdoti et al., 1995; Piscaglia et al., 1997). Flow characteristics and their changes in liver blood vessels are well detectable in doplerographic examinations. Veins of portal systems - *v.portae, v.mesenterica sup., v.lienalis,* as well as hepatic artery and liver veins are well visible in approximately 93-95% of patients undergoing liver sonography (Zwiebel & Pellerito, 2005).

A number of parameters and indexes are offered to assess and detect portal hypertension. They are: diameter of the portal vein, change of the size of *v.portae* and *v.lienalis* during the respiratory cycle, flow rate and direction in the portal vein, pulsitility of Doppler spectral waveform as well as congestation index, respectively: ratio between cross-sectional area of the portal vein and the flow velocity within it, the resistance index in the hepatic artery, portal and hepatic artery velocity rate, etc. Many studies have been performed regarding utility of all these parameters in diagnostics of liver cirrhosis, however the results are still controversial.

One of the signs of liver cirrhosis and portal hypertension is hepatofugal flow in the portal vein, i.e., the flow away from the liver. This sign is found in 3–23% of cirrhosis patients (Kawasaki et al., 1989; Gaiani et al., 1991; Taourel et al., 1998; von Herbay et al., 2001). Incidence of this symptom depends on the severity of the disease. The flow direction in the portal vein is influenced also by development of the paraumbilical shunts, retaining the hepatopetal flow in cirrhosis patients. Hepatofugal flow can also be found in patients with extrahepatic shunts (splenorenal, oesophageal, retroperitoneal, etc.).

The portal flow velocity, which is an easily assessable measure, is a variable parameter. In healthy subjects in various studies it ranges from 13.7 cm/s to 22 cm/s (O'Donohue et al., 2004; Walsh et al., 1998; Bernatik et al., 2002). With the development of liver cirrhosis it declines. For the diagnosis of liver cirrhosis using a cut-off value of 13 to 15 cm/s the sensitivity is 74.5% to 88%, the specificity - 53% to 96% (Zironi et al., 1992; Schneider et al., 2005; Iwao et al., 1997). In precirrhotic stages there is no significant difference in velocity of the portal flow from healthy subjects (Bernatik et al., 2002; Schneider et al., 2005).

Under normal conditions the flow in the portal vein is continuous and hepatopetal but its velocity is slightly pulsatile during the heart cycle. These pulsations cause a pressure change in the right atrial flow initiated by fluctuations in the lower vena cava which through the liver veins and sinusoides are transmitted to *v.portae*. Pronounced pulsations in the portal vein in patients with right heart diseases serve as the evidence of such explanation of the pulsation mechanism (Görg et al., 2002). Besides, there is also influence of the adjacent hepatic artery pulsations and respiratory cycle phases. Presinusoidal obstruction, collagenisation of the Disse space and enlargement of hepatocytes due to liver fibrosis and cirrhosis may prevent the transmission of pulsations from the heart and liver veins. Flatened Doppler waveform of the portal vein could therefore be a sign of liver fibrosis and cirrhosis. Undulating Doppler waveform of the portal vein in healthy subjects is found in 63.8%-100% of cases. The degree of pulsatility of the portal vein quantitatively is characterized by two indexes: the ratio between minimal and maximal flow velocity as well as pulsation index (PI) in which the maximal flow rate is extended to the difference between the minimum and the maximum flow rate. The minimum and maximum velocity ratio >0.54 for healthy subjects is higher than 90% of cases (Gallix et

al., 1997). In liver cirrhosis patients reduced hepatic vein pulsatility is found significantly more often than in patients with lower degrees of fibrosis or in healthy subjects, however, the incidence in different studies varies considerably. Distinguishing between various degrees of severity of fibrosis in this manner fails (Schneider et al., 2005; Barkat, 2004; Maktanir et al., 2005).
In a number of studies the measurement of size of the portal vein is used as one of the methods of detecting portal hypertension. In most cases in healthy subjects the portal vein is smaller than in patients suffering from cirrhosis and various degrees of liver fibrosis, although these differences are not statistically significant and a large overlap of values is found (O'Donohue et al., 2004; Lim et al., 2005; Kutlu et al., 2002). Similar results were gained when determining the liver congestation index, calculated by extending v.portae diameter to the average blood flow velocity in it (Walsh et al., 1998; Lim et al., 2005), although some studies provide evidence of the ability of this feature to differentiate liver cirrhosis from other conditions (Kutlu et al., 2002).
As the sinusoidal resistance increases and the portal flow decreases there is a compensatory increment of the flow in the liver artery. Since the increase of resistance also affects the arterial system, changes occur in haemodynamic parameters recordable in Doppler waveform as well as increase of the resistance index and growth of the volume. Under normal conditions a Doppler waveform of hepatic artery of healthy subjects is of low pulsitility with antegrade flow within whole diastole. Resistance index (RI), determined by extending the peak systolic and end-diastolic velocity difference to the peak systolic velocity in healthy subjects ranges from 0.5 to 0.7 (Vilgranin, 2001). In cirrhotic patients RI within different studies ranges from 0.68 to 0.98, in precirrhotic stages of the disease - from 0.58 to 0.73 (O'Donohue et al., 2004; Bernatik et al., 2002; Haktanir et al., 2005; Lim et al., 2005; Pierce&Sewell, 1990). The overlap of these parameters significantly limits the use of dopplerographic parameters of hepatic arteries in diagnostics. No studies have yielded results that would reliably differentiate various degrees of fibrosis from each other.
In some trials a number of other arterial flow factors have been used, as the mean flow velocity (cm/s), minute volume flow (ml/min), liver perfusion index (hepatic artery and common liver flow ratio), however, they have not gained wide acceptance.
One of the most widely used liver vascular ultrasound examination is hepatic vein dopplerography. In most cases liver veins are easily visible tubular structure, with diameter changing during the respiratory cycle. In healthy subjects 2 cm away from the inflow to *v. cava inferior* it is 4-6 mm but less than 1 cm (Bolondi et al., 1991). In cases of various diseases, such as the right heart diseases, circulatory congestion in the large vasculatory circle, severe liver steatosis, Budd-Chiary syndrome, etc. vein size may vary. Blood flow in liver veins is markedly pulsating, changing directions with different phases of the cardiac cycle. During the diastole of the heart atria and ventriculi it is antegrade, respectively towards the heart, or away from the liver. During the atrial systole the flow is retrograde or towards the liver. Healthy liver is elastic and easily responds to the pressure changes in liver veins during heart cycle phases. In the Doppler waveform of liver veins these fluctuations are reflected as two antegrade waves followed by a single retrograde wave. Haemodynamics of the liver veins is detailed in the L.Bolondi study in 1991. (Fig.1)

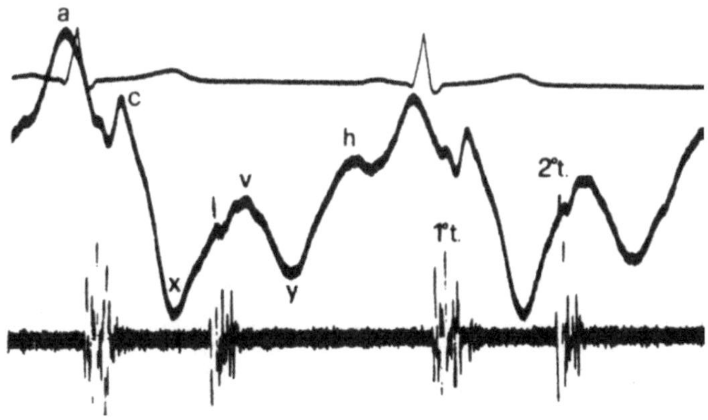


Fig. 1. Mechanism of wave formation in VHDx Doppler waveform. Simultaneous record of ECG, phonocardiogram and Doppler waveform of the jugular vein (adapted from Bolondi L et al, Radiology 1991; 178:513-516.)

Wave A (+) - atrial systole. Retrograde flow in VCI and VH. Wave C (+) - a small positive wave in the descendent part or the A wave which is caused by closing of tricuspidal valves. Wave X (-) - ventricular systole and atrial relaxation (diastole). Antegrade flow during filling of the atrium. Wave V (+) - atrial filing. The peak of the wave shows opening of tricuspidal valves at the begininning of ventricular diastole. Wave Y (-) - ventricular diastole. Atrial emptying towards ventriculi.

In order to assess the Doppler waveform of hepatic veins a number of methods are recommended. The most widespread method was introduced by Bolondi. He advised to divide all curves into 3 groups: triphasic, showing a positive wave due to retrograde flow during the atrial systole, biphasic, with no positive wave, but with saved pulsations, and fully flattened or monophasic appearance. This method is simple, easy to use and reproducible.

Flow type of hepatic veins, respectively, shape of Doppler waveform of liver veins, is dependent on a number of diseases and conditions. Incidence of flattened curve significantly increases during pregnancy and increases as pregnancy progresses (Roobottom et al., 1995). In case of regurgitation and insuficience of tricuspidal valves during ventricular systole the blood is pushed backwards to atria and - further - to *v.cava inferior* and to hepatic veins. In their Doppler waveform the systolic wave X reduces, disappears and becomes retrograde and interacts with wave A (Abu-Yousef, 1991). Also, in case of constrictive pericarditis changes in hepatic vein Doppler waveform are seen (von Birbra et al., 1989).

Pathological processes within liver veins themselves, as Budd-Chiari syndrome and veno-occlusive disease or sinusoidal obstruction syndrome, are seen and diagnosed by B-mode and Doppler ultrasound methods. Unlike Budd-Chiari syndrome, in cases of veno-occlusive disease main liver veins can be patent (Desser et al., 2003).

Flow in liver veins is influenced by intra-abdominal and intrathoracic pressure. In patients with triphasic waveform during deep inspiration and Valsalva test the waveform often paves and becomes monophasic or biphasic (Techgraber et al., 1997). Due to this reason liver vein examination is held during mild, superficial inspiration or mild expiration following mild inspiration.

One of the basic factors influencing the type of liver flow is the physical condition of the liver, its hardness and elasticity. With increase in hardness and decrease in elasticity liver tissue looses compliance with hepatic venous pulsations caused by variations in pressure within them. Haemodynamically it is expressed as loss of changing of flow direction during atrial systole in v.cava inferior and hepatic veins what can be registered by Doppler ultrasound. The feasibility that the hepatic veins Doppler waveform assesses changes in liver structure, resp., fibrosis and cirrhosis, has been investigated by many researchers, and the results are generally better than in other hepatic circulatory dopplerographic measurements, although not very clear.

Flattened, resp., biphasic or monophasic hepatic vein Doppler waveforms in liver cirrhosis patients with varying forms of cirrhosis, occur in 50% (Bolondi et al., 1991) to 85% (Barkat, 2004) cases. With increasing severity of cirrhosis, the frequency of flattened curves increases (von Herbay et al., 2001; Barkat, 2004). The sensitivity and specificity of the method to detect cirrhosis are 37%-75% and respectively 41%-100%, respectively (Colli et al., 2003; Schneider et al., 2005; Arada et al., 1997). In precirrhotic stages of the disease with increase of fibrosis stage the incidence of flattened waveform tends to increase. In some studies this increase is statistically significant (O'Donohue et al., 2004; Schneider et al., 2005), while in others it is insignificant, there is overlap between the results (Bernatik et al., 2002; Lim et al., 2005). This leads to critical assessment of hepatic vein Doppler ultrasound ability to detect the precirrhotic forms or differentiate between degrees of fibrosis, while the diagnosis of cirrhosis flattened Doppler waveform is a key symptom. (Fig.2, 3)

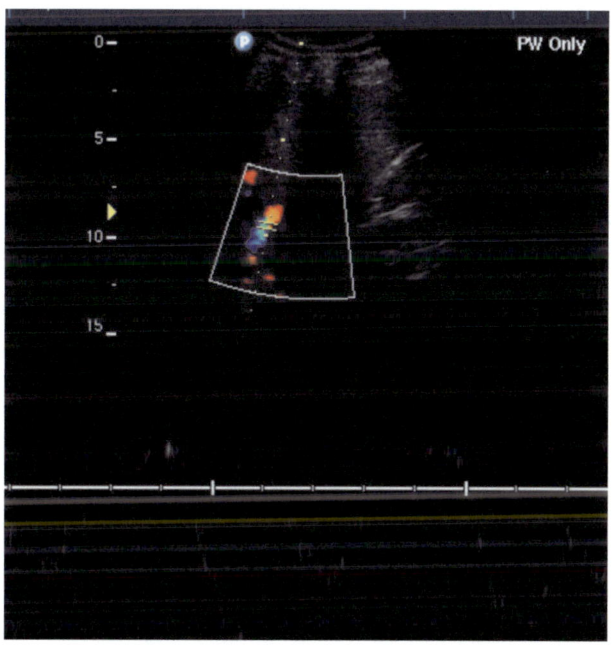


Fig. 2. Triphasic VHDx Doppler waveform in 29 y.o. patient with mild (Knodell F1) liver fibrosis and without liver steatosis (S-0).

Liver steatosis also should be taken into account when assessing liver veins Doppler ultrasound results. The increased fat in the liver increases the pressure on the hepatic veins and reduces liver tissue compliance to venous pulsations. In patients with severe liver steatosis

(> 66% of hepatocytes affected by fat) flattened hepatic vein Doppler waveform is found significantly more frequently than in patients without steatosis or those with mild forms in respectively 90% vs. 5% -20% of cases (Schneider et al., 2005). Sensitivity of the method in detecting severe steatosis is 88%, specificity 74% (Schneider et al., 2005). It should be noted that appearance of liver steatosis in B-Mode ultrasound image has been researched much, however, its effect on blood flow types in hepatic veins, the dependence on the morphological forms of steatosis (macrovesicular or microvesicular) has been assessed much less frequently. (Fig.4)

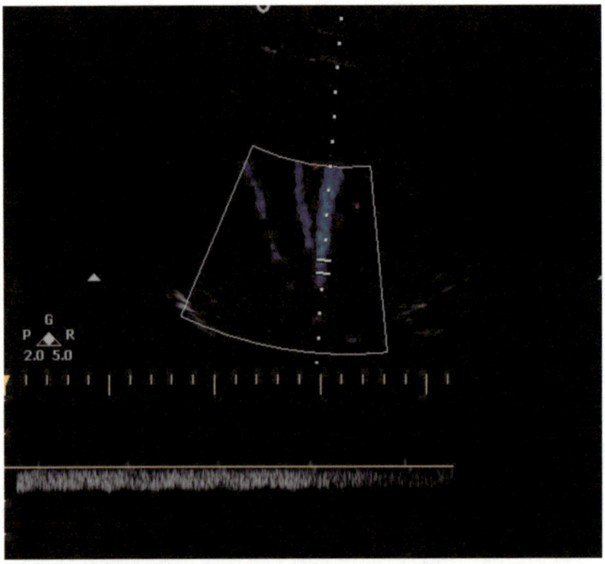


Fig. 3. Monophasic VHDx Dopler waveform in 53 y.o. patient with moderate severity of liver fibrosis (Knodell F-3) and severe mixed type (macro - microvesiculare) steatosis (S3). There are no typical steatosis signs in B- mode image

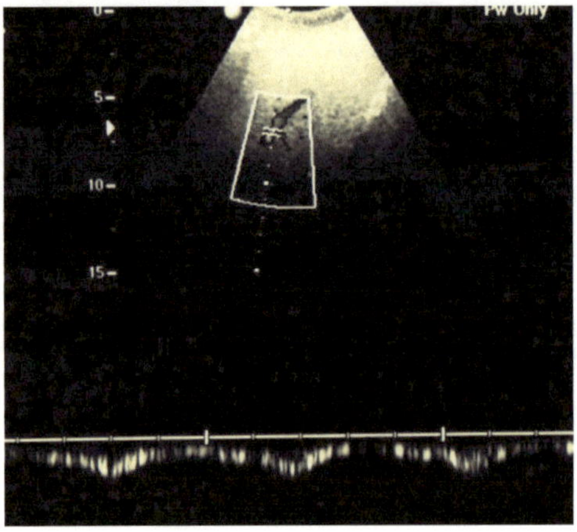


Fig. 4. Biphasic VDHx waveform in 44 y.o. patient with moderate liver steatosis (S-2) and mild fibrosis (F-1). In B-Mode image appearance of expressed steatosis is visible: increased liver exhogenicity, impaired visualization of deeper tissues and diaphragmal line.

## 4. Conclusion

Evaluation of apoptosis by estimating CK-18 neoepitope level should be included into hepatitis virus infection and toxic liver damage management algorithm. Apoptosis, not only necrosis, is essentially involved in liver damage development mechanisms in acute and chronic HBV and HCV infection. Monitoring of serum apoptotic CK-18 neoepitope level might be useful for the appropriate estimation of liver diseases therapy efficacy and open new approach to apoptosis therapeutic regulation.

If in alcoholic hepatitis apoptosis may be a principal cause of cell death, then in acute hepatitis B cell death would be associated with both cell apoptosis and cell necrosis.

As fibrotic process is dynamic, serum hyaluronic acid levels may show fibrogenesis rather than developed and formed fibrosis. Circulating HA measurement has been proposed for operative monitoring of fibrotic lesion dynamics in acute and chronic liver damages.

The punctual identification of immunogenetic factors may prove to be useful in predicting disease evolution, in guiding the appropriate therapy for patients with poor prognosis, and in encouraging the development of untherapeutic strategies.

As regards to the potential of US to assess the diagnosis of diffuse liver disease, it must be concluded that the method is applied to the detection of manifest cirrhosis. In detection of precirrhotic stages and differentiation between them the options are greatly restricted and the liver biopsy cannot be replaced. Liver vein Dopplerography can be applied in liver screening examinations to detect occult liver diseases. It can be also applied in follow-up of diffuse liver diseases, however, this suggestion still requires further studies.

## 5. Acknowledgement

This study was financially supported by the Project No 9.1. of National Program No 4.

## 6. References

Abu-Youset, M.M. (1991). Duplex Doppler Sonography of the Hepatic vein in Tricuspid Regurgitation. *AJR*, Vol.156, pp.79-83

Afdhal, N.H. & Nunes, D. (2004). Evaluation of liver fibrosis: a concise rerview. *Am. J. Gastroenterol.*, Vol.99, pp.1160-1174

Arada, K., Ofelli, M., Calikoglu, U. et al. (1997). Hepatic vein Doppler waveform changes in early stage (Child-Pugh A) chronic liver parenchimal diseases. *J.Clin.Ultrasound*, Vol.25, pp.15-19

Barkat, M. (2004). Non-pulsatile hepatic and portal vein waveforms in patients with liver cirrhosis: concordant and disconcordant relationships. *British J Radiology*, Vol.77, pp.547-550

Bedossa, P.&Poynard, T. (1996). An algorithm for the grading of activity in chronic hepatitis C. The METAVIR Cooperative Study Group. *Hepatology*, Vol.24, No.2, pp.289-293

Bedossa, P.&Carrat, F. (2009). Liver biopsy: the best, not the gold standard. *J. Hepatology*, Vol.50, No.1, pp.1-3

Bedossa, P. (2009). Assessment of hepatitis C: non-invasive fibrosis markers and/or liver biopsy. *Liver international*, Vol.29, S.1, pp.19-22

Bennett, M.R. (2002). Apoptosis in the cardiovascular system. – *Heart*, Vol.87, No.5, pp.480-487

Bernatik, T., Strobel, D., Hahn, E.G.&Becker, D. (2002). Doppler measurements: a surrogate marker of liver fibrosis? *European Journal of Gastroenterology and Hepatology*, Vol.14, pp.383-387

Bialecki, E.S.&Bisceglie, A.M. (2005). Diagnosis of hepatocellular carcinoma. *HPB*, Vol.7, pp.26 - 34

Bolondi, L., Bassi, S.L. et al. (1991). Liver cirrhosis: changes of Doppler waveform of hepatic veins. *Radiology*, Vol.178, pp.513-516

Bottero, J., Lacombe, K., Guéchot, J., Serfaty, L., Miailhes, P., Bonnard, P., Wendum, D., Molina, J.-M., Lascoux-Combe, C. & Girard, P.-M. (2009). Performance of 11 biomarkers for liver fibrosis assessment in HIV/HBV co-infected patients. *J. Hepatology*, Vol.50, No.6, pp.1074-1083

Bravo, A.A., Sheth, S.G.&Chopra S. (2001). Liver biopsy. *N Engl J Med*, Vol.344, No.7, pp.495 - 500

Brown, K.E., Janney, C.G.&Brunt, E.M. (2000). Liver biopsy: indications, technique, complications, and interpretation. In: *Liver disease: diagnosis and management*. Bacon, B.R.; DiBisceglie, A.M. (Eds.) 47-75, Churchill Livingstone, New York

Burton-Opitz R. (1911). The vascularity of the liver: the influence the portal blood flow upon the flow in the hepatic artery. *Experimental Physioloy*, Vol.4, pp.93-102

Carpenter, H.A.&Czaja, A.J. (2002). The role of histoogic evaluation in the diagnosis and management of autoimmune hepatitis and its variants. *Clin Liver Dis*, Vol.6, No.3, pp.685 - 705

Caturelli, E., Castellano, L., Fussili, S. et al. (2003). Coarse nodular pattern in hepatic cirrhosis: risk for hepatocelular carcinoma. *Radioloogy*, Vol.226, pp.691-697

Churukian, C.L. Pigments and minerals. (2002). In: *Theory and practice of histological techniques, 5th ed.* Ed by Bancroft, J.D. and Gamble, M. (Ed.) 243-268, Churchill Livingstone, Edinburgh (International edition)

Clark, P., Britton, L.J., Powell, L.W. (2010). The diagnosis and management of hereditary haemochromatosis. *Clin Biochem Rev*, Vol.31, pp.3 - 8

Colli, A., Fraquelli, M., Andreoletti, M. et al. (2003). Severe Liver Fibrosis or Cirrhosis: Accuracy of US for Detection - Analysis of 300 Cases. *Radiology*, Vol.227, pp.89-94

Colli, A.&Fraquelli, M. (2009). What is the actual role of diagnosis and how to assess it? *J of hepatology*, Vol.50, No.4, pp.827-829

Colloredo, G., Guido, M., Sonzogni, A. & Leandro, G. (2003). Impact of liver biopsy size on histological evaluation of chronic viral hepatitis: the smaller the sample, the milder the disease. *J. Hepatology*, Vol.39, pp.239-244

Couinaud C. Parabiliary venous sistem. (1988). *Surg Radiol Anat*, Vol.10, pp.311-316

Czaja, A.J.&Carpenter, H.A. (2003). Histologic features associated with relapse after corticosteroid withdrawal in type 1 autoimmune hepatitis. *Liver Int*, Vol.23, No.2, pp.116 - 123

Desmet, V.J.&Rosai, J. (2004). Liver. In: *Rosai and Ackerman's surgical pathology, 9th ed.* Rosai J. Mosby (ed.), 917-1034, Edinburgh (International Edition)

Desser, T.S., Sze, D.Y.&Brook, J.R. (2003). Imaging and intervention in the hepatic veins. *AJR*, Vol.180, pp.1583-1591

Di Lelio A., Cestari, C., Lomazzi, A., Beretta, L. (1989). Cirrhosis: diagnosis with sonographic study of the liver surface. *Radiology*, Vol.172, pp.389-392

Dioguardi, N., Grizzi, F., Fiamengo, B.&Russo, C. (2008). Metrically measuring liver biopsy: A chronic hepatitis B and C computer-aided morphologic description. *World J Gastroenterol*, Vol.14, No.48, pp.7335 - 7344

Feld, J.J. (2005). Autoimmune hepatitis: effect of symptoms and cirrhosis on natural history and outcome. *Hepatology*, Vol.42, No.1, pp.53 - 62

Gaiani, S., Bolondi, L., Bassi, L. et al. (1991). Prevalence of spontaneous hepatofugal flow in liver cirrhosis: clinical and endoscopic correlation in 228 patients. *Gastroenterology*, Vol.100, pp.160-167

Gaiani, S., Grammantieri, L., Venturoli, N. et al. (1997). What is the criterion differentiating chronic hepatitis from compensated cirrhosis: a prospective study comparing ultrasonography and percutaneous liver biopsy. *J of Hepatology*, Vol.27, pp.979-985

Gallix, B.P., Taovrel, P., Dauzat, M. et al. (1997). Flow pulsatility in the portal venous system: a study of Doppler sonography in the healthy adults. *AJR*, Vol.169, pp.141-144

Gamble, M.&Wilson, I. (2002). The hematoxylins and eosin. In: *Theory and practice of histological techniques, 5th ed.* Bancroft, J.D. and Gamble, M. (Ed.), 125-138, Churchill Livingstone, Edinburgh (International edition)

Giorgio, A., Amoroso, P., Lettieri, G. et al. (1986). Chirrosis: value of caudate to right lobe ratio in diagnosis with US. *Radiology*, Vol.161, pp.443-445

Görg, C., Riera-Knorrenschild, J.&Diterich, J. (2002). Colour Doppler ultrasound patterns in the portal venous system. *British J of Radiology*. Vol.75, pp.919-929

Haktanir, A., Songul, B., Celenk, C. et al. (2005). Value of Doppler sonography in assessing the progression of chronic viral hepatitis and in the diagnosis and grading of cirrhosis. *J Ultrasound Med.*, Vol.24, pp.311-321

Hamato, N., Moriyasu, F., Someda, H., Nishikawa, K., Chiba, T. et al. (1997). Clinical aplication of hepatic venous hemodinamics by Doppler ultrasonography in chronic liver disease. *Ultrasound Med Biol*, Vol.23, pp.829-835

Hayashi, P.H., Trotter, J.F., Forman, L., Kugelmas, M., Steinberg, T., Russ, P. et al. (2004). Impact of pretransplant diagnosis of hepatocellular carcinoma on cadaveric liver allocation in the era of MELD. *Liver Transpl*, Vol.10, pp.42 - 48

Hohenester, S., Oude-Elferink, R.P.J.&Beuers, U. (2009). Primary biliary cirrhosis. *Semin Immunopathol*, Vol.31, pp.283 - 307

Holmgren, L., O'Reilly, M.S. & Folkman, J. (1995). Dormancy of micrometastases: balanced proliferation and apoptosis in the presence of angiogenesis suppression. *Nat. Med.*, Vol.1, pp.149-153

Hultcrantz, R.&Gabrielsson, N. (1993). Patients with persistent elevation of aminotransferases: investigation with ultrasonography, radionuclide imaging and liver biopsy. *J Intern Med*, Vol.233, pp.7 - 12

Ishak, K., Baptista, A., Bianchi, L., Callea, F., De Groote, J., Gudat, F., Denk, H., Desmet, V., Korb, G., MacSween, R.N. et al. (1995). Histological grading and staging of chronic hepatitis. *J Hepatol*, Vol.22, No.6, pp.696 - 699

Iwao, T., Toyonaga, A., Oho, K. et al. (1997). Value of portal Doppler ultrasound parameters of portal vein and hepatic artery in diagnosis of cirrhosis and poral hypertnesion. *Am J Gastroenterology*, Vol.92, pp.1012-1017

Jones, M.L. (2002). Connective tissues and stains. In: *Theory and practice of histological techniques, 5th ed*. Bancroft, J.D.&Gamble, M. (Eds.), 139-162, Churchill Livingstone, Edinburgh (International edition)

Kawamoto, M., Mizuquchi, T., Katsuramaki, T., Nagayama, M., Oshima, H., Kawasaki, H., Nobuoka, T., Kimura, Y. & Hirata, K. (2006). Assessment of liver fibrosis by non invasive method of transient elastography and biochemical markers. *World J. Gastroenterol.*, Vol.12, No.27, pp.4325-4330

Kawasaki, T., Moryasu, F., Nishida, O. et al. (1989). Analysis of hepatofugal flow in portal venous system using ultrasonic Doppler duplex system. *Am J Gastroenterology*, Vol.148, pp.47-49

Knodell, R.G., Ishak, K.G., Black, W.C., Chen, T.S., Craig, R., Kaplowitz, N., Kiernan, T.W., Wollman, J. (1981). Formulation and application of a numerical scoring system for assessing histological activity in asymptomatic chronic active hepatitis. *Hepatology*, Vol.1, No.5, pp.431 - 435

Kock, N.G., Hahnloser, P., Roding, B. et al. (1972). Interaction between portal venous and hepatic arterial blood flow: an experimental study in the dog. *Surgery*, Vol.72, pp.414-419

Kumagi, T.&Heathcote, E.J. (2008). Primary biliary cirrhosis. Orphanet Journal of Rare Diseases; 3:1. Doi: 10.1186/1750-1172-3-1

Kutlu, R., Karman, I., Akbulut, A. et al. (2002). Quantitative Doppler evaluation of the splenoportal venous system in various stages of cirrhosis: Differences between right and left portal veins. *J Clin Ultrasound*, Vol.30, pp.537-543

Lackner, C., Struber, G., Liegl, B., Leibl, S., Ofner, P., Bankuti, C., Baner, B. & Stanber, R.E. (2005). Comparison and validation of simple noninvasive tests for predication of fibrosis in chronic hepatitis C. *Hepatology*, Vol.100, pp.868-873

Lafortune, M., Matricardi, Lm, Dens, A., Favret, M. et al. (1998). Segment 4 (quadrate lobe): barometer of cirrhotic liver disease at US. *Radiology*, Vol.206, pp.157-160

Lim, A.K.P., Patel, N., Eckersley, R.J. et al. (2005). Can Doppler sonography grade the severity of hepatic C-related liver disease? *AJR*, Vol.184, pp.1848-1853

Manning, D.S. & Afdhal, N.H. (2008). Diagnosis and quantitation of fibrosis. *Gastroenterology*, Vol.134, pp.960-974

Matsui, O., Kadoya, M., Yoshikava, J. et al. (1995). Aberant gastric venous drainage in cirrhotic liver: Imaging findings in focal area of liver parenhima. *Radiology*, Vol.197, pp.345-34

Mehta, S.H., Lau, B., Afdol, N.H. & Thomas, D.L. (2009). Exceeding the limits of liver histology markers. *J. Hepatology*, Vol.50, No.1, pp.36-41

Montano-Loza, A.J., Carpenter, H.A.&Czaja, A.J. (2007). Consequences of treatment withdrawal in type 1 autoimmune hepatitis. *Liver Int*, Vol.27, No.4, pp.507 - 515

Needleman, L., Kurtz, A.B., Rifkin, M., Cooper, H.S. et al. (1986). Sonography of diffuse benign liver disease: accuracy of pattern recognition and grading. *AJR*, Vol.146, pp.1011-1015

Nishiura, T., Vatanabe, H., Matsuoka, Y et al. (2005). Ultrasound evaluation of fibrosis stage in chronic liver disease by simultaneous use of low and high frequency probes.*The British J Radiology*, Vol.78, No.927, pp.189-197

O'Donohue, J., Chaan, N.G., Catnach, Ng.C. et al. (2004). Diagnostic value of Doppler assessment of the hepatic and portal vesels and ultrasound of the spleen in liver disease. *Eur J Gastroenterol Hepatol*, Vol.16, pp.147-155

Oo, Y.H., Hubscher, S.G., Adams, D.H. (2010). Autoimmune hepatitis: new paradigms in the pathogenesis, diagnosis, and management. Hepatol Int, Vol. 4, pp.475 - 493

Pierce, M.E.&Sewell, R. (1990). Identification of hepatic cirrhosis by duplex Doppler ultrasound value of the hepatic artery resistive index. *Australian Radiology*, Vol.34, pp.331-333

Piscaglia, F., Gaiani, S., Zironi, G. et al. (1997). Intra and extrahepatic arterial resistances in chronic hepatitis and liver cirrhosis. *Ultrasound Med Biol*, Vol.23, pp.675-682

Poff, J.A., Coakley, F.V., Qayyum, A., Yeh, B.M. et al. (2008). Frequency and histopathologic basis of hepatic surface nodularity in patients with fulminant hepatic feilure. *Radiology*, Vol.249, pp.518-523

Poynard, T., Imbert-Bismut, F., Munteanu, M., Messous, D., Myers, R.P., Thabut, D., Ratziu, V., Mercadier, A., Benhamou, Y.&Hainque, B. (2004). Overview of the diagnostic value of biochemical markers of liver fibrosis (FibroTest, HCV FibroSure) and necrosis (ActiTest) in patients with chronic hepatitis C. *Comparative Hepatology*, 3:8 doi:10.1186/1476-5926-3-8

Reed, J.C. (2000). Warner-Lambent/Parke-Davis awards lecture: mechanisms of apoptosis. *Am. J. Pathol.*, Vol.157, pp.1415-1430

Reddy, K.R. & Schiff, E.R. (2002). Sampling error and intraobserver variation in liver biopsy in patients with chronic HCV infection. *Am. J. Gastroenterol.*, Vol.97, pp.2614-2618

Roobottom, C.A., Hunter, J.D., Westson, M.J. et al. (1995). Hepatic venous Doppler waveforms: changes in pregnancy. *J Clin Ultrsound*, Vol.23, pp.477-482

Rousselet, M.C., Michalak, S., Dupre, F., Croué, A., Bedossa, P., Saint-André, J.P. & Cales, P. (2005). Sources of variability in histological scoring of chronic viral hepatitis. *Hepatology*, Vol.41, pp.257-264

Ryder SD and on behalf of the Trent Hepatitis C Study Group. (2004). Progression of hepatic fibrosis in patients with hepatitis C: a prospective repeat liver biopsy study. *Gut*, Vol.53, No.3, pp.451 - 455

Sacerdoti, D., Merkel, C., Bolognesi, M. et al. (1995). Hepatic arterial resistance in cirrhosis with and wihout portal vein trombosis: relationships with portal haemodynamics. *Gastroenterology*, Vol.108, pp.1152-1158

Schattenbeg, J.M., Galle, P.R. & Schuchmann, M. (2006). Apoptosis in liver disease. *Liver International*, Vol.26, No.8, pp.904-911

Scheuer, P.J. (1991). Classification of chronic viral hepatitis: a need for reassessment. *J Hepatol*, 1991; Vol.13, No.3, pp. 372 - 374

Schinoni, M.I., Paraná, R. & Cavalcante, D. (2006). Apoptosis and progression of hepatic fibrosis in hepatitis C patients. *Braz. J. Infect. Dis.*, Vol.10, No.2, pp.117-121

Schneider, A.R.J., Teuber, G., Kriener, S.&Caspary, W.F. (2005) Noninvasive asseessment of liver steatosis, fibrosis and inflamation in chronic hepatitis C virus infection. *Liver international*, Vol.25, pp.1150-1155

Shiha, G., Sarin, S.K., Ibrahim, A.E., Omata, M., Kumar, A., Lesmana, L.A., Leung, N., Tozun, N., Hamid, S., Jafri, W., Maruyama, H., Bedossa, P., Pinzani, M., Chawla, Y., Esmat, G., Doss, W., Elzanaty, T., Sakhuja, P., Nasr, A.M., Omar, A., Wai, C.T., Abdallah, A., Salama, M., Hamed, A., Yousry, A., Waked, I., Elsahar, M., Fateen, A.,

Mogawer, S., Hamdy, H., Elwakil, R. (2009). Liver fibrosis: consensus recommendations of the Asian Pacific Association for the study of the liver (APASL). *Hepatol Int*, Vol.3, pp.323 - 333

Silveira M.G.&Lindor, K.D. (2008). Primary sclerosing cholangitis. *Can J Gastroenterol*, Vol.22, No.8, pp689 - 698

Silveira, M.G.&Lindor KD. (2008). Clinical features and management of primary sclerosing cholangitis. *World J Gastroenterol*, Vol.14, No.2, pp.3338 - 3349

Skripenova, S., Trainer, T.D., Krawitt, E.L.&Blaszyk, E. (2007). Variability of grade and stage in simultaneously paired liver biopsies in patients with hepatitis C. *J Clin Pathol*, Vol.60, pp.321 - 324. Doi: 10.1136/jcp2005.036020

Standish, R.A., Cholongitas, E., Dhillon, A., Burroughs, A.K.&Dhillon, A.P. (2006). An appraisal of the histopatological assessment of liver fibrosis. *Gut*, Vol.55, pp.569 - 578

Suzuki, A., Mendes, F. & Lindor, K. (2005). Diagnostic model of esophageal varices in alcoholic liver disease. *Eur. J. Gastroenterol. Hepatol.*, Vol.17, No.3, pp.307-309

Taourel, P., Blanc, P., Dauzat, M., Pradel, J. et al. (1998). Doppler study of mesenteric, hepatic and portal circulation in alcoholic cirrhosis: relationship between quantitative Doppler measurements and severity of portal hypertension and liver failure. *Hepatology*, Vol.28, pp.932-936

Techgraber, U.K., Gebel, M., Benter, T. et al. (1997). Effect of respiration exercises and food intake on hepatic vein circulation. *J Ultrasound Med*, Vol.16, pp.549-554

Totty, B.A. (2002). *In: Theory and practice of histological techniques, 5th ed.* Bancroft, J.D.&Gamble (Eds.), 163-200, M. Churchill Livingstone, Edinburgh (International edition)

Vigano, M., Visentin, S., Aghemo, M. et al. (2005). US features of liver surface nodularity as a predictor of severe fibrosis in chronic hepatitis C. *Radiology*, Vol.234, pp.641

Vilgrain, V. (2001). Ultrasound of diffuse liver disease and portal hypertension. *Eur Radiology*, Vol.11, pp.1563-77

von Birbra, H., Schober, K., Jenni, R. et al. (1989). Diagnosis of constrictive pericarditis by pulsed Doppler echocardiography of hepatic vein. *Am J Cardiol*, Vol.63, pp.483-488

von Herbay, A., Frieling, T. et al. (2001). Association between duplex Doppler sonographic flow pattern in right hepatic vein and various liver diseases. *J Clin Ultrasound*, Vol.29, pp.25-30

Walsh, K.M., Leen, E., Mac Sween, R.N. et al. (1998). Hepatic blood flow changes in chronic hepatitis C measured by duplex Doppler color sonography: relationship to histological features. *Dig Dis Sci*, Vol.43, No.12, pp.2584-90

Yokoyama, S.C., Finegold, M.J., Sturniolo, G.C., Kim, K., Mescoli, C., Rugge, M.&Medici, V. (2010). Wilson disease: histopathological correlations with treatment on follow-up liver biopsies. *World J Gastroenterol*, Vol.16, No.12, pp.1487 - 1494

Zironi, G., Gaiani, S., Fenyves, D., Rigamonti, A., Bolondi, L. et al. (1992). Value of measurement of mean portal flow velocity by Doppler flowmetry in the diagnosis of portal hypertension. *J of Hepatology*, Vol.16, pp.298-303

Zwiebel, W.&Pellerito, J.S. (2005). *Introduction to vascular ultrasound*. Elsevier Suonders. 5th ed. pp.585-590

13

# Noninvasive Alternatives of Liver Biopsy

Květoslava Aiglová
*II. internal department, FN Olomouc*
*Czech Republic*

## 1. Introduction

Liver biopsy is considered the gold standart for the diagnosis of cirrhosis, it has important limitations ,such as being invasive,having the potential for complications and false-negative results or underestimating disease severity due to sampling error.
Liver biopsy is recomended in patiens with abnormal liver tests,for evaluation of chronic hepatitis, of alcohol liver disease, icterus of unknown origin, hepatomegaly,splenomegaly, ascites, cholestatic liver disease, toxic liver damage,metabolic disorders.Liver biopsy has limitations including small but significant morbidity and mortality rates,inter- and intra-observer variation in patology reporting. The most important contraindications of liver biopsy are trombopenia, abnormal parameters of hemocoagulation, important ascites, liver hemangioma and cysts, acute cholangitis, biliary obstruction ,severe obesity, respiratory insufficiency, heart failure,Chilaiditi´s sy, uncooperative patient.(1)
Complication of liver biopsy and their incidence:
Pain (0,056 -22%)-pleural, peritoneal, diaphragmatic
Bleeding-intraperitoneal(0,03-0,7%).
- intrahepatic or subcapsular ( 0,059-23%)
- hemobilia(0,059-0,2%)

Biliary peritonitis(0,03-0,22%)
Bacteriemia
Sepsis(0,088 %) and liver absces
Pneumothorax or pleural effusion (0,08-0,28%)
Hemothorax (0,18-0,49%)
Arteriovenous fistula (5,4%)
Subcutaneous emphysema(0,014%)
Reaction to anaestetic (0,029 %)
Beakage of needle (0,02-0,059%)
Biopsy of other organs:
- lungs (0,001-0,014%).
- gallbladder(0,034-0,117%),
- kidney ( 0.029-0,096%)
- colon (0.0038 0,011%)

Death (0,0088-0,3%)
Noninvasive methods of investigation of liver offer an atractive alternative to the liver biopsy, as they are less invasive than liver biopsy,repeatable.

Noninvasive approaches to assess histology in liver disease include clinical symptoms and signes, routine laboratory tests, serum markers of fibrosis and inflammation, quantitative assay of liver function and radiologic imaging methods.None of these tests or markers alone is accurate or reliable in predicting histology, in particular, liver fibrosis.
An ideal noninvasive ,diagnostic test should be simple, readily available, inexpensive and accurate.

## 2. Serum tests

Serum tests are used for assessment of steatosis, hepatitis, cirrhosis, metabolic and autoimmune disorders for prediction of liver fibrosis.
The group of routine tests includes liver enzymes- ALT, AST, ALP, GMT, level of bilirubin, platelets count, markers of infectious diseases, autoantibodies.
Results of serum tests and derived mathematical models are always compared with histological findings.

### 2.1 Markers of liver fibrosis

Markers of the I st class, non-routine, are based on knowledge about fibrogenesis, they are components of extracellular matrix, which are overproduced by activated stellate cells.

#### 2.1.1 Non-routine markers

*Hyaluronic acid*

Hyaluronic acid (HA) concentrations have been shown to be higher in cirrhotic and fibrotic patients, sensitivity is 88 %, specificity 78% for cirrhosis.
Most of hyaluronic acid in the blood is produced in the stellatae cells of the liver and is also cleared by the liver. Only small fraction of HA is eliminated via the kidneys and spleen. It is extracted from sinusoidal endothelial cells within 2-9 minutes. Its concentration in a normal liver tissue is low, but in fibrotic liver is 2 to10-fold increased.(2)
HA serum concentrations rise significantly in case of cirrhosis. The cutoff is 60μg/L.
HA is not suggested to replace liver biopsy, but is useful for long-term monitoring of disease progression.
Non- routine tests,which reflect fibrosis ,are extracellular matrix remodeling markers: amino-terminal propeptide of type III collagen(PIIIP),matrix metalloproteinase(MMP),tissue inhibitor of matrix metalloproteinase(TIMP),type IV collagen(CL-4).Markers are used alone or in combination with serum chemistries.
Index of PIIIP/MMP-1 significantly correlates with fibrosis score and is considered better than hyaluronic acid and TIMP-1.

*Laminin*

Laminin -a major,noncollagenous,high mollecular-mass glycoprotein of basement membranes, increases in fibrotic liver. Increases in laminin concentration are positively correlated with the extent of fibrotic transition of the liver.
Discrimination between fibrotic and cirrhotic stages of chronic liver diseases by means of laminin assay is better than the aminoterminal propeptide of type III procollagen.The increase of laminin is relatively independent of etiology of the disease(3)

*YKL-40*

YKL-40 can be used for diagnosing liver fibrosis,mild stage of fibrosis(value $< 186,4$), severe stage of fibrosis($186,4 < \text{value} < 284,8$) and F4 ($284,8 < \text{value}$).(3)

YKL-40 is thought to contribute to tissue remodeling or degradation of the extracellular matrix.(4)

*Alpha-2-macroglobulin*

Alpha-2-macroglobulin (A2M) is a proteinase inhibitor and acute–phase protein.Cells synthetising A2M are hepatocytes, activated Ito cells and granuloma cells.Fibrosis is associated with an increase of A2M,which is considered very informative marker.A2M is included in Fibrotest,Actitest, PGAA index,Patel score,Fibrometer, Hepascore.

*Amino-terminal propeptide of type III collagen*

Amino-terminal propeptide of type III collagen(PIIIP) is marker of deposition rate of type III collagen. The serum concentration of PIIINP reflects the turnover of type IIIcollagen.

*Matrix metalloproteinase(MMP)*

Changes of MMP reflect „pathologic" matrix degradation in liver. The most important enzymes are MMP -2(also called gelatinase A or 72-kDa type IV collagenase) and MMP-9(gelatinase B or 92-kDa type IV collagenase), which reflects type IV collagen. Markedly increased expression of MMP-2 is characteristic of cirrhosis.(5)

*Tissue inhibitor of matrix metalloproteinase(TIMP)*

Significant increases of TIMP 1 and TIMP 2 have been observed in chronic liver disease at any stage of the fibrotic process.(5)

*Type IV collagen(CL-4)*

CL-4 is a sensitive marker for active fibrosis and the elevation of serum type IV-collagen level reflects the enhancement of type IV-collagen synthesis and deposition in the liver tissue at the stage of active fibrosis in liver disease.

Elevated serum amino-terminal propeptide of type III collagen ,prolylhydroxylase(PH), collagen type IV and matrix metalloproteinase-1 were seen in cirrhosis of various cause, laminin and CL-IV in alcoholic hepatitis, hyaluronic acid,tissue inhibitor of metalloproteinase TIMP-1and TIMP-2, in chronic hepatitis. Serum CL-IV, MMP-2 and TIMP-1(but not laminin, MMP-1or MMP-3) were elevated in hereditary hemochromatosis, and only CL-IV and MMP -2 correlated with severity of hepatic fibrosis.

Prolylhydroxylase is marker of collagen synthesis, reflects the grade of fibrosis.

*Type VI collagen*

Type VI collagen is a minor but essential matrix component in the liver.Type VI collagen gene expression, together with other connective tissue components, including type I collagen, is activated in the early stages of the fibrotic process. Type VI collagen accumulation may contribute to the distorted architecture and functional impairment of the liver in hepatic fibrosis.(6)

*Tenascin*

is the extracellular matrix glycoprotein .A significant correlation was observed between the serum tenascin levels and serum levels of various extracellular matrix proteins such as type III procollagen N –aminoterminal peptide(PIIIP), laminin and the 7Sdomain of type IV collagen. A strong positive correlation was observed between the serum tenascin levels and histological findings,particullarly in the degree of hepatic fibrosis (7)

*Undulin*

Undulin is a constituent of the hepatic extracellular matrix of normal human liver. Undulin is distributed as densely packed fibers in portal tract stroma, and as fine fibers along sinusoids,and around central veins.Undulin ribonucleic acid expression is low in normal liver,and confined to mesenchymal cells of portal tract stroma, vessel walls and perisinusoidal space. In fibrotic liver , undulin deposition and gene expression are enhanced in fibrotic stroma and area of fibrogenesis identified by the presence of active septa and inflammatory infiltrate.Undulin participates in rearrangement of connective tissue occuring in hepatic fibrosis.(8)

*Fibronectin*

Fibronectin plays a role in liver fibrosis, which was studied in Egyptian patiens with chronic HCV infection.The efficiency of fibronectin for disciminating patiens with liver fibrosis from those with non fibrosis livers was 75%.Serum fibronectin can differentiate HCV infected patiens with liver fibrosis from patiens with non fibrosis(9).

| Marker | Serum | Urine | Biopsy | Method | Clinical application |
|---|---|---|---|---|---|
| Prolylhdroxylase | + | - | + | REA, RIA | (+) |
| Monoaminoxidase | + | - | (+) | Enzymatic | - |
| Lysyloxidase | + | - | + | RIA | - |
| Lysylhydroxylase | + | - | - | RIA | - |
| Galaktosylhydroxylysylglukosyltransferase | + | - | + | RIA | - |
| Collagenpeptidase | + | - | + | Enzymatic | - |
| N-acetyl-beta-D-glukosaminidase | + | + | + | Enzymatic | (+) |
| **Collagen typ I** | | | | | |
| N-terminal propeptide (PINP) | + | - | + | ELISA | - |
| C-terminal propeptide (PICP) | + | - | + | RIA | - |
| **Collagen typ III** | | | | | |
| Intact procollagen | + | - | - | | |
| N-terminal propeptide (PIIINP) | | | | | |
| Globular domain of propeptide (Col-1) | + | - | - | RIA | + |
| **Collagen typ IV** | | | | | |
| NC1-fragment [C-terminal] (PIVP) | + | + | - | ELISA, RIA | (+) |
| 7S domain (7S collagen) | + | + | - | RIA | (+) |
| **Collagen typ VI** | + | + | + | RIA | - |
| Laminin, P1-fragment | + | - | - | RIA, EIA | (+) |
| Undulin | + | - | - | EIA | - |
| Vitronectin | + | - | - | EIA | - |
| Tenascin | + | - | - | ELISA | - |
| YKL-40 | + | - | + | RIA, ELISA | (+) |
| (pro) MMP-2 | + | - | - | ELISA | (+) |
| TIMP-1, TIMP-Ě | + | - | - | ELISA | (+) |
| Hyaluronic acid | + | - | - | RLA, ELISA | ++ |

Fig. 1. Non-routine tests of liver fibrosis (30)

### 2.1.2 Routine tests

ALT,AST have been the most often used enzymes indicating hepatocellular damage.Activity of ALT is higher than AST,the exception is in alcohol liver disease and Rey´s syndrom.

Aminotransferases are elevated 3-20 fold in acute and chronic hepatitis, toxic liver damage.Elevation less than3-fold is in steatosis. nonalcoholic steatohepatitis, chronic hepatitis.Mild elevation is in cholestatic liver disease, liver cirrhosis.

AST/ALT ratio(de Ritis index) is usefull in alcohol liver disease,because AST/ALT > 2 is specific test for alcohol liver disease. AST/ALT < 1 is typical for viral hepatitis, but increase > 1 indicates progresssion to cirrhosis.

Single markers often correlate with fibrosis in large groups of patients, but do not sufficiently assess the amount of fibrosis in a single individual,especially in longitudinal use over time.

*Haptoglobin*

is a plasma glycoprotein which specially binds hemoglobin and is synthesized in the liver.Haptoglobin is the acute-phase protein and is strongly and negatively associated with fibrosis

*Apolipoprotein A1*

is synthesized by the liver and is responsible for cholesterol transport. It is included in extracellular matrix and its level is decreased at increasing stages of fibrosis.

*Total bilirubin*

is formed during decomposition of hemoglobin in the cells of the reticuloendothelial system especially in the spleen and Kupfer cells of the liver. Increase in its level suggests hepatocellular failure,except case of hemolysis.

*Apolipoprotein A1, haptoglobin,bilirubin are components of mathematical models for prediction of liver fibrosis.*

Forns index was developed to discriminate patiens with and without significant fibrosis with a noninvasive method.The cohort included 476 consecutive untreated patiens with chronic hepatitis C who underwent a liver biopsy.The study was designed to assess the accuracy of noninvasive method aimed to discriminate between patiens with and without significant liver fibrosis(stages 2-4 versus 0-1) The model consisted of combination of 4 variables identified by comparative analysis of patients with and without significant fibrosis: age,gamaglutamyltransferase, platelet count,cholesterol level(10). With these variables were constructed a simple score adressed to select patients at very low risk of having significant fibrosis.

*7,811-3,131.ln(platelet count)+0,781.ln(GMT)+3,467.ln(age) 0,014.(cholesterol).*

Two cutoff values were chosen to identify absence (less than 4,21)and presence (greater than6,9) of significant fibrosis.A score below 4,2 identified patiens at very low risk of having significant fibrosis with a96% certainty.

The age as a marker of liver fibrosis was used, because fibrosis progression is time dependent. The duration of HCV infection would be a more precise indicator of fibrosis than age. A low platelet count is a marker of severe fibrosis. Thrombocytopenia in patiens with advanced liver disease seems to be related to the development of portal hypertension and the decreased production of thrombopoetin. In this study ,increased GGT was an independent predictor of bile duct damage, because HCV infection frequently cause bile duct damage and steatosis. Patiens with bile duct lesions have significantly higher fibrosis score.

Wai et al. considered platelet count and AST level as the most important predictors of fibrosis and analyse the relationship between these two factors and the stage of hepatic fibrosis.(11)

Regression formula for prediction of signifiant fibrosis:

$$\text{Risk score} = 2.318 + 0{,}274.\ln(\text{AST level}[/\text{ULN}])-0{,}375.\ln(\text{platelet count } [10^9/\text{L}])$$

Regression formula for prediction of cirrhosis:

$$\text{Risk score}=2{,}411+ 0{,}100.\ln(\text{AST level}[/\text{ULN}])-0{,}436.\ln(\text{platelet count } [10^9/\text{L}])$$

$$\text{APRI} = \frac{\text{AST}(/\text{ULN})}{\text{PLT}(10^9/\text{L})} \times 100$$

The APRI was accurate in predicting both fibrosis and cirrhosis,with area under ROC of 0,8 and 0,898 in the training set, and 0,88 and 0,94 in the validations set.

The study of Wai included 270 patients.APRI predictive model consists of objective and readily available laboratory variables. The finding of decreased platelet count and increased AST level with progression of liver fibrosis has been reported in many studies.With increasing fibrosis and worsering portal hypertension, there are increased sequestration and destruction of platelets in the enlarging spleen.Progression of liver fibrosis may reduce the clearance of AST, leading to increased serum AST levels.The APRI was accurate in predicting both signifiant fibrosis and cirrhosis.with area under ROC of 0,80 and 0,89 in the training set,and 0,88 and 0,94 in the validation set. Although was not definied one single cut-off value to predict the only study endpoint, using values below the lower cut-off level and above the higher cut-off level, a prediction of absence of cirrhosis could be made in 81 % of patients.Similary, a prediction of absence or presence of significant fibrosis could be made in 51 % of patiens.The major advantage of the APRI is its simplicity. APRI can be determined in the clinic or bedside without the help of a calculator.

*FibroTest*

is a patented biomarker test that uses the results of six blood serum tests to generate a score that is correlated with the degree of liver damage in people with variety of liver disease. FibroTest has the same prognostic value as a liver biopsy.

FibroTest was presented in 2002. Study included 125 patients with chronic hepatitis C.Serum tests were taken at time of biopsy.The score was computed from age, sex and serum alpha2 macroglobulin,bilirubin, gamaglutamyltransferase activity, apolipoprotein A1 and haptoglobin.(12)

The equation for calculating FibroTest is

$$z = 4{,}467 \times \log10\,[\text{alpha2macroglobulin}(g/L)] - 1{,}357 \times \log 10\,[\text{haptoglobin}(g/L)] + 1{,}017 \times \log10[\text{GMT}(IU/L)] + 0{,}0281 \times [\text{age(years)}] + 1{,}737 \times \log10[\text{bilirubin}(\mu mol/L)] - 1{,}184 \times [\text{apolipoprotein A1}(g/L)] + 0{,}301 \times \text{sex(female=0,male=1)} - 5{,}54$$

At the recommended cutoff values, the negative predictive value of a FibroTest score < 0,1 for the presence of fibrosis stages F2 toF4 was 85%, the positive predictive value of a score >0,6 was78% and a score of 0,6 gave a likehood ration of 6,4.

The laboratory or physician connects to the BioPredictive website for calculation of the test results and prints the results sheet, which is available immediately and is accompanied by an interpretation aid and precautions for use.

In clinical practice it has been suggested that the FibroTest score might be applied to patiens who either have contraindications or risk liver biopsy for the management of their HCV.FibroTest score could not accurately predict either the presence or absence of significant fibrosis and cold not reliably be used to reduce the need for liver biopsy.

Other tests derived from FibroTest are:

ActiTest-diagnostic for necrotico-inflammatory hepatitis

SteatoTest -diagnostic for liver steatosis

NashTest-diagnostic for NASH inflammation

AshTest diagnostic for Alcoholic liver disease inflammation
FibroTest is independent of ethnic origin,sex,genotypes,viral load,transaminases or the presence of comorbidities. The test has been validated for the general population,including children,patiens with renal insufficiency, hemophiliacs, patiens with chronic inflammatory disease.
The test is not applicable in 1 to5% of cases, in patiens with acute viral hepatitis A,B,C,D,E,drug-induced hepatitis, extrahepatic cholestasis, severe hemolysis, Gilbert´s syndrome with high unconjugated hyperbilirubinemia,acute inflammatory syndrome.
FibroTest has comparable diagnostic value as 25 mm biopsy,while being noninvasive and easily repeatable.
ActiTest includes parameters of FibroTest plus the level of ALT.
SteatoTest was constructed using a combination of the 6 components of FibroTest-ActiTest plus body mass index,serum cholesterol,triglycerides and glucose adjusted for age and gender.(13)
NashTest was developed using patented algorithms combining 13 parameters: age,sex,heigh,weight,and serum levels of triglycerides,cholesterol, A2M,apolipoproteinA1, haptoglobin, GMT, ALT, AST, total bilirubin.(14)
AshTest is calculated using A2M, haptoglobin, apolipoprotein A1, total bilirubin, GMT, ALT and AST,with parameters adjusted for patienst´s gender and age.
FibroMAX is used for monitoring liver health in patients with viral, metabolic or alcoholic hepatitis when symptoms or risk factors are difficult to interpret. FibroMAX is a combination of five algorithm tests – FibroTest, ActiTest, SteatoTest,NashTest, and AshTest. FibroMAX uses a unique combination of serum marker tests and other patient ´s data including age, gender, weight and height. The test results and patient´s data are entered into patented algorithms, which accurately determine the level of liver disease. Serum markers measured by FibroMax include Alpha 2-macroglobulin, Haptoglobin, Apolipoprotein A1, Total bilirubin, Gamma Glutamyl Transpeptidase (GGT), Alanine Amino Transferase (ALT), Aspartate aminotransferase (AST), Fasting Glucose, Triglycerides, total cholesterol. The serum marker levels are analysed using BioPredictive algorithms to create the FibroMAX Test Report.
As FibroMax includes a Fasting Glucose test, fasting is required before sample collection.

*Fib-4*

combines standard biochemical tests-platelets,ALT,AST and age.The Fib 4 test was studied in cohort of 847 HCV patiens, also was performed liver biopsy and FibroTest. An Fib4 index value higher than 3,25 had a positive predictive value to confirm the existence of signifiant fibrosis F3-F4 of 82,1% with with a specificity of 98,2%. An Fib -4 index lower than 1,45 had a negative predictive value of 94,7 % to exclude severe fibrosis with a sensitivity of 74,3%. The FIB-4 index was strongly correlated to the FibroTest results for a score <1.45 or >3.25.
For values outside 1,45-3,25 the Fib-4 index is a simple,accurate and inexpensive method.(15)

*Hepascore*

is based on serum levels of alpha2macroglobulin, hyaluronic acid, gammaglutamyltransferase, total bilirubin, along with age and sex.(16)
The logistic regression model of:

$$y = \exp [-4,185818-(0,0249 \times age) + (0,7464 \times sex) + (1,0039xA2M) + (0,032 \times hyaluronic\ acid) + (0,0691 \times bilirubin) -(0,0012x\ GGT)]$$

The Hepascore was calculated from the following equation:

$$y/1+y$$

Hepascore higher than 0,5 is 67 % sensitive and 92 % specific for the presence of significant fibrosis, score lower than 0,5 is 88% sensitive and 74 % specific for excluding advanced fibrosis. The cutoff point of 0,84 was applied for detection of cirrhosis.
Hepascore has been shown to be accurate as liver biopsy in patiens with hepatitis C virus infection. Hepascore is applicable to the assessment of fibrosis in alcoholic and non-alcoholic fatty liver disease. Hepascore will allow more frequent monitoring to detect progression of liver disease and also response to therapy.

*PGA*

is a simple biological index combining a specific test for severe liver disease-protrombin time, a sensitive test of alcoholic liver disease-serum gammaglutamyl transpeptidase,and a test for liver fibrosis-serum apolipoprotein A1.The test was evaluated in a training sample of 333 drinkers and validated in 291 other drinkers.All patiens underwent a liver biopsy.The PGA index varied from 0 to12. When PGA was less than or equal to 2, the probability of cirrhosis was 0% and the probability of normal liver or minimal changes 83%.When PGA was greater than or equal to 9, the probability of normal liver or minimal changes was 0% and the probability of cirrhosis 86 %.
The diagnostic accuracy of this index was later improved by the addition of alpha2macroglobulin.(17)

*PGAA*

includes protrombin time,gamaglumatyltranspeptidase, apolipoprotein A 1 and alpha2macroglobulin.

*Fibrometer*

generates a score of fibrosis with an equivalence in F Metavir stage.
FibroMeters are blood tests for liver fibrosis with several specificities:two main diagnostic targets(fibrosis stages and area of fibrosis),adaptation to specific causes, and results confirmed by an expert system.
FibroMeters comprise six different tests: on effort paging and on effort quantitation of liver fibrosis in each of the free main cause of chronic liver disease- chronic viral hepatitis, alcoholic liver disease and nonalcoholic fatty liver disease.
There are 6 different main Fibrometers.
FibroMeter V(Band C virus and co-infection HCV/HIV)
score of fibrosis: age,gender,alpha2macroglobulin, prothrombin time, platelets,AST,urea, GGT,ALT
score of cirrhosis: age, gender,alpha2macroglobulin,prothrombin time, platelets,AST,urea, GGT,ALT
activity: alpha2macroglobulin, prothrombin time,platelets, ALT
Fibrometer A(alcohol)
score of fibrosis: age, gender,alpha2macroglobulin, hyaluronic acid,prothrombin time
percentage of fibrosis: alpha2macroglobulin,hyaluronic acid, platelets, hyaluronic acid
FibroMeter S(metabolic steatosis)
score of fibrosis: age,grade, patiens weight, platelets, AST,ALT,ferritin,glucose
percentage of fibrosis: hyaluronic acid, prothrombin time, platelets, AST, ALT, glucose
FIBROspect II was first described for hepatitis C patients in 2004. Fibrospect uses three serum markers, alpha 2 macroglobulin, hyaluronic acid and Tissue inhibitor of matrix

metalloproteinase, to calculate a score. When applied to 696 patients with hepatitis C, a score <0.36 excluded significant fibrosis with a negative predictive value of 76% and a score >0.36 detected significant fibrosis with a positive predictive value of 74%.

*Fortunato*

The test is based on concenrations of six biochemical markers- fibronectin, prothrombin, pseudocholinesterase, ALT, manganese superoxid dismutase, N- acetyl- beta-glucosaminidase.(18)

Following equation was developed

$$\text{discriminant score} = \text{PCHE}(\mu\text{kat/L}) \times 0{,}00011 + \text{fibronectin}(\text{mg/L}) \times 0{,}039 + \ln \text{prothrombin activity}(\%) \times 3{,}51 + \ln \text{ALT}(\mu\text{kat/L}) \times 0{,}49 - \ln \text{beta NAG}(\mu\text{kat/L}) \times 0{,}51 - \ln \text{MnSOD}(\mu\text{kat/L}) \times 1{,}29 - 9{,}41$$

Fortunato et al. studied two cohorts-54 patients with chronic hepatitis and 49 patients with cirrhosis.All patiens underwent percutaneous liver biopsyand laboratory tests.

The cutoff value was -0,22 (less than -0,22 indicated cirrhosis, greater than -0,22 indicated chronic hepatitis).

Prothrombin activity and PCHE are markers of liver protein synthetic activity, which is gradually impaired during the cirrhotic evolution of chronic hepatitis.

b-NAG and fibronectin are markers of fibrosis . The increase in serum b-NAG activity in cirrhotic patients is attributable to the increased accumulation of collagen typical of the disease. b-NAG is known to be important for the collagen pathways . By contrast, the reduction of circulating fibronectin in cirrhotic patients is likely related to the impaired protein synthesis that occurs in cirrhotic liver . Mn-SOD is located mainly in the mitochondrial matrix, a site of reactive oxygen species production; it is involved in the antioxidative pathways of human cells .

Mn-SOD mRNA concentrations in peripheral blood mononuclear cells and serum Mn-SOD concentrations are higher in patients with hepatitis C viral infections than inhealthy controls. Serum ALT could be considered a signal of liver cytolysis, which differs in chronic hepatitis and cirrhosis.

Fibronectin, ALT, PCHE, prothrombin activity, Mn-SOD, and b-NAG blood concentrations are easily and rapidly analyzed

*Patel*

developed the model using levels of extracellular matrix remodeling proteins. Study included 294 patients with chronic hepatitis C and was validated in an external cohort of 402 patients. The aim of this study was to evaluate the diagnostic accuracy of a panel of these markers in chronic hepatitis C patients develop a predictive algorithm that differentiates no/mild (METAVIR F0-F1) from moderate/severe ( F2-F4) fibrosis,and valid the model in external cohort.(19)

Hyaluronic acid, TIMP -1 and alpha2macroglobulin were selected as having the best accuracy for F2-F4 fibrosis. At an index cut-off >0.36 and prevalence for F2–F4 of 52%, results in all 696 patients indicated positive and negative predictive values of 74.3 and 75.8% with an accuracy of 75%.

Pohl score

Positive : AAR $\geq 1$ and platelet count $<150 \times 10^9$/L

AAR = AST/ALT

*Cirrhosis disciminant score*

The CDS was developed by Bonacini.The CDS includes platelets.ALT/AST ratio, and prothrombin time. The CDS of 8 or higher had a sensitivity of 46% and specificity of 98% for diagnosis of histological fibrosis scores of 3 or 4.(20,21)

| | |
|---|---|
| CDS | Platelet count (×109/L): >340 = 0; 280–339 = 1; 220–279= 2; 160–219 = 3; 100–159 = 4; 40–99 = 5; <40 = 6<br>ALT/AST ratio: >1.7 = 0; 1.2–1.7 = 1; 0.6–1.19 = 2;<0.6 = 3<br>INR: <1.1 = 0; 1.1–1.4 = 1; >1.4 = 2<br>CDS is the sum of the above (possible value 0–11). |
| AP index | Age (years): <30 = 0; 30–39 = 1; 40–49 = 2; 50–59= 3; 60–69 = 4; ≥70 = 5<br>Platelet count (×109/L): ≥225 = 0; 200–224 = 1; 175–199= 2; 150–174 = 3; 125–149 = 4; <125 = 5<br>AP index is the sum of the above (possible value 0–10).<br>AP index of 6 or higher is significant for advanced fibrosis |

*Enhanced liver fibrosis (ELF) test*

originaly combined age and three markers of liver fibrosis-hyaluronic acid, aminoterminal propeptide of type III collagen and tissue inhibitor of matrix metalloproteinase 1.The test was investigated on international multicenter cohort study. Subsequently the ELF team have established that Age could be omitted from the algorithm to generate the Enhanced Liver Fibrosis test or ELF Test. Performance was excellent for alcoholic liver disease and non alcoholic fatty liver disease.(22)

Combinations of serum markers for fibrosis calculated by algorithms, which give a discriminant score for fibrosis, represent a new group of liver function tests, which provide an alternative to an invasive liver biopsy. Providing they are properly validated, scores generated from combinations of serum tests represent a method for medical laboratory science to add value to laboratory reports. Clinicians must interpret conventional liver function tests carefully with only the individual reference ranges customarily provided by the laboratory for guidance. Experienced clinicians learn to make judgements and interpretations of conventional liver function tests, which are well beyond the scope of the reference ranges, and often difficult for less experienced clinicians. An advantage of algorithm-based scores is that a properly validated score represents evidence-based medicine as it incorporates clinical experience in the presentation of the reset.

*ELFGA index*

Includes parameters: age, aminoterminal propeptide of type IIIcollagen, haptoglobin, tissue inhibitor of matrix metalloproteinase 1.

*FibroIndex*

combines aspartate aminotransferase(AST), platelet count and gamaglobulin measurements.

Koda et al developed the FibroIndex to predict significant fibrosis.The authors collected clinical data on 402 consecutive patiens with chronic HCV-liver biopsy and blood samples taken no more than three days before the biopsy. Patiens were excluded if they had HIV or hepatitis B co-infection,drank more than10g of alcohol per day,had other liver disease, previous interferon therapy, or clinical evidence of cirrhosis, such as gastroesophageal varices, ascites, or hepatic encephalopathy.The investigators used multivariate logistic regression analysis to identify independent risk factors for fibrosis.(24)

$$\text{FibroIndex} = 1{,}738 - 0{,}064(\text{plateles}[\times 10^4/\text{mm}^3]) + 0{,}005(\text{AST}[\text{IU/L}]) + 0{,}463(\text{gamma globulin}[\text{g/dl}])$$

The index was tested in two validation sets.The investigators found that the areas under the receiver operating characteristic curves of the FibroIndex for predicting significant fibrosis were 0,83 and 0,82 for the validation set.The predictive value of the FibroIndex was better than either the Forns index or the aminotransferase to platelet ratio index.

*Fibrosis Probability Index*

FPI includes age, AST, past alcohol intake,cholesterol insulin rezistence,which was calculated from fasting serum insulin and plasma glucose determinations using the homeostasis model assessment(HOMA-IR) method:

fasting insulin(mU/mL) x plasma glucose (mmol/L).

An FPI was constructed using these independent predictors to determine the probability (0,0-1,0) of patient having signifiant fibrosis.

*SHASTA index*

Kelleher et al.developed a biomarker assay in a cohort of 95 HIV/HCV co-infected patients utilising Serum Hyaluronic acid, AST and Albumin (SHASTA). As with other biomarker assays, optimal results were noted in the extreme categories. Using a cutoff of 0.8 resulted in a specificity of 100% and a positive predictive value of 100% but this applied to less than 5% of patients. At the other end of the spectrum a cutoff of <0.30 was associated with a sensitivity of >88% and a negative predictive value of >94%. Overall 42% of patients could be correctly classified at either extreme but 58% would not be classifiable with scores between 0.3 and 0.8. The SHASTA index in HIV/HCV has similar accuracy to FibroTest and in this study performed significantly better than the APRI test(25)

*The Sequential Algorithm for Fibrosis Evaluation*

(SAFE) combines the APRI and Fibrotest-Fibrosure tests . In a large multicenter study validating this algorithm to detect significant fibrosis (stage F2 or greater by the F0–F4 METAVIR scoring system), its accuracy was 90.1%, the area under the receiver operating characteristic curve was 0.89 (95% CI 0.87–0.90), and it reduced the number of liver biopsies needed by 46.5%. When the algorithm was used to detect cirrhosis, its accuracy was 92.5%, the area under the curve was 0.92 (95% CI 0.89–0.94), and it reduced the number of liver biopsies needed by 81.5%.

*FibroFast*

A simple noninvasive score (FibroFast) was developed and evaluated on the basis of several simple blood biomarkers (ALT:AST ratio, albumin, alcaline phosphatase, and platelets count) that can be easily used by clinicians to predict severe fibrosis or cirrhosis in patients with chronic HCV infection . The validation of 1,067 cases from several international centers (Egypt, Italy, Brazil, Romania, and UAE) showed that the sensitivity of FibroFast was 61.5%, specificity 81.1%, positive predictive value 59%, and negative predictive value 82.6%. New cut-off scores of FibroFast were developed that allow the diagnosis of cirrhosis (F4) and F0–

F3 with the highest possible accuracy (>95%). FibroFast with the new two cut-off scores could be an alternative to liver biopsy in about one-third of the patients, with sensitivity 95% and specificity 95% .

| Index, score | Parameters | Disease | Senzitivity % | Specificity % |
|---|---|---|---|---|
| PGAA | Prothrombin time, GGT, apolipoprotein A1, alfa-2-macroglobulin | Alcohol | 79 | 89 |
| Bonacini | Ratio ALT/AST, INR, platelet count | HCV | 46 | 98 |
| De Ritis | Ratio AST/ALT | HCV | 53 | 100 |
| PGA | Prothrombin time, GGT, apolipoprotein A1 | Mixed | 91 | 81 |
| Fortunato | Fibronectin, prothrombin time, PCHE, ALT, Mn-SOD, beta-NAG | HCV | | 94 |
| Fibrotest | Haptoglobin, alfa-2-macroglobulin, apolipoprotein, A1, GGT, bilirubin | HCV, HBV | 75 | 85 |
| Pohl | Ratio AST/ALT, platelet count | HCV | 41 | 99 |
| Actitest | Fibrotest + ALT | HCV | | |
| Forns | Age, platelet count, GGT, cholesterol | HCV | 94 | 51 |
| WAI (APRI) | AST, ALP, platelet count | HCV | 89 | 75 |
| Rosenberg ELF-test | PIIINP, hyaluronic acid, TIMP-1 | Mixed | 90 | 41 |
| Patel | Hyaluronic acid, TIMP-1, alfa-2-macroglobulin | HCV | 77 | 73 |
| Sud (fibrosis probability index, FPI) | Age, AST, cholesterol, insulin resistence (HOMA), past alcohol intake | HCV | 96 | 44 |
| Leroy | PIIINP, MMP-1 | HCV | 60 | 92 |
| Fibrometer | Platelet count, prothrombin index, AST, alfa-2-macroglobulin, hyaluronic acid, urea, age | Mixed | 81 | 84 |
| Hepascore | Bilirubin, GGT, alfa-2-macroglobulin, hyaluronic acid, age, gender | HCV | 63 | 89 |
| Testa | Ratio platelet count/spleen diameter | HCV | 78 | 79 |
| FIB-4 | Platelet count, AST, ALT, age | HCV, HIV | 70 | 74 |

Fig. 2. Routine tests of liver fibrosis (30)

## 3. Imaging methods

### 3.1 Ultrasound

Ultrasound has been used for noninvasive investigation of liver, for detection of focal lesions, assessment the degree of liver fibrosis, description of trombosis of portal vein. Ultrasonographic parameters may represent an alternative to serum markers for the noninvasive assessment of liver disease severity and stage by finding signs of portal hypertension as splenomegaly, ascites, or a patent umbilical vein, and by examining the size, nodular liver surface, echogenicity and echotexture of the liver parenchyma.

The sensitivity of liver ultrasound scans in the diagnosis of fatty liver is almost 100 %. The correlation of fatty liver in ultrasound scans and liver biopsy tissue examination is 73.6 %. So, the degree of fatty infiltration observed in ultrasound scans is significantly correlated with degree of fatty accumulation of liver.

Some studies have shown an association between ultrasonography score and detection of cirrhosis with sensitivities ranging 87,5% to 100% and specificities ranging from 81,5% to 93,5%.

**Contrast-enhanced ultrasound (CEUS)** is the application of ultrasound contrast mediumto traditional medical sonography. Ultrasound contrast agents rely on the different ways in which sound waves are reflected from interfaces between substances. This may be the surface of a small air bubble or a more complex structure. Commercially available contrast media are gas-filled microbubbles that are administered intravenously to the systemic circulation. Microbubbles have a high degree of echogenicity, which is the ability of an object to reflect the ultrasound waves. The echogenicity difference between the gas in the microbubbles and the soft tissue surroundings of the body is immense. Thus, ultrasonic imaging using microbubble contrast agents enhances the ultrasound backscatter, or reflection of the ultrasound waves, to produce a unique sonogramwith increased contrast due to the high echogenicity difference. Contrast-enhanced ultrasound can be used to image blood perfusion in organs, measure blood flow rate in the heart and other organs, and has other applications as well.(26)

Vyas found that portal venous blood flow(PVBF), portal flow velocity(PFV) and gastric mucosal blood flow(GMBF) were all significantly slower in cirrhotic patiens and PVBF and PFV were lower in Child class B/C than class A.

Schneider et al. found that Doppler ultrasound alone was unable to discriminate between degrees of fibrosis, but portal venous undulations could predict liver cirrhosis with increased sensitivity(76,5%).(27)

Hirata et al. derived an arterio-portal(A/P)ratio by evaluating hepatic hemodynamics, which was higher in patients with cirrhosis compared with controls and demonstrated statistically significant differences in A/P ratio when comparing severe-to-mild or moderate fibrosis.

Hepatic vein transit times(HVTT) is using an ultrasound microbubble contrast agent as a tracer and has been investigated for grading liver disease.

Abbatista found that HVTT was significantly shorter in cirrhotic patients than in non - cirrhotic patients and distinguished between these patients with high accuracy

These results show that unenhanced Doppler ultrasound in not reliable in discrimination of varying degree of fibrosis, but that results can be improved with additional measurements such as heart pulsation at the liver surface and portal venous flow measurements.

High-resolution ultrasound of liver surface(LSS) can be used for investigation of liver cirrhosis. Liver surface is studied at the left liver lobe and is scored as smooth, irregular,

nodular. The smooth liver surface excludes cirrhosis, in case of irregular surface the results are indeterminate, the diagnosis of cirrhosis is when the surface is nodular.
The result can be improved with quantification,when the liver surface is semi-automatically measured.
The combination of ultrasonography and laboratory tests can improved the discrimination of patients with severe fibrosis and cirrhosis. Festa et al. investigated the cohort of 1143 patients with chronic hepatitis C, who underwent liver biopsy, laboratory tests and US.
All indices had specificity rate of > or =90% in excluding bridging fibrosis/cirrhosis, whereas sensitivity was acceptable (51%) for only platelet counts <140 000/μL. None of the ultrasonographic parameters singularly evaluated and reached an acceptable sensitivity rate. For ruling cirrhosis in or out, specificity rate was > or =82% for all tests, with the highest value reported by portal vein size. Low platelet counts plus nodular liver surface had the best sensitivity.
Ratio platelet/spleen diameter can be also beneficial
*Acoustic radiation force impulse elastography*
ARFI imaging technology involves the mechanical excitation of tissue using short-duration acoustic pulses (push pulses) in a region of interest chosen by the examiner, producing shear waves that spread away from the region of interest, generating localized, micron-scale displacements in the tissue . Simultaneously, detection waves of lower intensity than that of the push pulse are generated. The push pulse uses a few hundred cycles and different voltage compared to the short cycle B-mode pulse. The moment of interaction between the shear waves and detection waves marks the period of time elapsed between the generating of shear waves and their entire crossing of the region of interest. By recording the shear wave front at several locations and correlating these measurements with the elapsed time, the shear wave velocity (m/s) can be quantified; generally, the stiffer a region in the tissue, the greater the shear wave velocity as it travels through this region.
ARFI elastography has a good accuracy of diagnosis of liver fibrosis in chronic liver disease,might be available for the prediction of chronic liver disease related events such as hepatocellular carcinoma, esophageal varix.(28)

### 3.2 Elastography

Elastography is a noninvasive method measuring the mean stiffness of hepatic tissue ,a parameter, which correlates hihgly with liver fibrosis.
Transient elastography -FibroScan, Echosens, France , is equipped with a probe consisting in an ultrasonic transducer mounted on the axis of the vibrator. The probe is placed between two ribs in intercostal positions (sixth-eight intercostal area) on the right lobe of liver.A region of the liver selected for the test must be free from blood vessels structures of greater than 5 mm in diameter and should be homogenous.The sensor is focused at the zone of 25-65 mm from the surface of the skin. Vibrations of mild amplitude and low frequency are transmitted from the vibrator to the tissue by the transducer itself. This vibration induces an elastic shear wave , which propagates through the tissue. In the meantime, pulse-echo ultrasonic acquisitions are performed to follow the propagation of the shear wave and measure its velocity ,which is directly related to the tissue stiffness. The harder the tissue, the faster the shear wave propagates. After correct installation of the sensor,10 reliable measurements are taken and based on thein results, the software calculates the value of hepatic elasticity. The results are expressed in kilopascals(kPA) and median values are representative of liver stiffness.Following the previous studies TE was considered to exclude

cirrhosis at<12 kPa, indeterminate at 12-18 kPa, and to diagnose cirrhosis if >18kPa. FibroScan provides accurate prediction of hepatic fibrosis in patiens with chronic viral hepatitis,chronic cholestatic disease, provides accurate prediction of cirrhosis and its severity in patiens with chronic liver disease.

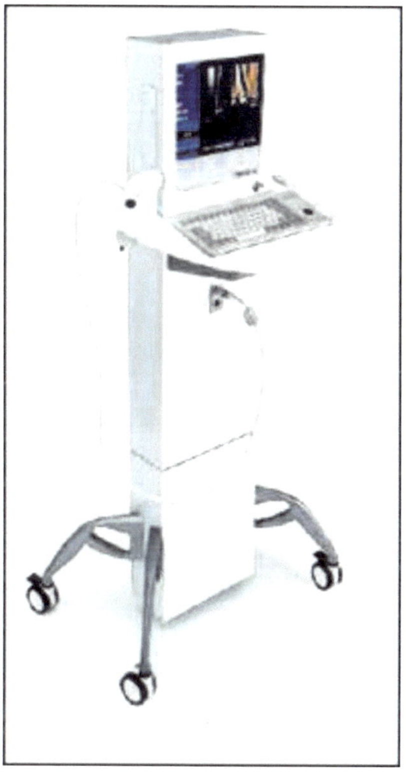

Fig. 3. Fibroscan (31)

### 3.3 Magnetic resonance imaging

Magnetic resonance imaging has been used for description of focal lesions- hemangiomas, liver tumors, malignant and also liver adenomas, focal nodular hyperplasia, for evaluation of liver fibrosis, for description of portal vein as MR splenoportography.
In MRI investigation is also often necessary using of contrast medium. Sensitivity of MRI for detection of liver focal lesions is 80-100%, sensitivity is higher than sensitivity of US or CT, specificity is more than 96%.
As contrast medium is often used gadollinium, superparamagnetic iron oxide(SPIO). Sequential administration of gadolinium and SPIO is used for investigation of liver fibrosis.Although SPIO-based images were highly accurate(85%) for detectiong fibrosis compared with histopatological features, the combination of gadolinium-based and SPIO contrast agents yielded even greater accuracy (93%) overall.
Diffusion weighted magnetic resonance imaging (DWMRI) has been widely used in brain imaging for the evaluation of acute ischemic stroke. With the advent of the echo-planar MRI technique, it became possible to be applied in the abdomen for the characterization of focal hepatic lesions. Recently, using DWMRI to measure the apparent diffusion coefficient

(ADC) of water, a parameter that is dependent on the tissue structure, has been introduced in the assessment of liver fibrosis. The ADC value is lower in livers with heavier fibrosis because of the restriction of water diffusion in fibrotic tissue. Lewin et al. assessed the performance of DWMRI in 54 patients with chronic HCV infection with reference to several other non-invasive methods.In discriminating significant fibrosis, the area under the curve (AUC) values were 0.79 for DWMRI, 0.87 for transient elastography, 0.68 for the FibroTest, 0.81 for aspartate aminotransferase to platelet ration index, 0.72 for the Forns index and 0.77 for hyaluronate. DWMRI performed better in discriminating between patients staged F3–F4, when the AUC value increased to 0.92, the same as in transient elastography. But besides fibrosis, it seems that ADC values might also reflect the intensity of inflammation, necrosis and steatosis. However, DWMRI still benefits from the intrinsic advantages of MRI. (29)

*MR Spectroscopy*

Based on its anatomical location and increased metabolic demands, the liver is considered an ideal organ for MR spectroscopy investigation.

*In vivo* MRspectroscopy is most commonly used to assess signals from hydrogen (1H) and phosphorus (31P). Although 1H-based MR spectroscopy allows for quantification of certain metabolites and lipids, 31P-based MR spectroscopy provides insights on processes including cell turnover and energy state based on substantial concentrations

within hepatocytes. Within the spectrum of 31P compounds, 6 discrete signals have frequently been analyzed by MR spectroscopy in human subjects, including (1) phosphomonoesters (PME), (2) inorganic phosphate, (3)phosphodiesters (PDE), (4) adenosine triphosphate (ATP), alpha-ATP, and beta-ATP. The chemical precursors phosphocholine, phosphoethanolamnine, adenosine monophosphate, and glycolytic intermediates,such as glucose-6-phosphate contribute to the PME peak. Glycerophosphorylcholine, glycerophosphorylethanolamine and mobile phospholipids from the endoplasmic reticulum are the main components of the PDE peak. Both PME and PDE appear to provide information on cellular degradation.The methodology used for performing MR spectroscopy has varied over time and between studies. MR spectroscopy of the liver is performed using a whole body MRI system at field strengths of 1.5 Tesla (T) or higher.

After a standard MR imaging for localization, special MR pulse sequences are applied to generate spectroscopic data within the appropriate anatomical location and volume (defined by voxels) of interest. As with diffusion-weighted imaging, an examination will take 45 to 60 minutes.

The spectral analysis of data requires processing to reduce noise and perform analysis. Metabolite concentrations can be expressed in absolute or relative terms. In general, the peak area of a metabolite signal is directly related to its concentration. Because the absolute quantitation of metabolites is difficult to achieve *in vivo,* many studies have used metabolite ratios for assessing spectral profiles.Peak areas in a spectrum are referenced to standards for correlation with MR signal intensities. An internal standard such as adenosine triphosphate (ATP) can be used, given its natural occurrence in tissue.

MR spectroscopy is recomended for investigation of diffuse liver disease, such as chronic hepatitis, steatosis non alcoholic fatty liver disease, for quantifying liver fat.There are also studies about the use of liver MR spectoroscopy for tumor assessment.The principal metabolite that has been targeted in focal liver disease is choline. Choline is elevated in tumors,because Choline is cell membrane compoment and increased cell turnover is associated with malignancy

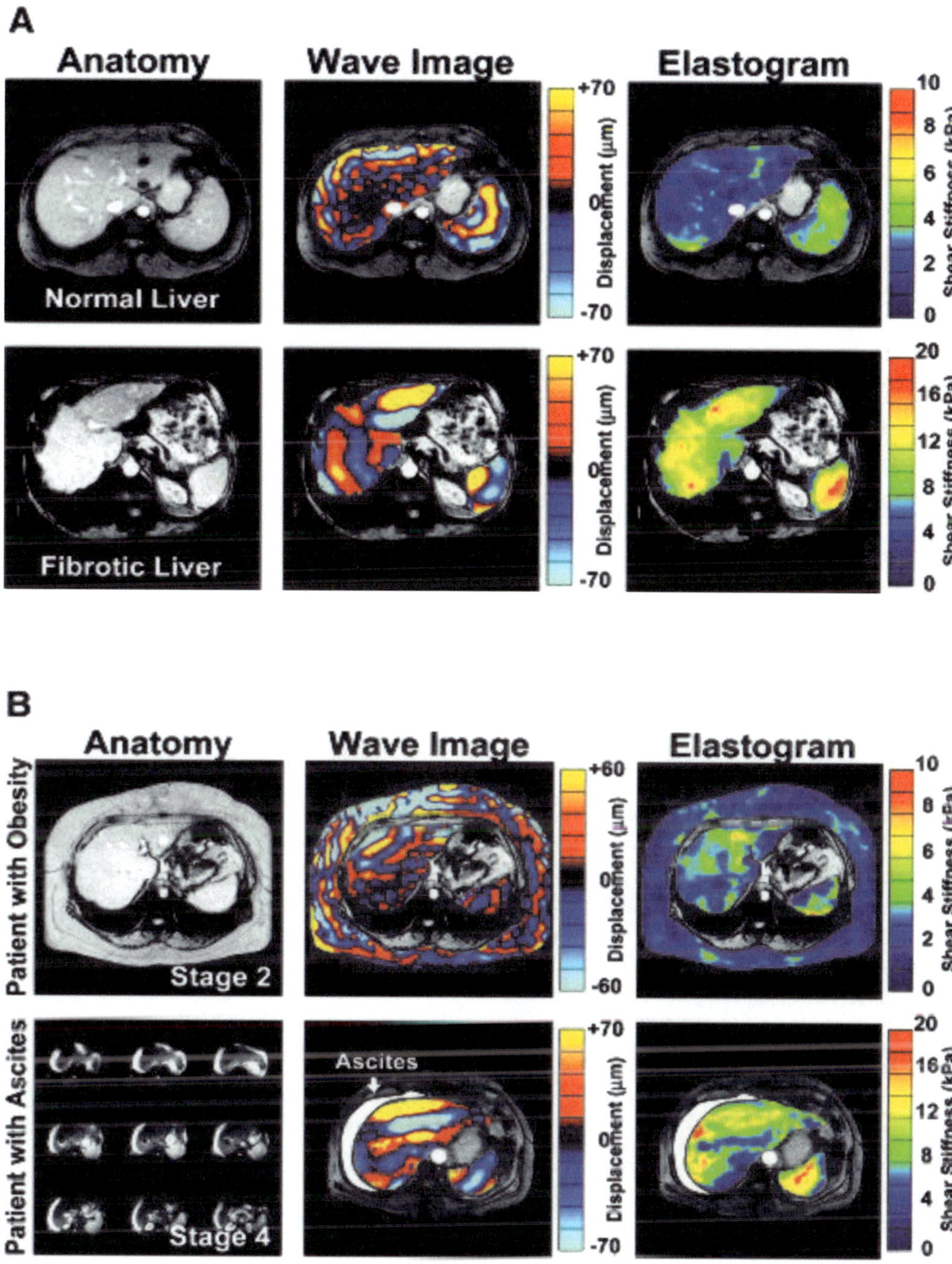
A
Anatomy
Wave Image
Elastogram
Normal Liver
Fibrotic Liver
+70
0
-70
Displacement (µm)
Shear Stiffness (kPa)
10
8
6
4
2
0
20
16
12
8
4
0
B
Patient with Obesity
Patient with Ascites
Stage 2
Stage 4
Ascites
+60
-60

Fig. 4.

(A) MR elastography of the liver in a healthy volunteer and a patient with cirrhosis. The middle column of images shows wave image data in the liver and spleen, superimposed on the corresponding anatomical images. The resulting elastograms are shown in the far right column. Elastograms show a higher mean stiffness of the fibrotic liver compared with the normal liver (12.1 ± 1.2 kPa versus 1.8 ± 0.3 kPa, respectively). (Adapted from Yin M, Talwalkar JA, Glaser KJ, Manduca A, Grimm RC, Rossman PJ, et al. Assessment of hepatic fibrosis with magnetic resonance elastography. Clin Gastro Hepatol 2007. In press).
(B) MR elastography of the liver in patients with obesity and ascites. The top row demonstrates a patient with obesity (BMI = 36) and stage 2 fibrosis on liver biopsy with a mean liver stiffness of 3.2 ± 0.8 kPa. The bottom row illustrates a patient with ascites. Excellent shear wave illumination of the liver was obtained, and the mean liver stiffness was 11.3 ± 2.8 kPa. (Adapted from Yin M, Talwalkar JA, Glaser KJ, Manduca A, Grimm RC, Rossman PJ, et al. Assessment of hepatic fibrosis with magnetic resonance elastography. Clin Gastro Hepatol 2007;5:1207-1213.e2.)

*MR elastography(MRE)*

is used for evaluation of the degree of liver fibrosis. The technic use is simile to that used in ultrasound elastography in that it uses a vibrafon device to induce a shear wave in the liver.The wave is detected by a modified magnetic resonance paging machine, and a color - coded image is generated that depicts the wave velocity,and hence stiffness,throughout the organ. MRE demonstrated that patients with hepatic fibrosis have higher liver stiffness measurements than healththy volunteers and that those with mild fibrosis were also able to be differentiated form those with moderate to advanced fibrosis,with mean hepatic shear elasticity being 2,24±0,23kPa in patiens with F0-F1 fibrosis, 2,56 ±0,24 kPa with F2-F3 fibrosis and 4,68 ±1,61 kPa in patiens with F4 fibrosis. MRE was found to have a higher technical succes rate than US elastography.

*Computed tomography*

CT imaging of liver provides specific method of noninvasive diagnosis of diffuse liver disease and also focal lesions of liver.Hepatic steatosis can be definied with a 76 % predictive value. Density of liver in steatosis is lower than density of intrahepatal vessels.CT imaging does not provide any information on the stage of fibrosis.CT imaging helps in diagnosis of cirrhosis according the nodular,irregular margin of liver.Pathological accumulation of iron increases density of liver parenchyma, but accumulation of copper does not change the density.

*Single photon emission computed tomography(SPECT)*

SPECT was tested in HIV-HCV co-infected patients,also in cirrhotic patients, in an effort to correlate histological severity of liver fibrosis with SPECT results.Cirrhotic patients showed a signifiant decrease of total liver uptake and a signifiant increase in total spleen uptake.Spleen volume was best at detecting liver cirrhosis, but total liver uptake correlated better with chronic liver disease severity.

## 4. Breath tests

There are several 13C breath tests for non-invasive investigation of hepatocellular function.
13 C-methacetin breath test (MBT) is essentially a microsomal liver function test. The patient ingest 75g 13C-methacetin dissolved in 200 ml water. Breath samples are collected at baseline and 15 min after ingestion of substrate. During the test period,the patient is in rest

and fasts to avoid influences due to variations in $CO_2$ production and food intake. 13C-methacetin is rapidly metabolised by healthy liver cells into acetaminophen and by a single dealkylation, and the increase of CO in breath samples can be quantified by isotope ratio mass spectrometry or nondispersive isotope-selective infrared spectroscopy. The 13 C-methacetin -breath test is more expensive than biochemical markers,but is also widely available.The breath samples can be sent to specialized centres or can be directly analysed as bedside test by nondispersive isotope-selective infrared spectrometers. The 13 C methacetin-breath test is more practicable than other 13 C based liver function tests because it can be performed as a simple two-point measurements as known from the 13C urea breath test. The rapid metabolism of methacetin allows a short sampling interval for the breath test.Methacetin undergoes a high hepatic extraction rate,which makes the methacetin breath test susceptible to variations in hepatic blood flow. (27)

13C methacetin-breath tests measure the functional metabolit capacity of residual hepatic cells and indirectly reflex how many hepatic cells are already lost .MBT has high sensitivity (93,5-95 %) and specificity (95-96,7%) for identifying cirrhotic patients, but can not differ patiens with early fibrosis and advanced fibrosis as determined by liver biopsy.

Another breath test is the 13C-aminopyrine breath test (ABT), where the aminopyrine is another substrate for labelling with the 13C isotope, much like the MBT.

## 5. Conclusion

Liver biopsy is curerrently the most beneficial method in diagnostic of liver dieases.Non-invasive methods of assessment of liver fibrosis,cirrhosis, steatosis are not able to replace liver biopsy because of their limitations.Increasing application of serum tests, imaging methods and breath tests is based on their advantages as absence of pain,of risk of complications, easy repeatability.

## 6. References

[1] Ehrmann J,Hůlek P.Aiglová K. Hepatologie,Grada 2010,116-118,ISBN 978-80-247-3118-6

[2] SaitouY et al., Noninvasive estimation of hepatic fibrosis.*World Journal of Gastroenterology*, Vol.11No.4,(2005),pp.476-481, ISSN: 1007-9327

[3] Kropf J. Efficacy of serum Laminin Measurement for Diagnosis of Fibrotic Liver Disease. *Clinical Chemistry*,Vol.34,No.10,(1998),pp.2026-2030, ISSN: 0009-9147

[4] Esmat G,Metwally M,Zalata KR,Shahinaz G.Evaluation of serum biomarkers of fibrosis and injury in Egyptian patiens with chronic hepatitis C. *Journal of Hepatology*, Vol.46, No.4,(2007),pp.620-627, ISSN: 0168-8278

[5] Pereira TN,Lewindon PJ,Smith JL,Murphy TL,Lincoln D.Serum markers of hepatic fibrogenesis in cystic fibrosis liver disease.*Journal of Hepatology*, Vol. 41, No.4, (2004), pp. 576-583, ISSN: 0168-8278

[6] Takahara T, Sollberg S,Muona P, Uitto J. Type VI collagen gene expression in experimental liver fibrosis: quantitation and spatiale distribution of mRNAs,and immunodetection of the protein. *Liver* ,Vol.15,No.2,(April1995),pp. 78-86, ISSN:0106-9543

[7] Yamanouchi M,Mizuhara Y, Maezawa Y, Toda G.Serum tenascin levels in chronic liver disease. *Liver* ,Vo.14,No.3,(June 1994),pp.148-53, ISSN:0106-9543

[8] Milani S,Grappone C, Pellegrini G, Schoppan D, Herbst H, ClabróA,Casini A: Undulin RNA and protein expression in normal and fibrotic human liver. *Hepatology,* Vol.20,(October 1994),pp.908-16, ISSN: 0270-9139

[9] Attallah AM,ZahranF., Ismail H.,Omran MM,El-DosokyI., Shiha GE. Immunochemical identification and detection of serum fibronectin in liver fibrosis patiens with chronic hepatitis C. *Journal of .Immunoassay and Immunochemistry*. Vol. 28, No. 4, (2007), pp.331-42, ISSN: 1532-1819

[10] Forns X, Ampuradanes S, Llovet J, Aponte J,Quintó L, Martínek-Bauer E. Identification of chronic hepatitis C patiens without hepatis fibrosis by a simple predictive model. *Hepatology*, Vol 36,No 4,(2002),pp. 986-992, ISSN: 0270-9139

[11] Wai C,Greenson J, Fontana R, Kalbfleisch J,Marrero J, Conjeeveram H, Lok A. A simple noninvasive index can predict both significant fibrosis and cirrhosis in patiens with chronic hepatitis C. *Hepatology*,Vol. 38,No. 2,(2003),pp.518-526,ISSN: 0270-9139

[12] RossiE, Adams L, Prins A, Bulhara M, De Boer B, Garas G, Mac Quillan G,Speers D,Jeffrey G. Validation of the FibroTest biochemical Markers score in assessing in liver fibrosis in hepatitis C patiens. *Clinical Chemistry* ,Vo.49,No.3,(2003),pp.450-454, ISSN: 0009-9147

[13] Poynard T,RatziuV,Naveau S,Thalud D,CharlotteF, Messous D,Capron D,Abella A. The diagnostic value of biomarkers(SteatoTest) for the prediction of liver steatosis. *Comparative Hepatology* ,Vol.4,No.10,(December2005), ISSN: 1476-5926

[14] Poynard T,Ratziu V,Charlotte F,MessousD, Munteanu M,Imbert-Bismut F.Diagnostic value of biochemical marker(NashTest) for prediction of nonalcoholo steatohepatitis in patiens with non alcoholic fatty liver disease.*BMC Gastroenterology* ,Vol. 6,No.34,(November 2006), ISSN: 1471-230X

[15] Vallet-Pichard A,Mallet V, Nalpas B,Verkarre V, Nalpas A,Dhalluin-Vernier V,Fontaine H. Fib-4:an inexpensive and accurate marker of fibrosis in HCV infectioncomparison with liver and fibrotest. *Hepatology*.Vol.47,No.2,(February2008) pp.762-3, ISSN: 0270-9139

[16] Adams L,Bulsara M, Rossi E, DeBoer B, Speers D, Greoge J, Kench J,Farrell G, McCaughan G, Hepascore: An accurate validated predictor of liver fibrosis in chronic hepatitis C infection. *Clinical Chemistry* , Vol.51(2005),pp.1867-1873, ISSN: 0009-9147

[17] Poynard T,Aubert A, Bedossa P, Abella A,Naveau S, Paraf F, Chaput JC.A simple biological index for detection of alcoholic liver disease in drinkers. *Gastroenterology,*Vol.100,*(May* 1991),pp.1397-402, ISSN: 0016-5085

[18] Fortunato G,Castaldo G,Cerini R, Intrieri M, Gentile I,Borgia G,Piazza M, Salvatore F.Multivariate Discriminant Function Based on Six Biochemical Markers in Blood Can Predict the Cirrhotic Evolution of Chronic Hepatitis. *Clinical Chemistry* ,Vol.47,No.9 ,(2001),pp.1696–1700 , ISSN: 0009-9147

[19] Patel K,GordonS.C, JacobsonI,Hézode Ch, SmithK.M,nPawlotsky J-M, Mc-Hutchinson J.G .Evaluation of a panel of non-invasive serum markers to differentiate mild from moderate-to-advanced liver fibrosis chronic hepatitis C patiens. *Journal of Hepatology,* Vol.41,No.6,(December 2004),pp. 935-942,ISSN: 0168-8278

[20] Lackner C,Struber G,LieglB,LeiblS,Ofner P, Bankuti C,Bauer B, Stauber R. Comparison and validation of simple noninvasive tests for predistion of fibrosis in chronic hepatitis C. *Hepatology,* Vol.41,No.6,(June 2005),pp.1376-1382, ISSN: 0270-9139

[21] Bonacini M,Hadi G,Govindarajan S, Lindsay KL. Utility of a discriminant score for diagnosing advanced fibrosis or cirrhosis in patiens with chronic hepatitis C virus infection. *American Journal of Gastroenerology* ,Vol.92,No.8,(August 1996),pp.,1302-4, ISSN: 0002-9270

[22] Rosenberg WM, Voelker M, Thiel R, et al. Serum markers detect the presence of liver fibrosis: a cohort study. *Gastroenterology.* Vol.127,(2004,)pp.1704–13, ISSN: 0016-5085

[23] Koda M,Matunaga Y,Kawakami M,Kishimoto Y,Suou T,Murawakai Y. Fibroindex, a practical index for predicting significant fibrosis in patiens with chronic hepatitis C. *Hepatology.*Vol.46,No.1.,(July 2007),pp.280-1, ISSN: 0270-9139

[24] Sud A., Hui JM,Farrell GC. Improved prediction of fibrosis in chronic hepatitis C using measures of insulin rezistence in a probability index. *Hepatology,* Vol.39,No.5,( May2004), pp. 1239-1247, ISSN: 0270-9139

[25] Kelleher T, Mehta S, Bhaskar R, Sulkowski M, Astemborski J., Thomas DL. *et al.*, Prediction of hepatic fibrosis in HIV/HCV co-infected patients using serum fibrosis markers: the SHASTA index, *Journal of Hepatology* Vol.43, (2005), pp. 78–84, ISSN: 0168-8278

[26] Iacobellis A.,Fussili S,Magnia A, Clemente R,Festa V,Giaccobe A, Facciorusso D,Niro C,Conoscitore A. Ultrasonographic and biochemical parameters in the non-invasive evaluation of liver fibrosis in hepatitis C virus chronic hepatitis. *Alimentary Pharmacology and Therapeutics* ,Vol.22,No.9,(November 2005),pp.:769-74, ISSN: 0269-2813

[27] Smith JO,Sterling RK. Systematic review:non-invasive methods of fibrosis analysis in chronic hepatitis C.*Alimentary Pharmacology and Therapeutics* Vol. 30,No. 6,(September 2009), ,pp. 557 576, ISSN: 0269-2813

[28] Bota S,Sporea I,Sirli R,Popescu A, Spleen assessment by Acoustic Radiation Force Impulse Elastography (ARFI) for prediction of liver cirrhosis and portal hypertension , *Medical Ultrasonography,*, Vol. 12, No. 3, (2010),pp.213-217, ISSN: 1844-4172

[29] Lewin M, Poujol-Robert A, Boelle PY *et al* . Diffusion-weighted magnetic resonance imaging for the assessment of fibrosis in chronic hepatitis C. *Hepatology* Vol.46,(2007),pp. 658–65, ISSN: 0270-9139

[30] GressnerOA,Weiskirchen R,Gressner AM:Biomarkers of liver fibrosis:Clinical translation of molecular pathogenesis or based on liver-dependent malfunction tests.*Clinica Chimica Acta* Vol..381,(2007).pp. 107-113, ISSN: 0009-8981

[31] http://www.biopredictive.com/ru/current-applications-of-elastometry-and-fibro-and-acti-test-for-diagnostics-of-hepatic-fibrosis

14

# Can We Replace Liver Biopsy with Non-Invasive Procedures?

Carmen Fierbinteanu Braticevici[1], Raluca Papacocea[2], Laura Tribus[1] and Anca Badarau[2]

[1]*Medical Clinic II and Gastroenterology, University Hospital Bucharest,*
[2]*Physiology Department I,*
*"Carol Davila" University of Medicine and Pharmacy Bucharest,*
*Romania*

## 1. Introduction

Liver fibrogenesis is the consequence of all hepatic lesions, regardless of etiology. Progressive scars, which are the response to constant liver injuries lead to cirrhosis, disorganize the normal liver architecture through fibrosis bands, parenchyma nodules and blood vessel distortions. For this reason, liver fibrosis is a central parameter which expresses the severity of liver diseases, regardless of etiology; it is a key element which predicts the evolution of liver diseases towards cirrhosis.

Irrespective of the cirrhosis etiology, the clinical evolution is similar, towards major complications such as: portal hypertension and hepatocellular insufficiency. Due to these complications, cirrhosis is the seventh death cause within general mortality. Cirrhosis also encourages the development of hepatocellular carcinoma, an aggressive neoplasm which causes death in a few months in the absence of early diagnosis. That is why liver fibrosis is a major criterion in initiating the etiologic treatment of chronic liver diseases.

A long time ago, liver fibrosis was deemed irreversible. This axioma has been discarded for quite some time; at present, fibrosis is considered to be a bidirectional dynamic phenomenon: fibrogenesis and fibrinolysis. Thus, it is possible to reshape the scar healing tissue. Due to this dynamic process, it is necessary to quantify fibrosis in order to set the therapeutic decision and especially to monitor the efficiency of anti fibrotic treatments.

There are several methods to diagnose liver fibrosis: liver biopsy, serum biomarkers, breath tests and hepatic elastography. Liver biopsy is currently essential in diagnosis of inflammatory and metabolic liver diseases. It provides particularly invaluable informations for disease diagnosis and patient monitoring.

The role of liver biopsy is still a controversial issue being an invasive method with well-known risks and complications. Although liver biopsy is considered the golden standard for chronic liver diseases, it is worth mentioning that the histological tested fragment is however a small part of the liver, and the scar lesions, which are secondary to chronic inflammatory processes are unevenly distributed in the liver mass. Thus, liver biopsy is a method neither ideal nor sufficient to diagnose and determine the stage of liver fibrosis. In this context, a noninvasive method to assess liver fibrosis is more than welcome.

Noninvasive tests can be classified in several ways based on the modality of the test (serum blood tests or imaging) or the constituents of the tests (direct markers versus indirect markers of fibrosis). With the evolution of noninvasive tests, the performance can improve particularly with the use of combination or serial noninvasive tests.
In this chapter the role of liver biopsy and non-invasive tests to assess liver fibrosis and to manage the treatment of patients with chronic liver disease is discussed.

## 2. Liver biopsy

Liver biopsy was first described by Paul Ehrlich, 130 years ago, as a diagnostic tool of the chronic liver disease. It can be performed using blind percutaneous technique, computer tomography or ultrasound-guided, transjugular, open surgical, laparoscopic and even endoscopic approaches.
Microscopic examination of liver tissue often provides the definitive diagnosis and leads to effective management of the liver disorders. Because fibrosis is tissue damage, biopsy is by definition the only direct tool to assesses liver fibrosis.

### 2.1 When is liver biopsy useful?

The major indication for performing a liver biopsy is to clarify the nature of liver disease. In some instances, liver biopsy is performed to establish the effect of the treatment in known liver disease. In chronic viral hepatitis, the knowledge of liver fibrosis stage is important for prognosis and for decision about the antiviral treatment. Significant fibrosis ($F \geq 2$) in these patients is an indication for antiviral treatment.
In patients with alcoholic liver diseases, the clinical features and the values of serum aminotransferases are poorly correlated with the liver diseases stage and the long-term prognosis strictly depends on the severity of histological lesions. In alcoholic liver disease, the biopsy can reveal fatty liver infiltration, large shape of hepatocytes, the presence of Mallory bodies, or polimorfonuclear infiltrates in portal spaces, and also histological features specific to cirrhosis. On the other side, fatty liver infiltration occurs in various etiologic situations: obesity, diabetes, consumption of alcoholic beverages, chronic HCV infection and the liver biopsy may provide distinct etiologic information.
In patients with chronic hepatitis C there is a low correlation between symptoms, serum aminotransferases and histological modifications; thus, serum aminotransferases may have normal values, but liver histology is suggestive for severe fibrosis or cirrhosis. Liver biopsy ensures a certain diagnosis in more than 90% of the patients with unexplainable increase of serum aminotransferases. In the same time, it is useful in evaluating infectious complications, drug toxicity or the reoccurrence of the primary disease in the transplanted liver.
In patients who present space replacing liver formations, the indication of liver biopsy is still debatable. It is useful to establish the origin of metastasis when the primary tumor is not known, to confirm the metastases in case of diagnosed cancers before and after surgical resection. It is also able to certify the benign nature of liver formations.
In patients with nonresected hepatocellular carcinoma, echographic guidance allows specific therapeutically approach like: alcoholization, radiofrequency, chemoembolization.
In conclusion, liver biopsy is recommended in diagnosis of:
**Infiltrative liver diseases**:tuberculosis, sarcoidosis, lymphoma, amyloidosis;
**Hereditary disorders:** Wilson disease (determining the amount of intrahepatocyte copper deposits), hemochromatosis (determining the amount and quality of intrahepatocyte iron deposits), alpha-1 antitrypsin deficiency;

**Liver cholestasis**: primary billiary cirrhosis, primary sclerosing cholangitis;.
**Diagnostic uncertainty** (abnormal liver tests with no clear etiology: the increase of serum aminotransferases, bilirubin, alkaline phosphatase or ϒglutamiltranspeptidase.
**Coexisting disorders**: Human immunodeficiency virus [HIV] and hepatitis C virus infection, alcoholic liver disease and hepatitis C
**Overlap syndrome**: Primary biliary cirrhosis with autoimmune hepatitis.
**Fatty liver**: liver biopsy can distinguish between benign steatosis and progressive steatohepatitis;
**Space replacing processes** discovered by chance during a routine imagistic check up.
Periodic needle biopsy is also valuable in the management of a few diseases.
**In autoimmune hepatitis,** monitoring the plasma cell score on liver biopsy may help predict relapse;
**Liver transplantation:** possible complications occurring after the liver transplant rejection or the disease recurrence (Carey & Carey, 2010).

### 2.2 The liver biopsy interpretation

Histologic assessment of a liver biopsy specimen remains the "gold standard" for quantifying fibrosis that is essential to guide management and predict prognosis in patients with chronic liver injury .

There is a wide range of methods used to interpret a liver biopsy. For morphological analysis of liver liver biopsy is necessary to use either ordinary staining (hematoxilin-eozin), or special ones: Masson's trichrome stain (for fibrosis), Pass stain (for glycogen), Pearls stain (for intrahepatocyte iron deposits) and rhodamin (for hepatocyte copper). Immunohistochemical and in situ mRNA hybridization methods to identify specific matrix components can be employed for experimental aim and have some utility in assessing fibrosis progression.

The most important role of liver biopsy is the assessment of necroinflammation (grade) and fibrosis (stage). The morphological features of chronic viral hepatitis are portal fibrosis, portal and periportal mononuclear inflammation and necroinflammatory changes within the parenchyma with a an irregular distribution between one lobule and another. There is also regenerative activity in an irregular distribution. The degree of necrosis depends on the disease activity –more severe during exacerbations and lesser in quiescent stages. Fibrosis progresses to cirrhosis and the periseptal inflammatory activity continues with cirrhosis .

A number of numerical scoring systems have been used to evaluate the amount of inflammation and degree of fibrosis in liver biopsy specimens from patients with chronic liver disease. Histological scores such as Metavir, Knodell, Ishak and Desmet/ Scheuer systems were created to standardize the interpretation of liver biopsies. The Knodell system was the first staging system, having a total of 18 for necroinflammation and a total of 4 for fibrosis (0-4). However, this system is noncontiguous and no longer used. Instead, the Ishak system had more details for necroinflammation (0-18) and expanded scores for fibrosis(0-6) This may be helpful in clinical studies when fine gradations of fibrosis pattern are required to demonstrate change, but this system is not commonly used in clinical practice. These scores are semi- quantitative scales for evaluation of a complex pathobiological process: fibrosis, necroinflammation and finally nodule formation. The Metavir system is simpler with a combination score for inflammation including periportal and lobular activity (A0-A3) and a fibrosis score on a scale of F0-F4. Metavir is the most used system in clinical practice today. The accuracy of grading and staging is dependent on the adequacy of the specimen and the experience of the pathologist.

Bedossa considers that the advantages of using the scores for liver biopsy interpretation consist in :an increase of reproducibility between pathologists, a standardization of biopsies reports, an homogeneity between liver centers, and a better comparison of consecutive biopsies for monitoring disease follow-up . The scores also serve as reference for choosing and validation of non invasive methods for liver fibrosis assessment.

| Appearance | Ishak stage:<br>Categorical description | ISHAK | METAVIR |
|---|---|---|---|
|  | No fibrosis (Normal) | 0 | F0 |
| 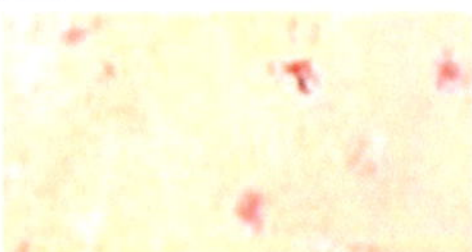 | Fibrosis expansion of some portal areas ± short fibrous septa | 1 | F1 |
| 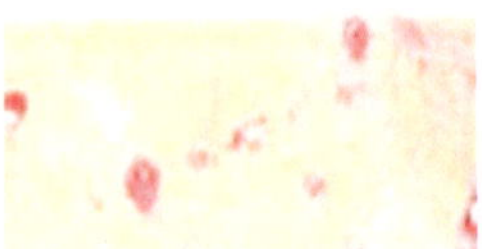 | Fibrosis expansion of most portal areas ± short fibrous septa | 2 | F2 |
| 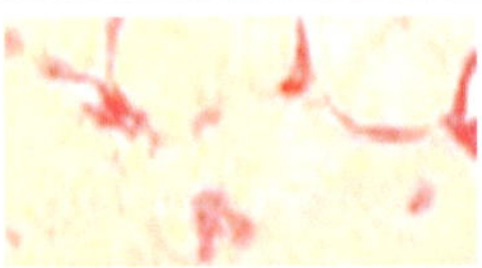 | Fibrosis expansion of most portal areas with occasional portal to portal(P-P) bridging | 3 | |
| 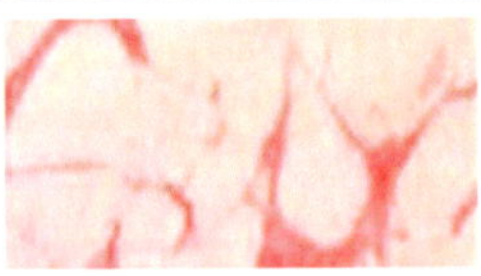 | Fibrosis expansion of portal areas with marked portal to portal(P-P) bridging as well as portal to central( P-C) | 4 | F3 |
| 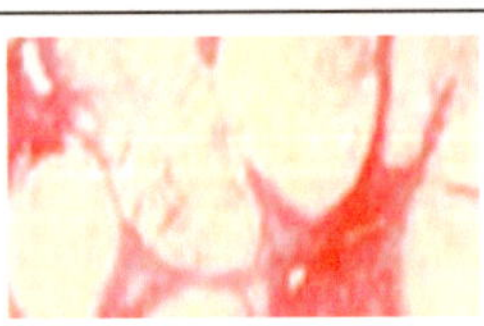 | Marked bridging (P-P and/or P-C) with occasional nodules (incomplete cirrhosis) | 5 | |
| 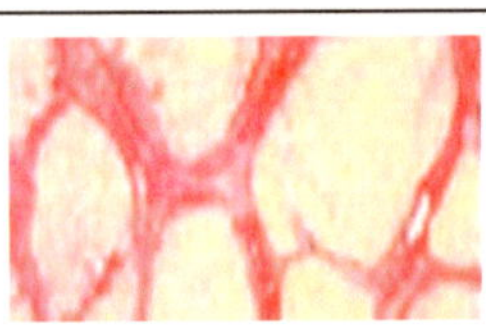 | Cirrhosis, probable or definite | 6 | F4 |

Table 1. Scoring systems in liver fibrosis.( Standish RA et al.,2006)

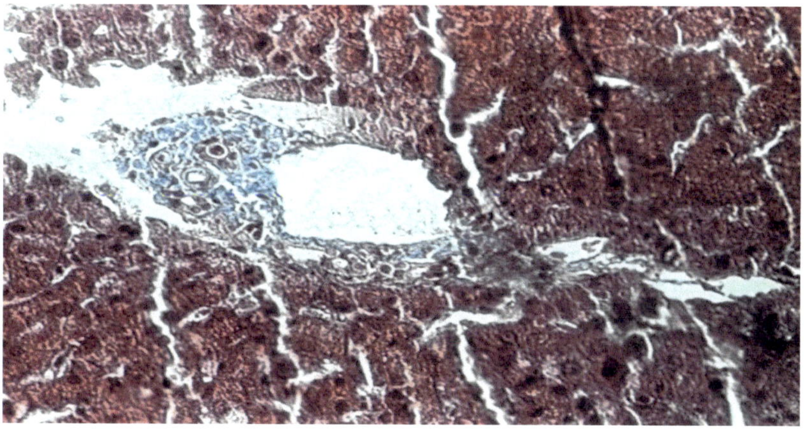

Fig. 1. Fibrosis stage 1

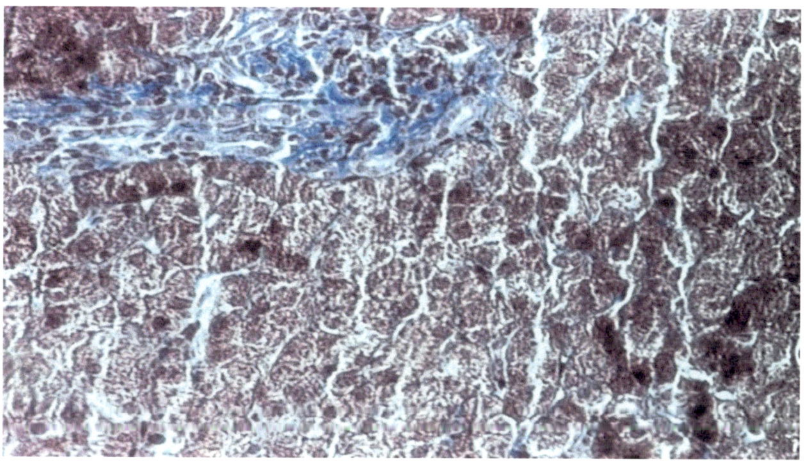

Fig. 2. Fibrosis stage 2

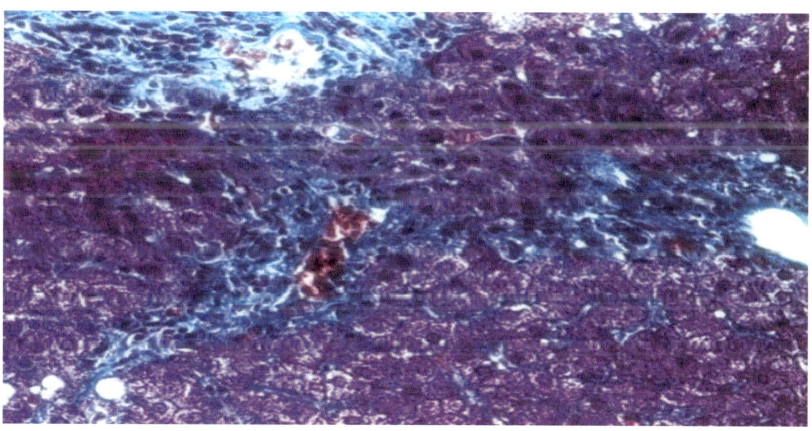

Fig. 3. Fibrosis stage 3.

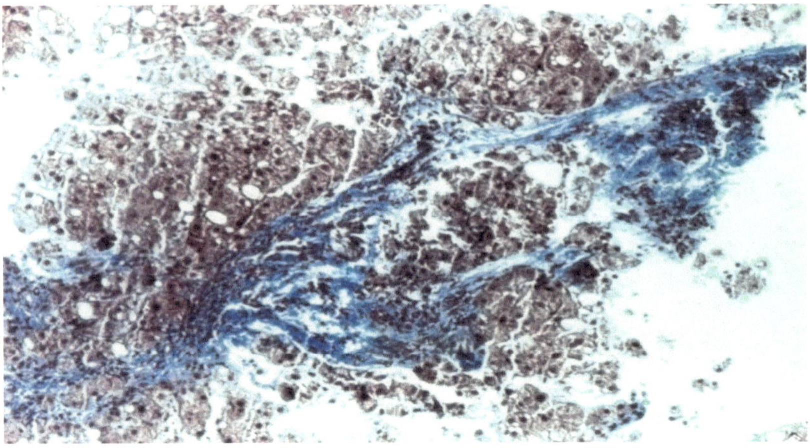

Fig. 4. Fibrosis stage 4

### 2.3 Complications of liver biopsy

Liver biopsy is a safe procedure if it is carried out by experienced gastroenterologists. Froehlich et al noticed a lower rate of complications in the case of doctors who performed over 50 biopsies in a year. Although the liver is a highly irrigated organ, complications after the biopsy are rarely. Thus, it was noted that over 60% of the complications occur within two hours and over 90% within the first 24 hours after the procedure. Within out patients who present complications, 1-3% require hospitalization, often after Tru-cut type needle use.

Complications may be minor (pain or vagal reactions, blood hypotension) or major. Significant complications, defined as those resulting in hospital admission or prolonged hospitalisation, occur in 1-5% of patients. The mortality rate is reported between 1:1000 and 1:10000. The complications of liver biopsy and their frequency are indicated in table no. 2

### 2.4 Limits of liver biopsy

The hepatic function is compromised to a minimum until the development of cirrhosis. The presence of clinical manifestations such as ascites and encephalopathy are clear evidences of the advanced disease.

So far, only liver biopsy has been able to determine the severity of pre-cirrhotic stages. However, the role of liver biopsy as a "golden standard" in diagnosing liver diseases seems to be controversial due to the development of modern imagistic techniques: ultrasonography, computer tomography, nuclear magnetic resonance and the appearance of noninvasive serum markers.

Liver biopsy may be the "golden standard" in assessing liver fibrosis, but it is not 24 karat gold. We have to mention that the biopsy needle takes a small fragment from the liver. It is important to take into account that a biopsy is merely a sample of the entire liver and the scarring in chronic liver disease is typically irregularly distributed in the liver. For this reason, the perfect liver biopsy should remove a fragment into a known area of the disease or multiple fragmentes in many areas of a diseased liver.

| **Complications of liver biopsy** | |
|---|---|
| Pain at the right hypochondrium, shoulder | 0.056-83% |
| Arterial hypotension | |
| Hemorrhagic complications | sub capsular hematoma: 0.05%<br>intrahepatic hematoma: 0.05%<br>intraperitoneal bleeding: 0.03%<br>hemobilia: 0.05% |
| Bacteriemia | 0.08% |
| Death | 0.001-0.0001% |
| Bile peritonitis | 0.03-0.22% |
| Pneumothorax, hemothorax | 0.08-0.28% |
| Subcutaneous emphysema | 0.014% |
| Subphrenic abscess | |
| Anaphylactic shock (hydatid cyst) | |
| Break of the biopsy needle | 0.02% |
| Biopsy of other organs | lungs-0.001%<br>bile -0.003%<br>colon-0.003%<br>kidneys-0.09% |

Table 2. The complications of liver biopsy

The liver biopsy removes only about 1/50 000$^{th}$ of the liver and can miss the diagnosis of cirrhosis in 20% to 30% of patients. That is why, many investigators recommend a biopsy length at least 15 mm, containing sixt or eight portal tracts, to improve the diagnostic accuracy. Both the size of the biopsy and the number of biopsies taken have a major effect on diagnosis accuracy. Although widely used, liver biopsy can be a source of errors given by the small size of the samples or the inappropriate sizes of the needle.The length of the fragment is proportional to the length of the needle used (18 gauge) and the size of the liver fragment is essential in assessing the hepatic architecture. There are several studies which revealed a decrease of diagnosis accuracy in biopsies smaller than 2 cm. In a study which comprised 10.000 virtual biopsies, Bedossa and collaborators showed that the staging of liver fibrosis is accurate in 65% of the cases when the analyzed biopsy fragment was at least 15 mm long, in 75% of the cases when the fragment was at least 25 mm length and that the best length should be 40 mm. The same study, in which laparoscopic biopsies were collected from both lobes of patients with chronic hepatitis C, estimated that biopsy specimens with a minimum 4 cm or greather in length would reliably avoid sampling error. However, in many specialized hepatology centers, the biopsy fragment does not meet the best criteria for an accurate histological analyse. Surgical wedge biopsy provides adequate tissue volume to overcome this problem.

Another limitation of the liver biopsy is that is very sensitive to analysis errors. Several studies have investigated the interobserver and intraobserver variability in the histological diagnosis of liver diseases. To minimize the analysis errors and to standardize the histological evaluation, staging scores for fibrosis, such as the METAVIR, Ishak and Scheuer systems, were created. Nevertheless, liver biopsy is associated with error in fibrosis staging in up to 20% of patients and a misdiagnosis of cirrhosis in up to 15 % of patients. In example of the resulting sampling errors that can occur, were considered the two most common chronic liver diseases: hepatitis C and fatty liver disease. Regev et al (2002) performed laparoscopically guided biopsy of the right and left hepatic lobes in a serie of 124 patients with chronic hepatitis C. The two fragments of the same patient were interpreted by the same anatomopathologist who was not awared about the identity of the biopsy fragment. Differences of more than one Metavir stage of fibrosis was present in 33,1% of cases and more than 2 stages in 2.4%. In 14.5%, cirrhosis was diagnosed in one lobe but not the other. As regards liver diseases of other etiologies than the viral one, differences were even bigger. In a study on patients with nonalcoholic fatty liver disease, Ratziu et al found that differences of more than one stage Metavir was present in approximately 40% of paired liver biopsy; in the patients with primary sclerosing cholangitis or primary biliary cirrhosis, ≥1 fibrosis stage discordances occurred in up to 60% of paired liver biopsy.

Clearly, needle liver biopsy is far from an ideal test. For these reasons it is necessary to develop some semi-automated systems to assess additional histological and immunohistochemical features.

Another limit of the liver biosy is related to slow rate of fibrosis progression; from normal liver to cirrhosis it takes more than 20 years. Follow-up biopsy is too insensitive to detect changes in fibrosis progression or regression within weeks to months and even years.

From another point of view, liver biopsy is an invasive procedure with certain unavoidable risks and complications. For both, the physician and the patient, the decision to proceed with liver biopsy is not a trivial one. There is an urgent need for a noninvasive diagnostic procedure for liver fibrosis because this is currently the main limitation of antifibrotic drug testing in clinical trials.

## 3. Noninvasive methods for the evaluation of liver fibrosis

Liver biopsy has been used in more than a century for the staging and diagnosis of acute or chronic liver diseases. In order to monitor patients with chronic liver diseases, liver biopsy has been increasingly less used because of the sampling and interpretation errors, the patient's high emotional cost and especially because it captures only one moment in a diffuse and evolutive hepatic process. In this context, the identification of a noninvasive method for the evaluation of liver fibrosis is a challenging option.

Noninvasive testes are an attractive alternative to liver biopsy for staging and monitoring of chronic liver diseases. A noninvasive method which provides the same information as liver biopsy is also desirable in cases when the latter is not possible.

The purpose of any noninvasive technique is to replace liver biopsy. These methods have the advantage of representing the liver in its entirely unlike puncture which analyzes only a limited fragment of liver. They also provide information related to the hepatic function: secretion, bile excretion or endothelial uptake.

Considering the slowly evolution of chronic liver diseases, the information provided through liver puncture is not enough to monitor the disease at short time intervals ue to the minimal histological changes. Noninvasive tests have to be sensitive enough to detect the minor changes of the dynamic fibrosis process.

Another indication of noninvasive tests is that they evaluate the efficiency of antifibrotic treatments, which cannot be performed through repeated hepatic punctures. It is important to have safe and efficient methods to objectify liver fibrosis from several perspectives. In the first place, patients with liver fibrosis are part of a high risk group as regards liver diseases mortality. In the second place, the prognosis of chronic liver diseases depends on the severity and related risk factors. In the third place, when the etiologic factor can be removed, it is important to introduce the antifibrotic therapy as soon as possible to reverse the hepatic lesions.

The criteria used in evaluating the severity of liver diseases through other procedures than liver biopsy are not specified yet. That is why, for now, potential noninvasive methods must be relatively well correlated with the biopsy. The errors of this histological method prevent the perfect correlation between the biopsy and noninvasive tests in the diagnosis and staging of liver fibrosis. The best correlation occurs in biopsies > de 2.5 cm, the correlation index (r) being 0.85. For the interpretation of noninvasive tests, it is important to consider the fact that liver biopsy may fail in 20% of the cases, especially for intermediary forms of liver fibrosis. This is the reason why many experts believe that the noninvasive methods whose ROC (Receiver Operator Characteristic) curve is 0.85-0.90 are as effective as the histological exam in the accurate staging of liver fibrosis.

The two major categories of noninvasive tests include: serum fibrosis markers and hepatic elasticity imaging (elastography).

The results of noninvasive tests will be interpreted in the clinical context; in case of discrepancies, liver biopsy is recommended.

### 3.1 Serum fibrosis markers

The physiopathology's knowledge of liver fibrosis has determined a high number of biomarkers used to diagnose it. Depending on the elements they represent, there are two marker categories: direct (representing components of extracellular matrix) or indirect (reflecting hepatic inflammation and function).

In order to be sensitive and specific, therefore ideal for the diagnosis of liver fibrosis, Afdhal N.H (2007) considers that biomarkers have to meet the following requirements:

- they should be specific hepatic tests;
- the results should not be influenced by the alteration of the hepatic, renal or reticuloendothelial function;
- they should reflect fibrosis regardless of etiology;
- they should be reproducible and easy to perform;
- they should be sensitive enough to differentiate among various fibrosis stages;
- the risks for patients should be minimum;
- the cost should be low.

Due to the high number of molecules involved in liver fibrosis efforts were made to compile the serum markers within panels for clinical use. More indicators and sophisticated scores utilizing direct and indirect markers have been developed to enhance the detecting and noninvasive staging of liver fibrosis. The most widely known of these are listed in table no.3.

| Panel | Liver Disease | Se | Sp | PPV | NPV |
|---|---|---|---|---|---|
| AST/ALT ratio | AST/ALT | 53% | 100% | 100% | 81% |
| Forns test | Platelets, GGT, Cholesterol | 94% | 51% | 40% | 96% |
| APRI Index | AST, Platelets | 41% | 95% | 88% | 64% |
| PGA Index | Platelets, GGT, apo A | 91% | 81% | 85% | 89% |
| FibroTest | GGT, haptoglobin, bilirubin, apoA, alpha$_2$-macroglobulin | 87% | 59% | 63% | 85% |
| Fibrospect | Hyaluronic acid, TIMP-1, alpha$_2$-macroglobulin | 83% | 66% | 72% | 78% |
| FPI | AST, Cholesterol, HOMA-IR | 85% | 48% | 70% | 69% |
| ELF | ECM proteins and proteinases | 90% | 41% | 35% | 92% |

Abbreviations: Se, sensitivity, Sp, specificity, PPV, positive predictive value, NPV, negative predictive value, AST, aspartate aminotransferase, ALT, alanine aminotransferase, GGT, Gamma glutamyl transferase, apoA, apolipoprotein $A_1$, TIMP-1, tissue inhibitors of metalloproteinase 1, HOMA-IR, homeostasis model assessment of insulin resistance, EMC, extracellular matrix molecules

Table 3. Diagnostic performances of serum markers panels for hepatic fibrosis compared to the referenced standard of liver biopsy (Adapted from Rockey DC& Bissel DM, 2006).

The serum markers of fibrosis are an attractive, noninvasive and affordable alternative, replacing at least part of the liver biopsies used in clinical practice. Crockett et al (2006) made a comparison between liver biopsy and serum markers, considering the advantages and disadvantages of the two methods used alternatively to diagnose and stage liver fibrosis.

| Factor | Liver biopsy | Serum markers |
|---|---|---|
| Cost | 2200$ | Laboratory cost |
| Risks | Significant | Minimal |
| Contraindications | Multiple: bleeding diathesis, morbid obesity, ascites, extrahepatic biliary obstruction | Conditions with high rate of false positivity |
| Accuracy | 80% | 60-80% |
| System requirements | Operator, pathology laboratory, pathologist | Clinical laboratory, phlebotomy, materials. |
| Specimen adequacy | Length of liver fragment at least 15 mm with 6-8 portal tracts | Blood sample |
| False positives | Interobserver variability | Sepsis, nonhepatic inflammation, hemolysis, trombocitopenia |
| False negatives | Sampling variability | Varies per test |
| Time for results | 24-72 hours minimum | 1-2 hours minimum |

Table 4. Comparison of liver biopsy and serum markers of fibrosis

The ability of serum tests of fibrosis are similar, with area under the receiver operating characteristic curve 0.8-0.85. Compared to biopsy, current serum biomarkers represent the whole liver, permit only crude staging sparing about 30-40% patients for biopsy and reflect also liver function (secretion, endotelial uptake).Although their accuracy value are improving they cannot supplant direct analysis of the liver. They have some limitatios:

- They reflect the rate of matrix turnover and tend to be more elevated when there is high inflammatory activity;
- None of the molecules is liver specific, so concurrent sites of inflammation may contribute to serum level;
- Serum levels are influenced by clearance rates;

The clinical usefulness of serological tests is to set quickly whether fibrosis is mild or severe, being less efficient in intermediary fibrosis stages. Most serum markers are more efficient in identifying fibrosis that in infirming it. That is why, when fibrosis is severe, regardless of the invasive or noninvasive diagnosis method, patients without signs of portal hypertension should start etiologic treatment.

So far, there is no ideal noninvasive test. Serum markers are based on probability calculations and thus they are less specific. Their diagnosis performances increase through the combined use of several serum markers tests.

Using the algorithms based on the sequential combination of serum markers, diagnosis accuracy in detecting significant fibrosis can increase to 93-95%, and the liver biopsies could be avoided in 50% of the patients with chronic liver diseases. As clinical experience accumulates we shall expect that serum markers will begin to replace many of the liver biopsies used today for prognostic and treatment purpose.

Are serum markers ready for the first line fibrosis diagnosis? Overall, the serum assay approach remains promising, in part because these tests may represent an "integrated readout of liver activity rather than a minute sampling of the type obtained by conventional liver biopsy. Initially established as a niche especially in patients who have a high risk of complications from liver biopsy, by continued refinement, biomarkers are very close to become first line method for the diagnosis and monitoring of liver fibrosis. (Schiff, 2007).

### 3.2 Elastography imaging

Elastography is a much simpler method used to stage liver fibrosis than the X ray methods which are commonly used. This technique is quick and noninvasive. It helps to determine the stiffness of the hepatic tissue. It is well-known that the stiffness of the hepatic tissue is closely related to the stage of liver fibrosis. Touching the firm edge of the liver is a clinical parameter used for many years to diagnose cirrhosis.

#### 3.2.1 Transient Elastography (TE)

Fibro scan is a device which measures hepatic stiffness through transient elastography. It determines the elasticity of a hepatic volume equal to a cylinder with the diameter of 1 cm and the length of 4 cm, being thus 100 times larger than the standard biopsy fragment and, as such, more representative for the entire hepatic parenchyma.

Fibro scan uses an ultrasound transducer fixed on the axes of a vibrator which induces a low frequency vibration (50 MHz). The vibration transmitted to the hepatic tissue produces an elastic wave which propagates inside the liver. The propagation of this wave is followed by an ultrasound impulse and the measurement of its speed determines, through direct correlation, the tissue stiffness. The more rigid the liver, the higher the propagation speed. The results are expressed as kilopascal. Since a larger area of hepatic tissue is studied,

diagnosis errors related to the sample size which occur in standard liver biopsy are eliminated, even in disorders with focal liver fibrosis.
This technology has many of the features of a noninvasive ideal method in evaluating liver fibrosis, with a series of advantages: it is quick, reproducible, painless and safe.
Transient elastography is a relative new method. The first clinical data related to this technology were published in 2002. Numerous studies on patients with chronic hepatitis C demonstrated that elastography is a safe method for detecting severe fibrosis (Casterra, 2010). Although it is limited in differentiate the intermediary fibrosis stages, its major advantage is that it accurately detects persons with significant fibrosis.
Usually, 10 measurements are carried out for each patient, the total exam duration being 5-10 minutes. The success rate is automatically calculated by the machine as a ratio between the number of successful measurements and the total number of measurements. The recommendations of the manufacturers of this technology are that transient elastography can only be validated if there are 10 measurements with a success rate of at least 60%. However, recent studies have suggested that 3 validated measurements have the same value as 10 measurements for cirrhosis diagnosis; the minimum number of measurements for significant fibrosis has still to be set. It is considered that 10 validated measurements and a success rate of at least 60% can be obtained in 90% of exams.
Transient elastography is easy to interpret; the coefficient of concordance for the same examiner is 96-98% (the correlation coefficient in the same class) and between examiners, the coefficient of concordance is of 89-98%. Measurements validation depends on the IQR (interquartile range), <30%) and the success rate of measurements, >60%.
The largest study of hepatic elastography evaluated 327 patients with chronic infection C (Ziol et al, 2005) . For each patient, fibrosis was staged by means of 2 methods: Fibro scan and liver biopsy. Metavir scoring system for histological staging of liver fibrosis served as reference. The conclusion was that elastography is a reliable tool to detect significant fibrosis or cirrhosis. Table no. 5 indicates the diagnosis performance of Fibro scan in detecting significant fibrosis, as well as the authors who reported these results.

| **Study** | **Liver disease** | **No patients** | **Prevalence of significant fibrosis** | **AUROC** | **Limit KPa** | **Se/Sp** |
|---|---|---|---|---|---|---|
| Gomez-Dominguez et al. | Mixt | 94 | 82 | 0.74 | 4.0 | 94/33 |
| Fraqelli et al | Mixt | 200 | 50 | 0.86 | 7.6 | 81/76 |
| Chang et al | Mixt | 120 | 44 | 0.86 | 9.0 | 83/85 |
| Castera et al | HCV | 183 | 74 | 0.83 | 7.1 | 67/89 |
| Ziol et al | HCV | 251 | 65 | 0.79 | 8.8 | 56/91 |
| Yoneda et al | NAFLD | 67 | 49 | 0.87 | 6.6 | 83/81 |

Abbreviations: HCV, hepatitis virus C, Se, sensitivity, Sp,specificity, NAFLD - non alcoholic fatty liver disease

Table. 5. Fibroscan performance in detecting significant fibrosis (Guha & Rosenberg,2008)

When comparing with liver biopsy, TE is non-invasive, easy to repeat, reproducible, without contraindications, highly performant technique for detecting cirrhosis. Its disadvantage is that unlike liver biopsy, TE is unable to discriminate between intermediate stages of fibrosis. Comparing with serum markers, TE has lower applicability: failure in 5% of cases and unreliable results in 15% of cases.( Casterra, 2010). The known limits of this method are: the impossibility to conduct measurements in case of ascites (elastic waves do not propagate in liquids) and in patients with narrow intercostals spaces (it is necessary to insert the probe in the intercostals space). Another significant limiting factor is obesity (body mass index >28Kg/m$^2$) due to the diminishing of the surface fat tissue signal. False positive results appear in case of acute hepatitis, extra hepatic cholestasis and congestive heart failure (Casterra, 2010). The combination between TE and serum markers increases diagnostic accuracy for liver fibrosis.

### 3.2.2 Magnetic Resonance Elastography

Magnetic resonance elastography (MRE) has the same basic principles as sonographic elastography. By using a probe (pneumatic or electromagnetic), placed directly on the patient's abdominal wall, a shear wave is created. A specialized system of magnetic resonance measures the sequential propagation of the shear wave and transforms the data analyzed as an elastogram (color - encoded images). The analysis contains the liver in its entirety and allows assessing of fibrosis distribution, which is usually heterogeneous. Although until now the number of publications related to this method has been reduced, the results look promising. A study which compared MRE with the APRI index in patients with viral or alcoholic liver diseases has shown that MRE is more sensitive in detecting moderate and severe fibrosis than the APRI index. Among 96 patients with liver biopsy and noninvasive examinations the reproducibility of both TE and MRE were excellent. The elasticity imaging techniques had greater diagnostic accuracy than APRI for detecting liver fibrosis. MRE was also found to be more accurate than TE for significant fibrosis (F≥2) and for cirrhosis diagnosis (Huwart 2008).
The problems related to this technique refer to the increased exposure time (the exam takes 60 minutes), the significant capital invested in the equipment and the computerized analysis system, the standardized measurement threshold and method reproducibility. In contrast with TE, MRE can be successfully performed in obese patients (BMI > 40 kg/m$^2$ ). Furthermore, MRE had in part higher diagnostic accuracy in detecting significant fibrosis (F≥2) as compared with TE by examining of larger liver parenchyma areas (Huwart, 2008).
Although modern magnetic resonance technique is not the most pragmatic noninvasive methods it is a promising method as regards the diagnosis potential of liver fibrosis. The acknowledgment of its diagnosis sensitivity still requires large population studies.

### 3.2.3 Acoustic Radiation Force Imaging (ARFI)

A new technique used to determine liver elasticity is ARFI elastography. The elastographic analysis model combines two technologies, 'Virtual Touch tissue imaging™' and 'Virtual Touch tissue quantification™', which allow the quantitative and qualitative analysis of liver elasticity. Using the Virtual Touch application, the tissue gets compressed via acoustic energy. It enables the physician to evaluate the mechanical characteristics of deep tissue and tissue changes. ARFI imaging (Virtual Touch tissue quantification ) measures liver stiffness within a defined region of interest (central window of 5mm axial by 4mm width), while performing real-time B-mode imaging. Transmission of short-duration (~262 sec) longitudinal acoustic pulses with a fixed transmit frequency of 2.67 MHz leads micron-scale displacements in liver tissue, which results in a shear -wave propagation, away from the

region of excitation. Maximum movement is estimated by ultrasound detection fascicles adjacent to the central acoustic pulse. By measuring the maximum movement amplitude as compared to the time of each side fascicle, the shear - wave speed of the tissue can be reconstructed. Results expressed in meters per second are displayed by the machine (Friedrich-Rust, 2009).
Preliminary results indicate that ARFI imaging technology is a promising method for the diagnosis of significant fibrosis in patients with chronic hepatitis C.( Friedrich-Rust, 2009, Fierbinteanu-Braticevici, 2009). The benefits of ARFI imaging as compared with Fibro scan consist in: lesser time consuming (new software allowed to the 12 measurements per 1min) and successful measurements in difficult patients (obese) because of subcostal scanning. Another advantage of ARFI imaging is that it is integrated into a conventional ultrasonography (US) system and can thus be performed during standard US examinations of the liver, which are routinely performed in patients with chronic liver disease. Further studies on large number of patients are needed in order to specify the role of ARFI elastography for noninvasive staging of liver fibrosis.

### 3.3 Breath tests

Taking into account that the liver has a complex and high metabolic capacity, translated into detoxification, synthesis, metabolization, storage, a unique classical test may not reflects all these sides. More, each function may be different affected in various stages of the liver disease, so that the determination of the reserve capacity of the liver appears to reflect a global functional image. During the last decade, several dynamic tests have been proposed to improve the functional diagnosis of liver diseases. Although numerous tests which explore a specific hepatic function have been used, these methods were not introduced in the clinical practice.
The introduction of breath tests that use marked carbon ($C^{13}$) attached to various substrata (aminopyrin, phenylalanin, methacetine, phenacetyne, galactose) was due to the need to have a quick and practical test to determine the functional hepatic reserve. While neither of these tests allows quantification of a global liver function, each has been shown to reflect the most important partial liver functions i.e. cytosolic, microsomal or mitochondrial function.
The principle of breath tests is simple. An ingested substrate attached to $C^{13}$ or $C^{14}$, administered orally or parenterally is converted by the liver in $^{13}CO_2$ or $^{14}CO_2$. The marked $CO_2$ is collected at different time intervals in an alkaline environment which serves as a trap. The hepatic metabolism of the bonding substrate may be determined from a semi quantitative perspective by multiplying the specific $CO_2$ activity in the exhaled air within a given time interval. An ideal compound for this purpose is metabolized solely by the liver and therefore reflects liver function.
In the beginning, breath tests required sophisticated and expensive mass spectrometers that were no longer used. $^{13}C$ can now be measured with non dispersive infrared spectrometry, a simple and cost-saving method which provides information correlated with those of the mass spectrometry. Functional hepatic tests, including breath tests, together with clinic scores, had been proved to be helpful in diagnosis and prognosis of the patients with advanced hepatic disease. As regard the role of methacetin breath test (MBT) in the assessement of fibrosis in patients with chronic hepatitic C, our study indicated that the methacetin breath test parameters didn't allow differentiation of patients without fibrosis from those with mild fibrosis (F1). This limit was overcome by the fact that MBT was highly

correlated with significant fibrosis (≥ F2) which is considered the hallmark of progressive liver disease and a stronger indication for treatment.
Additional studies are required to assess the role of these tests as an alternative to liver biopsy in the diagnosis and follow-up of hepatic injury in patients with chronic liver diseases.

## 4. Conclusion

Liver biopsy remains an important tool in the evaluation and management of liver disease. However it is invasive, can cause significant complications and clearly, needle liver biopsy is far from an ideal test. Even though it is an imperfect "gold standard", liver biopsy remains an important tool in the evaluation and management of liver disease.
For this reason, the efforts to estimate the hepatic lesion stage through noninvasive methods are justified. Noninvasive investigations, such as various biomarkers, fibrosis scoring panels, imaging techniques and breath tests offer considerable promise in their ability to detect and to stage liver fibrosis. Until now, not even one noninvasive test can be considered enough sensitive to predict by itself the severity of acute or chronic liver diseases. That is why combining various noninvasive tests is promising and many times they can avoid liver biopsy. Further testing and validation are needed for these noninvasive procedures to refine their role of clinical practice and supplant the need for liver biopsy in chronic liver diseases.
Now, when many non - invasive procedures have been studied, the question is if that do we still need a liver biopsy? We think that the answer is „yes", because despite its limitations, the liver biopsy remains an invaluable procedure of the clinician, whenever the etiology of liver disease is in impass. Liver biopsy is still needed if laboratory testing and imaging studies are inconclusive. It may take many years, if at all, until liver biopsy will be fully replaced.

## 5. References

Carey E , Carey W. (2010). Noninvasive tests for liver disease, fibrosis, and cirrhosis: Is liver biopsy obsolete? *Cleaveland clinic journal of medicine,* 77 (8), 527. ISSN: 0891-1150

Castera I, Pinzani M. (2010). Biopsy and non-invasiv e methods for the diagnosis of liver fibrosis does it take two to tango?, *Gut*, 59, 861-6, ISSN: 0017-5749

Friedrich-Rust M, et al. (2009). Liver Fibrosis in Viral Hepatitis: Noninvasive Assessment with Acoustic Radiation Force Impulse Imaging versus Transient Elastography. *Radiology*, 597-604, ISSN 0033-8419

Fierbinteanu-Braticevici C, Andronescu D, Usvat R,et al .(2009). Acoustic radiation force imaging sonoelastography for noninvasive staging of liver fibrosis. *World Journal of Gastroenterology*, 15, 5525-5532, ISSN: 1007-9327

Huwart L, et al. (2008). Magnetic resonance elastography for the noninvasive staging of liver fibrosis. *Gastroenterology*,135, 32-40, ISSN: 0016-5085

Knodell RG, Ishak KG, et al. (1981). Formulation and application of a numerical scoring system for assessing histological activity in asymptomatic chronic active hepatitis. *Hepatology*,1, 431-435, ISSN, 1665-2681

Metavir Cooperative Study Group. (1994). Intraobserver and interobserver variations in liver biopsy interpretation in patients with chronic hepatitis C. The French METAVIR Cooperative Study Group. *Hepatology*,20, 15-20, ISSN: 1665-2681

Schiff E, SorrellM, Maddrey W, (2007). *Schiff's diseases of the liver*,Lippincott-Williams&Wilkins, 10th edition ISBN, 10-7817-60-40-2,Philadelphia,USA

Desmet VJ, Scheuer PJ et al. (1994) Classification of chronic hepatitis: diagnosis, grading and staging. *Hepatology,* 19, 6, 1513-20, ISSN: 1665-2681

Standish R. A. et al, (2006) An appraisal of the histopathological assessment of liver fibrosis *Gut*, 55, 569-578, ISSN: 0017-5749

Bedossa P.(2011). How pathological scores can be improved?. EASL, *Monothematic Conference*, Nice.

Regev A et al. (2002). Sampling error and intraobserver variation in liver biopsy in patients with chronic HCV infection. *American Journal of Gastroenterology*, 97, 2614-2618, ISSN: 0002-9270

Ratziu V et al. (2005). Sampling variability of liver biopsy in nonalcoholic fatty liver disease.*Gastroenterology*, 128, 7, 1898-906 ISSN: 0016-5085

Afdhal N.H.(2007).Non-biopsy methods to determine hepatic fibrosis, *Postgraduate Course*, AASLD, 91-94

Rockey DC, Bissell DM. (2006) Noninvasive measures of liver fibrosis. *Hepatology*. 43,2, Suppl 1, S113-20. ISSN: 1665-2681

Ziol M, et al. (2005). Noninvasive assessment of liver fibrosis by measurement of stiffness in patients with chronic hepatitis C. *Hepatology*, 41,1, 48-54,ISSN: 1665-2681

Guha IN. Rosenberg WM. (2008).Noninvasive Assessment of Liver Fibrosis: Serum Markers, Imaging, and Other Modalities. *Clinical Liver Disease*, 12, 883–900, ISSN : 1590-8658

Crockett S.D. et al (2006). Do will still need a liver biopsy? Are the serum fibrosis tests ready for prime time? *Clinics in liver disease*,10, 513-534, ISSN:1089-3261,ISBN:1-4160-3553-2

# 15

# The Current Status of Non-Invasive Assessment of Liver Fibrosis: Real Time Tissue Elastography

Hiroyasu Morikawa and Norifumi Kawada
*Department of Hepatology, Graduate School of Medicine, Osaka City University, Japan*

## 1. Introduction

Liver biopsy has long been an important tool for assessing the degree of liver fibrosis. Currently, there are many reports and approaches to evaluate the staging of hepatic fibrosis by using noninvasive imaging methods. The main modalities are based on ultrasonography (US) and magnetic resonance imaging (MRI). Among these techniques, Transient Elastography (TE, Fibroscan) has taken a leading role in the noninvasive assessment of liver stiffness at current clinical medicine in Europe. The principal of TE is simple: TE measures the propagation speed of elastic shear wave within the liver parenchyma. The velocity of the wave propagation correlates directly to tissue stiffness; that is, the harder the tissue is, the faster the shear wave spread.

In this chapter, we introduce a new US-based approach for non-invasive assessment of liver fibrosis using real-time tissue elastography (RTE) that can be performed simultaneously with conventional ultrasound probes during routine US examination. RTE is technically different from TE: echo signals representing tissue strain before and under mild compression are compared and analyzed. RTE was developed in Japan for the visual assessment of tissue elasticity integrated in a sonography machine. The technique is based on the Combined Autocorrelation Method that calculates the relative hardness of tissue rapidly from the degree of tissue distortion and displays this information as a color image [Shiina T, 2002]. The distortion of tissue is transferred to a color-coded image according to its magnitude and superimposed translucently on the conventional B-mode image. Such a simultaneous display of tissue elasticity and B-mode images enables us to evaluate the anatomical correspondence between these modalities. The RTE image is constructed by the amount of displacement of the reflected ultrasound echoes under compression. Although US-based elastography is unable to demonstrate physical elasticity directly, it shows the relative degree of tissue strain when subtle compression is applied. In hard tissue, the amount of displacement of the reflected ultrasound echoes is low, whereas, in soft tissue, the amount of displacement is high because soft tissue can be compressed more than hard tissue.

This technology has already been proved to be diagnostically valuable in detecting space occupying lesions in the breast, prostate, and pancreas. In 2007, Friedrich-Rust applied this technique to measure liver stiffness and reported its usefulness for the detection of significant fibrosis (≧F2, area under the receiver operating characteristic curve; AUC 0.93) in combination with AST to platelet ratio index (APRI). In 2010, we reported that AUC for no significant

fibrosis (F0-1) was 0.89 and 0.92 in RTE and TE, respectively, and AUC for cirrhosis (F4) was 0.93 and 0.95 in RTE and TE, respectively, in 101 patients with chronic hepatitis C.
We report here an update of the RTE system as a tool for the noninvasive assessment of liver stiffness together with an overview of recent advancement in this area in the literature.

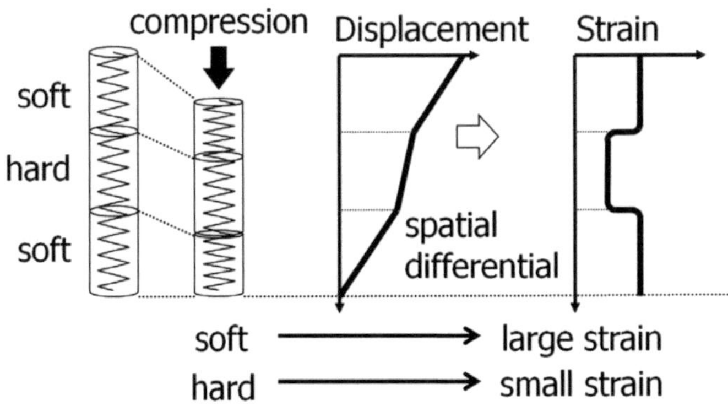


Fig. 1. The principle of real time tissue elastography, illustrated here by a spring model.

## 2. Methods

### 2.1 Real-time tissue elastography

The principle underlining RTE is shown in Figure 1, which indicates a spring model [Ophir J, 1991]. When a spring is compressed, displacement in each section of the spring depends on the stiffness of the spring: a soft spring compresses more than a hard spring. The strain distribution can be measured by spatially differentiating the displacement at each location. Although the tissue displacement is usually generated by manual compression and relaxation of the probe in practice, we were able to improve the acquisition of RTE images representing the distortion of liver tissue as a result of the beating of the heart or pulsing of the abdominal aorta.
RTE is carried out using a high-end model of Hitachi ultrasound system (Hitachi Medical, Chiba, Japan). The developed software with a complex algorithm is able to process all the data coming from the lesion as radiofrequency impulses in a very short time and minimize the artifacts due to lateral dislocations, allowing accurate measurement of the degree of tissue distortion. We used Hitachi EUB-8500 and an EUP-L52 Linear probe (3–7 MHz; Hitachi Medical) for RTE.
This system is currently commercially available for the diagnosis of mammary neoplasm. Patients were examined in a supine position with the right arm elevated above the head, and were instructed to hold their breath. The examination was performed on the right lobe of the liver through the intercostal space, and liver biopsy and Fibroscan were also performed at the same site. The RTE equipment displays two images simultaneously; one shows the regions of interest (ROI) as a colored area and the other indicates the conventional B-mode image (Fig. 2A). We chose an area where the tissue was free from large vessels and near the biopsy point. The measurement was fixed to a rectangle 30 mm in length and 20 mm in breadth placed 5-10 mm below the surface of the liver (Fig. 2A). The color in the ROI was graded from blue (representing hard areas) to red (representing soft areas) (Fig. 2A). We stored the RTE images as moving digital images for 20–40 s. Ten static images captured by the observer at random from the moving images using AVI2JPG v6.10 converter software

(Novo, Tokyo, Japan) were analyzed using the novel software Elasto_ver 1.5.1,which was developed and donated by Hitachi Medical, on a personal computer. Numerical values of pixels were from 0 to 255 (256 stepwise grading) according to color mapping from blue (0) to red (255), and a histogram of the distribution was generated (Fig. 2B). The scale ranged from red for components with the greatest strain (i.e., softest components) to blue for those with no strain (i.e., hardest components). Green indicated average strain in the ROI, and therefore intact liver tissue was displayed as a diffuse homogeneous green pattern. An appearance of unevenness in the color pattern was considered to reflect a change in the liver stiffness. For quantification, all pixel data in the colored image were transferred into a histogram and binary image (Fig. 2B).

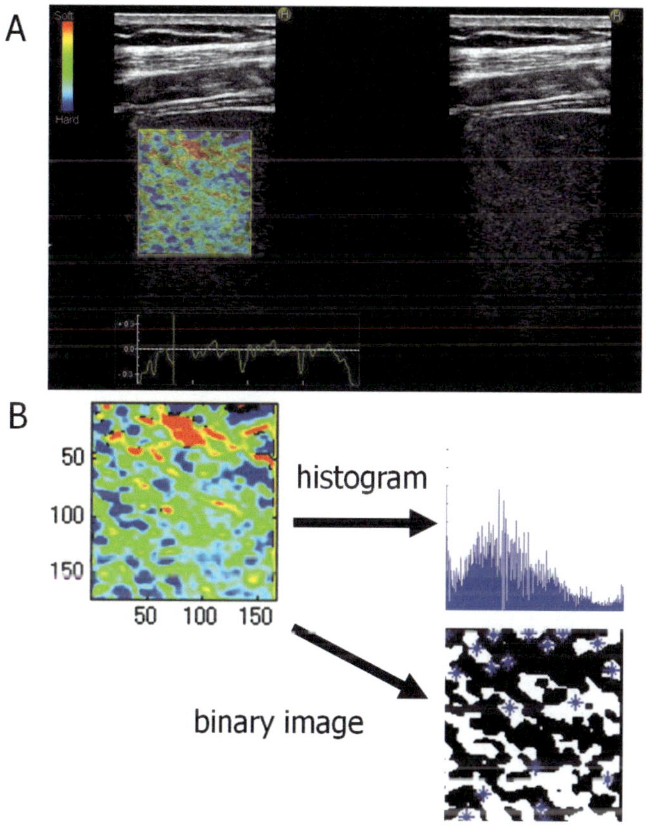


Fig. 2. Procedure of image analyses for real-time tissue elastography.
(A) The ROI was fixed to a rectangle of approximately 20-30 mm length x 20 mm breadth with a 400–600 $mm^2$ area placed 5-10 mm below the surface of the liver. Left; RTE image, right, B-mode image. (B) The color-coded images from the ROI of RTE were analyzed by the software Elasto ver1.5.1. The colors ranged from blue to red indicating the relative gradients from hardness to softness. Mean and Standard deviation were calculated by a histogram, which was generated by 256 stepwise grading derived from the color image. Area and Complexity were calculated from the binary image. Area was derived from the percentage of white regions (asterisks, i.e. hard area). Complexity was calculated as $periphery^2$/Area. Median value of the data were kept as representative of RTE parameters.

Colored RTE images are usually classified into several patterns in the diagnosis of breast disease. We paid attention to the pattern change of RTE color images according to the progression of fibrosis. We proposed three patterns for representing the stages of liver fibrosis: a diffuse soft pattern, an intermediate pattern, and a patchy hard pattern (Fig. 3). The diffuse soft pattern indicated a homogeneously light-green colored image. The intermediate pattern represented a partially mottled and dotted image with blue spots on a light green background. The patchy hard pattern comprised mixed images with a patchwork effect of light green, red, and blue. Normal or minimally fibrotic liver exhibited a homogeneous RTE image that was colored light green (diffuse soft pattern). According to the progression of liver fibrosis, the homogeneous pattern transitioned to a patchy pattern consisting of a blue-colored area (patchy hard pattern), which may suggest a decrease of homogeneity.

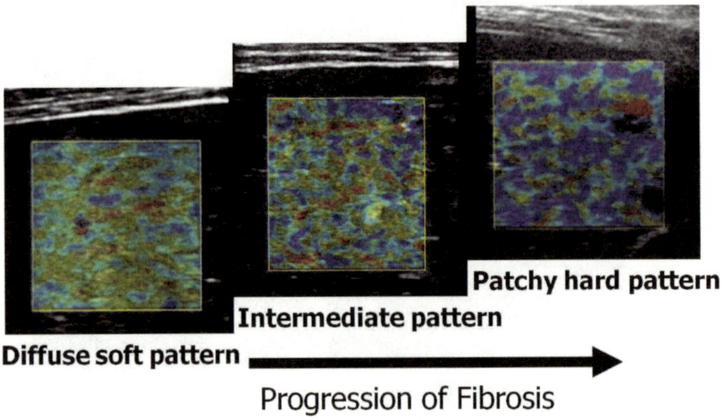


Fig. 3. Representative colored images of real-time tissue elastography according to the progression of liver fibrosis.

Normal or minimally fibrotic liver exhibited a homogenous RTE image that was colored light green. According to the progression of liver fibrosis, the homogenous pattern transitioned to a patchy pattern consisting of a blue-colored area, which may suggest a collapse of homogeneity. A relatively homogeneous light green image indicated a diffuse soft pattern in RTE. A partially mottled and dotted image with blue and red spots in the light green background indicated an intermediate pattern. A mixed image with light green, blue, and red colors indicated patchy hard pattern.

### 2.2 Transient elastography

Liver stiffness was also measured by TE (Fibroscan; Echosens SA, Paris, France). Briefly, patients were placed in a horizontally supine position and a probe was placed on the skin above the right intercostal space. The velocity of shear waves, which were generated temporarily and passed though the liver, was combined with Young's modulus for the automated calculation of elasticity [Yeh WC, 2002]. The measurement depth was between 25 and 65 mm. The results that were obtained in ten valid measurements with a success rate of at least 60% and an interquartile range under 30% were considered successful. Failure was defined as when less than ten valid measurements were obtained. A median of 10 valid measurements was regarded as the liver stiffness for a given subject and expressed in kilopascals (kPa).

## 3. Results

### 3.1 Our results

Our results were expressed as Mean and Standard Deviation (SD), which indicates the mean and the standard deviation of the histogram, respectively. In another analysis, the data were transformed into a binary image and the results were described as Area, which indicates the percentage of hard tissue and represents the hard tissue domain divided by the ROI and Complexity (complex ratio of the shape of an extracted hard tissue domain in the ROI calculated as periphery$^2$/area of the hard tissue domain). The four image features were calculated automatically by Elasto_ver 1.5.1 (Hitachi Medical). Mean, SD, and Complexity were described in arbitrary units [a.u.].

Figure 4 shows box plots of the RTE values corresponding to fibrosis stage in 126 patients with chronic hepatitis C. The Mean decreased in proportion to the increase of fibrosis score (Jonckheere-Terpstra test, $p<0.0001$). SD, Area, and Complexity increased in proportion to the increase of fibrosis score (Jonckheere-Terpstra test, $p< 0.0001$). The significant differences between each fibrosis stage were as follows: F1 versus F3 and F4, and F2 versus F4 for every parameter; F1 versus F2 and F2 versus F3 for Mean; and F3 versus F4 for Complexity (Tukey-Kramer test, $p<0.05$). No significant difference was found between the activity of chronic hepatitis and the fibrosis stages for any parameters (Tukey-Kramer test). The AUC of RTE parameters for no significant fibrosis (F0-1) and cirrhosis (F4) in 121 patients who were also examined successfully by TE, together with the corresponding sensitivities, specificities, and positive and negative predictive values are presented in Table 1.

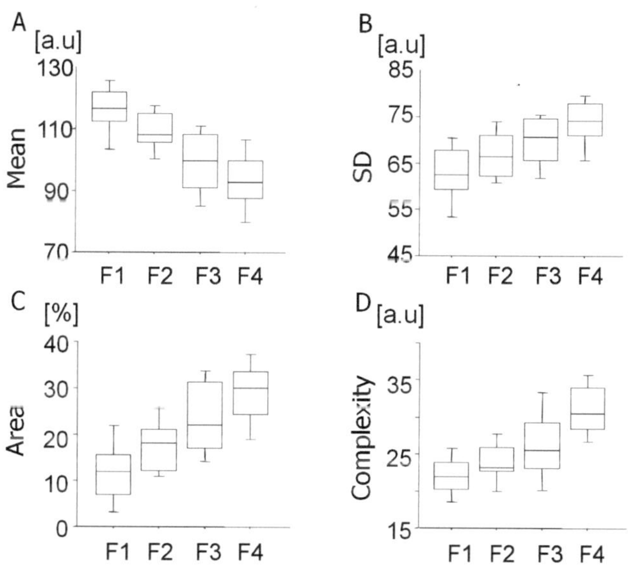


F1, n=62. F2, n=19. F3, n=19. F4, n=20. F scale was divided by METAVIR score.

Fig. 4. Parameter analyses measured by real-time tissue elastography for each fibrosis stage. Box plots of each value of RTE corresponding to fibrosis stages F1-4. The top and bottom of the boxes indicate the 1st and 3rd quartiles. The length of the box represents the interquartile range within which 50% of values are located. The lines through the middle of the boxes represent the median. A) Mean, B) SD, C) Area, and D) Complexity.

| | F=0-1 | | | | | F=4 | | | | |
|---|---|---|---|---|---|---|---|---|---|---|
| | Mean | SD | Area | Complexity | TE | Mean | SD | Area | Complexity | TE |
| Cut-of | 110.1 | 61.2 | 25.8 | 23.2 | 10.1 | 106.9 | 63 | 29.5 | 24.9 | 13.3 |
| **AUC** | **0.89** | **0.81** | **0.87** | **0.81** | **0.92** | **0.91** | **0.84** | **0.91** | **0.93** | **0.95** |
| Sensitivity [%] | 84.1 | 70.5 | 81.8 | 77.3 | 88.6 | 82.8 | 75.9 | 79.3 | 79.3 | 89.7 |
| Specificity [%] | 82.7 | 73.1 | 80.8 | 75 | 86.5 | 85.1 | 77.6 | 80.6 | 80.6 | 86.6 |
| Accuracy [%] | 83.3 | 71.9 | 81.3 | 76 | 87.5 | 84.4 | 77.1 | 80.2 | 80.2 | 87.5 |

TE, transient elastography.

Table 1. Results of comparisons between four image features of real time tissue elastography and transient elastography.

### 3.2 Search results

A PubMed search was conducted in February 2011 for full papers published in journals written in English in the past 5 years. The following keywords were used in combination: "real-time tissue elastography" and "liver". The first author' names, patient's selection critera, patient number, and diagnostic accuracies are summarized in Table 2. The primary outcome was the identification of the degree of fibrosis defined as stages F1 to F4 according to the METAVIR score.

Two articles were reported by Friedrich-Rust in 2007 and 2009, one article was from China, and three articles including ours were from Japan. Three of the articles described studies conducted in patients with chronic liver disease, one article limited the subjects to those with chronic hepatitis B, and two articles including our report included only subjects with chronic hepatitis C. There are two ways to calculate the results of RTE: one is the ratio of strain distribution between the ROI of liver parenchyma and that of other areas, and the other is the analysis of color images in ROI. Koizumi's report showed the best sensitivity and specificity until now; 83.8 % and 90.9 %, respectively for F1, and 90.9% and 91.5 %, respectively, for F4. They used the ratio between the tissue compressibility of the liver parenchyma and that of intrahepatic small vessel. Only two articles Friedrich-Rust's in 2009 and ours in 2010 compared the diagnostic value of RTE with TE. Others compared the value of RTE with serum fibrosis markers represented by APRI.

## 4. Discussion

Liver biopsy has long been the gold standard for the assessment of hepatic fibrosis and will remain important in the diagnosis of liver disease with unknown etiology. However, because of complications, sampling error, and interobserver variability, the role of liver biopsy in the assessment and quantification of fibrosis in viral liver diseases is thought to be less valuable. Many modern noninvasive tests including serum markers and imaging methods are expected to become increasingly important in the near future.

A large number of serum markers have been identified for the assessment of hepatic fibrosis. In clinical practice, type IV collagen 7s, type III procollagen N-terminal peptide (P-III-P), and hyarulonic acid are commonly utilized as direct serum markers for human liver fibrosis, although it is difficult to distinguish each pathological fibrosis stage using one of these extracellular matrix products. On the other hand, the European Liver Fibrosis (ELF) study reported a marker composed of the combination of P-III-P, hyarulonic acid, and tissue inhibitor of metalloproteinases, which achieved the diagnostic power of AUC 0.80 for Scheuer 3-4 [Guha IN, 2008.]. Reported indirect serum markers of liver fibrosis include AAR (AST/ALT ratio), APRI (AST-to-platelet ratio index), Forns score, FibroTest, and the HALT-C model, which are composed of several parameters commonly measured in clinical practice. FibroTest is currently the most carefully evaluated noninvasive serum fibrosis marker panel that is commercially available. FibroTest is an algorithm composed of 6 parameters, including haptoglobin, α2-macroglobulin, apolipoprotein-A1, γ-glutamyltransferase, bilirubin, and γ-globulin, and its diagnostic power for ≧F2 was reported to be AUC 0.87 [Imbert-Bismut F, 2001.]. While the diagnostic accuracy was high, the FibroTest costs more than APRI and the Forns score, and requires two uncommon parameters. In APRI, using the cutoffs proposed by Wai et al. [Wai CT, 2003.], approximately 50% of patients could be correctly classified as having cirrhosis without a liver biopsy. With the Forns score, the AUC for the prediction of significant fibrosis (Scheuer classification, F2) was 0.86 in the test set and 0.81 in the validation set [Forns X, 2002]. Although direct, indirect, and combined serum marker systems consist of multiple biomarkers, they are all characterized by an AUC for the ROC clustering around 0.85 in recent studies. [Afdhal NH and Curry M, 2007].

| Author, year | Patients selection | Patients | Control | Calculation | Fibrosis stage | AUC | Sensitivity [%] | Specificity [%] | PPV [%] | NPV [%] |
|---|---|---|---|---|---|---|---|---|---|---|
| Friedrich-Rust M, 2007 | viral hepatitis | 79 | 20 | elasticity score, stepwise multivariate logistic regression | F=1<br>F=4 | 0.75<br>0.69 | 80<br>29.2 | 61.1<br>90.7 | 63.2<br>50 | 78.6<br>80 |
| Friedrich-Rust M, 2009 | chronic liver disease | 134 | | Japanese Elasticity score, 256 stepwise of color mapping | F=1<br>F=4 | 0.64<br>0.63 | | | | |
| Kanamoto M, 2009 | underwent an operation | 41 | | Elastic ratio, ratio of liver for the intercostal muscle | F=1<br>F=4 | | 96.2<br>93.3 | 73.3<br>73.1 | 86.2<br>66.7 | 91.7<br>95 |
| Wang J, 2010 | chronic hepatitis B | 55 | 20 | Elastic index, principal components analysis | F=1<br>F=4 | 0.93<br>0.66 | 87.3<br>71.4 | 85<br>80 | 94.1<br>93.8 | 70.8<br>40 |
| Koizumi Y, 2011 | chronic hepatitis C | 70 | | Elastic ratio, ratio of liver for the small hepatic vein | F=1<br>F=4 | 0.89<br>0.95 | 83.8<br>90.9 | 90.9<br>91.5 | 98<br>83.3 | 50<br>95.6 |
| Our report | chronic hepatitis C | 101 | 10 | Mean | F=1<br>F=4 | 0.89<br>0.91 | 84.1<br>85.7 | 82.7<br>82.9 | 80.4<br>46.2 | 86<br>97.1 |

Table 2. Diagnostic accuracy of real time tissue elastography in individual studies.

Standard US, CT, and MRI have long been used to survey liver morphology. These modalities are able to detect changes in the liver parenchyma when there is early cirrhosis and signs of portal hypertension. However, these methods are not useful to identify the presence of mild fibrosis. In this regard, elastography is sensitive for evaluating liver fibrosis based on the fact that, as the liver becomes progressively fibrotic, it becomes harder and less elastic. The technique based on US and MRI easily and noninvasively measures the relative values of liver stiffness. TE has been used most frequently worldwide and has established a role in clinical practice for detecting advanced fibrosis instead of liver biopsy. A pioneering report from Castera in 2005 showed that the AUC of TE was 0.84 for the diagnosis of F1 and 0.94 for the diagnosis of cirrhosis. Although MR elastography (MRE) was shown to be superior to APRI and TE for determining the stage of fibrosis in patients with underlying liver diseases [Huwart L, 2008], MRE cannot be performed on patients with an iron overloaded liver because of background noise. In addition, MRE takes more time and costs more than the US-based elastographies.

Four published reports have compared the diagnostic accuracy of RTE with serum markers including APRI. RTE was shown to be superior to APRI in determining the stage of liver fibrosis in all of these studies except for the first report by Friedrich-Rust in 2007. It is believed that the more sensitive probes have been developed which could mitigate the deep attenuation of the ultrasound image and without requiring external stress. Accordingly, we were able to avoid the influence of the liver surface inside the ROI which is hard and therefore assessed as a harder area and to improve the acquisition of the color image representing the distortion of liver tissue due to the heartbeat or the pulse of the abdominal aorta without interobserver variability.

Although Friedrich-Rust (2009) reported that RTE was inferior in determining the stage of liver fibrosis compared to TE, our results presented in Table 1 indicated that the performance of RTE compares favorably with that of TE for detecting the degree of liver fibrosis in patients with chronic hepatitis C. TE has been reported to have several limitations and disadvantages in evaluating patients with obesity and ascites. In fact, in our study, we achieved successful evaluation of all patients with RTE, while five patients (F1, 2; F3, 1; F4, 2) failed to receive TE measurements due to obesity and liver atrophy. Koizumi also reported that RTE could be employed in patients with BMIs greater than 30 $kg/m^2$.

Although the results from RTE were conducted by the image of color map, the results were calculated by either the ratio of strain distribution between ROI of the liver parenchyma and that of another area or by the image analysis of ROI. The method of Kanamoto which was used intercostal muscle as the reference for the ratio was inferior to the other method, since the area is considered to be influenced by instability of tissue distortion of subcutaneous fat and by the liver surface which is one of the hardest areas in liver parenchyma. In contrast, Koizumi adopted the hepatic vein as a reference and obtained the best sensitivity and specificity for characterizing the stage of fibrosis in related articles. Other studies utilized image analysis using exclusive software and reported different results. Thus the best method for the analysis and unit of RTE remains unclear, but may be revealed by future multicenter studies using larger patient cohorts.

In the future, the combination of image modalities with serological parameters will further improve the accuracy in differentiating fibrosis stages. Interestingly, Castera reported that the best results were achieved by a combination of TE with the FibroTest. Although acoustic radiation force impulse, which is a most recent technology, TE, and MRE are all based on shear wave propagation, RTE is constructed by an original theory which is based on tissue distortion. Friedrich-Rust reported in 2007 that the best diagnostic accuracy was obtained by combining the variables used for the calculation of the RTE elasticity score with the platelet count and GGT.

Elastography will be applicable to the screening of hepatocellular carcinoma (HCC) and the complication of cirrhosis. In the METAVIR and Desmet's histological scoring systems, cirrhosis is classified as a single category, F4. However, the degree of fibrosis that indicates the amount of extracellular matrix materials including collagen that may be closely associated with the function of hepatocytes and portal hypertension may vary among patients with cirrhosis. Foucher reported in 2006 that liver stiffness (kPa) measured by TE in cirrhotic patients correlates well with clinical parameters indicating the severity of cirrhosis; 27.5 kPa was the cutoff value for the presence of esophageal varices stage 2 or 3, 37.5 kPa for liver function Child B or C, 49.1 kPa for a past history of ascites, and 62.7 kPa for bleeding from esophageal varices. Masuzaki prospectively observed that, in 866 patients with chronic hepatitis C, HCC developed in 77 cases within 3 years of observation, and 0.4% of HCC was detected in patients whose liver stiffness at entry was less than 10 kPa and 38.5% of it was more than 25 kPa, indicating the usefulness of liver stiffness measurement as a tool for predicting the development of HCC. Because RTE is expected to stage cirrhosis in greater detail with clinical relevance, it may be useful for detecting and assessing the risk of cirrhotic complications and the development of HCC.

Although noninvasive assessment of liver fibrosis is already established in patients with chronic hepatitis C, it is still necessary to improve assessment in other highly prevalent diseases, such as non-alcoholic fatty liver disease/non-alcoholic steatohepatitis (NASH). We reported that the AUC of AAR, age-platelet index, APRI, and cirrhosis discriminant score for predicting cirrhosis were 0.81, 0.87, 0.79, and 0.95, respectively, in 50 patients with NASH and 0.56, 0.65, 0.76, and 0.78, respectively, in 100 patients with chronic hepatitis C [Fujii H 2009]. RTE will be expected to play a major role in elastography for these patients, since it is not influenced by obesity or BMI.

## 5. Conclusion

We have described a convenient and noninvasive procedure, RTE, for the visual assessment of liver stiffness. The performance of RTE compared favorably to TE for detecting the degree of liver fibrosis in patients with chronic hepatitis C. We suggest that RTE could also be used as a routine imaging method to evaluate the degree of liver fibrosis in patients with liver diseases other than chronic hepatitis C. Future studies on larger patient cohorts will be necessary for the validation of RTE analysis, and the combination of RTE parameters with other clinical values including serum biomarkers will enable improvement of accuracy in assessing hepatic fibrosis.

## 6. Acknowledgment

We thank Ms. Akiko Tonomura and Mr. Junji Warabino, Hitachi Medical Co., for the technical support for RTE. Hiroyasu Morikawa was supported by a research grant from Osaka City University (2009). Norifumi Kawada was supported by Research on Hepatitis, Health and Labour Science Research Grants from the Ministry of Health, Labour and Welfare of Japan (2008–2009) and by a Thrust Area Research Grant from Osaka City University.(2008–2009).

## 7. References

Afdhal NH and Curry M (2007) Technology evaluation: a critical step in the clinical utilization of novel diagnostic tests for liver fibrosis. J Hepatol 46: 543–54

Castera L, Vergniol J, Foucher J, Le Bail B, Chanteloup E, Haaser M. (2005) Prospective comparison of transient elastography, Fibrotest, APRI, and liver biopsy for the assessment of fibrosis in chronic hepatitis C. Gastroenterology. 2005;128:343–50.

Forns X, Ampurdane`s S, Llovet JM, Aponte J, Quinto´ L, Marti´nez-Bauer E, et al. Identification of chronic hepatitis C patients without hepatic fibrosis by a simple predictive model. Hepatology. 2002;36:986–92.

Foucher J, Chanteloup E, Vergniol J, Caste´ra L, Le Bail B, Adhoute X. (2006) Diagnosis of cirrhosis by transient elastography (FibroScan): a prospective study. Gut. 2006;55:403–8

Friedrich-Rust M, Ong MF, Herrmann E, Dries V, Samaras P, Zeuzem S, Sarrazin C. (2007) Real-time elastography for noninvasive assessment of liver fibrosis in chronic viral hepatitis. AJR Am J Roentgenol. 2007;188:758-64.

Friedrich-Rust M, Schwarz A, Ong M, Dries V, Schirmacher P, Herrmann E, Samaras P, Bojunga J, Bohle RM, Zeuzem S, Sarrazin C. (2009) Real-time tissue elastography versus FibroScan for noninvasive assessment of liver fibrosis in chronic liver disease. Ultraschall Med. 2009 ;30 :478-84.

Fujii H, Enomoto M, Fukushima W, Ohfuji S, Mori M, Kobayashi S, Iwai S, Morikawa H, Tamori A, Sakaguchi H, Ikura Y, Ueda M, Kawada N. (2009) Noninvasive laboratory tests proposed for predicting cirrhosis in patients with chronic hepatitis C are also useful in patients with non-alcoholic steatohepatitis. J Gastroenterol. 2009;44 :608-14

Guha IN, Parkes J, Roderick P, et al. Noninvasive markers of fibrosis in nonalcoholic fatty liver disease: Validating the European Liver Fibrosis Panel and exploring simple markers. Hepatology. 2008;47:455-460.

Huwart L, Sempoux C, Vicaut E, Salameh N, Annet L, Danse E. (2008) Magnetic resonance elastography for the noninvasive staging of liver fibrosis. Gastroenterology. 2008;135:32–40

Imbert-Bismut F, Ratziu V, Pieroni L, Charlotte F, Benhamou Y, Poynard T, et al. Biochemical markers of liver fibrosis in patients with hepatitis C virus infection: a prospective study. Lancet.2001;357:1069–75.

Kanamoto M, Shimada M, Ikegami T, Uchiyama H, Imura S, Morine Y, Kanemura H, Arakawa Y, Nii A. (2009) Real time elastography for noninvasive diagnosis of liver fibrosis. J Hepatobiliary Pancreat Surg. 2009;16(4):463-7.

Koizumi Y, Hirooka M, Kisaka Y, Konishi I, Abe M, Murakami H, Matsuura B, Hiasa Y, Onji M. (2011) Liver fibr osis in patients with chronic hepatitis C: noninvasive diagnosis by means of real-time tissue elastography--establishment of the method for measurement. Radiology. 2011 ;258 :610-7.

Masuzaki R, Tateishi R, Yoshida H, Goto E, Sato T, Ohki T, Imamura J, Goto T, Kanai F, Kato N, Ikeda H, Shiina S, Kawabe T, Omata M. (2009) Prospective risk assessment for hepatocellular carcinoma development in patients with chronic hepatitis C by transient elastography. Hepatology. 2009 ;49 :1954-61.

Morikawa H, Fukuda K, Kobayashi S, Fujii H, Iwai S, Enomoto M, Tamori A, Sakaguchi H, Kawada N. (2010) Real-time tissue elastography as a tool for the noninvasive assessment of liver stiffness in patients with chronic hepatitis C. J Gastroenterol. 2010 Aug 10. [Epub ahead of print]

Ophir J, Céspedes I, Ponnekanti H, Yazdi Y, Li X. (1991) Elastography: a quantitative method for imaging the elasticity of biological tissues. Ultrason Imaging. 1991;13:111-34.

Shiina T, Nitta N, Ueno E, Bamber JC. (2002) Real time tissue elasticity imaging using the combined autocorrelation method. J Med Ultrason 2002;29:119–128.

Wai CT, Greenson JK, Fontana RJ, Kalbfleisch JD, Marrero JA, Conjeevaram HS, et al. A simple noninvasive index can predict both significant fibrosis and cirrhosis in patients with chronic hepatitis C. Hepatology. 2003;38:518–26.

Wang J, Guo L, Shi X, Pan W, Bai Y, Ai H. (2011) Real-time elastography with a novel quantitative technology for assessment of liver fibrosis in chronic hepatitis B. Eur J Radiol. 2011 Jan 6. [Epub ahead of print]

Yeh WC, Li PC, Jeng YM, Hsu HC, Kuo PL, Li ML. (2002) Elastic modulus measurements of human liver and correlation with pathology. Ultrasound Med Biol. 2002; 28 : 467–74.

# 16

# Noninvasive Alternatives for the Assessment of Liver Fibrosis

Lungen Lu and Kun Zhou
*Department of Gastroenterology, Shanghai First People's Hospital, Shanghai Jiaotong University School of Medicine*
*China*

## 1. Introduction

Chronic liver diseases (CLD) are common and may lead to fibrosis, cirrhosis, and hepatic malignancy. Detection and staging of liver fibrosis is crucial for management of patients with CLD. At present, liver biopsy is the standard method for staging fibrosis, but biopsies are poorly tolerated because they are invasive and associated with some discomfort and complications. In addition, limitations of biopsy include intra- and inter-observer variation and sampling error[1,2]. In recent years, a great interest and many studies have been dedicated to the development of noninvasive tests to substitute liver biopsy for fibrosis assessment and follow-up. Unfortunately, all of them have limitations and pitfalls. To discuss their advantages and deficiencies will be helpful in scientific research and clinical practice.

## 2. Invasive measurements

### 2.1 Liver biopsy

Liver biopsy has been considered as the gold standard to confirm the clinical diagnosis, to assess the severity of necro-inflammation and fibrosis, to identify cofactors and comorbidities, and to monitor the efficacy of treatments since the first liver biopsy was performed by Paul Ehrlich in 1883 [3]. The procedure is particularly useful for diagnosing the earlier stages of fibrosis and identifying patients at high risk of progressing fibrosis, but it has also a number of limitations. The patient acceptance is pretty low because biopsy is expensive, invasive and associated with some discomfort and complications. Pain appears in about one fourth of patients, other complications including bleeding, biliary peritonitis, pneumothorax and a mortality rate about 0.01% [4]. Sampling error of at least 24% is reported usually because of specimen fragmentation or inadequate length. Colloredo *et al* concluded that an optimum specimen should be at least 20 mm in length with 11 complete portal tracts[1]. Even with adequate-sized biopsies, the interpretation might be unreliable, because the distribution of necro-inflammation and fibrosis is not homogeneous, and liver biopsy samples only 1:50 000th of the mass of the liver.

Several semi-quantitative scoring systems have been proposed to describe and quantify the necro-inflammation, steatosis and fibrosis in the liver, particularly for chronic viral hepatitis. These include the Knodell histological activity index (HAI) first proposed in 1981, then modified to the Scheuer system, the METAVIR system and the Ishak modified HAI [5]. However, all the scoring systems could only provide qualitative descriptors to stage fibrosis, and the staging of certain histopathological changes differ in different systems (Table 1). This could cause considerable intra- and inter-observer variation and difficulty in comparison [2].

| Pathologic Features | Knodell | Scheuer | METAVIR | Ishak |
|---|---|---|---|---|
| No fibrosis | 0 | 0 | 0 | 0 |
| Enlargement of some portal tracts | 1 | 1 | 1 | 1 |
| Enlargement of most portal tracts | 1 | 1 | 1 | 2 |
| Periportal septa | 1 | 2 | 1 | 2 |
| Occasional portal-portal septa | 3 | 2 | 2 | 3 |
| Numerous septa (portal-portal and/or portal-central) | 3 | 3 | 3 | 4 |
| Occasional nodules | 4 | 4 | 4 | 5 |
| Definite cirrhosis | 4 | 4 | 4 | 6 |

Table 1. Scoring systems for staging fibrosis

Using computerized digital image analysis, the amount of fibrosis in liver biopsy specimens can be evaluated by a quantitative score [6-9]. Though it is thought to be less reliable in determining early stage fibrosis, recent advances such as a higher resolution digital camera can improve discrimination between the varying stages of liver fibrosis, including mild fibrosis [8]. It may be a more precise method than semi-quantitative histological stages for monitoring fibrosis progression or regression during clinical therapeutic trials [9]. Considering the irregular shape of specimens, fractal and spectral dimension analysis can also be used to improve accuracy [10].
The detection of genes correlated with fibrosis from biopsy samples regains interest for liver biopsy. The changes in liver gene expression can indicate fibrosis progression precisely at an early stage [11]. Genetic studies have identified possible genetic polymorphisms that influence the progression of liver fibrosis [12]. The identification of panels of key genes correlating with differences in the progression of CLDs could lead to establishing excellent prognostic/diagnostic tools.

### 2.2 Hepatic venous pressure gradient

Hepatic venous pressure gradient (HVPG), as an expression of intrahepatic resistance, does not exceed 5 mmHg in absence of significant fibrotic evolution. The measurement of HVPG is a validated, safe and highly reproducible technique. It may be considered as a dynamic marker of disease progression in patients with HCV and an end point in antiviral therapy, irrespective of antiviral response [13]. However, the technique is invasive, expensive, requires technical expertise, and has low patient acceptance.

## 3. Serological tests

The limitations of liver biopsy led to the searching of noninvasive tests for assessment of liver fibrosis. Afdhal and Nunes *et al* [14] suggest the following criteria for an ideal marker of liver fibrosis: it should be liver specific; should not be influenced by alterations in liver, renal, or reticuloendothelial function; should measure one or more of the processes related to fibrosis (stage of fibrosis, activity of matrix deposition, or activity of matrix removal); and should be easy to perform.

### 3.1 Direct serum markers

The key step in the pathophysiology of liver fibrosis is the balance between ECM deposition and removal. Accumulation of ECM results from both increased synthesis and decreased degradation. The principal ECM constituents are synthesized by activated HSCs, while broken down by a family of enzymes known as matrix metalloproteinases (MMPs). Many studies have been dedicated to find serum ECM markers for fibrosis assessment.

Hyaluronic acid (HA), a glycosaminoglycan distributed in the connective tissue, is a component of the liver extracellular matrix, which is synthesized and degraded in the liver sinusoidal cells. The high levels of HA observed in patients with chronic liver disease, have been related with a decreased function of the endothelial sinusoidal cells. Many studies showing a close relationship between liver fibrosis and HA levels.

These similar markers of fibrosis incuding: (1) collagens: N-terminal peptide of type Ⅲ pro-collagen (PⅢNP), type Ⅳ collagen 7s domain(Ⅳ-7S) [15], (2) proteoglycans: hyaluronic acid (HA) [16], (3) glycoproteins: laminin (LN) [17], human cartilage glycoprotein 39 (YKL-40) [18], (4) collagenases and their inhibitors: MMPs, tissue inhibitor of metalloproteinases (TIMPs) [19], (5) cytokines: transforming growth factor β1 (TGF-β1), platelet-derived growth factor (PDGF), tumor necrosis factor β (TNF-β).

The clinical applications of such markers appear innovative, they are useful to assess the speed of liver fibrogenesis and estimate the response to anti-viral therapies or anti-fibrotic drugs. But most of them are insensitive in milder fibrosis, and it must be stressed that these markers reflect fibrogenesis and fibrolysis more than fibrosis itself. In other words, there may be a highly active fibrotic process in the liver, although fibrotic tissue has not yet been developed, or there may be heavy fibrosis in the liver but fibrotic activity is temporarily discontinued.

### 3.2 Serum marker panels

Since present direct markers could not satisfy the clinical need of measuring the fibrosis yet, an alternative approach turns out to be combining a number of serum markers to generate algorithms capable of evaluating fibrosis. A large number of panels have been suggested by groups worldwide [20-49] (Table 2).

These panels are mainly based on two kinds of markers, direct and indirect. Direct markers are those directly linked to the modifications in ECM metabolism, such as HA and PⅢNP. Indirect markers include a broad range of blood tests which have no direct link with liver fibrosis. They reflect liver dysfunction or other phenomena caused by fibrosis rather than fibrosis per se. Generally speaking, indexes including direct markers, such as the Fibrometer, may perform a higher accuracy, but indexes composed by only indirect markers are effective as well, and usually more useful because they are based on routine blood tests easy to be performed in a hospital general laboratory.

The diagnostic value of the models was assessed by calculating the area under the receiver operating characteristic curves (AUROC). Most studies reported an AUROC >0.80 in differentiating significant fibrosis (fibrosis spread out the portal tract with septa) from no/mild fibrosis (no fibrosis or portal fibrosis without septa), improved performance with a higher AUROC value was showed in differentiating between no cirrhosis and cirrhosis. But it must be underlined that the AUROC values in table 2 came from each different designed study and are not suitable to make a comparison.

| Index, Author, year, reference | Patients no. | CLDs | markers in panel | AUROC(T-V) [a] |
|---|---|---|---|---|
| AAR, Williams, 1988 [20] | 177 | Mixed | AST/ALT-ratio (AAR) | n/a |
| PGA index, Poynard , 1991 [21] | 624 | Alcohol | PT, GGT, apoA1 | n/a |
| PGAA index, Naveau , 1994[22] | 525 | Alcohol | PT, GGT, apoA1, A2M | n/a |
| CDS index, Bonacini, 1997 [23] | 75 | HCV | PLT, AAR, PT | n/a |
| AP index, Poynard 1997 [24] | 620 | HCV | Age, PLT | 0.763-0.690 |
| BAAT score, Ratziu 2000 [25] | 93 | NAFLD | Age, BMI, ALT, TG | 0.84 |
| Fortunato, 2001 [26] | 103 | HCV | Fibronectin, prothrombin, ALT, PCHE, Mn-SOD, β-NAG | n/a |
| Pohl, 2001 [27] | 211 | HCV | AAR, PLT | n/a |
| FibroTest, Imbert-Bismut, 2001 [28] | 339 | HCV | A2M, Hpt, GGT, ApoA1, bilirubin | 0.836-0.870 |
| Kaul 2002 [29] | 264 | HCV | PLT, AST, sex, spider naevi | n/a |
| Forns index, Forns, 2002 [30] | 476 | HCV | Age, GGT, cholesterol, PLT | 0.86-0.81 |
| APRI, Wai, 2003 [31] | 270 | HCV | AST, PLT | 0.80-0.88 |
| ELF-score, Rosenberg, 2004[32] | 1021 | Mixed | Age, HA, PⅢNP, TIMP-1 | 0.804 |
| FIBROSpect II, Patel, 2004 [33] | 696 | HCV | HA, TIMP-1, A2M | 0.831-0.823 |
| FPI, Sud, 2004 [34] | 302 | HCV | Age, AST, TC, HOMA-IR, past alcohol intake | 0.84-0.77 |
| MP3, Leroy, 2004 [35] | 194 | HCV | PⅢNP, MMP-1 | 0.82 |
| HALT-C, Lok, 2005 [36] | 1141 | HCV | PLT, AAR, INR | 0.78-0.81[d] |
| Hepascore, Adams, 2005 [37] | 221 | HCV | Bilirubin, GGT, HA, A2M, age, sex | 0.85-0.82 |
| Fibrometer, Cales, 2005 [38] | 383 | Mixed | PLT, PI, AST, A2M, HA, urea, age | 0.883-0.892 |
| SHASTA index, Kelleher, 2005 [39] | 95 | HCV/HIV | HA,AST and albumin | 0.878 |
| Sakugawa, 2005 [40] | 112 | NAFLD | Ⅳ-7S, HA | n/a |
| Hui,2005 [41] | 235 | HBV | BMI, PLT, albumin, TB, ALP | 0.803-0.765 |
| SLFG, Zeng, 2005 [42] | 372 | HBV | A2M, age, GGT, HA | 0.84-0.77 |
| FIB-4, Sterling, 2006 [43] | 832 | HCV/HIV | Age, AST, ALT, PLT | 0.765[b] |
| Virahep-C, Fontana, 2006 [44] | 399 | HCV | age, AST, ALP,PLT | 0.837-0.851 |
| Mohamadnejad, 2006 [45] | 276 | HBV | HBV DNA levels, ALP, albumin, PLT, | 0.91-0.85 |
| FibroIndex, Koda, 2007 [46] | 402 | HCV | PLT, AST, γ- globulin | 0.828-0.835 |
| Alsatie, 2007 [47] | 286 | HCV | diabetes mellitus, PLT, AST, INR, bilirubin | 0.79-0.75[c] |
| Esmat, 2007 [48] | 220 | HCV | HA, age | 0.84[b] |
| NAFLD fibrosis score, Angulo, 2007 [49] | 733 | NAFLD | Age, BMI, PLT, albumin, AAR, hyperglycemia | 0.88-0.82 |

[a] The area under the receiver operating characteristic curves (AUROC) for the diagnosis of significant fibrosis (stage 2-4 by the METAVIR or Scheuer classification, 3-6 by the Ishak score). T-V means the AUROC values of training group and validation group.

[b] Differentiation advanced fibrosis (Ishak 4-6) from mild to moderate fibrosis (Ishak 0-3).

[c] Differentiation advanced hepatic fibrosis (defined as F3-F4 by METAVIR) from milder (F0-F2).

[d] Differentiation cirrhosis from no cirrhosis.

*Abbreviations used:* CLD, Chronic liver disease; ROC, receiver operating characteristic; AUROC, area under the ROC curve; AAR, AST/ALT-ratio; AST, aspartate aminotransferase; ALT, alanine aminotransferase; PT, prothrombin time; GGT, γ-glutamyltransferase; apoA1, apolipoprotein A1; A2M, α2-macroglobulin; PLT, platelet count; TG, triglycerides; PCHE, pseudocholinesterase; Mn-SOD, manganese superoxide dismutase; β-NAG, N-acetyl β-glucosaminidase; Hpt, haptoglobin; HA, hyaluronic acid; PⅢNP, N-terminal peptide of type Ⅲ pro-collagen; TIMP-1, tissue inhibitor of metalloproteinase 1; TC, total cholesterol; HOMA-IR, Homeostasis Model Assessment insulin resistance(fast glucose×plasma gluc/22.5); MMP-1, metalloproteinase 1; INR, international normalized ratio; PI, Prothrombin index; Ⅳ-7S, type Ⅳ collagen 7s domain; BMI, body mass index; TB, total bilirubin; ALP, alkaline phosphatase.

Table 2. Studies of serum markers panels for assessment of liver fibrosis

Chronic hepatitis B (CHB) is the most frequent infectious cause of CLD worldwide. More than 400 million people are chronically infected with HBV. The virus is responsible for more than 300,000 cases of liver cancer every year and for similar numbers of gastrointestinal haemorrhage and ascites [50]. Predictive models designed specially for CHB patients have been proposed by the Shanghai Liver Fibrosis Group (SLFG) [42], Hui et al [41] and Mohamadnejad et al [45]. But few of these models mentioned above has been widely validated and implemented in clinical practice. In our study of the S index [51], a simpler noninvasive model based on routine laboratory markers, we compare its diagnostic value with that of some typical models (Fig. 1), We noticed that the SLFG model and Hepascore performed better in identifying significant fibrosis than the Forns score and APRI, but the superiority was not so significant in identifying advanced fibrosis or cirrhosis. The result was similar to a validation study in CHC patients [52], indicating that such special tests might improve the sensitivity of a diagnostic model in predicting early fibrosis. But including tests unavailable in daily practice makes standardization, validation and routine bedside use difficult.

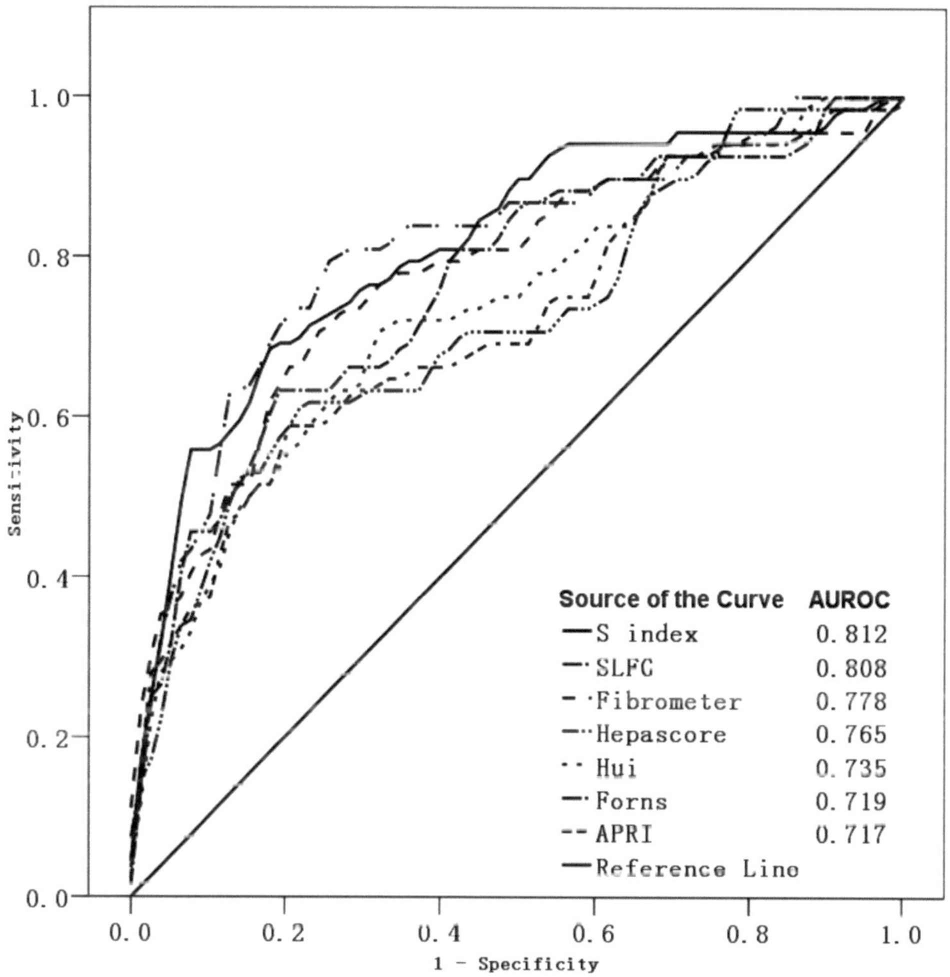


Fig. 1. ROC curves in the prediction of significant fibrosis

There are still some limitations of these marker panels to be considered. First, the design of every study differed in population characteristic, patient selection, significant fibrosis prevalence, blood test inclusion, biochemical measurement and liver histological assessment, resulted in various panels with different markers and parameters. The agreement among these indexes is poor and validation study is needed to choose a proper panel and cutoff value for clinical use. Second, none of the studies controlled for degree of necro-inflammatory activity, most of the panels include markers likely to reflect or be affected by inflammation in the liver, which is much more mobile than fibrosis stage. Third, the formulae are easy to fail because many markers included will be influenced by extrahepatic diseases or conditions such as inflammation, haemolysis, cholestasis, hypercholesterolaemia and renal failure. Finally, few of the studies include treated patients. It is not clear whether these indexes are suitable for assessing treatment response. However, a few studies by Poynard *et al* suggested that Fibrotest could also be used as surrogate markers of the histological impact of treatments in patients infected by HCV and HBV [53, 54]. These indexes, in their current form, are not able to give us the exact stage of fibrosis in most studies. Their main value is to reduce the need for liver biopsy by distinguishing significant fibrosis from no/mild fibrosis, and telling the presence of cirrhosis. It does not seem appropriate to completely replace liver biopsy with serum marker panels at the present time, but it can be anticipated that these indexes will become very useful in the clinical management of CLDs by offering an attractive alternative to liver biopsy, as they are noninvasive, convenient, inexpensive, and may allow dynamic assessment of fibrosis. Validation in larger cohorts of patients with different CLDs is needed before an index will be proposed for extensive clinical use.

### 3.3 Proteomics and glycomics

Over the last 5-6 years, it was reported that the use of proteomic patterns in serum to distinguish individual stages of fibrosis could achieve perfect diagnostic sensitivity and specificity. Using a proteome-based fingerprinting model generated by surface-enhanced laser desorption/ ionization time-of-flight (SELDI-TOF) ProteinChip arrays, Poon *et al* [55] achieved an AUROC of 0.93 in identifying significant fibrosis. Another proteomic index combining eight peaks established by Morra *et al* [56] could diagnosis advanced fibrosis with an AUROC of 0.88, significantly greater than the FibroTest AUROC of 0.81. Besides, The SELDI-TOF ProteinChip technology is useful for the early detection and prediction of HCC in patients with chronic HCV infection [57]. Similar technologies were also used to generate profiles of serum N-glycan profile for identifying liver fibrosis [58, 59]. Further studies identifying the altered peaks in these models to understand their origins may help to find new biomarks for fibrosis, or even improve our understanding in the mechanism of liver fibrosis.

## 4. Radiological tests

Since significant structural changes are present only in advanced CLDs, the routine examinations by Ultrasound (US), computed tomography (CT) and magnetic resonance imaging (MRI) could bring specific findings, but with very limited sensitivity. Thus, persistent efforts were made to search for technological developments.

### 4.1 Perfusion examinations

MR and Doppler US techniques are studied to find sensitive perfusion changes in the progression of fibrosis [60]. For example, the circulatory changes will result in a decrease of hepatic vein transit time (HVTT), which can be measured by microbubble-enhanced US [61]. Using HVTT measurements, Lim *et al* achieved 100% sensitivity and 80% specificity for diagnosis of cirrhosis, and 95% sensitivity and 86% specificity for differentiation of mild hepatitis from more severe liver disease [62]. Progressive liver fibrosis gradually obliterates normal intrahepatic vessels and sinusoids and slows passage of blood through the parenchyma. In addition, as portal hypertension develops, portal venous flow to the liver decreases, hepatic arterial flow increases, and intrahepatic shunts form. These physiologic alterations can be detected with kinetic models of dynamic image data sets acquired rapidly after bolus intravenous injection of paramagnetic extracellular contrast agents. Several perfusion parameters can be estimated by MR perfusion imaging, a recent study applied a dual-input kinetic model for the noninvasive assessment of liver fibrosis. The dual-input approach models two sources of blood flow into the liver, via the he patic artery and portal vein, and assumes a single tissue compartment. Significant differences were found in several perfusion parameters between patients with and without advanced fibrosis [63].

### 4.2 Liver stiffness measurement

In chronic liver disease, progressive deposition of interconnecting collagen fibers throughout the liver produces a lattice-like framework that increases parenchymal rigidity. Because liver stiffness cannot be reliably assessed with external physical palpation, an imaging approach is required. There are two main imaging methods for measuring hepatic stiffness. One is US-based transient elastography; the other is MR elastography.

The FibroScan, a new medical device based on one-dimensional transient elastography [64], which assesses fibrosis through liver stiffness measurement (LSM). A special probe generates an elastic shear wave propagating through the liver tissue, the harder the tissue, the faster the shear wave propagates. Transient elastography could accurately predict different stages of fibrosis or cirrhosis (AUROC: 0.79 for $F \geq 2$, 0.91 for $F \geq 3$, and 0.97 for $F = 4$. by the METAVIR scoring system) [65].

The major advantage of transient elastography compared with serum markers and marker panels is that it measures directly on the liver and there is no interference from extrahepatic diseases or conditions. Further more, the test is standardized and completely noninvasive. Though assessing earlier fibrosis is the common shortcoming of various noninvasive tests, Colletta *et al* reported that the agreement between transient elastography and liver biopsy was much better than FibroTest in normal transaminases HCV carriers with early stages of fibrosis[66].

Compared to liver biopsy, transient elastography is painless, rapid, has no risk of complications, and is therefore very well accepted. Transient elastography measures liver stiffness of a volume which is 100 times bigger than the biopsy specimen. The high reproducibility (intra- and inter-observer agreement intraclass correlation coefficient was 0.98 [67]) and acceptance of transient elastography makes it an attractive alternative to biopsy for individual follow-up.

There are also some physical limitations of transient elastography. The signal penetrates only 25-65 mm, makes obesity (particularly the fatness of the chest wall) the most important cause of failure[68]. But new technological developments may overcome the limitation. Additional limitations include a narrow intercostal space and ascites. The main reason that transient elastography can not totally replace liver biopsy is that it is only a means to stage disease. It is unable to diagnose liver disease by distinguishing subtle diagnostic differences. Nor can transient elastography identify cofactors and comorbidities or grade necro-inflammation and steatosis. But it represents a totally different approach to assess fibrosis and therefore could be combined with other noninvasive modalities to better assess liver fibrosis. The combined use of transient elastography and FibroTest to evaluate liver fibrosis could avoid a biopsy procedure in most patients with chronic hepatitis C [69].

Magnetic resonance elastography (MRE) is a technique using a modified phase-contrast magnetic resonance imaging sequence to image propagating shear waves in tissue [70]. The technique has been previously applied to quantitatively assess the viscoelastic properties of the breast, brain, and muscle in humans. Several recent studies showed that MRE is also a feasible method to assess the stage of liver fibrosis. Liver stiffness as measured with MR elastography increases as the stage of fibrosis advances. The differences in stiffness between patients with early stages of fibrosis (F0 vs F1 vs F2) are small and there is overlap between groups, but the differences between groups with higher stages (F2 vs F3 vs F4) are large, with little overlap between groups[71]. MRE has several potential advantages compared with ultrasound transient elastography. It can be performed in obesity patients. It can assess larger volumes and provide full three-dimensional information about the viscoelastic parameters of tissues. With MR techniques, a comprehensive examination of the liver can be performed, including MRE, contrast-enhanced MRI to detect hepatocellular carcinomas and perfusion MRI to assess liver function.

### 4.3 Real-time elastography

Real-time elastography is another ultrasound technique developed by Hitachi Medical Systems that can reveal the physical property of tissue using conventional ultrasound probes during a routine sonography examination. In the first study assessing real-time elastography for the detection of liver fibrosis [72], the AUROC was 0.75 for the diagnosis of significant fibrosis. Much higher diagnostic accuracy (AUROC = 0.93) was obtained by a mathematic combination of the elasticity score and two routine laboratory values (platelet count and GGT), which provided a more superior way to combine serological and radiological tests together.

### 4.4 Double contrast material-enhanced magnetic resonance imaging

The conspicuity of gadolinium-enhanced lesions is increased in the setting of decreased signal intensity from the uninvolved liver parenchyma following superparamagnetic iron oxide (SPIO) injection. This MRI technique has been used to improve detection of focal hepatic lesion and hepatocellular carcinoma [73, 74]. Recently, Aguirre *et al* [75] examined 101 CLD patients who underwent double-enhanced MR imaging to detect hyperintense reticulations, which are postulated to represent septal fibrosis. They achieved an accuracy of greater than 90% for the diagnosis of advanced hepatic fibrosis compared with histopathological analysis. Clinical trials are currently under way to prospectively assess fibrosis staging with this technique.

### 4.5 Diffusion weighted magnetic resonance imaging

Diffusion weighted magnetic resonance imaging (DWMRI) has been widely used in brain imaging for the evaluation of acute ischemic stroke. With the advent of the echo-planar MRI technique, it became possible to be applied in the abdomen for characterization of focal hepatic lesions [76]. Recently, using DWMRI to measure the apparent diffusion coefficient (ADC) of water, a parameter that is dependent on the tissue structure, is introduced in the assessment of liver fibrosis [77]. The ADC value is lower in livers with heavier fibrosis because of the restriction of water diffusion in fibrotic tissue. Lewin *et al* assessed the performance of

DWMRI in 54 patients with chronic HCV infection with reference to several other noninvasive methods [78]. In discriminating significant fibrosis patients, the AUC values were 0.79 for DWMRI, 0.87 for transient elastography, 0.68 for FibroTest, 0.81 for APRI, 0.72 for the Forns index, and 0.77 for hyaluronate. DWMRI performed better in discriminating patients staged F3-F4, the AUC value increased to 0.92, the same as transient elastography. But besides fibrosis, it seems that ADC values might also reflect the intensity of inflammation, necrosis and steatosis. Because technical factors lead to differences in estimated ADC, reported ADCs are variable, with considerable overlap between normal and abnormal ranges. Thus, there is a need to develop site- and technique-specific normal ranges and to standardize methods across imaging centers.
Several other MR techniques have also been introduced in the area of fibrosis assessment, such as ultrashort echo time (UTE) MRI [79] and magnetic resonance spectroscopy (MRS) [80]. New MR imaging contrast agents that specifically target collagen or other extracellular matrix macromolecules may be developed. A collagen-specific MR imaging contrast agent could act as a fibrosis-imaging agent, and these agents may have higher efficacy for fibrosis assessment than the current methods [81]. All such data may provide valuable information for guiding antifibrotic therapy development and monitoring patients in clinical trials.

## 5. Conclusion

The increasing of potentially effective managements for CLDs such as antiviral and antifibrotic therapies has led to an urgent need for a rapid, safe and repeatable tool to assess fibrosis of CLDs and to follow-up progression or regression of fibrosis during treatment. Liver biopsy has been the gold standard for the assessment of hepatic fibrosis, but the invasive procedure has considerable limitations and fails to satisfy the current needs. Many noninvasive methods have been proposed with the aim of substituting liver biopsy. The numerous advances in serological, radiological techniques and their combinations have allowed to satisfactorily identify patients without a liver biopsy. But each of them has some deficiencies and the liver biopsy will still have an important role to play. Applying new techniques for the detection of fibrosis may potentially circumvent the pitfalls and deficiencies of the existing surrogates mentioned above. These include serum proteomics, glycomics and new imaging techniques such as molecular imaging technique for the imaging of cellular biochemical processes [82], diffraction-enhanced imaging technique for the imaging of soft tissues [83], photonic imaging technique for three-dimensional whole-body images [84]. However, further studies are needed to develop or validate noninvasive tests that can accurately reflect the full spectrum of hepatic fibrosis in CLDs. But an incorrigible defect in our studies will be the questionable gold standard we have to use. More errors are due to the histological staging [85]. Mathematical modeling suggested that assuming either 80% or 90% diagnostic accuracy of liver biopsy, noninvasive tests cannot achieve an AUROC better than 0.9 and are likely to perform between 0.75 and 0.9 [86], exactly where they are today. We may find a better surrogate for liver biopsy, but how can we prove it will be a question. Laparoscopic biopsy can decrease sampling error and increases the reliability of histopathologic assessment [87]. Using automated image analysis to assess texture features and shape representation of the fibrosis structural expansion can turn the current semiquantitative methods of liver fibrosis assessment into real quantitative ones with significant reduction in variability and subjectivity [88]. Validating noninvasive tests against not only histological stage scores but also digital image analysis and clinical outcomes may also be a better choice.

## 6. References


[1] Colloredo G, Guido M, Sonzogni A, Leandro G. Impact of liver biopsy size on histological evaluation of chronic viral hepatitis: the smaller the sample, the milder the disease. *J Hepatol.* 2003; 39: 239-44.

[2] The French METAVIR Cooperative Study Group. Intraobserver and interobserver variations in liver biopsy interpretation in patients with chronic hepatitis C. *Hepatology.* 1994; 20: 15-20.

[3] Bravo AA, Sheth SG, Chopra S. Liver biopsy. *N Engl J Med.* 2001; 344: 495-500.

[4] McGill DB, Rakela J, Zinsmeister AR, Ott BJ. A 21-year experience with major hemorrhage after percutaneous liver biopsy. *Gastroenterology.* 1990; 99: 1396-400.

[5] Brunt EM. Grading and staging the histopathological lesions of chronic hepatitis: the Knodell histology activity index and beyond. *Hepatology.* 2000; 31: 241-6.

[6] Chevallier M, Guerret S, Chossegros P, Gerard F, Grimaud JA. A histological semiquantitative scoring system for evaluation of hepatic fibrosis in needle liver biopsy specimens: comparison with morphometric studies. *Hepatology.* 1994; 20: 349-55.

[7] Pilette C, Rousselet MC, Bedossa P, *et al.* Histopathological evaluation of liver fibrosis: quantitative image analysis vs semi-quantitative scores. Comparison with serum markers. *J Hepatol.* 1998; 28: 439-46.

[8] Lazzarini AL, Levine RA, Ploutz-Snyder RJ, Sanderson SO. Advances in digital quantification technique enhance discrimination between mild and advanced liver fibrosis in chronic hepatitis C. *Liver Int.* 2005; 25: 1142-9.

[9] Goodman ZD, Becker RL, Jr., Pockros PJ, Afdhal NH. Progression of fibrosis in advanced chronic hepatitis C: evaluation by morphometric image analysis. *Hepatology.* 2007; 45: 886-94.

[10] Dioguardi N, Franceschini B, Aletti G, Russo C, Grizzi F. Fractal dimension rectified meter for quantification of liver fibrosis and other irregular microscopic objects. *Anal Quant Cytol Histol.* 2003; 25: 312-20.

[11] Asselah T, Bieche I, Laurendeau I, *et al.* Liver gene expression signature of mild fibrosis in patients with chronic hepatitis C. *Gastroenterology.* 2005; 129: 2064-75.

[12] Bataller R, North KE, Brenner DA. Genetic polymorphisms and the progression of liver fibrosis: a critical appraisal. *Hepatology.* 2003; 37: 493-503.

[13] Burroughs AK, Groszmann R, Bosch J, *et al.* Assessment of therapeutic benefit of antiviral therapy in chronic hepatitis C: is hepatic venous pressure gradient a better end point? *Gut.* 2002; 50: 425-7.

[14] Afdhal NH, Nunes D. Evaluation of liver fibrosis: a concise review. *Am J Gastroenterol.* 2004; 99: 1160-74.

[15] Murawaki Y, Ikuta Y, Koda M, Kawasaki H. Serum type III procollagen peptide, type IV collagen 7S domain, central triple-helix of type IV collagen and tissue inhibitor of metalloproteinases in patients with chronic viral liver disease: relationship to liver histology. *Hepatology.* 1994; 20: 780-7.

[16] Pares A, Deulofeu R, Gimenez A, *et al.* Serum hyaluronate reflects hepatic fibrogenesis in alcoholic liver disease and is useful as a marker of fibrosis. *Hepatology.* 1996; 24: 1399-403.

[17] Walsh KM, Fletcher A, MacSween RN, Morris AJ. Basement membrane peptides as markers of liver disease in chronic hepatitis C. *J Hepatol.* 2000; 32: 325-30.

[18] Saitou Y, Shiraki K, Yamanaka Y, *et al.* Noninvasive estimation of liver fibrosis and response to interferon therapy by a serum fibrogenesis marker, YKL-40, in patients with HCV-associated liver disease. *World J Gastroenterol.* 2005; 11: 476-81.
[19] Kasahara A, Hayashi N, Mochizuki K, *et al.* Circulating matrix metalloproteinase-2 and tissue inhibitor of metalloproteinase-1 as serum markers of fibrosis in patients with chronic hepatitis C. Relationship to interferon response. *J Hepatol.* 1997; 26: 574-83.
[20] Williams AL, Hoofnagle JH. Ratio of serum aspartate to alanine aminotransferase in chronic hepatitis. Relationship to cirrhosis. *Gastroenterology.* 1988; 95: 734-9.
[21] Poynard T, Aubert A, Bedossa P, *et al.* A simple biological index for detection of alcoholic liver disease in drinkers. *Gastroenterology.* 1991; 100: 1397-402.
[22] Naveau S, Poynard T, Benattar C, Bedossa P, Chaput JC. Alpha-2-macroglobulin and hepatic fibrosis. Diagnostic interest. *Dig Dis Sci.* 1994; 39: 2426-32.
[23] Bonacini M, Hadi G, Govindarajan S, Lindsay KL. Utility of a discriminant score for diagnosing advanced fibrosis or cirrhosis in patients with chronic hepatitis C virus infection. *Am J Gastroenterol.* 1997; 92: 1302-4.
[24] Poynard T, Bedossa P. Age and platelet count: a simple index for predicting the presence of histological lesions in patients with antibodies to hepatitis C virus. METAVIR and CLINIVIR Cooperative Study Groups. *J Viral Hepat.* 1997; 4: 199-208.
[25] Ratziu V, Giral P, Charlotte F, *et al.* Liver fibrosis in overweight patients. *Gastroenterology.* 2000; 118: 1117-23.
[26] Fortunato G, Castaldo G, Oriani G, *et al.* Multivariate discriminant function based on six biochemical markers in blood can predict the cirrhotic evolution of chronic hepatitis. *Clin Chem.* 2001; 47: 1696-700.
[27] Pohl A, Behling C, Oliver D, Kilani M, Monson P, Hassanein T. Serum aminotransferase levels and platelet counts as predictors of degree of fibrosis in chronic hepatitis C virus infection. *Am J Gastroenterol.* 2001; 96: 3142-6.
[28] Imbert-Bismut F, Ratziu V, Pieroni L, Charlotte F, Benhamou Y, Poynard T. Biochemical markers of liver fibrosis in patients with hepatitis C virus infection: a prospective study. *Lancet.* 2001; 357: 1069-75.
[29] Kaul V, Friedenberg FK, Braitman LE, *et al.* Development and validation of a model to diagnose cirrhosis in patients with hepatitis C. *Am J Gastroenterol.* 2002; 97: 2623-8.
[30] Forns X, Ampurdanes S, Llovet JM, *et al.* Identification of chronic hepatitis C patients without hepatic fibrosis by a simple predictive model. *Hepatology.* 2002; 36: 986-92.
[31] Wai CT, Greenson JK, Fontana RJ, *et al.* A simple noninvasive index can predict both significant fibrosis and cirrhosis in patients with chronic hepatitis C. *Hepatology.* 2003; 38: 518-26.
[32] Rosenberg WM, Voelker M, Thiel R, *et al.* Serum markers detect the presence of liver fibrosis: a cohort study. *Gastroenterology.* 2004; 127: 1704-13.
[33] Patel K, Gordon SC, Jacobson I, *et al.* Evaluation of a panel of non-invasive serum markers to differentiate mild from moderate-to-advanced liver fibrosis in chronic hepatitis C patients. *J Hepatol.* 2004; 41: 935-42
[34] Sud A, Hui JM, Farrell GC, *et al.* Improved prediction of fibrosis in chronic hepatitis C using measures of insulin resistance in a probability index. *Hepatology.* 2004; 39: 1239-47.
[35] Leroy V, Monier F, Bottari S, *et al.* Circulating matrix metalloproteinases 1, 2, 9 and their inhibitors TIMP-1 and TIMP-2 as serum markers of liver fibrosis in patients with chronic hepatitis C: comparison with PIIINP and hyaluronic acid. *Am J Gastroenterol.* 2004; 99: 271-9.

[36] Lok AS, Ghany MG, Goodman ZD, *et al.* Predicting cirrhosis in patients with hepatitis C based on standard laboratory tests: results of the HALT-C cohort. *Hepatology.* 2005; 42: 282-92.

[37] Adams LA, Bulsara M, Rossi E, *et al.* Hepascore: an accurate validated predictor of liver fibrosis in chronic hepatitis C infection. *Clin Chem.* 2005; 51: 1867-73.

[38] Cales P, Oberti F, Michalak S, *et al.* A novel panel of blood markers to assess the degree of liver fibrosis. *Hepatology.* 2005; 42: 1373-81.

[39] Kelleher TB, Mehta SH, Bhaskar R, *et al.* Prediction of hepatic fibrosis in HIV/HCV co-infected patients using serum fibrosis markers: the SHASTA index. *J Hepatol.* 2005; 43: 78-84.

[40] Sakugawa H, Nakayoshi T, Kobashigawa K, *et al.* Clinical usefulness of biochemical markers of liver fibrosis in patients with nonalcoholic fatty liver disease. *World J Gastroenterol.* 2005; 11: 255-9.

[41] Hui AY, Chan HL, Wong VW, *et al.* Identification of chronic hepatitis B patients without significant liver fibrosis by a simple noninvasive predictive model. *Am J Gastroenterol.* 2005; 100: 616-23.

[42] Zeng MD, Lu LG, Mao YM, *et al.* Prediction of significant fibrosis in HBeAg-positive patients with chronic hepatitis B by a noninvasive model. *Hepatology.* 2005; 42: 1437-45.

[43] Sterling RK, Lissen E, Clumeck N, *et al.* Development of a simple noninvasive index to predict significant fibrosis in patients with HIV/HCV coinfection. *Hepatology.* 2006; 43: 1317-25.

[44] Fontana RJ, Kleiner DE, Bilonick R, *et al.* Modeling hepatic fibrosis in African American and Caucasian American patients with chronic hepatitis C virus infection. *Hepatology.* 2006; 44: 925-35.

[45] Mohamadnejad M, Montazeri G, Fazlollahi A, *et al.* Noninvasive markers of liver fibrosis and inflammation in chronic hepatitis B-virus related liver disease. *Am J Gastroenterol.* 2006; 101: 2537-45.

[46] Koda M, Matunaga Y, Kawakami M, Kishimoto Y, Suou T, Murawaki Y. FibroIndex, a practical index for predicting significant fibrosis in patients with chronic hepatitis C. *Hepatology.* 2007; 45: 297-306.

[47] Alsatie M, Kwo PY, Gingerich JR, *et al.* A multivariable model of clinical variables predicts advanced fibrosis in chronic hepatitis C. *J Clin Gastroenterol.* 2007; 41: 416-21.

[48] Esmat G, Metwally M, Zalata KR, *et al.* Evaluation of serum biomarkers of fibrosis and injury in Egyptian patients with chronic hepatitis C. *J Hepatol.* 2007; 46: 620-7.

[49] Angulo P, Hui JM, Marchesini G, *et al.* The NAFLD fibrosis score: a noninvasive system that identifies liver fibrosis in patients with NAFLD. *Hepatology.* 2007; 45: 846-54.

[50] Lai CL, Ratziu V, Yuen MF, Poynard T. Viral hepatitis B. *Lancet.* 2003; 362: 2089-94.

[51] Zhou K, Gao CF, Zhao YP, *et al.* Simpler score of routine laboratory tests predicts liver fibrosis in patients with chronic hepatitis B. *Journal of Gastroenterology and Hepatology.* 2010; 25: 1569-77.

[52] Bourliere M, Penaranda G, Renou C, *et al.* Validation and comparison of indexes for fibrosis and cirrhosis prediction in chronic hepatitis C patients: proposal for a pragmatic approach classification without liver biopsies. *J Viral Hepat.* 2006; 13: 659-70.

[53] Poynard T, McHutchison J, Manns M, Myers RP, Albrecht J. Biochemical surrogate markers of liver fibrosis and activity in a randomized trial of peginterferon alfa-2b and ribavirin. *Hepatology.* 2003; 38: 481-92.

[54] Poynard T, Zoulim F, Ratziu V, *et al.* Longitudinal assessment of histology surrogate markers (FibroTest-ActiTest) during lamivudine therapy in patients with chronic hepatitis B infection. *Am J Gastroenterol*. 2005; 100: 1970-80.

[55] Poon TC, Hui AY, Chan HL, *et al.* Prediction of liver fibrosis and cirrhosis in chronic hepatitis B infection by serum proteomic fingerprinting: a pilot study. *Clin Chem*. 2005; 51: 328-35.

[56] Morra R, Munteanu M, Bedossa P, *et al.* Diagnostic value of serum protein profiling by SELDI-TOF ProteinChip compared with a biochemical marker, FibroTest, for the diagnosis of advanced fibrosis in patients with chronic hepatitis C. *Aliment Pharmacol Ther*. 2007; 26: 847-58.

[57] Kanmura S, Uto H, Kusumoto K, *et al.* Early diagnostic potential for hepatocellular carcinoma using the SELDI ProteinChip system. *Hepatology*. 2007; 45: 948-56.

[58] Callewaert N, Van Vlierberghe H, Van Hecke A, Laroy W, Delanghe J, Contreras R. Noninvasive diagnosis of liver cirrhosis using DNA sequencer-based total serum protein glycomics. *Nat Med*. 2004; 10: 429-34.

[59] Kam RK, Poon TC, Chan HL, Wong N, Hui AY, Sung JJ. High-throughput quantitative profiling of serum N-glycome by MALDI-TOF mass spectrometry and N-glycomic fingerprint of liver fibrosis. *Clin Chem*. 2007; 53: 1254-63.

[60] Annet L, Materne R, Danse E, Jamart J, Horsmans Y, Van Beers BE. Hepatic flow parameters measured with MR imaging and Doppler US: correlations with degree of cirrhosis and portal hypertension. *Radiology*. 2003; 229: 409-14.

[61] Albrecht T, Blomley MJ, Cosgrove DO, *et al.* Non-invasive diagnosis of hepatic cirrhosis by transit-time analysis of an ultrasound contrast agent. *Lancet*. 1999; 353: 1579-83.

[62] Lim AK, Taylor-Robinson SD, Patel N, *et al.* Hepatic vein transit times using a microbubble agent can predict disease severity non-invasively in patients with hepatitis C. *Gut*. 2005; 54: 128-33.

[63] Miyazaki S, Yamazaki Y, Murase K. Error analysis of the quantification of hepatic perfusion using a dual-input single-compartment model. *Physics in Medicine and Biology*. 2008; 53: 5927-46.

[64] Sandrin L, Fourquet B, Hasquenoph JM, *et al.* Transient elastography: a new noninvasive method for assessment of hepatic fibrosis. *Ultrasound Med Biol*. 2003; 29: 1705-13.

[65] Ziol M, Handra-Luca A, Kettaneh A, *et al.* Noninvasive assessment of liver fibrosis by measurement of stiffness in patients with chronic hepatitis C. *Hepatology*. 2005; 41: 48-54.

[66] Colletta C, Smirne C, Fabris C, *et al.* Value of two noninvasive methods to detect progression of fibrosis among HCV carriers with normal aminotransferases. *Hepatology*. 2005; 42: 838-45.

[67] Fraquelli M, Rigamonti C, Casazza G, *et al.* Reproducibility of transient elastography in the evaluation of liver fibrosis in patients with chronic liver disease. *Gut*. 2007; 56: 968-73.

[68] Foucher J, Castera L, Bernard PH, *et al.* Prevalence and factors associated with failure of liver stiffness measurement using FibroScan in a prospective study of 2114 examinations. *Eur J Gastroenterol Hepatol*. 2006; 18: 411-2.

[69] Castera L, Vergniol J, Foucher J, *et al.* Prospective comparison of transient elastography, Fibrotest, APRI, and liver biopsy for the assessment of fibrosis in chronic hepatitis C. *Gastroenterology*. 2005; 128: 343-50.

[70] Muthupillai R, Lomas DJ, Rossman PJ, Greenleaf JF, Manduca A, Ehman RL. Magnetic resonance elastography by direct visualization of propagating acoustic strain waves. *Science*. 1995; 269: 1854-7.

[71] Yin M, Talwalkar JA, Glaser KJ, *et al.* Assessment of Hepatic Fibrosis With Magnetic Resonance Elastography. *Clinical Gastroenterology and Hepatology.* 2007; 5: 1207-13.e2.

[72] Friedrich-Rust M, Ong MF, Herrmann E, *et al.* Real-time elastography for noninvasive assessment of liver fibrosis in chronic viral hepatitis. *AJR Am J Roentgenol.* 2007; 188: 758-64.

[73] Kim MJ, Kim JH, Chung JJ, Park MS, Lim JS, Oh YT. Focal hepatic lesions: detection and characterization with combination gadolinium- and superparamagnetic iron oxide-enhanced MR imaging. *Radiology.* 2003; 228: 719-26.

[74] Kwak HS, Lee JM, Kim CS. Preoperative detection of hepatocellular carcinoma: comparison of combined contrast-enhanced MR imaging and combined CT during arterial portography and CT hepatic arteriography. *Eur Radiol.* 2004; 14: 447-57.

[75] Aguirre DA, Behling CA, Alpert E, Hassanein TI, Sirlin CB. Liver fibrosis: noninvasive diagnosis with double contrast material-enhanced MR imaging. *Radiology.* 2006; 239: 425-37.

[76] Ichikawa T, Haradome H, Hachiya J, Nitatori T, Araki T. Diffusion-weighted MR imaging with a single-shot echoplanar sequence: detection and characterization of focal hepatic lesions. *AJR Am J Roentgenol.* 1998; 170: 397-402.

[77] Koinuma M, Ohashi I, Hanafusa K, Shibuya H. Apparent diffusion coefficient measurements with diffusion-weighted magnetic resonance imaging for evaluation of hepatic fibrosis. *J Magn Reson Imaging.* 2005; 22: 80-5.

[78] Lewin M, Poujol-Robert A, Boelle PY, *et al.* Diffusion-weighted magnetic resonance imaging for the assessment of fibrosis in chronic hepatitis C. *Hepatology.* 2007; 46: 658-65.

[79] Chappell KE, Patel N, Gatehouse PD, *et al.* Magnetic resonance imaging of the liver with ultrashort TE (UTE) pulse sequences. *J Magn Reson Imaging.* 2003; 18: 709-13.

[80] Lim AK, Patel N, Hamilton G, Hajnal JV, Goldin RD, Taylor-Robinson SD. The relationship of in vivo 31P MR spectroscopy to histology in chronic hepatitis C. *Hepatology.* 2003; 37: 788-94.

[81] Caravan P. Protein-targeted gadolinium-based magnetic resonance imaging (MRI) contrast agents: Design and mechanism of action. *Accounts of Chemical Research.* 2009; 42: 851-62.

[82] Margolis DJ, Hoffman JM, Herfkens RJ, Jeffrey RB, Quon A, Gambhir SS. Molecular imaging techniques in body imaging. *Radiology.* 2007; 245: 333-56.

[83] Meuli R, Hwu Y, Je JH, Margaritondo G. Synchrotron radiation in radiology: radiology techniques based on synchrotron sources. *Eur Radiol.* 2004; 14: 1550-60.

[84] Ntziachristos V, Ripoll J, Wang LV, Weissleder R. Looking and listening to light: the evolution of whole-body photonic imaging. *Nat Biotechnol.* 2005; 23: 313-20.

[85] Poynard T, Munteanu M, Imbert-Bismut F, *et al.* Prospective analysis of discordant results between biochemical markers and biopsy in patients with chronic hepatitis C. *Clin Chem.* 2004; 50: 1344-55.

[86] Afdhal NH, Curry M. Technology evaluation: a critical step in the clinical utilization of novel diagnostic tests for liver fibrosis. *J Hepatol.* 2007; 46: 543-5.

[87] Pagliaro L, Rinaldi F, Craxi A, *et al.* Percutaneous blind biopsy versus laparoscopy with guided biopsy in diagnosis of cirrhosis. A prospective, randomized trial. *Dig Dis Sci.* 1983; 28: 39-43.

[88] Matalka, II, Al-Jarrah OM, Manasrah TM. Quantitative assessment of liver fibrosis: a novel automated image analysis method. *Liver Int.* 2006; 26: 1054-64.

# 17

# Non-Invasive Assessment of the Liver – Serum Markers and Imaging Techniques

Anna Mania, Paweł Kemnitz, Katarzyna Mazur-Melewska,
Magdalena Figlerowicz and Wojciech Służewski
*Department of Infectious Diseases and Child Neurology,
University of Medical Sciences, Poznan,
Poland*

## 1. Introduction

Management and prognosis of the liver diseases highly depends on the advancement of the liver lesions. It is particularly important to distinguish patients at greatest risk of developing liver cirrhosis, liver failure and hepatocellular carcinoma. Liver biopsy remains the gold standard for evaluating the liver tissue. It allows not only for establishing the grade of inflammatory activity and the stage of fibrosis, but also for more accurate differential diagnosis and detection of coexisting liver diseases. Needle biopsy removes, however, only about 1/50,000 of the liver tissue and carries the risk of sampling error. Furthermore, the specimen should be sufficient in length (20-25 mm), width, fragmentation and number of complete portal tracts (at least 11) [Cholongitas et al., 2006]. Moreover, liver assessment is affected by significant interpretative error and interobserver variability of histological interpretation. Besides, many patients are reluctant to experience repeated biopsies, which limits the ability to monitor disease progression and the effects of treatments.

Search for new non-invasive approaches have been initiated as a result of the limitations of the liver biopsy. Non-invasive tests for the assessment of the severity of chronic liver diseases seem to be an attractive option designed to replace liver biopsy in the near future.

Ideal non-invasive marker of particular liver lesion should be reliable, liver specific, inexpensive and easy to perform. In addition, it should allow not only to diagnose particular liver problem but also to monitor its progression. Recently extensive research is performed to evaluate non-invasive techniques for the detection of liver fibrosis, necroinflammatory activity and steatosis in various liver diseases. This chapter revises currently used non-invasive techniques of liver assessment.

## 2. Serum biochemical markers

### 2.1 Serum markers of fibrosis in hepatitis

The progression of liver fibrosis is a complex wound-healing process, that involves various types of cells and their mediators that eventually leads to the deposition and accumulation of various extracellular matrix (ECM) components.

Serum biochemical tests including direct and indirect markers of fibrosis have been most widely investigated. Certain markers, especially cytokines, growth factors, metaloproteinases and their inhibitors may reflect balance or imbalance between fibrogenesis and fibrinolysis, revealing information about the progression of the disease.

## 2.2 Direct markers

Direct markers include profibrotic cytokines as transforming growth factor beta-1 (TGF beta-1), ECM components - glycoproteins as hyaluronan (HA), laminin, metaloproteinases their tissue inhibitors and others. Some of them demonstrated associations with liver fibrosis.

Fibryl-forming collagens accumulate in the process of liver fibrosis being important components of extracellular matrix. The most extensively studied collagen is PIIINP, an aminotreminal peptide of procollagen III, that is cleaved from procolagen III during its secretion by fibroblasts. Therefore, it is mainly considered to be a marker of fibrogenensis, rather than fibrosis. PIIINP was found proportional to the liver fibrosis in several studies. However, this parameter should be validated in further studies, as it is too early to recommend its use as a single marker [Leroy et al., 2004].

Transforming growth factor beta 1 (TGF-beta 1) is a cytokine that activates fibrogenesis and inhibits fibrinolysis. This protein stimulates mesenchymal cells and increases production of ECM components. TGF-beta 1 was found to be related to the liver fibrosis in patients with CHC and CHB [Marek et al., 2003].

Laminin is a glycoprotein of ECM consisting of 3 different polipeptide chains $\alpha$, $\beta$, and $\gamma$. Laminins take part in the cellular adhesion, stimulate cellular growth and act as cellular mediators. This protein is also considered to be a marker of the liver fibrosis. In various studies it was found to be related to the degree of the liver fibrosis in patients with CHC [Walsh et al., 2000].

Hyaluronic acid (HA) a glycosaminoglycan produced by fibroblasts that seems to be a major component of extracellular matrix. Liver sinusoidal cells are responsible for degradation of its particles. Therefore elevated HA serum levels may reflect endothelial dysfunction associated with the progression of fibrosis. Several studies proved correlation between HA serum levels and hepatic fibrosis, it has, however limitations in distinguishing exact stages [Patel et al., 2003]. HA was validated in HCV, HBV and HCV/HIV coinfected patients. Serum concentrations of HA were found to be related to the level of fibrosis. However, in lower fibrosis stages serum HA levels may overlap, therefore the parameter is more reliable in advanced stages of fibrosis [Resino et al., 2010]. HA< 60 ug/l exclude fibrosis and extensive fibrosis, whereas values >110 ug/l predicted cirrhosis [McHutchinson et al., 2002].

Metaloproteinases (MMPs) and their tissue inhibitors (TIMPs) are proteins involved in the regulation of fibrogenesis and fibrinolysis. MMPs are secreted by fibroblasts and Kupfer cells in inactive form that requires further cleavage for functional capability. They are involved in degradation of extracellular matrix components and are regulated by tissue inhibitors (TIMPs). MMP-2 is an enzyme up-regulated by collagen type II, that was found to be positively related to the liver fibrosis. Similar correlations were found for TIMP-1 and TIMP-2. Moreover, TIMP-1 was found to be very sensitive and displayed good specificity for the detection of liver cirrhosis [Boeker et al., 2002]. In combination with HA and PIIINP, TIMP-1 showed good accuracy for the diagnosis of extensive fibrosis and cirrhosis [Leroy et al., 2004].

Although direct markers are less expensive than the liver biopsy, they are still costly and are not available in most clinical settings. Therefore, none of those biomarkers is until now in frequent use except for research studies.

### 2.2.1 Indirect markers

Indirect markers associated with fibrosis, such as routine biochemistry, platelets, and alpha-2-macroglobulin, are widely available in daily clinical practice. Biochemical tests mainly include aspartate (AST) and alanine aminotransferase (ALT) activity and prothrombine time. They are either tested alone or in combination, which enhances their value. Prothrombine time, a well-known marker of hepatic dysfunction, was negatively correlated to fibrosis even in its earlier stages [Croquet et al. 2002]. Thrombin is believed to be trapped by the hepatic sinusoidal capillary network and bind to the receptors on the surface of activated hepatic stellate cells.

AST levels usually increase in patients with liver fibrosis as a result of reduced clearance by sinusoidal capillary network. AST/ALT ratio was found related to the presence of liver cirrhosis with high predictive values for ratio exceeding 1. Nevertheless, not all studies confirm such results. Diagnostic value of AST/ALT ratio was improved by its combination with platelet count below 150 G/l. Number of platelets declines with the progression of liver fibrosis as a consequence of sequestration in the spleen but also reduced thrombopoetin production.

Indirect markers are cost-free, thus they have not been tested in less advanced cases of liver fibrosis. Recent studies combine these markers to produce valuable scores. Several indirect markers and have been incorporated into composite panels that have been developed to evaluate the presence hepatic necroinflammation and fibrosis.

FibroTest- Acti-Test consisting of the panel of selected biochemical markers was designed to evaluate liver fibrosis and necroinflammatory activity in chronic hepatitis C (CHC) [Poynard et al., 2002; Myers et al., 2003]. The test consist of six biochemical markers: alfa2-macroglobulin (A2-M), haptoglobin (HPT), gamma glutamyltranspeptidase (GTP), total bilirubin, apolipoprotein A1 (ALP-A1) and ALT that are adjusted to the patient age and gender in a patented algorithm. No single blood test possesses sufficient negative or positive predictive value to substitute for liver biopsy, especially for the diagnosis of moderate fibrosis (F2). Each of the components adds complementary value to, the estimation of fibrosis and necroinflammatory activity. A2-M is a protein synthesized by hepatocytes, stellate cells and granulomas, which serum concentration increases during stellate cell activation in the course of fibrogenesis. As proteinases inhibitor it can increase fibrosis by inhibiting the breakdown of extracellular matrix proteins. HPT is a protein synthesized by the liver which serum level decreases with fibrosis. This decline does not depend on hemolysis or hepatic insufficiency. In the circumstances of the liver fibrosis HPT synthesis is decreased by hepatic growth factor. ALP-A1 is a protein synthesized by hepatocytes, responsible for the transport of the cholesterol. In liver fibrosis, its release is hampered by the ECM collagen fibers, moreover its transcription is equally reduced. Serum apolipoprotein A1 levels declines in the presence of fibrosis. Bilirubin is a pigment resulting from the degradation of hemoglobin, which in normal conditions is taken up from the blood, conjugated and excreted in bile. Bilirubin increases in liver fibrosis. Hepatitis C virus infection modifies the transporters of bilirubin that could explain the increase observed in the early stages of fibrosis. GTP is an enzyme synthesized by hepatocytes, which increases with fibrosis on unknown mechanisms, that are independent of the growth in aminotransferases and bilirubin. It is believed that epidermal growth factor stimulates the synthesis of GTP during of fibrogenesis. ALT is an enzyme synthesized by hepatocytes, which increases in serum when necrosis and hepatic tissue inflammation occur. Fibrotes-Actitest was proven to have high predictive value in CHC patients before and after antiviral treatment [Poynard et al., 2001], in patients with persisting normal ALT activity [Colletta et al., 2005], coinfected with HIV [Myers et al., 2003]. The test was also found useful in chronic hepatitis B (CHB) [Myers et al., 2003], alcoholic liver disease [Naveau et al., 2005], nonalcoholic fatty liver disease (NAFLD) [Ratziu et al., 2006] and hemochromatosis [Adhoute X et al., 2006]. The test was also confirmed to other single direct and indirect markers as well as the test panels. Its main disadvantage are false positive results induced by ribavirin treatment on HPT levels. Numerous publications were released concerning this method of assessment in various liver diseases. It enables direct extrapolation from the results of the test to the stages of fibrosis in different scoring systems (Table 1). The test is available on commercial bases. Thus, the chief researcher involved in validation of the test has financial interests in its manufacturing company.

| Fibrotest | METAVIR fibrosis stage estimate | Knodell fibrosis stage estimate | Ishak fibrosis stage estimate |
|---|---|---|---|
| 0.75-1.00 | F4 | F4 | F6 |
| 0.73-0.74 | F3-F4 | F3-F4 | F5 |
| 0.59-0.72 | F3 | F3 | F4 |
| 0.49-0.58 | F2 | F1-F3 | F3 |
| 0.32-0.48 | F1-F2 | F1-F3 | F2-F3 |
| 0.28-0.31 | F1 | F1 | F2 |
| 0.22-0.27 | F0-F1 | F0-F1 | F1 |
| 0.00-0.21 | F0 | F0 | F0 |

Table 1. Conversion between the results of FibroTest and fibrosis stages in METAVIR, Knodell and Ishak scoring systems. Fibrosis scoring systems.

Beside Fibrotest-Actitest, more panels of direct and indirect markers were developed.

FibroSpect evaluates liver fibrosis by analyzing the following parameters: hyaluronic acid, tissue-inhibited matrix metalloproteinase inhibitor-1 and α-2 macroglobulin [Patel et al., 2004]. The score is licensed and commercially available in the USA. Validated in several studies, the test was proven to be effective for excluding significant fibrosis and cirrhosis. Positive predictive values for detecting fibrosis were found much lower than negative values for excluding significant fibrosis or cirrhosis [Zaman et al., 2007].

Fibrosure combines quantitative results of the following parameters: A2-M, HPT, GTP, total bilirubin, ALP-A1 and ALT with a patient's age and gender in a patented artificial intelligence algorithm to create a measure of fibrosis and necroinflammatory activity in the liver. The test is an American form of Fibrotest and provides continuous numerical assessment of liver fibrosis and necroinfalmmatory activity corresponding to METAVIR scoring system. Values <0.48 exclude significant fibrosis while a score >0.78 is highly predictive for the liver cirrhosis. Values <0.36 indicate minimal activity, while scores>0.62 a specific for severe necroinflammatory activity [Poynard et al., 2004].

Hepascore includes bilirubin, GTP, A-2M, HA, age and gender [Adams et al. 2005]. A score >0.5 indicated significant fibrosis with 92% of specificity and 67% of sensitivity. While scores <0.5 had 74% specificity and 88% sensitivity to exclude advanced fibrosis. A cutoff of 0.84 had a 71% specificity and 89% of sensitivity for the prediction of liver cirrhosis. However, there was a significant overlap between patients with mild and moderate fibrosis.

Fibroindex was a proposed score that includes: platelets, AST levels and gammaglobulin according to the formula: Fibroindex=1.738 - 0.064 x platelets ($10^4/mm^3$) + 0.005 x AST (IU/l) + 0.463 x gammaglobulin (g/dl). Two threshold were proposed for the diagnosis of significant fibrosis. A score >1.25 confirmed fibrosis with 94% of specificity and >2.25 with 97% of specificity [Koda et al. 2007].

Forns score combines: age, GTP, cholesterol level, platelet count according to the formula: Forns score=7.811-3.131 x ln platelets (g/l) +0.781 x ln GTP(IU/l)+3.647 x ln age(years)-0.014 x cholesterol [Forns et al. 2002]. A score <4.2 excluded and a score>6.9 confirmed significant fibrosis. The main limitation of the scale is that the result is indefinite in many patients and no thresholds were created for the diagnosis of extensive fibrosis or cirrhosis. Thus, lipid abnormalities observed in hepatitis patients raise concerns related to the utility of the scale and requires further validation for the use in routine clinical practice.

APRI score is AST/platelets ratio calculated as (AST/upper normal limit X 100/platelet count) [Wai et al 2003] originally proposed for hepatitis C patients. In original study a score <0.5 ruled out significant fibrosis, a score <1.0 excluded cirrhosis and a score >2.0 suggested cirrhosis with good predictive value. Nevertheless, subsequent studies in hepatitis C and HIV coinfected patients had much poorer outcome. This score was found to be useful to exclude significant fibrosis and particularly cirrhosis with around 90% certainty also in HCV infected hemodialysis patients [Schiavon et al., 2007]. The results were, however much worse in alcoholic patients as alcohol may have direct effects on AST activity and platelet count. Therefore this limitation should be taken into account in daily clinical practice [Trabut et al., 2009]. APRI may be used as an easy first-line investigation, however, not as the only tool as it has moderate diagnostic utility for the prediction of fibrosis in HCV-infected patients. Its major role appears to be the exclusion of significant fibrosis and cirrhosis, which can be achieved with acceptable accuracy in at least one third and three quarters of patients, respectively [Shaheen and Myers, 2007].

FIB-4 uses the following formula: $(\text{age X AST/platelets X ALT})^{1/2}$ [Vallet-Pichard et al., 2007]. Values <1.45 ruled out extensive fibrosis and >3.25 confirmed the diagnosis with around 90% of accuracy in comparison to the histological results in the Ishak scoring system. Significant proportion of patients fell into indeterminate range of results.

Although these test give promising results in detecting advanced fibrosis their ability to replace liver biopsy is still not probable as some of them have not been sufficiently validated [Bourliere 2006]. Some of the scores like APRI may be influenced by other factors like for example alcohol abuse that may influence on the level of indirect markers in the scale. Diagnostic panels were presented in Table 2.

| Score | Parameters involved | Formula | Reference |
|---|---|---|---|
| Fibrotest-Actitest | alfa2-macroglobulin<br>haptoglobin<br>GTP<br>total bilirubin<br>apolipoprotein A1<br>ALT<br>Age<br>gender | Patented and commercially used | Poynard et al. 2002 |
| FibroSpect | hyaluronic acid<br>tissue-inhibited matrix metalloproteinase inhibitor-1<br>α-2 macroglobulin | Licensed and commercially used | Patel et al. 2004 |
| FibroSure | alfa2-macroglobulin<br>haptoglobin<br>GTP<br>total bilirubin<br>apolipoprotein A1<br>ALT | The USA patented form of Fibrotest-Actitest | Poynard et al 2004 |
| Hepascore | Bilirubin<br>GTP<br>α-2 macroglobulin<br>hyaluronic acid<br>age<br>gender | Hepascore=y/1+y;<br>y=exp [4.185818 –(0.0249 x age +(0.7464 x sex + 1.0039 x α2-macroglobulin +(0.0302x_ hyaluronic acid)+(0.0691 x bilirubin)-(0.0012 x GGT)] | Adams et al. 2005 |
| Fibroindex | PLT<br>AST<br>gammaglobulin | Fibroindex= 1.738 – 0.064 x PLT ($10^4$/mm$^3$) + 0.005 x AST (IU/l) + 0.463 x gammaglobulin (g/dl) | Koda et al. 2007 |
| APRI | AST<br>PLT | APRI = AST level (/ULN) x100<br>PLT ($10^9$/L) | Wai et al. 2003 |
| FIB-4 | Age<br>AST<br>ALT<br>PLT | FIB-4= (age X AST/PLT X ALT)$^{1/2}$ | Vallet-Pichard et al. 2007 |

Abbreviations: AST – aspartate aminotransferase, ALT – alanine aminotransferase, GTP- gamma glutamyltranspeptidase, UNL – upper normal limit, PLT – platelet count

Table 2. Serum diagnostic panels of direct and indirect markers.

### 2.3 Serum markers of steatosis

Several studies proposed various tests to distinguish between simple steatosis and NASH in patients with NAFLD. The most important parameters are acute phase proteins as they enable to establish NASH. Several markers of inflammation were extensively studied in relation to fatty liver disease. C-reactive protein (CRP) is an acute phase parameter that is produced in the liver and increases in various inflammatory conditions. The evaluation of serum CRP levels was found to be associated with NASH and helps to differentiate this

condition from simple steatosis. Furthermore, high levels of high-sensitivity CRP were found to be associated with extensive liver fibrosis in NASH [Yoneda et al. ,2007].
Nevertheless, study conducted in children with liver steatosis revealed that fatty liver itself may not be a cofactor in stimulating inflammatory markers in obese patients. Obese children with NAFLD may have simple steatosis and their increased inflammatory markers are therefore compatible with those expected in obesity [Neuman et al. ,2010].
Another acute phase protein used to distinguish NASH from non-NASH patients is plasma pentraxin-3 (PTX 3) a novel marker that seems to be promising in assessing the severity of fibrosis. Plasma PTX-3 levels were, however, found increased not only in NASH, but also in other cardiovascular and inflammatory conditions and vasculites [Yoneda et al., 2008].
Interleukin-6 seems to be another marker playing an important role in fatty liver disease. This biomarker is a cytokine synthesized in hepatocytes, endothelial cells, adipocytes and cells of the immune system, that rises in NAFLD and indicates inflammatory activity and liver fibrosis [Wieckowska et al. , 2008].
Tumor necrosis factor-alpha (TNF-alpha) is another proinflammatory cytokine which role in NASH was clearly established. As levels of TNF-alpha are increased in NASH, anti-TNF-alpha therapy was found effective in the improvement of liver histology and normalization of aminotransferase levels.
Cytokeraitn-18 is a marker of hepatic apoptosis and is utility in the detection of NASH is based on the observation that apoptosis is prominent in NASH and absent in simple steatosis. Its use is, however, so far limited to research areas [Wieckowska et al. , 2008].
As oxidative stress has been found to play an important role in NASH pathogenesis several parameters were evaluated in various studies: vitamin E levels, glutathione peroxidase activity and superoxide dismutase activity [Hardwick et al.,2010]. None of these markers reflect liver histology in NASH, therefore its clinical value is still questionable and were not entirely defined yet. The assessment of the liver fibrosis is an important component in the evaluation of NASH as end stage liver disease is constantly present in this state. Several matrix components have been studied in various trials: HA, TGF beta-1, TIMP and other markers. Nevertheless so far none of them entered clinical use.
To avoid liver biopsy several noninvasive panels of serological markers have been developed to assess the presence of hepatic necroinflammation and steatosis. SteatoTest is a quantitative test designed to estimate liver steatosis especially in patients with metabolic syndrome [62]. NASH test is a variation of SteatoTest and ActiTest for the differentiation of simple steatosis from NASH and should be performed only if SteatoTest is positive. The scores combine various parameters. The NASH test combines total bilirubin, GGT, α2-macroglobulin, apolipoprotein A1, haptoglobin and ALT, and is adjusted for age and gender plus weight, height, AST, serum glucose, triglycerides, cholesterol and SteatoTest.
NASH FibroSURE is the USA patented algorithm combining quantitative results of 10 biochemical parameters, including A2M, HPT, ALP-A1, bilirubin, GTP, ALT, AST, total cholesterol, triglycerides, and fasting glucose, in relation to the age, gender, height, and weight. The registered algorithm provides quantitative alternate markers for liver fibrosis, hepatic steatosis, and NASH. Markers of fibrosis are corresponding to METAVIR scoring system. Marker of hepatic steatosis varies from S0 to S3 and is corresponding to 0% to >66%. In a study conducted on patients with significant (>5%) steatosis score a value >0.5 confirmed steatosis with high sensitivity and specificity [Poynard et al., 2005]. The test also provides a diagnostic assessment of the presence of NASH using three broad categories N0-N2 corresponding to "Not NASH," "Borderline NASH," and "NASH" per the Kleiner classification [Kleiner et al.;2005].

Other tests combine both direct and indirect markers or other clinical parameters: age, gender, BMI, AST, AST/ALT ratio, hyaluronan [Palekar et al., 2006] or adiponectin and collagen type IV [Shimada et al., 2007].
Various test panel were compared with one another. The results are, however, ambiguous and vary from study to study. Although patented commercial tests seem to present a higher diagnostic value, simply non-patented panels are much easier available.

## 3. Transient elastography

Non-invasive assessment of the liver fibrosis is also possible by transient elastography. The technique is performed by device called Fibroscan that enables the assessment of the liver stiffness. The device holds an ultrasound probe in a vibrating piston that induces elastic vibrations propagating through the liver. The reflected waves captivated by a transducer enable to measure the liver elasticity that is inversely related to the speed of the waves [Sandrin 2003]. After several measurements, calculated mean value enables the exact assessment of liver fibrosis. This method was proven precise enough when compared to the liver biopsy and evaluates a portion of the liver 500 times bigger than conventional method [Castera 2005]. Transient elastography is described in detailed in another chapter of this book.
It was also used in combination with serum markers of fibrosis. The Fibro-Stiffness index is a panel consisting of liver stiffness measured by Fibroscan, platelet count and prothrombin time. The method demonstrated superior diagnostic performance to liver stiffness obtained by elastography alone, the APRI, the Forns score and the FibroIndex for significant and severe fibrosis and liver cirrhosis. The diagnostic value of the Fibro-Stiffness index for liver cirrhosis was increased by combination with serum HA levels [Ichino et al., 2010].
Various test panles were validated either compared to elastography or used simultaneously with this method. The most promising results were obtained were both serum markers and elastography were used together.

## 4. Imaging techniques

Conventional imaging techniques that include ultrasound with Doppler, CT and MRI can be used to evaluate advanced liver cirrhosis. Their ability to detect minor lesions is, however, limited [Hussain 2005].

### 4.1 Hepatic ultrasound

Ultrasonography is simple, inexpensive, easy to reproduce and can be repeatedly used to assess changes over time. It is a first-line imaging technique, a simple non-invasive method, that is widely used in clinical practice to detect fatty infiltration of the liver. It assesses the presence of steatosis detecting a hyperechogenic parenchyma of the liver displayed as "bright liver " or "blurring of the vascular margins". An ultrasound index for quantitative assessment of the liver steatosis is the hepato-renal contrast. Normal liver shows an echostructure similar to renal parenchyma. In liver steatosis the increased echogenity forms hepato-renal contrast. Severity of liver steatosis was assessed according to a discrepancy in ultrasonographic liver-kidney densities. The hepato-renal index was supposed to quantify the severity of liver steatosis to a lower limit of 5% [Webb et al. , 2007].
Spleen longitudinal parameter is another simple, noninvasive and easy to perform parameter, that could differentiate between NAFLD and NASH better than serum markers with values exceeding 11.6 cm for predicting NASH.

When the degree of steatosis is less than 30%, sensitivity of this technique is low. Moreover, it is impossible to detect inflammatory changes of the hepatic parenchyma and to differentiate between simple steatosis and staeatohepatitis. Therefore, it is very difficult to distinguish between the liver steatosis and liver fibrosis as both changes look similar on ultrasound.

The biggest limitation of this technique is morbid obesity as ultrasonographic examination is difficult to perform in such patients. Ultrasonography is, however, insufficient for detecting early and intermediate stages of fibrosis.

### 4.1.1 Doppler ultrasound

Doppler ultrasound is another helpful tool in the diagnosis of steatosis. Hepatic parenchyma perfusion abnormalities were observed in NASH. Altered hepatic hemodynamics can be described by various parameters including, among others, hepatic vein Doppler pattern and Doppler perfusion index (DPI), which is a ratio between hepatic arterial blood flow and total liver blood flow. DPI allows for the detection of overt liver metastatic disease and helps to differentiate between benign and malignant focal hepatic lesions [Kyriakopoulou et al. ,2008]. DPI was also found predictive of the liver steatosis in patients with NAFLD in the study conducted on a small group of patients, therefore it requires further evaluation [Dugoni et al. 2007]. Conventional Doppler ultrasound examination of hepatic vasculature is, unfortunately not a good tool to evaluate mild and moderate fibrosis. Data reporting the use of hepatic vein blood flow pattern assessment suggests improvements in detecting advanced fibrosis and cirrhosis [Bertzigotti et al., 2010].

### 4.1.2 Contrast-enhanced ultrasonography

This technique allows to overcome limitations of simple ultrasonography. Hepatic vein transit times (HVTT) were evaluated with microbubble contrast agent and were found to predict disease severity in patients with hepatitis C. The uptake of another contrast agent levovist was decreased in NASH due to cell injury, when compared to NAFLD. The study was, however conducted on a small group of patients and should be validated on a larger cohort to establish the role of this technique in clinical practice.

## 4.2 Computed tomography

Computed tomography (CT) provides improved resolution of early liver cirrhosis in the absence of portal hypertension but remains unhelpful in a detection of fibrosis. Even more advanced variations as helical and multidetector row CT reveal early morphological changes with cirrhosis but do not identify fibrosis.

Nevertheless, this conventional technique is a helpful tool in detecting steatosis. Moreover, non-contrast enhanced CT is the best way to identify and characterize hepatic steatosis. Changes in signal sensitivity are related to the liver density, therefore as liver density decreases, the liver steatosis increases. Although abdominal ultrasound is more sensitive in the diagnosis of fatty liver disease, CT scans are more adequate when the fat deposition is focal. They may also be used to evaluate thickened abdominal fatty tissue and to measure the fat in the liver [Davidson et al., 2006]. CT scans may also be used to visualize enlarged spleen and portal hypertension, which may suggest advanced fibrosis. Calculation of the liver-to-spleen attenuation ratio allows grading of steatosis [Park et al., 2006]. As the images appear enhanced, non-contrast CT is chosen for detecting steatosis. Focal fatty lesions may

be detected by dual-energy CT scans or by contrast enhanced CT. Figure 1 provides picture of multiple fatty lesions in the liver.
However the difficulty to identify intermediate fibrotic stages and the uselessness in the follow-up of the patients due to the exposure to radiation are major limitations of CT.

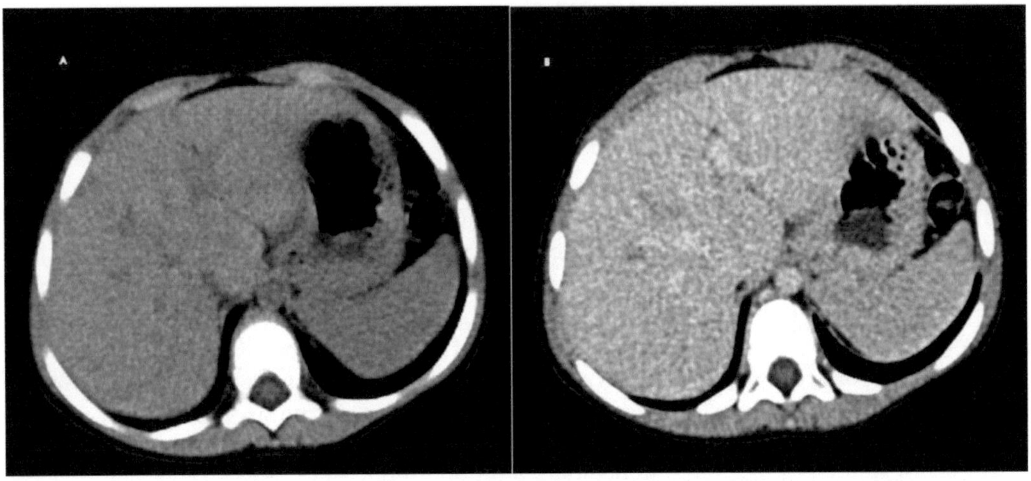


Fig. 1. Computed tomography with multiple focal lesions in the liver (A) of lower density than the liver parenchyma after contrast-enhancement (B) corresponding to hemangiomas.

### 4.3 Magnetic resonance imaging

Magnetic resonance imaging (MRI) reliably identifies cirrhosis but does not show earlier stages of fibrosis. Specific features on MRI including hepatic vein narrowing, caudate to right lobe ratio, and expanded gallbladder fossa, reliably identify cirrhosis but remain absent in earlier stages of fibrosis [Numminen et al., 2005]. This technique provides an accurate and fast evaluation of the liver steatosis even if the degree is low (around 3%). Good correlation between liver steatosis, MRI and liver biopsy have also been recently demonstrated [Hussain 2005]. Phase-contrast imaging is used for the quantitative assessment of fatty infiltrations in various liver diseases. Lower intensity in T1-weighted images may be used in the detection of focal fat depositions [Szczepaniak et al., 2005].
Significant number of technological advances in developing clinical applications for MRI of the liver have been made over the past decade. Recent improvements focused on using the physiological and biomechanical properties of human liver tissue to improve the detection of focal and diffuse pathological conditions of this organ. New techniques such as magnetic resonance (MR) spectroscopy, diffusion-weight MR, MR elastography are evaluated to examine fibrosis [Talwalkar 2008].

#### 4.3.1 Contrast-enhanced magnetic resonance imaging

The development of contrast-enhanced imaging of the liver have been enabled by the introduction of gadolinium chelates to clinical practice. Changes in hepatic parenchyma were described in various studies after contrast-enhanced imaging by MRI [Gandhi et al., 2006]. Early irregular enhancement corresponds to the increased necroinflammatory activity in the liver histology due to higher numbers of macrophages. Whereas, a postponed, heterogeneous enhancement is related to hepatic fibrosis as a result of bright-appearing reticulations. This finding may be explained by a reduced distribution of gadolinium in extracellular spaces of the liver [Semelka et al., 2001]. Contrast enhancement depends on the contrast agents. Supermagnetic iron oxide (SPIO) contrast media result in hypointensity within hepatic parenchyma as they accumulate in reticulo-endothelial cells [Yamashita et al., 1996]. The most interesting findings were, however, obtained by sequential administration of gadolinium followed by SPIO contrast agents. Highly accurate SPIO-based images were even improved in accuracy for the detection of liver fibrosis architecture [Aguirre et al., 2006]. Further validation of semi quantitative fibrosis criteria is required to verify the diagnostic performance of this technique.

#### 4.3.2 Magnetic resonance spectroscopy

Magnetic resonance spectroscopy (MRS) has been available for the last twenty years allowing evaluation of metabolism of various tissues. The liver is considered to be an ideal organ for MRS due to its anatomical location and increased metabolic demands. MRS is usually used to evaluate signals from hydrogen, which allows for quantitative assessment of lipids and from phosphorus, which reflects cellular turnover and energy state [Solga et al., 2005]. MRS of the liver is performed after a standard MR imaging for localization. Special MR pulse sequences are used to produce spectroscopic data within the suitable anatomical location and volume of interest. Peak area of metabolite signal is directly related to its concentration, which may be expressed in absolute or relative conditions. As the absolute quantification is difficult to obtain in vivo, many studies use metabolite ratios for the evaluation of spectral profiles. Peak areas of the spectrum are compared to standards for correlation with the strength of MR signal. The most widely used standard is adenozyne triphosphate (ATP), taking into account its natural distributions in the tissues. Changes in phospholipids metabolism, reflected in increased phosphomonoesters signal or increased phopsphomonoesters/phosphodiesters ratio in patients with liver cirrhosis, are believed to be associated with regenerating activity - extensive membrane remodeling.
MRS represents useful method for highly accurate noninvasive measurement of liver steatosis [Friedrich-Rust 2010]. This technique measures the fat proton fraction and hepatic trigliceryde level. Concentration exceeding 5% is a limit of the detection of steatosis. MRS describes metabolic processes of cellular regeneration, therefore it can assess the disease severity in NASH. This technique is probably more accurate for the diagnosis of NAFLD but it requires further validation in humans.
The studies have to be, however, repeated and validated on the larger number of patients with various liver diseases using unified methods.

#### 4.3.3 Diffusion weight magnetic resonance imaging

Diffusion-weighted magnetic resonance imaging (DWI) has been widely used for the early detection of cerebral ischemia. This technique measures the freedom of water proton diffusion in tissues and was recently facilitated to be used for abdominal imaging [Naganawa et al., 2005]. As collagen is not reach in unbound water, therefore in the liver fibrosis the amount of water proton diffusion is restricted in affected tissue. DWI produces a signal inversely related to the freedom of water proton diffusion. Tissues with reduced distribution are brighter than normal. The strength of diffusion weighting is described by "b" value of the sequence, which rises with time and amplitude of the gradients responsible for the diffusion. Apparent diffusion coefficient (ADC) of water proton in tissues may be calculated from DWI images. It is determined by the grade of the log intensity set against b value [Girometti et al., 2007]. Possibility to display the calculated ADC values as images enable the quantitative analysis by the measurements of the mean values within region of interest. This measurement is usually performed in the right hepatic parenchyma, where major vessels are not present.

Patients with liver cirrhosis were found to have lower ADC compared to healthy individuals. Nevertheless, the results of the studies in patients with various stages of fibrosis are ambiguous with respect to demonstrating a specific relationship between ADC values and fibrosis stage [Koinuma et al., 2005].

Before the DWI becomes more widely used in clinical practice, the studies would have to be conducted on a larger number of patients and properly validated in relation to different hardware and sequencing profiles as currently comparisons are difficult. It was also detected that significant hepatic iron accumulation may considerably reduce signal intensity making DWI impossible in patients with hemochromatosis [Aube et al., 2004]. Fat suppression techniques are necessary in DWI performed in the liver steatosis as otherwise imaging is seriously affected.

### 4.3.4 Magnetic resonance elastography

Many pathological processes as malignancies and liver fibrosis result in increased liver stiffness, which may be detected by physical examination on palpation. Normal liver tissue is similar to fatty tissue on palpation, whereas cirrhotic liver is much harder. Recent reports suggest that the stiffness of hepatic matrix may influence continued differentiation of hepatic stellate cells and the production of fibrosis. Beside ultrasonography-based elastography, a MR-based elastography was described for evaluation of the stiffness of various tissues. The technique uses a phase-contrast method to display the propagation characteristics of acoustic sheer waves generated within the organ of interest [Kruse et al., 2000]. Elastography is usually added to a conventional MR examination of the abdomen with pneumatic or electromechanical driver placed on abdominal wall in the supine patient. The device is used to generate mechanical waves that propagate in the liver at various frequencies [Yin et al., 2007]. A specialized phase contrast MRI sequence, is subsequently used to image the propagating waves in the liver with motion-encoding gradients that are oscillated along with applied movements enabling clear imaging of the waves with very small amplitudes. Provided images represent displacement generated by shear wave propagation in the tissue. They are subsequently processed using a particular inversion algorithm to produce quantitative images describing the tissue stiffness called elastograms. The imaging allows for the measurement of mean elasticity values within the liver, presented in in kilopascals, as in the case of ultrasound-based transient elastography.

Mean liver stiffness in patients with chronic liver diseases was found significantly increased, compared to healthy volunteers in various studies [Klatt et al., 2006]. A quadratic relationship between histological fibrosis stage and elasticity measurements were observed in the studies using ultrasound-based transient elastography. MR elastography was detecting stages 2 to 4 with good sensitivity and specificity. Thus, no relationship between hepatic steatosis and liver stiffness was found. MR elastography was a useful tool to exclude the presence of the liver fibrosis suggesting that this technique could be valuable in finding indications for the liver biopsy [Yin et al., 2007].

Several advantages of this method were observed in relation to its potential use in different populations: potential assessment of entire hepatic parenchyma, operator independence and the ability to obtain a conventional abdominal MRI at the same time. Correspondingly to other techniques, the equipment and sequences have to be standardized in order to increase the accuracy of the results and enable comparison of different studies. Further assessment is also necessary to characterize the procedure including its reproducibility among patients with progressive liver disease.

#### 4.3.5 Multi-echo magnetic resonance

Multi-echo MRI allows simultaneous T2 and fat content evaluation. This method can be used to define the fat-to-water ratio as well as T2 values [O'Regan et al., 2008].

#### 4.3.6 Magnetic resonance cholangiopancreatography

Magnetic resonance cholangiopancreatography (MRCP) is a well-established non-invasive imaging method that creates images of the biliary tree and pancreatic duct without the necessity of intravenous contrast. The images are corresponding to those from endoscopic retrograde cholangiopancreatography (ERCP). The most common indications for this technique include choledocholithiasis, primary sclerosing cholangitis or stricture of bile ducts and others. MRCP also plays an important role in other conditions involving cholangiohepatitis, inborn malformations, tumors and other cysts. The biggest advantage of this technique is the lack of contrast administration, relative operator independence and possibility to evaluate both sides of obstructed ducts with exact stricture size and morphology. Example of MRCP imaging was presented in Figure 2.

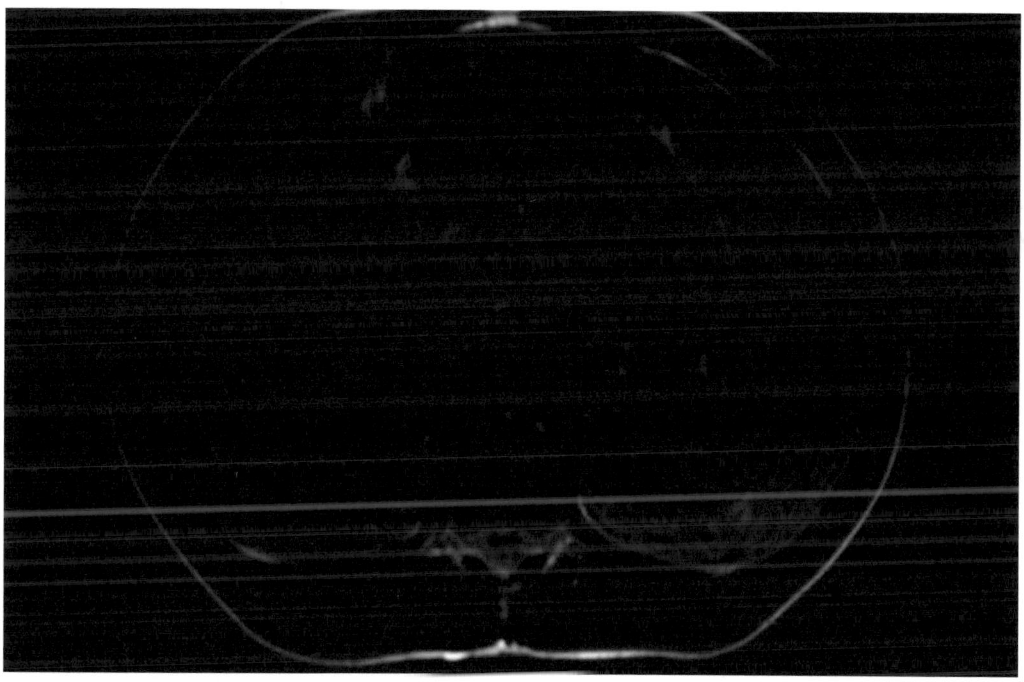

Fig. 2. MRCP image showing the liver of patient with primary sclerosing cholangitis and numerous fibrous septa within the liver with coexisting splenomegaly.

A reliable and valuable noninvasive method to assess hepatic fibrosis would be a very useful clinical tool. Several MR techniques or their combinations are still evaluated to meet

these requirements and are very promising. Further research is, however necessary to create true functional hepatic imaging.
Clinical utility of imaging techniques is still under evaluation. Advanced MRI techniques are available in tertiary medical centers and it will probably take time before they become widely available. Furthermore, even with this technique some patients may be unable or unwilling to undergo the examination.

## 5. Conclusions

Combination of non-invasive methods like Fibro-test and elastography may substitute the liver biopsy in a near future. They are reliable in patients either with no or progressed fibrosis. Evaluation of intermediate states is, however, difficult. For this reason the liver biopsy remains a most valuable tool in evaluation of the liver and according to current guidelines treatment decisions should be made after liver biopsy. Thus, non-invasive methods may be still an option for patients with contraindications to the liver biopsy or a helpful monitoring tool for those who are reluctant or unable to undergo repeated biopsies.

## 6. Acknowledgements

This paper was supported by a grant from The Ministry of Science and Higher Education No -NN407 012036 to A. Mania

## 7. References

Adams LA, Bulsara M, Rossi E, DeBoer B, Speers D, George J, Kench J, Farrell G, McCaughan GW & Jeffrey GP. Hepascore: an accurate validated predictor of liver fibrosis in chronic hepatitis C infection. Clin Chem. 2005;51:1867-73

Adhoute X, Foucher J, Castera L, Lovato B, Laharie D, Bertet J, Couzigou P & de Ledinghen V. Is liver stiffness mesurement useful in genetic hemochromatosis and hepatosiderosis? J Hepatol. 2006; 44: S242

Aguirre DA, Behling CA, Alpert E, Hassanein TI & Sirlin CB. Liver fibrosis: noninvasive diagnosis with double contrast material-enhanced MR imaging. Radiology 2006;239:425-437

Aube C, Racineux PX, Lebigot J, Oberti F, Croquet V, Argaud C, Cales P, Caron C. Diagnosis and quantification of hepatic fibrosis with diffusion weighted MR imaging: preliminary results. J Radiol 2004;85:301-306

Berzigotti A, Nicolau C, Bellot P, Abraldes JG, Gilabert R, García-Pagan JC & Bosch J. Evaluation of Regional Hepatic Perfusion (RHP) by Contrast-ENHANCED Ultrasound in Patients with Cirrhosis. J Hepatol. 2010 Dec 14. [Epub ahead of print]

Boeker KH, Haberkorn CI, Michels D, Flemming P, Manns MP & Lichtinghagen R. Diagnostic potential of circulating TIMP-1 and MMP-2 as markers of liver fibrosis in patients with chronic hepatitis C. Clin Chim Acta. 2002;316:71-81

Bourliere M, Penaranda G, Renou C, Botta-Fridlund D, Tran A, Portal I, Lecomte L, Castellani P, Rosenthal-Allieri MA, Gerolami R, Ouzan D, Deydier R, Degott C & Halfon P. Validation and comparison of indexes for fibrosis and cirrhosis prediction in chronic hepatitis C patients: proposal for a pragmatic approach classification without liver biopsies. J Viral Hepat. 2006;13:659-70

Castera L, Vergniol J, Foucher J, Le Bail B, Chanteloup E, Haaser M, Darriet M, Couzigou P & De Ledinghen V. Prospective comparison of transient elastography, Fibrotest, APRI, and liver biopsy for the assessment of fibrosis in chronic hepatitis C. Gastroenterology 2005; 128: 343-350

Cholongitas E, Senzolo M, Standish RA, Marelli L, Quaglia A, Patch D, Dhillon AP & Burroughs AK. A systemic review of the quality of liver biopsy specimens. Am J Clin Pathol 2006; 125: 710–21

Colletta C, Smirne C, Fabris C, Toniutto P, Rapetti R, Minisini R & Pirisi M. Value of two noninvasive methods to detect progression of fibrosis among HCV carriers with normal aminotransferases. Hepatology. 2005;42:838-45

Croquet V, Vuillemin E, Ternisien C, Pilette C, Oberti F, Gallois Y, Trossaert M, Rousselet MC, Chappard D & Calès P. Prothrombin index is an indirect marker of severe liver fibrosis. Eur J Hepatol 2002;14:1133-41

Davidson LE, Kuk JL, Church TS & Ross R. Protocol for measurement of liver fat by computed tomography. J Appl Physiol. 2006;100:864-8

Dugoni M, Miglioli L, Borelli L, Anderlini R, Bedogni G, Mariano M, Battistini N, & Bellentani S. Doppler perfusion index (DPI) and homa are highly predictive of fatty liver in patients with NAFLD. Dig Liver Dis 2007;40:A39.

Forns X, Ampurdanès S, Llovet JM, Aponte J, Quintó L, Martínez-Bauer E, Bruguera M, Sánchez-Tapias JM & Rodés J. Identification of chronic hepatitis C patients without hepatic fibrosis by a simple predictive model. Hepatology. 2002;36:986-92

Friedrich-Rust M, Müller C, Winckler A, Kriener S, Herrmann E, Holtmeier J, Poynard T, Vogl TJ, Zeuzem S, Hammerstingl R & Sarrazin C. Assessment of liver fibrosis and steatosis in PBC with FibroScan, MRI, MR-spectroscopy, and serum markers. J Clin Gastroenterol. 2010;44:58-65

Gandhi SN, Brown MA, Wong JG, Aguirre DA & Sirilin CB. MR contrast agents for liver imaging: what, when, how. Radiographics 2006;26:1621-1636

Girometti R, Furlan A, Bazzocchi M, Soldano F, Isola M, Toniutto P, Bitetto D & Zuiani C. Diffusion-weighted MRI in evaluating liver fibrosis: a feasibility study in cirrhotic patients. Radiol Med 2007;112:394-408

Hardwick RN, Fisher CD, Canet MJ, Lake AD & Cherrington NJ. Diversity in antioxidant response enzymes in progressive stages of human nonalcoholic fatty liver disease. Drug Metab Dispos 2010;38:2293-301

Hussain SM & Semelka RC. Hepatic imaging: comparison of modalities. Radiol Clin North Am 2005;43:929-947

Klatt D, Asbach P, Rump J, Papazoglou S, Somasundaram R, Modrow J, Braun J & Sack I. In vivo determination of hepatic stiffness using steady-state free precision magnetic resonance elastography. Invest Radiol 2006;41:841-848

Kleiner DE, Brunt EM, Van Natta M, Behling C, Contos MJ, Cummings OW, Ferrell LD, Liu YC, Torbenson MS, Unalp-Arida A, Yeh M, McCullough AJ & Sanyal AJ; Nonalcoholic Steatohepatitis Clinical Research Network. Design and validation of a histological scoring system for nonalcoholic fatty liver disease. Hepatol. 2005 ; 41:1313-1321

Koda M, Matunaga Y, Kawakami M, Kishimoto Y, Suou T & Murawaki Y. Fibroindex, a practical index for predicting significant fibrosis in patients with chronic hepatitis C. Hepatology 2007;45:297-306

Koinuma M, Ohashi I, Hanafusa K & Shibuya H. Apparent diffusion coefficient measurements with diffusion-weighted magnetic resonance imaging for evaluation of hepatic fibrosis. J Magn Reson Imaging 2005;22:80-85

Kruse SA, Smith JA, Lawrence AJ, Dresner MA, Manduca A, Greenleaf JF & Ehman RL. Tissue characterization using magnetic resonance elastography: preliminary results. Phys Med Biol 2000;45:1579-1590

Kyriakopoulou K, Antoniou A, Fezoulidis IV, Kelekis NL, Dalekos GN & Vlychou M. The role of Doppler Perfusion Index as screening test in the characterization of focal liver lesions. Dig Liver Dis. 2008;40:755-60.

Leroy V, Monier F, Bottari S, Trocme C, Sturm N, Hilleret MN, Morel F & Zarski JP. Circulating matrix metalloproteinases 1, 2, 9 and their inhibitors TIMP-1 and TIMP-2 as serum markers of liver fibrosis in patients with chronic hepatitis C: comparison with PIIINP and hyaluronic acid. Am J Gastroenterol. 2004;99:271-9

Marek B, Mazurek U, Janczewska-Kazek E, Strzałka B, Beniowski M, Kos-Kudła B, Kajdaniuk J, Niedziołka D, Ostrowska Z, Borgiel-Marek H, Siemińiska L, Nowak M, Pakuła D, Gatnar A, Gnot R & Filipczyk P. Serum aminoterminal peptide of type III procollagen (PIIINP) and transforming growth factor-beta1 (TGF-beta1) levels in patients with chronic hepatitis B and C. Pol Arch Med Wewn. 2003 ;109:603-8

McHutchinson JG, Blatt LM, de Medina M, Craig JR, Conrad A, Shiff ER & Tong MJ. Measurement of serum hyaluronic acid levels in patients with chronic hepatitis C and its relationship to the liver histology. Consensus Interferon Study Group. J Gastroenterol Hepatol 2000;15:945-51

Myers RP, Benhamou Y, Imbert-Bismut F, Thibault V, Bochet M, Charlotte F, Ratziu V, Bricaire F, Katlama C & Poynard T. Serum biochemical markers accurately predict liver fibrosis in HIV and hepatitis C virus-coinfected patients. AIDS 2003; 17: 721-25

Myers RP, Tainturier MH, Ratziu V, Piton A, Thibault V, Imbert-Bismut F, Messous D, Charlotte F, Di Martino V, Benhamou Y & Poynard T. Prediction of liver histological lesions with biochemical markers in patients with chronic hepatitis B. J Hepatol. 2003;39:222-30.

Naganawa S, Kawai H, Fukatsu H, Sakurai Y, Aoki I, Miura S, Mimura T, Kanazawa H & Ishigaki T. Diffusion-weighted imaging of the liver: technical challenges and prospects for the future. Magn Reson Med Sci 2005;4:175-186

Naveau S, Raynard B, Ratziu V, Abella A, Imbert-Bismut F, Messous D, Beuzen F, Capron F, Thabut D, Munteanu M, Chaput JC & Poynard T. Biomarkers for the prediction of liver fibrosis in patients with chronic alcoholic liver disease (ALD). Clin Gastroenterol Hepatol. 2005; 3: 167-74

Neuman G, Sagi R, Shalitin S & Reif S. Serum inflammatory markers in overweight children and adolescents with non-alcoholic fatty liver disease. IMAJ 2010; 12: 410–415

Numminen K, Tervahartiala P, Halavaara J, Isoniemi H & Hockerstedt K. Non-invasive diagnosis of liver cirrhosis: magnetic resonance imaging presents special features. Scand J Gastroenterol 2005;40:76-82

O'Regan DP, Callaghan MF, Wylezinska-Arridge M, Fitzpatrick J, Naoumova RP, Hajnal JV & Schmitz SA. Liver fat content and T2*: simultaneous measurement by using breathhold multiecho MR imaging at 3.0 T--feasibility. Radiology 2008; 247: 550-557

Palekar NA, Naus R, Larson SP, Ward J & Harrison SA. Clinical model for distinguishing nonalcoholic steatohepatitis from simple steatosis in patients with nonalcoholic fatty liver disease. Liver Int. 2006;26:151-6

Park SH, Kim PN, Kim KW, Lee SW, Yoon SE, Park SW, Ha HK, Lee MG, Hwang S, Lee SG, Yu ES & Cho EY. Macrovesicular hepatic steatosis in living liver donors: use of CT for quantitative and qualitative assessment. Radiology 2006; 239: 105-112

Patel K, Lajoie A, Heaton S, Pianko S, Behling CA, Bylund D, Pockros PJ, Blatt LM, Conrad A & McHutchison JG. Clinical use of hyaluronic acid as a predictor of fibrosis change in hepatitis C. J Gastroenterol Hepatol. 2003;18:253-7

Patel K, Gordon SC, Jacobson I, Hézode C, Oh E, Smith KM, Pawlotsky JM & McHutchison JG. Evaluation of a panel of non-invasive serum markers to differentiate mild from moderate-to-advanced liver fibrosis in chronic hepatitis C patients. J Hepatol. 2004 ;41:935-42

Poynard T, Imbert-Bismut F, Ratziu V, Chevret S, Jardel C, Moussalli J, Messous D & Degos F; GERMED cyt04 group. Biochemical markers of liver fibrosis in patients infected by hepatitis C virus: longitudinal validation in a randomized trial. J Viral Hepatitis. 2002; 9:128-33

Poynard T, McHutchison J, Manns M, Myers RP & Albrecht J. Biochemical surrogate markers of liver fibrosis and activity in a randomized trial of peginterferon alfa-2b and ribavirin. Hepatology. 2003; 38: 481-92

Poynard T, Imbert-Bismut F, Munteanu M, Messous D, Myers RP, Thabut D, Ratziu V, Mercadier A, Benhamou Y & Hainque B. Overview of the diagnostic value of biochemical markers of liver fibrosis (FibroTest, HCV FibroSure) and necrosis (ActiTest) in patients with chronic hepatitis C. Comp Hepatol. 2004; 3:8-19

Poynard T, Ratziu V, Naveau S, Thabut D, Charlotte F, Messous D, Capron D, Abella A, Massard J, Ngo Y, Munteanu M, Mercadier A, Manns M & Albrecht J. The diagnostic value of biomarkers (SteatoTest) for the prediction of liver steatosis. Comp Hepatol. 2005 Dec 23;4:10

Ratziu V, Massard J, Charlotte F, Messous D, Imbert-Bismut F, Bonyhay L, Tahiri M, Munteanu M, Thabut D, Cadranel JF, Le Bail B, De Ledinghen V & Poynard T, the LIDO Study Group and the CYTOL Study Group Diagnostic value of biochemical markers (FibroTest-FibroSURE) for the prediction of liver fibrosis in patients with non-alcoholic fatty liver disease. BMC Gastroenterology 2006, 6:6

Resino S, Bellón JM, Asensio C, Micheloud D, Miralles P, Vargas A, Catalán P, López JC, Alvarez E, Cosin J, Lorente R, Muñoz-Fernández MA & Berenguer J. Can serum hyaluronic acid replace simple non-invasive indexes to predict liver fibrosis in HIV/Hepatitis C coinfected patients?. BMC Infectious Diseases 2010 10:244

Sandrin L, Fourquet B, Hasquenoph JM, Yon S, Fournier C, Mal F, Christidis C, Ziol M, Poulet B, Kazemi F, Beaugrand M & Palau R. Transient elastography: a new noninvasive method for assessment of hepatic fibrosis. Ultrasound Med Biol. 2003;29:1705-13

Schiavon LL, Schiavon JL, Filho RJ, Sampaio JP, Lanzoni VP, Silva AE & Ferraz ML. Simple blood tests as noninvasive markers of liver fibrosis in hemodialysis patients with chronic hepatitis C virus infection. Hepatology. 2007;46:307-14

Semelka RC, Chung JJ, Hussain SM, Marcos HB & Woosley JT. Chronic hepatitis: correlation of early patchy and late linear enhancement patterns on gadolinium-enhanced MR images with histopathology initial experience. J Magn Reson Imaging 2001;13:385-391

Shaheen AA &, Myers RP Diagnostic accuracy of the aspartate aminotransferase to-platelet ratio index for the prediction of hepatitis C–related fibrosis: a systematic review. Hepatology 2007; 46:912-920

Shimada M, Kawahara H, Ozaki K, Fukura M, Yano H, Tsuchishima M, Tsutsumi M & Takase S. Usefulness of a combined evaluation of the serum adiponectin level, HOMA-IR, and serum type IV collagen 7S level to predict the early stage of nonalcoholic steatohepatitis. Am J Gastroenterol. 2007 ;102:1931-8

Solga SF, Horska A, Clark JM & Diehl AM. Hepatic 31P magnetic resonancespectroscopy: a hepatologist's user guide. Liver Int 2005;25:490-500

Szczepaniak LS, Nurenberg P, Leonard D, Browning JD, Reingold JS, Grundy S, Hobbs HH & Dobbins RL. Magnetic resonance spectroscopy to measure hepatic triglyceride content: prevalence of hepatic steatosis in the general population. Am J Physiol Endocrinol Metab 2005; 288: E462-E468

Talwalkar JA, Yin M, Fidler JL, Sanderson SO, Kamath PS & Ehman RL. Magnetic resonance imaging of hepatic fibrosis: emerging clinical applications. Hepatology. 2008; 47:332-42

Trabut JB, Mallet V & Pol S. Aspartate aminotransferase to platelet ratio index (APRI) score is inappropriate for assessment of liver fibrosis in HIV-infected patients with hazardous drinking. HIV Med. 2009;10:524

Vallet-Pichard A, Mallet V, Nalpas B, Verkarre V, Nalpas A, Dhalluin-Venier V, Fontaine H & Pol S. FIB-4: an inexpensive and accurate marker of fibrosis in HCV infection. comparison with liver biopsy and Fibrotest. Hepatology 2007;46:32-6

Wai CT, Greenson JK, Fontana RJ, Kalbfleisch JD, Marrero JA, Conjeevaram HS & Lok AS. A simple noninvasive index can predict both significant fibrosis and cirrhosis in patients with chronic hepatitis C. Hepatology. 2003;38:518-26

Walsh KM, Fletcher A, MacSween RN & Morris AJ. Basement membrane peptides as markers of liver disease in chronic hepatitis C.J Hepatol. 2000 ;32:325-30

Webb M, Hanny Yeshua H, Zelber-Sagie S, Santo M, Barazovski E, Katz R, Halpern Z & Oren R. Diagnostic value of a computerized hepatorenal index for sonographic quantification of liver steatosis. AJR Am J Roentgenol 2009 ;192:909-14

Wieckowska A, McCullough AJ & Feldstein AE. Noninvasive diagnosis and monitoring of nonalcoholic steatohepatitis: present and future. Hepatology 2007; 46: 582-589

Wieckowska A, Papouchado BG, Li Z, Lopez R, Zein NN & Feldstein AE. Increased hepatic and circulating interleukin-6 levels in human nonalcoholic steatohepatitis. Am J Gastroenterol 2008; 103: 1372-1379

Yamashita Y, Yamamoto H, Hirai A, Yoshimatsu S, Baba Y & Takahashi M. MR imaging enhancement with superparamagnetic iron oxide in chronic liver disease: influence of liver dysfunction and parenchymal pathology. Abdom Imaging 1996;21:318-323

Yin M, Talwalkar JA, Glaser KJ, Manduca A, Grimm RC, Rossman PJ, Fidler JL &, Ehman RL. Assessment of hepatic fibrosis with magnetic resonance elastography. Clin Gastro Hep 2007;5:1207-1213

Yoneda M, Mawatari H, Fujita K, Iida H, Yonemitsu K, Kato S, Takahashi H, Kirikoshi H, Inamori M, Nozaki Y, Abe Y, Kubota K, Saito S, Iwasaki T, Terauchi Y, Togo S, Maeyama S & Nakajima A. High-sensitivity C-reactive protein is an independent clinical feature of nonalcoholic steatohepatitis (NASH) and also of the severity of fibrosis in NASH. J Gastroenterol 2007; 42: 573-582

Yoneda M, Uchiyama T, Kato S, Endo H, Fujita K, Yoneda K, Mawatari H, Iida H, Takahashi H, Kirikoshi H, Inamori M, Nozaki Y, Kobayashi N, Kubota K, Saito S, Maeyama S, Sagara M, Aburatani H, Kodama T & Nakajima A. Plasma Pentraxin-3 is a novel marker for nonalcoholic steatohepatitis (NASH). BMC Gastroenterol 2008; 8: 53

Zaman A, Rosen HR, Ingram H, Corless CL, Oh E & Smith K. Assessement of Fibrospect II to detect hepatic fibrosis in chronic hepatitis C patients Am J Med 2007;120:280

# 18

# Transient Elastography for Assessment of Non-Alcoholic Fatty Liver Disease

Ludovico Abenavoli
*University "Magna Græcia" of Catanzaro, Italy*

## 1. Introduction

In 1958, Menghini published the first description of liver biopsy (LB) as it pertained to the study of fibrosis. Since then, LB has become the "gold standard" in the evaluation of liver fibrosis. However, the use of LB has several limitations, including physical and mental discomfort of patients, which may lead to a high percentage of refusals, non-negligible morbidity and occasional mortality. Fibrosis is evaluated by histological semiquantitative scores, among which the METAVIR fibrosis scoring system is the most used; it is able to detect different degrees of fibrosis, from absence of fibrosis (F0) to cirrhosis (F4), and shows a better intra- and inter-observer reproducibility than other scales (i.e., Brunt, Knodell, Ishak and Scheuer). However these scores do not provide a dynamic picture of the disease, but only information about diagnosis and prognosis, such as the necroinflammatory activity and the presence of steatosis (Abenavoli et al, 2007).

Non-alcoholic fatty liver disease (NAFLD) is a relevant issue in public health because of its epidemiologic burden (Argo & Caldwell, 2009). NAFLD is also not a new condition, but was not appreciated in early reports. It represents the most common chronic liver disease in the general population and is expected to increase in the future as a result of an ageing population, the improving control of other major causes of chronic liver disease and the epidemics of obesity and diabetes (Abenavoli et al, 2011). Steatosis consists of an accumulation of fat in the liver cells, and is not a disease in and of itself. It is an aggravating factor in certain pathological situations of varying degrees of gravity, and becomes dangerous when associated with inflammation or fibrosis. It is reversible, however, through diet and exercise. In fact NAFLD, may present as a spectrum ranging from asymptomatic steatosis with elevated or normal aminotransferases to steatohepatitis [non-alcoholic steatohepatitis (NASH)], all the way to cirrhosis with complications of liver function to hepatocellular carcinoma. NAFLD occurs in 60-95% patients with obesity, in 28-55% patients with type 2 diabetes mellitus (T2DM) and in 27-92% patients with dyslipidemia. Insulin resistance with compensatory hyperinsulinemia is the common denominator of obesity, T2DM and dyslipidemia and it can play a pathogenetic role in NAFLD. Accordingly, it has been reported that insulin resistance is the single laboratory finding most closely associated with NAFLD in a large series of patients, irrespective of body mass index (BMI), fat distribution, or glucose tolerance. Indeed, NAFLD has been recently proposed as an additional feature of the metabolic syndrome.

Currently liver steatosis, can be detected only by ultrasound (US) and quantified only by performing a biopsy. LB is still considered the "gold standard" for distinguishing between the broad range of NAFLD. However LB is not recommended in NAFLD patients, because of its cost, the potential risk of bleeding, and the absence of consensus regarding the histopatological criteria that firmly define NASH and differentiate between NAFLD entities. Due to the remarkable increase in the prevalence of NAFLD and the concomitant efforts in developing new therapies for fatty liver, non-invasive, simple, reproducible, and reliable non-invasive techniques are needed. In this way US is widely used in the diagnosis of patients with suspected liver disease because it is highly accurate, relatively inexpensive and non-invasive. Based on these characteristics, US has been the first-line imaging technique suitable both in the clinical setting and for epidemiological studies. In particular US is the least expensive modality for detecting changes associated with NAFLD. However, echography-based US techniques begin to become sensitive at moderately high levels of steatosis (33% or more) and suffer from low intra- and inter-operator repeatability (Schwenzer et al, 2009).

Vibration-controlled transient elastography ([VCTE], Fibroscan®, Echosens, Paris, France) is a non-invasive technique which measures liver stiffness, and allows the assessment of the extent of hepatic fibrosis. VCTE has been proposed for the measurement of liver stiffness, considered to be one of the direct consequences of the fibrotic evolution of chronic liver disease (Sandrin et al, 2003).

A few meta-analyses have suggested liver stiffness measurement (LSM) through VCTE to be a reliable tool to detect advanced liver fibrosis and early liver cirrhosis (Friedrich-Rust et al, 2008). In NAFLD patients, various degrees of hepatic steatosis may attenuate the elastic shear wave, but it does not change its underlying speed which is the parameter used for stiffness measurement. Literature showed a clearly positive correlation between liver stiffness and the severity of liver fibrosis in patients with NAFLD. Rapid, non-invasive estimation of the stage of fibrosis in NAFLD patients, especially NASH patients, is of major clinical interest because such patients have been shown to be at a high risk of developing complications. Recently, a new measurement technique, the controlled attenuation parameter (CAP®, EchoSens, Paris, France), which provides good accuracy with even low levels of steatosis in the liver has been introduced. Because of its sensitivity at early phases of steatosis. CAP could provide a means to monitor the progression or regression of steatosis.

The combination of the measurement of liver attenuation parameter (CAP) and liver stiffness (VCTE) could provide a means to follow NAFLD patients throughout the course of the disease and observe independently the effects of steatosis and liver injury effects that are signs of the worsening of the disease.

## 2. Transient elastography for staging liver disease

The development of non-invasive tools to evaluate liver disease stages, has emerged as a major clinical and research priority. The quest for accurate techniques to stage NAFLD stems from a variety of recent data. First, the prevalence of NAFLD has grown to epidemic proportions. It is currently one of the most common chronic liver diseases worldwide. It is strongly associated with metabolic syndrome and obesity, and may progress to cirrhosis and hepatocellular carcinoma. The prognosis depends heavily on histological severity. Although patients with simple steatosis have excellent prognosis, those with NASH tend to progress and have hepatic complications. In Western countries, one in three men and nearly every other woman is affected by NAFLD. Second, it is well reported that NAFLD exists as a spectrum consisting of two major phenotypes that have drastically different natural histories. The majority of patients present simple steatosis, which has a benign clinical course. However 10-20% of these individuals present NASH that can evolve into cirrhosis. Third, according to literature, several problems for the management of NAFLD patients in clinical practice still exist: how to diagnose NAFLD and its type, how to select patient candidates for treatment and how to treat the patients selected. Discovery and validation of new diagnostic tools for NAFLD have several potential benefits, including reduced risk, reduced cost, as well as insights into disease mechanisms and pathogenesis. More accurate detection and diagnosis of NAFLD will help focus service provision for what is already a very common condition.

The limitations of LB (invasive procedure, sampling errors, interobserver variability and non-dynamic evaluation) have stimulated the search for non-invasive approaches for the assessment of steatosis and liver fibrosis in patients with NAFLD. A variety of new methods, including serum markers, imaging techniques such as US, computed tomography, magnetic resonance imaging and VCTE, and more recently, CAP, have been proposed. In particular VCTE has shown excellent results for the diagnosis of severe fibrosis and cirrhosis and moderate results for the diagnosis of significant fibrosis in patients with NAFLD/NASH.

The stiffness of a body is defined as the ability of the body to deform itself under the action of a mechanical force (Abenavoli et al, 2007). The stiffness of a soft tissue can be estimated on the basis of the speed of propagation of a transverse shear elastic wave. The higher is the speed of propagation of that wave, the higher is the stiffness of the tissue. VCTE measures such speed of propagation in relatively homogenous organs like the liver, by using US pulses to localise the shear elastic wave at different times. The measuring device is equipped with a probe consisting of an ultrasonic transducer mounted on the axis of a vibrator. A low-frequency at 50 Hz and mild amplitude vibration, referred to as "shots", is transmitted from the vibrator to the tissue by the transducer itself. This vibration induces an elastic shear wave which propagates through the tissue. In the meantime, ultrasonic acquisitions are performed by an echographic transducer, using a frequency at 3.5MHz, to determine the propagation of the shear wave. The propagation speed is transformed into stiffness by a formula derived by the physics of the propagation of a transverse shear elastic wave of a given frequency (50 Hz) through the soft tissue and expressed in kiloPascals (kPa). The probe is applied perpendicularly to the skin (with a little gel film) through one of the right side intercostal spaces along the mid-axillary line. The measurement of the speed is taken along a cylinder of tissue ranging from 25 to 65 millimetres of depth under the skin. This corresponds to a volume of liver tissue approximately 100 times greater than an LB specimen and represents about 1% of the total organ volume. The examination is non-invasive and can be performed on ambulatory patients, in an outpatient setting or at the bedside of a hospitalized patient. VCTE can be performed indifferently by hepatologists or medical staff (physician, resident, medicine student, nurse) after a single training session provided by a specifically certified trainer. Results of the measurements range from 1.3 and 75.4 kPa. The manufacturer currently recommends that fibrosis score should be established from the median value of at least 10 successful acquisitions, with the rate of valid measures always higher than 50%. The intra- and inter-observer coefficients of variation are 3.2 and 3.3%, respectively, indicating very good reproducibility and operator independence.

## 3. Elastography assessment of fatty liver

A prospective study (Kim et al., 2007) aimed to assess the ability of VCTE to identify histologic parameters, including steatosis, in asymptomatic healthy individuals such as potential liver donors, and to compare these findings with results in liver disease patients. Forty-seven patients with abnormal liver function and/or hepatitis symptoms and 80 living related potential liver donors were consecutively enrolled, and LB and a LSM was performed in each subject. Histologic parameters were evaluated according to METAVIR score by a single pathologist. In liver disease patients, stiffness was significantly correlated with fibrosis stage ($P < 0.001$), and the optimal stiffness cut-off values for F≥2, F≥3, and F=4 were 7.35, 8.85, and 15.1 kPa respectively. In potential liver donors, stiffness was not correlated with fibrosis ( $P = 0.851$). In the latter group, the area under the receiver-operating characteristics curve (AUROC) was 0.70 (95%, confidence interval [CI], 0.58-0.81), and the optimal stiffness cut-off value was 4.00 kPa for F ≥ 2, which was lower than that in liver disease patients. Steatosis was not correlated with stiffness ($P = 0.463$) in potential liver donors. The Authors concluded that VCTE presets limited value for detecting steatosis in asymptomatic healthy individuals.

Nobili et al. (2008) have been assessed the value of VCTE in a cohort of pediatric patients with NASH. TE was performed in 50 consecutive biopsy-proven NASH patients age 13.6±2.44 years). The AUROC for the prediction of different degrees of liver fibrosis on the basis of Brunt score, were 0.977, 0.992, and 1, for respectively "any", significant and advanced fibrosis. Calculation of multilevel likelihood ratios shows that VCTE values <5, <7, and <9 kPa, suggest the presence of "any" fibrosis, significant fibrosis, and advanced fibrosis, respectively. VCTE values between 5 and 7 kPa predict a fibrosis stage of 1, but with some degree of uncertainty. VCTE values between 7 and 9 kPa predict fibrosis stages 1 or 2, but cannot discriminate between these two stages. VCTE values of at least 9 kPa are associated with the presence of advanced fibrosis. In summary this study reported the reliability of VCTE to predict the presence of "any" fibrosis, significant fibrosis, and advanced fibrosis in these special populations.

Yoneda et al. (2008) have been investigated the usefulness of LSM in the evaluation of liver fibrosis in NAFLD patients. VCTE was performed for liver stiffness measurement in 97 NAFLD patients. The Authors have also investigated the relationship between LSM and the serum levels of hyaluronic acid and type IV collagen 7s domain. Liver stiffness was well correlated with the different stage of METAVIR score ($P<0.0001$). The AUROC were 0.927 for ≥F1, 0.865 for ≥F2, 0.904 for ≥F3, 0.991 for ≥F4. Only fibrosis stage was strictly correlated with liver stiffness measurement by multiple regression analysis. Liver stiffness was also strongly correlated with the serum levels of type IV collagen 7s domain ($r=0.525$, $P<0.0001$) and hyaluronic acid ($r=0.457$, $P<0.0001$). These data show a significant correlation between liver stiffness measurement and fibrosis stage in NAFLD patients, as confirmed by the results of LB.

Lupsor et al. (2010) assess VCTE performance in NASH patients, as well as the factors determining the discordance between the VCTE-predicted and the fibrosis stage evaluated by the Brunt system. LB and VCTE were performed on 72 consecutive NASH patients. LSM ranged from 2.80 to 16.90 kPa. In the univariate analysis, LSM was correlated with fibrosis ($P<0.0001$), steatosis ($P<0.0001$), ballooning ($P=0.001$) and lobular inflammation ($P=0.002$). In multivariate analysis, only fibrosis significantly correlated with LS ($P<0.0001$). The median LSM values according to the fibrosis stages were: 4.90 kPa (range: 2.80-7.30) for F0; 6.15 kPa (4.80-12.50) for F1; 6.90 kPa (3.30-16.90) for F2 and 14.00 kPa (10.70-14.10) for F3, with significant difference between stages, except for F1-F2 ($P=0.249$). Cut-off values were calculated for predicting each fibrosis stage: 5.3kPa (AUROC=0.879) for F1; 6.8kPa (AUROC=0.789) for F2; and 10.4kPa (AUROC=0.978) for F3. Patients with false positive

results had a significantly higher ALT level than those with concordant results ($P$=0.039). These data show that steatosis degree, ballooning and inflammation do not influence LSM.
In NAFLD patients, various degrees of hepatic steatosis may attenuate the elastic shear wave, possibly leading again to an underestimation of liver damage. Wong et al. (2010) aimed to evaluate the accuracy of VCTE in the diagnosis of fibrosis and cirrhosis in patients with NAFLD and to study factors associated with discordance between LSM and histology. Two hundred forty-six consecutive patients from two ethnic groups had successful LSM and satisfactory liver biopsy specimens. The AUROC of VCTE for F3 or higher and F4 disease was 0.93 and 0.95, respectively, and was significantly higher than that of other prediction scores (e.g. aspartate aminotransferase-to-alanine aminotransferase ratio, aspartate aminotransferase-to-platelet ratio index, FIB-4, BARD, and NAFLD fibrosis scores). AUROC ranged from 0.62 to 0.81, $P < 0.05$ for all comparisons. At a cut-off value of 7.9 kPa, the sensitivity, specificity, and positive and negative predictive values for F3 or greater disease were 91%, 75%, 52%, and 97%, respectively. LSM was not affected by hepatic steatosis, necroinflammation, or body mass index. Discordance of at least two stages between VCTE and histology was observed in 33 (13.4%) patients. By multivariate analysis, a LB length less than 20 mm and F0-2 disease, rather than VCTE, were associated with discordance. Unsatisfactory LB specimens rather than VCTE account for most cases of discordance. However, when the diagnostic characteristics were compared using an "intention to diagnose" approach with the inclusion of subjects who had unsuccessful TE acquisition, the sensitivity and specificity values were not dissimilar from the clinical/biochemical models, although 95% CIs were not provided for statistical comparison.
Subsequently a prospective study by Gaia et al. (2011) assess the accuracy and the efficacy of VCTE for the detection of fibrosis in patients with liver disease of different etiology (chronic hepatitis B - CHB, C- CHC and NAFLD) and evaluate the effect of steatosis on LSM. VCTE was performed in 219 consecutive patients with chronic liver disease (35% CHC, 32% CHB, and 33% NAFLD) within 6 months of the liver biopsy. LSM was related to the fibrosis stage in each group (CHC: $P$=0.596, $P$<0.001; CHB: $P$ =0.418, $P$<0.001; NAFLD: $P$=0.573, $P$<0.001), but the correlation was less strong in CHB and NAFLD than in CHC patients. Median LSM values were 7 kPa (3.2–26) in HCV patients (n=77), 7.6 kPa (3.7–30.7) in HBV patients (n=70), 6.6 kPa (3.0–44.3) in NAFLD patients (n=72) compared to 4.35 kPa (range 2.6–7) in controls (n=40), ($P$<0.001). The median values of LSM according to fibrosis stage evaluated by METAVIR were in the 72 NAFLD patients: F0: 5.3 kPa (3.0–9.7), F1: 6.15 kPa (3.2–12.1), F2:7.75 kPa (4.3–13.9), F3:6.5 kPa (4.3–10.3), F4:11.9 kPa (7.9–44.3), ($P$=0.001). VCTE underestimated the stage of fibrosis in 75% of patients with F3 and steatosis >33%. At multiple logistic regression analysis, in CHC and CHB patients, LSM was the only predictive variable of severe fibrosis/cirrhosis (odds ratio [OR]=1.42, $P$=0.003 and OR=1.354, $P$=0.003, respectively), while in NAFLD subjects BMI and AST (OR=1.433, $P$=0.002 and OR=1.053, $P$=0.020, respectively) but not LSM were independently related with advanced fibrosis and cirrhosis. This study confirms that VCTE can be considered a valid support to detect fibrosis in chronic liver disease related to HCV but it should be interpreted cautiously in CHB and NAFLD patients.

## 4. Elastography assessment of NAFLD in obese patients

LSM can be influenced by metabolic syndrome even in the absence of biological features in NAFLD. It would be important to identify the rates and factors associated with unreliable

LSM or LSM failure, as the results may provide guidance to referral physicians regarding the optimal candidates for LSM. The knowledge would also assist clinicians to counsel patients before arranging LSM. However, studies have shown that BMI>28 is an independent risk factor for a LSM failure (Foucher et al, 2006). In a prospective pilot study on VCTE in NAFLD, de Lédinghen et al. (2010) aimed to assess the feasibility of LSM when using a new XL-probe on patients with a BMI≥30 kg/m$^2$ is used. In this study 99 patients (mean BMI 40.5 kg/m$^2$) were included. LSM was successful in 45% of the cases with the M probe, versus 76% of the cases with the XL-probe ($P<0.001$). Fifty-nine percent of those who could not be measured (<10 valid measurements) using the M-probe could successfully be measured using the XL-probe. In the 44 patients successfully measured with both probes, LSM was correlated with the platelet count, prothrombin time, gamma-glutamyltransferase, aspartate aminotransferase, fasting glucose, AST platelet ratio index, Forns score and FIB-4. The XL-probe allows providing a higher rate of LSM than the M-probe in patients with an increased BMI and shows promising results for the evaluation of liver fibrosis.

| Lead author | Yoneda (*N* 97)* | Nobili (*N* 50)° | Lupsor (*N* 72)° | Wong (*N* 246)° |
|---|---|---|---|---|
| **F≥ 2** | | | | |
| AUROC | 0.86 | 0.99 | 0.78 | 0.84 |
| Optimal cut-off (kPa) | 6.6 | 7.4 | 6.8 | 7.0 |
| Sensitivity (%) | 88 | 100 | 100 | 79 |
| Specificity (%) | 74 | 92 | 97 | 76 |
| PPV (%) | 79 | 80 | 71 | 70 |
| NPV (%) | 85 | 100 | 100 | 84 |
| **F≥ 3** | | | | |
| AUROC | 0.90 | 1.0 | 0.978 | 0.93 |
| Optimal cut-off (kPa) | 9.8 | 10.2 | 10.4 | 8.7 |
| Sensitivity (%) | 85 | 100 | 100 | 84 |
| Specificity (%) | 81 | 100 | 97 | 83 |
| PPV (%) | 64 | 100 | 71 | 59 |
| NPV (%) | 93 | 100 | 100 | 95 |
| **F≥ 3** | | | | |
| AUROC | 0.99 | - | - | 0.95 |
| Optimal cut-off (kPa) | 17.5 | | | 10.3 |
| Sensitivity (%) | 100 | - | - | 92 |
| Specificity (%) | 97 | - | - | 88 |
| PPV (%) | 75 | - | - | 46 |
| NPV (%) | 100 | - | - | 99 |

Table 1. Analysis of VCTE cut-off for the diagnosis of NAFLD in adult patients. (AUROC: area under receiver operative curve; PPV: positive predictive value; NPV: negative predictive value. Histological evaluation by *METAVIR and °Brunt score).

In this way Wong et al. (2011) have recently investigated the rates of unreliable LSM and LSM failure in patients suffering from chronic liver diseases. They also aimed to evaluate the factors including BMI and central obesity associated with unreliable LSM and LSM failure. Among 3205 Chinese patients with LSM, 370 (12%) with liver steatosis, 371 (11.6%) and 88 (2.7%) had unreliable LSM and LSM failure, respectively. The rates started to increase when BMI≥28.0 kg/m$^2$. Comparing patients with BMI≥28.0-29.9 kg/m$^2$ vs those with BMI≥30.0 kg/m$^2$, the rates of unreliable LSM (16.4% vs 18.9%; *P*=0.62) and LSM failure (11.8% vs 17.8%; *P*=0.16) were similar. BMI≥28.0 kg/m2 was the most important factor associated with unreliable LSM (OR=2.9, 95% CI=2.1–3.9, *P*<0.0001) and LSM failure (OR=10.1, 95% CI=6.4–14.2, *P*<0.0001). Central obesity, defined as waist circumference >80 cm in women and >90 cm in men, was another independent risk factor of unreliable LSM (OR=1.3, 95% CI=1.0–1.6, *P*=0.04) and LSM failure (OR=5.8, 95% CI=2.9–11.5, *P*<0.0001).

## 5. Controlled attenuation parameter and liver steatosis

Fat affects US propagation, however this is the most common liver imaging technique used to detect the presence of steatosis. In B-mode images, steatosis appears as an increased parenchymal echogenicity caused by the increased reflectivity induced by fatty accumulation. This increased echogenicity is determined by the sonographer, most of the time by comparison with kidney echogenicity. Such as procedure it is highly operator- and machine-dependant. Many studies have reported averaged specificity and sensitivity of the technique as around 60-70%. Other studies have reported better specificity and sensitivity up to 95%, and therefore its performance in clinical practice is still controversial. Another limitation of US is that it cannot quantify steatosis and can only detect steatosis from around 30% of fatty infiltration, where there is a clinical relevance to detect lower extent of liver fat.

Furthermore, some studies have shown that liver fibrosis can induce an increased liver echogenicity without posterior beam attenuation. It is therefore impossible to distinguish between increased echogenicity caused by an extensive fibrosis from increased echogenicity caused by fatty infiltration. A quantitative attenuation parameter can overcome this limitation.

Recently a new parameter has been developed to detect and quantify degree of liver steatosis. This parameter is based on the US properties of the radiofrequency backpropagated signals acquired by the VCTE. It is called controlled attenuation parameter (CAP), because it was devised to specifically target the liver (Sasso et al, 2010). This coefficient is an estimate of the total US (go-and-return path) at 3.5 MHz and is expressed in decibel per meters (dB.m$^{-1}$). CAP is evaluated using the same radio-frequency data and in the same region of interest than the ones used for LSM and it is only appraised if the acquisition is valid. CAP is VCTE guided and obtains an ultrasonic attenuation value of the liver only. Therefore, CAP can be assessed by an operator who does not have any ultrasound imaging skills. Furthermore, CAP has been designed to be immediate, reproducible and operator and machine-independent. Performance of CAP was evaluated by Sasso et al. on 115 patients, taking the histological grade of steatosis as reference. Among those patients, 42 were CHC, 17 CBV, 39 with alcoholic liver disease and 17 with NAFLD. Mean BMI was 25 ± 4 kg/m$^2$. CAP was significantly correlated to steatosis (*P*=10$^{-16}$). AUROC was equal to 0.91 and 0.95 for the detection of more than 10% and 33% of steatosis, respectively. These data show that CAP can efficiently separate several steatosis grades. CAP appears to be a promising diagnostic tool for non-invasive assessment and quantification of steatosis, enhancing the spectrum of the non-invasive method for the exploration and follow-up of patients with fatty liver. However validation of this novel indicator is ongoing in a large multi-etiology cohort study.

## 6. Conclusion

LB will still be part of clinical practice in the coming years, but progress in medicine will challenge previously entrenched assumptions and will change our current approach to liver diseases in the next future. Non-invasive assessment of liver fibrosis is currently a reality in patients with CHC. In other highly prevalent diseases, such as NAFLD there is still room for improvement, although in the next few years LB will likely be supplanted in most cases. Many imaging techniques can be used to identify liver steatosis, such as computed tomography scans, magnetic resonance imaging or proton nuclear magnetic resonance. However all of these imaging tools present some important limitations: they are not easily available and their costs are relatively expensive (Sasso et al, 2010).
VCTE is a simple, non-invasive and inexpensive method used to measure LS. The accuracy and reproducibility of VCTE score is excellent for the diagnosis of cirrhosis; it is probably the most accurate non-invasive method for the early detection of cirrhosis. It is a user-friendly technique that can be performed without any preparation in the less than five minutes in clinic or at the bedside, with immediate results and high patient acceptance, it is very likely that in future it will become the most widely used technique for staging liver disease. A panel discussion is in progress to define the role of VCTE in the staging of liver disease. In particular, there are a few methodological approaches that need to be implemented in future studies designed to further validate LSM. A new statistical approach is needed in order to obtain reliable and clinically useful information from LSM (Vizzuti et al, 2009). In fact, most of the published studies reported the cut-off values selected by binary measures, like sensitivity and specificity. However, it seems insufficiently informative to discriminate the optimal cut-off value in a wide range of values, specially in a context of liver steatosis. A new parameter measuring the US attenuation could be interesting and might be related to steatosis. This indicator, called CAP, has been developed to process the raw ultrasonic signals stored in the VCTE examination file. Performance of CAP has to be validated into specific etiologic groups. In addiction influence of the steatosis topography and other histologic constituents, specific to each etiology has to be considered. Large cohorts are required to determine appropriate threshold to detect and quantify steatosis.
Further technological improvements are requested for better application of this technique in specific populations, such as patients with increased BMI, along with efforts to improve and standardize the procedure and adequate operator training.

## 7. Acknowledgment

We would like to thank Emanuela Libri for the linguistic revision.

## 8. References

Menghini G.(1958). One-second needle biopsy of the liver. *Gastroenterology*. Volume 35, pp. 190-199.

Argo C.K. & Caldwell S.H. (2009). Epidemiology and natural history of non-alcoholic steatohepatitis. *Clin Liver Disease*. Volume 13, pp. 511-531

Abenavoli L., Corpechot C. & Poupon R. (2007). Elastography in hepatology. *Canadian Journal of Gastroenterology*. Volume 21, No. 12, pp. 839-842

Abenavoli L., Aviello G., Capasso R., Milic N. & Capasso F. (2011). Milk thistle for non-alcoholic fatty liver disease treatment. *Hepatitis Monthly*. Volume 11, No.3, pp. 173-177

Schwenzer N.F., Springer F., Schraml C., Stefan N., Machann J. & Schick F. (2009). Non-invasive assessment and quantification of liver steatosis by ultrasound, computed tomography and magnetic resonance. *Journal of Hepatology*. Volume 51, No. 3, pp.433–445.

Sandrin L., Fourquet B., Hasquenoph J.M., Yon S., Fournier C., Mal F., Christidis C., Ziol M., Poulet B., Kazemi F., Beaugrand M. & Palau R. (2003). Transient elastography: A new noninvasive method for assessment of hepatic fibrosis. *Ultrasound in Medicine and Biology*. Volume 29, No.11, pp.1705-1713.

Friedrich-Rust M., Ong M.F., Martens S., Sarrazin C., Bojunga J., Zeuzem S. & Herrmann E. (2008). Performance of transient elastography for the staging of liver fibrosis: a meta-analysis. Gastroenterology. Volume 134, No. 4 pp. 960-974.

Kim K.M., Choi W.B., Park S.H., Yu E., Lee S.G., Lim Y.S., Lee H.C., Chung Y.H., Lee Y.S., & Suh D.J. (2007). Diagnosis of hepatic steatosis and fibrosis by transient elastography in asymptomatic healthy individuals: a prospective study of living related potential liver donors. *Journal of Gastroenterology*. Volume 42, No. 5, pp. 382-388.

Nobili V., Vizzutti F., Arena U., Abraldes J.G., Marra F., Pietrobattista A., Fruhwirth R., Marcellini M. & Pinzani M. (2008). Accuracy and reproducibility of transient elastography for the diagnosis of fibrosis in pediatric nonalcoholic steatohepatitis. Hepatology. Volume 48, No. 2, pp. 42-48.

Yoneda M., Yoneda M., Mawatari H., Fujita K., Endo H., Iida H., Nozaki Y., Yonemitsu K., Higurashi T., Takahashi H., Kobayashi N., Kirikoshi H., Abe Y., Inamori M., Kubota K., Saito S., Tamano M., Hiraishi H., Maeyama S., Yamaguchi N., Togo S. & Nakajima A (2008). Noninvasive assessment of liver fibrosis by measurement of stiffness in patients with nonalcoholic fatty liver disease (NAFLD). *Digestive and Liver Disease*. Volume 40, No 5, pp. 371-378.

Lupsor M., Badea R., Stefanescu H., Grigorescu M., Serban A., Radu C., Crişan D., Sparchez Z., Iancu S. & Maniu A. (2010). Performance of unidimensional transient elastography in staging non-alcoholic steatohepatitis. *Journal of Gastrointestinal and Liver Diseases*. Volume 19, No. 1, pp. 53-60.

Wong V.W., Vergniol J., Wong G.L., Foucher J., Chan H.L., Le Bail B., Choi P.C., Kowo M., Chan A.W., Merrouche W., Sung J.J. & de Lédinghen V. (2010). Diagnosis of fibrosis and cirrhosis using liver stiffness measurement in nonalcoholic fatty liver disease. *Hepatology*. Volume 51, No 2, pp. 454-462.

Gaia S., Carenzi S., Barilli A.L., Bugianesi E., Smedile A., Brunello F., Marzano A. & Rizzetto M (2011). Reliability of transient elastography for the detection of fibrosis in non-alcoholic fatty liver disease and chronic viral hepatitis. *Journal of Hepatology*. Volume 54, No. 1, pp. 64-71.

Foucher J., Castéra L., Bernard P.H., Adhoute X., Laharic D., Bertet J., Couzigou P. & de Lédinghen V. (2006). Prevalence and factors associated with failure of liver stiffness measurement using FibroScan in a prospective study of 2114 examinations. *European Journal of Gastroenterology and Hepatology*. Volume 18, No 4, pp. 411-412.

de Lédinghen V., Vergniol J., Foucher J., El-Hajbi F., Merrouche W. & Rigalleau V. (2010). Feasibility of liver transient elastography with FibroScan using a new probe for obese patients. *Liver International.* Volume 30, No. 7, pp. 1043-1048.

Wong G.L., Wong V.W., Chim A.M., Yiu K.K., Chu S.H., Li M.K. & Chan H.L. (2011). Factors associated with unreliable liver stiffness measurement and its failure with transient elastography in the Chinese population. *Journal of Gastroenterology and Hepatology.* Volume 26, No. 2, pp. 300-305.

Sasso M., Beaugrand M., de Ledinghen V., Douvin C., Marcellin P., Poupon R., Sandrin L. & Miette V. (2010). Controlled attenuation parameter (CAP): a novel VCTE™ guided ultrasonic attenuation measurement for the evaluation of hepatic steatosis: preliminary study and validation in a cohort of patients with chronic liver disease from various causes. *Ultrasound in Medicine & Biology.* Volume 36, No 11, pp.1825-1835.

Vizzutti F., Arena U., Nobili V., Tarquini R., Trappoliere M., Laffi G., Marra F. & Pinzani M. (2009). Non-invasive assessment of fibrosis in non-alcoholic fatty liver disease. *Annals of Hepatology.* Volume 8, No. 2, pp. 89-94.

# 19

# Non-Invasive Assessment of Liver Fibrosis by Vibration-Controlled Transient Elastography (Fibroscan®)

Sandrin Laurent[1], Oudry Jennifer[1], Bastard Cécile[1],
Fournier Céline[1], Miette Véronique[1] and Mueller Sebastian[2]
[1]Echosens,
[2]University of Heidelberg,
[1]France
[2]Germany

## 1. Introduction

Chronic liver diseases result in fibrosis ultimately leading to cirrhosis, a liver end stage disease with high mortality and life threatening complications such as hepatocellular carcinoma. Thus far, no treatment options exist to cure and stop fibrosis progression except organ replacement by liver transplantation. This clinically unsatisfactory situation justifies the enormous interest in quantifying and monitoring fibrosis progression. Though liver biopsy remains the gold standard for assessing liver fibrosis, non invasive procedures are being developed for many years to overcome its complications (Bravo et al. 2001), sampling error and interobserver variability (Abdi et al. 1979; Bedossa et al. 2003; Cadranel et al. 2001). Fibrosis and activity marker scores based on several blood parameters from a simple blood test have been developed to assess liver fibrosis and activity as obtained by liver biopsy Many efforts have been invested to identify serum markers that allow the diagnosis of cirrhosis from simple blood tests (Poynard et al. 2004). However those scores are indirect and reflect the fibrogenetic activity. Thus they do not correlate with the absolute amount of fibrotic tissue within the liver.

It is now well established that fibrosis increases liver stiffness. Liver palpation (Fig. 1) is a routine medical practice that has been used since the beginning of medicine to assess liver stiffness. Though, palpation suffers from major limitations: it is highly subjective, very operator dependent and sometimes even impossible to perform. Recently, quantitative elastography emerged as a means to assess liver fibrosis non-invasively. Nowadays Vibration-Controlled Transient Elastography (VCTE™) is by far the most clinically validated quantitative elastography technique and VCTE™ based device, Fibroscan® (Echosens, France), has emerged as the reference tool for liver stiffness measurement. As a fact, Fibroscan® is more and more used in routine clinical practice as an alternative method to liver biopsy in patients with chronic liver diseases.

The chapter is organized as follows: Section 2 covers quantitative elastography; the main quantitative elastography techniques are described with a strong focus on the most clinically validated technique: VCTE™. Fibroscan® device is described in Section 3; the examination procedure is described. Advantages and limitations of the device are detailed. Applications of VCTE™ in hepatology are described in Section 4. The role of liver stiffness as a clinically relevant parameter will be pointed out. In Section 5, the pressure-stiffness-fibrosis sequence hypothesis is addressed. Eventually, discussion and conclusion are drawn in Section 6 and Section 7, respectively.

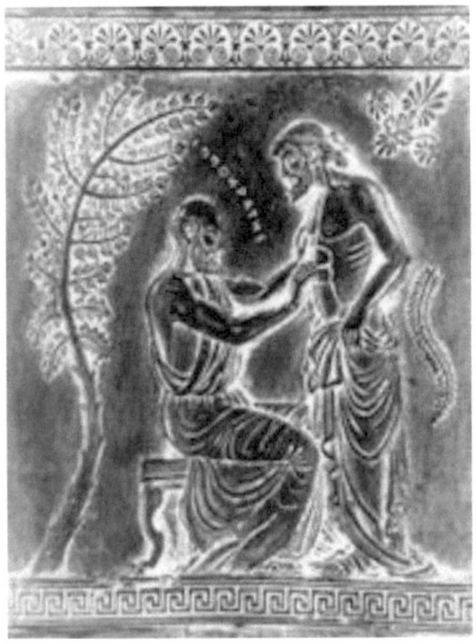

Fig. 1. Liver hand palpation: "The living are soft and yielding; the dead are rigid and stiff", Lao Tzu, (6th century BCE).

## 2. Quantitative elastography

### 2.1 Elastography techniques

It was a matter of time to see the development and emergence of sophisticated techniques such as elastography to quantitatively and non-invasively measure liver stiffness. Elastography is a recent field of research that started in the 80s to propose a reproducible and operator-independent alternative technique to hand palpation. Elastography techniques may be divided into two groups: qualitative elastography and quantitative elastography.

Qualitative elastography is now widely available on ultrasound scanners, it provides a qualitative color image that gives an interpretation of stiffness without providing any number. Basically, while the operator moves the ultrasound transducer at the skin surface of the body, the scanner measures the quasi static displacements within the tissues. A map representing the inverse of the displacement is displayed usually in color: the larger the displacement, the softer the tissue. While this technique may be helpful in radiology to identify focal lesions, it is definitively not adapted to quantify stiffness.

Quantitative elastography techniques rely on the use of low frequency shear waves. Indeed the velocity of these mechanical waves is directly related to the stiffness. Thus all quantitative elastography techniques combine a means to generate shear waves and an imaging technique to measure the propagation of the generated shear waves.

### 2.2 Physics of elastography

From a physical and mechanical point of view, stiffness can be defined as the shear modulus, $\mu$, or the Young's modulus, E. These moduli describe the mechanical response of a medium under shear stress and longitudinal stress, respectively. The theory of linear elasticity is based on this relationship between stress and strain and states that the deformation of a material is directly proportional to the applied stress, $\sigma = E\varepsilon$, where $\sigma$ is the stress applied to the material, and $\varepsilon$ is the strain induced in the material. The Young's modulus $E$ is expressed in kilopascals (kPa) and represents the resistance of material to deformation. This law, known as Hooke's law, gives the relationship between the strain $\varepsilon$, the Young's modulus and the stress $\sigma$. A rod, length L, of elastic material can be seen as a linear spring. Under a stress $\sigma$, it will experience an extension $\Delta L$:

$$\sigma = E\varepsilon$$
$$\Delta L = \frac{\sigma L}{E} \tag{2.1}$$

The relationship between the Young's modulus E, the Poisson coefficient $\upsilon$ and the Lamé coefficients $\lambda$ and $\mu$ (also known as compression and shear moduli), is given by:

$$E = \mu\frac{3\lambda + 2\mu}{\lambda + \mu}$$
$$\upsilon = \frac{\lambda}{2(\lambda + \mu)} \tag{2.2}$$

Biological tissues are mainly composed of water. The compression modulus $\lambda$ is several Giga Pascal; it is thus very large compared to the shear modulus of soft biological tissues (several kilo Pascal) (Sarvazyan et al. 1995). With $\lambda >> \mu$, it yields that $\upsilon \approx 0.5$ which is characteristic of a quasi-incompressible medium. Eventually, in soft medium, the Young's modulus $E$ simplifies to:

$$E = 3\mu \tag{2.3}$$

Interestingly, under some simplification hypothesis, the shear modulus can be deduced from the shear wave velocity, $V_s$, and the mass density, $\rho$:

$$\mu = \rho V_s^2$$
$$E = 3\rho V_s^2 \tag{2.5}$$

Since the soft body tissues mass density is almost constant (1000 kg/m³), the Young's modulus $E$ can be obtained by measuring the velocity of shear waves. Thus shear waves are the foundation of quantitative elastography techniques.

## 2.3 Background of quantitative elastography

Quantitative elastography techniques, also called dynamic elastography techniques, have the advantage of allowing a quantitative imaging and better resolution than the static elastography techniques. However, they require more complex equipment for the generation of shear waves (monochromatic, transient) and imaging devices (ultrafast ultrasound, magnetic resonance imaging) able to measure shear wave induced displacement with a high resolution. There are basically two groups of quantitative elastography techniques depending on the shear wave generation method: remote generation using radiation force and mechanical vibration. The shear wave frequency content may also be different: harmonic or transient.

In transient elastography techniques, the propagating shear wave results from a transient (impulsive or short tone burst) excitation of the tissue. Indeed, an important feature of transient elastography techniques is that the vibration be transient to avoid reflections and interferences occurring within the tissues. The transient shear wave travels through the tissues within tens of milliseconds which implies that the ultrasound-based imaging modality be ultrafast to follow its propagation. Harmonic elastography techniques are using a continuous vibration at a fixed frequency. Several quantitative elastography techniques (see Table 1) were proposed to assess liver stiffness as a marker of pathological state. Advantages and limitations of quantitative elastography techniques are summarized in Table 2.

| | Imaging modality | Shear wave generation mode | Frequency |
|---|---|---|---|
| Vibration-Controlled Transient Elastography (VCTE™) | Ultrasound | Mechanical vibration<br>Transient | Fixed<br>50 Hz |
| Magnetic Resonance Elastography (MRE) | Magnetic resonance imaging | Mechanical vibration<br>Harmonic | Fixed<br>60 Hz |
| Acoustic Radiation Force Impulse (ARFI) | Ultrasound | Radiation force<br>Transient | Wideband |
| Supersonic Shear Imaging (SSI) | Ultrasound | Radiation force<br>Transient | Wideband |

Table 1. Quantitative elastography techniques for liver stiffness measurement.

| | Advantages | Limitations |
|---|---|---|
| Vibration-Controlled Transient Elastography (VCTE™) | Ease of use<br>Highly standardized<br>Controlled shear frequency<br>Transient shear wave<br>Large clinical validation | Ascites |
| Magnetic Resonance Elastography (MRE) | Controlled shear frequency<br>Penetration depth<br>2D stiffness map | Cost |
| Acoustic Radiation Force Impulse (ARFI) | Image guidance<br>Transient shear wave | Absence of shear wave control<br>High intensity ultrasound<br>Penetration depth<br>Limited clinical validation |
| Supersonic Shear Imaging (SSI) | Image guidance<br>Transient shear wave | Absence of shear wave control<br>High intensity ultrasound<br>Penetration depth<br>Absence of clinical validation |

Table 2. Advantages and limitations of quantitative elastography techniques.

### 2.3.1 Radiation force based elastography

Radiation force based elastography uses high intensity ultrasound beams to induce displacements and tissue heating inside the liver remotely. Acoustic radiation force is applied to absorbing and/or reflecting materials in the propagation path of acoustic waves. This phenomenon is caused by a transfer of momentum from the acoustic wave to the propagation medium. The spatial distribution of the radiation force field is determined by both the acoustic excitation parameters and the tissue properties.

ARFI technique (Nightingale et al. 2003; Palmeri et al. 2008) involves the mechanical excitation of tissue using localized, focused, impulsive radiation force excitations. This results in shear-wave propagation away from the region of excitation. The mechanical excitation occurs along the acoustic wave propagation path and within the focal region of the acoustic beam. The resulting displacement response is ultrasonically tracked through time using an abdominal ultrasound transducer combined with a dedicated ultrasound scanner. Direct inversion methods are then applied to estimate the associated shear velocity.

Supersonic shear imaging (Bercoff et al. 2004; Muller et al. 2009) relies on the use of radiation force and a high frame rate ultrasound scanner (Sandrin et al. 2002). The medium is illuminated by a supersonic Mach cone: ultrasounds are focused successively at different increasing depths. The different spherical waves generated by each focus then interfere along a Mach cone in which the source is spreading faster than the shear wave generated and creates a plane wave front in the imaging plane. The ultrasound imaging system is then used to visualize the entire imaging plane with a good temporal resolution in a single acquisition typically 5000 to 20000 frames per second. Maps of the Young's modulus are estimated by inverse problems from the time of flight of the shear wave front.

Generating shear waves within the liver using radiation force requires high intensity ultrasound beams which induce liver tissue heating. Thermal safety issues related to incident radiation force pulses have been studied (Fahey et al. 2006; Palmeri & Nightingale 2004). It required the development of special cooling time sequences to prevent overheating of liver tissues. As a consequence of the relative low energetic transfer efficacy, the amplitude of the remotely induced displacements remains low and the penetration depth of radiation force based elastography technique is thus limited.

### 2.3.2 Mechanical vibration based elastography

Mechanical vibration based elastography techniques are using a mechanical vibrator to induce shear waves into the body. In Magnetic Resonance Elastography (MRE) (Muthupillai et al. 1995), a nuclear magnetic resonance imaging (MRI) method is used for quantitatively mapping the physical response of the tissues to an excitation of low frequency typically between 50 Hz and 80 Hz (Klatt et al. 2006, Rouviere et al. 2006). MRE showed promising results especially for 2D mapping of tissue stiffness.

Vibration-Controlled Transient Elastography (Castera et al. 2005; Sandrin et al. 2003; Sandrin et al. 2002; Ziol et al. 2005) is based on a single ultrasound transducer mounted on the axis of a mechanical actuator (Fig. 2). The ultrasound transducer (3.5 MHz) is used in pulse-echo mode to measure the displacements induced in a medium by the propagation of a low-frequency (50 Hz) shear wave. Interestingly the low frequency shear wave and the ultrasound are generated by the same piston-like transducer. The ultrasound beam coincides with the vibrator axis. Under the assumption of homogeneity, the symmetry considerations impose that the displacements on the axis of the transducer be purely longitudinal. Diffraction effects from the piston-like transducer result in longitudinally polarized shear wave on the axis of symmetry (Sandrin et al. 2004). The displacements induced by the shear wave in the medium are measured using cross-correlation of successive ultrasound lines acquired at high frame rate. A spatial-temporal strain map is computed from the recorded displacements. The shear wave speed is calculated based on the slope of the wave front visualized in the strain map.

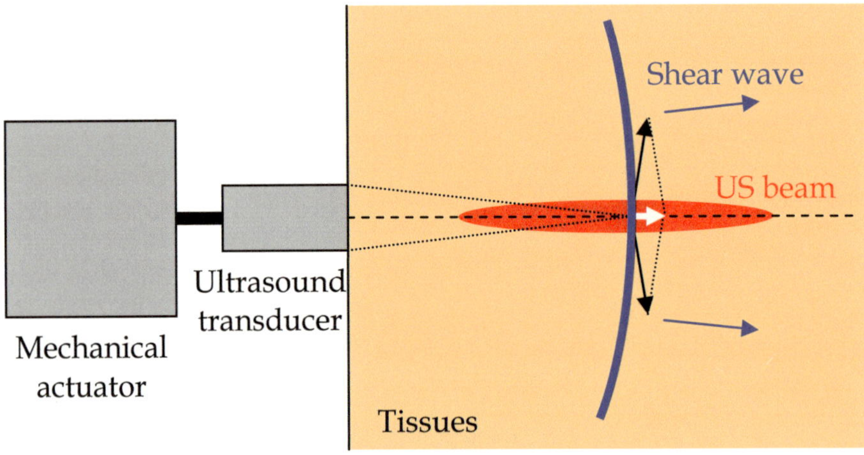


Fig. 2. The low frequency shear wave (blue) and the ultrasound beams (red) are generated by the same piston-like transducer. Under the assumption of homogeneity, the symmetry considerations impose that the displacements on the axis of the transducer be purely longitudinal (white arrow).

This technique is implemented in a standalone clinical device: Fibroscan®. It is the unique device that does not require integration into a conventional imaging system. Fibroscan® device is detailed in the next section.

### 2.4 The importance of the vibration control in quantitative elastography

The proper use of shear wave velocity analysis for clinical diagnosis requires the control of various physical parameters and in particular the control of the vibration to ensure an accurate, reliable and reproducible assessment of tissue stiffness. The control must be done on the shape, frequency and amplitude of the vibration. Of course, in VCTE™, the amplitude of the vibration may be adapted to the morphology of the patients to increase the penetration depth of the shear wave.

Furthermore, as stiffness value depends on shear wave frequency, the shape of the vibration must be controlled to obtain a consistent measurement that can be used for diagnostic purposes whatever the mechanical properties of the organ under investigation or the etiology of the patient. Provided that the shape of the vibration be constant, a reference frequency is obtained and a comparison of the shear wave propagation parameters can be performed independently of the organ conditions, etiology, patient and operator.

### 2.5 The difficult process of liver stiffness measurement standardization

The development and clinical validation of non-invasive methods for assessing liver fibrosis in patients with chronic liver diseases were eased by the fact that liver biopsy is not a perfect gold standard. However, standardization of elastography procedures is a challenging aspect of the success of elastography in the medical field and more precisely in hepatology.

Radiation force based elastography techniques such as ARFI and SSI are attractive techniques since they are intrinsically image-guided and do not require the use of an external vibrator. Actually these attractive aspects of the technology may result in significant loss of performances.

As a matter of fact, using an image guided system in which the operator has a full freedom of choice of the region of measurement will increase the operator dependency of the technique. While VCTE™ may look less sophisticated, it is based on a highly standardized procedure that can be followed not only by physicians but also by nurses. A short training is required before using Fibroscan®. This standardization favors the consistency of the results obtained whatever the operator, the studied population and the etiology of the patients.

Shear waves remotely generated using radiation force are wide band with frequencies ranging from 100 Hz to 500 Hz. Indeed with radiation force, the frequency of the shear waves can not be controlled precisely. Thus the frequency content of the generated shear wave will vary as a function of parameters such as the acoustic attenuation, the nature of reflecting materials, the mechanical properties of the tissues through which the ultrasound and shear waves travel, the depth of the region of measurement, etc. Some of these parameters are obviously etiology-dependent. As a consequence, measured stiffness will vary. Moreover, it is now well described that liver stiffness increases when the shear wave frequency increases (see Fig. 3). Thus, the higher the frequency is, the higher the measured stiffness will be.

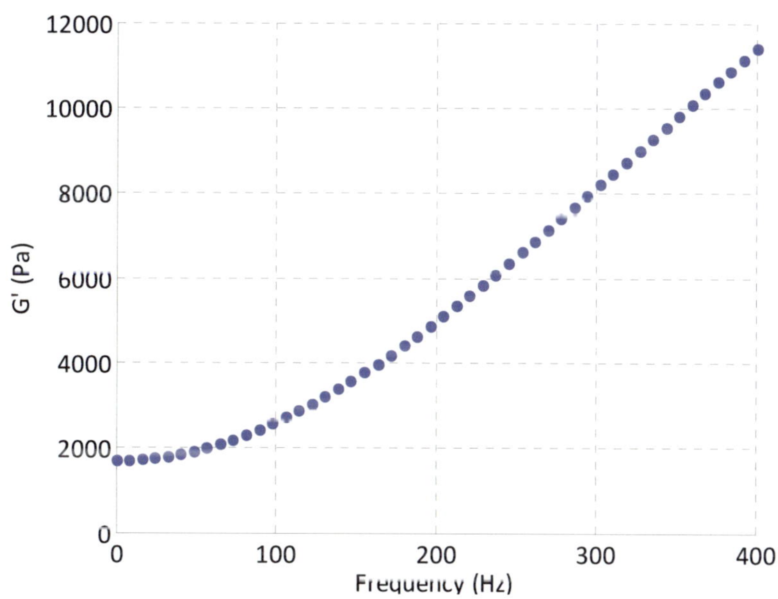


Fig. 3. Preliminary result: elastic modulus of a fresh pig liver sample as a function of frequency (courtesy of RheoLution inc).

Eventually, though a direct conversion of liver stiffness values measured with transient elastography techniques based on radiation force and mechanical vibration is tempting, this task might be a very challenging task. Indeed, theoretically Young's modulus as provided by VCTE™ could be deduced from the shear velocity as measured by radiation force-based technique (ARFI, SSI, etc.). However, this relationship is only valid at a given frequency:

$$E(f) = 3\rho V_S(f)^2 \tag{2.6}$$

As a matter of fact, while shear wave frequency in VCTE™ is 50 Hz, shear wave frequency using radiation force is not controlled. Thus, as the frequencies may be significantly different with these techniques, a direct conversion of radiation-force-based shear wave velocity to VCTE™ Young's modulus is not possible. The Young's modulus obtained with VCTE™ and radiation-force based elastograhy will differ. Therefore liver stiffness thresholds used for clinical decision support will have to be reevaluated.
The success of VCTE™ and the good performances reported in many studies all over the world is certainly due to its high standardization and high control of the shear wave shape.

## 3. Fibroscan® device

In this Section, the Fibroscan® device is described from a technical point of view. The operating principle is detailed with appropriate figures. Tables are included to provide parameters of the different probes available associated with measurement depths, operating ultrasound frequency, probe diameter, etc. A list of the special controls used in the Fibroscan® to ensure high performances is included. The examination procedure is described.

### 3.1 The device

Transient elastography measures shear wave velocity and thus determines tissue stiffness by using ultrasound to follow the propagation of a low frequency shear wave generated in a tissue by an external vibrator (Sandrin et al. 2002; Ziol et al. 2005). The Fibroscan® (Fig. 4) is composed of an integrated computer and dedicated electronics for ultrasound emission end reception, vibrator command and signal processing.

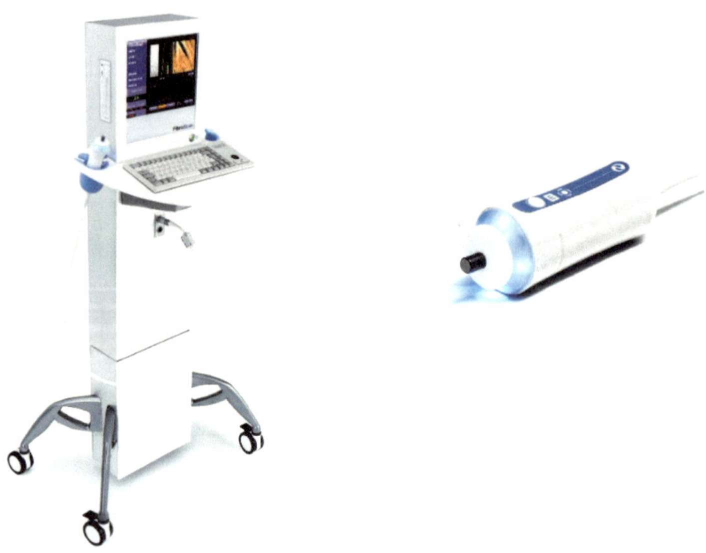

Fig. 4. The Fibroscan® and its M-probe.

The Fibroscan® probe contains an ultrasonic transducer used both as receiver and emitter which is mounted on a mechanical vibrator to generate a low frequency (50 Hz) shear wave. During the propagation of the low frequency shear wave, the radiofrequency (RF) data are acquired at a repetition frequency of 6000 Hz. The displacements induced in the medium are computed from the RF data using an autocorrelation method and derived versus depth in order to provide a strain rate image called elastogram (Fig. 5(c)). Analysis of the strain image yields the shear wave velocity and thus elasticity using the formula $E = 3\rho Vs^2$ where E, $\rho = 1000$ kg/m$^3$, and Vs are the Young's modulus, the mass density and the shear wave, respectively. In order to compute the shear wave velocity, a time-of-flight algorithm is used (Sandrin et al. 2003). The system enables to measure stiffness values (Young's modulus) between 1.5 kPa and 75 kPa.

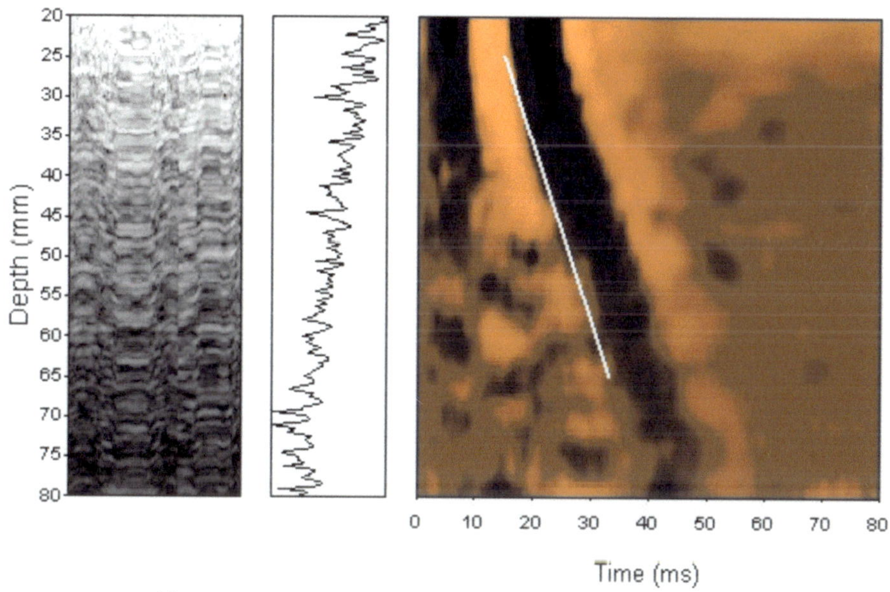


(a) (b) (c)

Fig. 5. (a) TM-mode, (b) A-mode and (c) elastogram images. The elastogram is a 2D graphical representation of the strain rates as a function of depth and time. The slope of the shear wave is represented by a white dotted line.

As shown in Table 3, four types of examination with specific depth and ultrasound frequency are available according to the morphology of the patient: skin-capsule distance (SCD) and thoracic perimeter (TP).

| Probe | Exam.Type | Criteria | Examination depth | Frequency |
|---|---|---|---|---|
| S | Small 1 (S1) | TP ≤ 45 cm | From 15 mm to 40 mm | 5 MHz |
| | Small 2 (S2) | 45 cm < TP ≤ 75 cm | From 20 mm to 50 mm | |
| M | Medium (M) | 75 cm < TP ≤ 110 cm and SCD < 2.5 cm | From 25 mm to 65 mm | 3.5 MHz |
| XL | XL | 2.5 cm ≤ SCD < 3.5 cm | From 35 mm to 75 mm | 2.5 MHz |

Table 3. Fibroscan® examination parameters.

### 3.2 Examination procedure

During the examination, the patient is lying in dorsal decubitus and the right arm in maximal abduction so as to enlarge the intercostals space in which the probe is placed (Fig. 6). The ribs play an important role since they prevent the application of large pressure on the liver by the probe. Indeed, biological tissues have a non linear elastic behavior when they are submitted to large strains. This nonlinearity would result in a biased measurement of the stiffness. This phenomenon also explains why elasticity measurements cannot be performed on the left lobe of the liver which is not protected by the ribs.

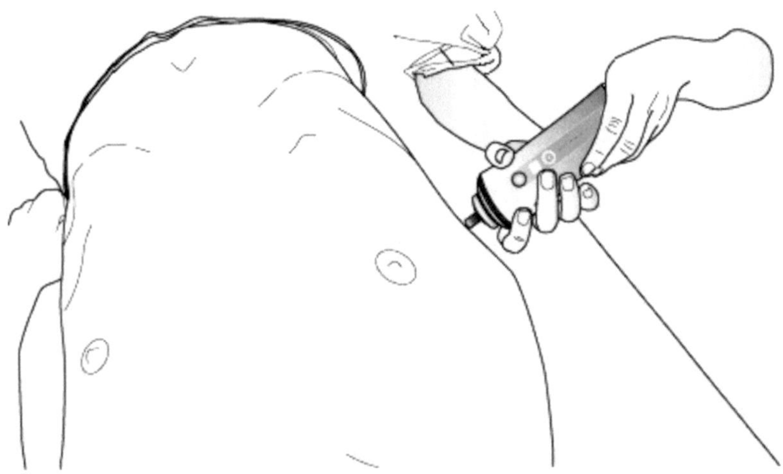

Fig. 6. During Fibroscan® examination, the patient is lying in dorsal decubitus and the right arm in maximal abduction so as to enlarge the intercostals space in which the probe is placed.

The probe should be placed between the rib bones opposite to the right lobe of the liver in the middle of the parenchyma far from the border of the liver. The measurement point should actually be similar to the location where the liver biopsy would be performed. Measurements performed too close to the borders the liver stiffness should be avoided as they will be overestimated.

The Fibroscan® device provides A-mode and M-mode images which should be used to find a liver portion suitable for the examination (Fig. 7). This liver area should be at least 60 mm deep and free of large vascular structures. In the case of a standard examination, the stiffness measurements are performed between 25 mm and 65 mm below the skin surface. The force applied by the probe on the skin is controlled during the whole examination and must be comprised between 4 N and 8 N in order to trigger a stiffness measurement.

During the examination, the operator should be careful about keeping the probe perpendicular to the skin surface or the liver stiffness may be overestimated (Fig. 8). The perpendicularity along both axes should be checked by looking at the probe. The operator should also check on the A-mode and TM-mode that the area is homogeneous and free of vessels structures (Fig. 9).

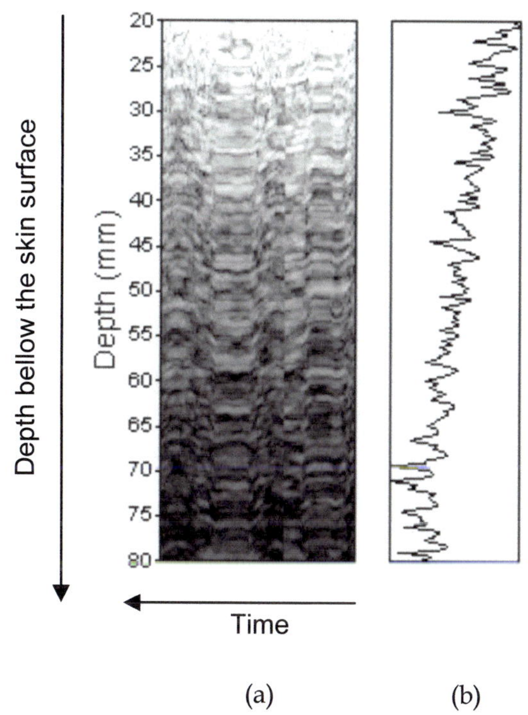


Fig. 7. The operator uses (a) TM-mode and (b) A-mode images to localize the measurement point. TM-mode represents the ultrasonic amplitude in log scale as a function of depth and time. A-mode is the real time ultrasonic line amplitude in log scale as a function of depth.

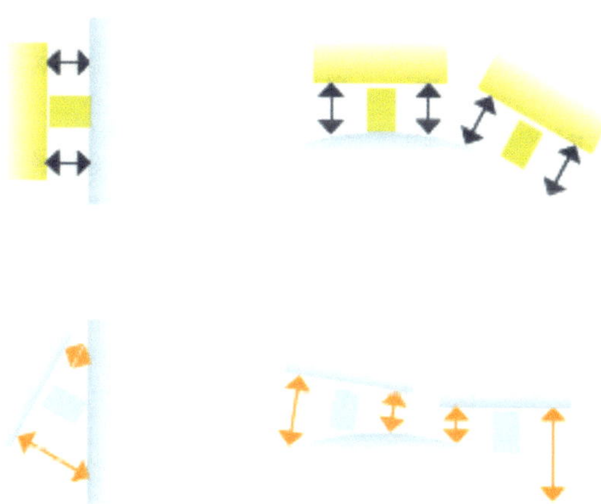

Fig. 8. During the examination, the operator should be careful about keeping the probe perpendicular to the skin surface or the liver stiffness may be overestimated.

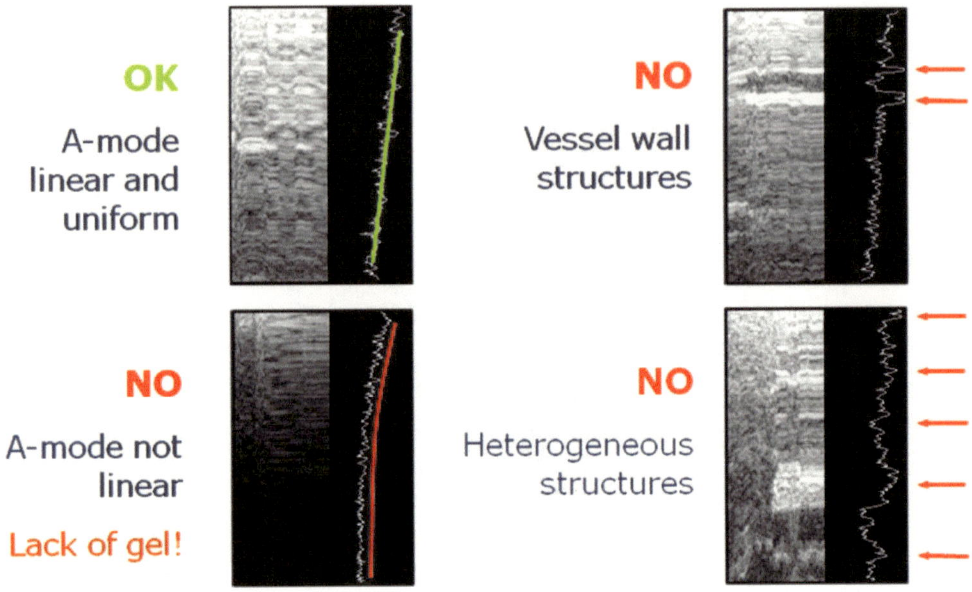


Fig. 9. The good window of acquisition is localized using A-mode and TM-mode displays.

When all the conditions mentioned above are met, the operator can trigger a measurement. An acquisition is almost instantaneous; it lasts a tenth of second. The software automatically rejects elastograms not fulfilling quality criteria and if the measurements are invalid, no result is displayed. The result of the examination is the median of all valid stiffness measurements within the current examination. The Inter Quartile Range (IQR) of all valid measurements and the success rate are also computed. Echosens recommends that a minimum of 8 valid measurements be obtained to get a consistent liver stiffness estimate.

Fibroscan® examination typically lasts between 2 and 5 minutes with recent devices. The liver explored volume by VCTE™ can be roughly approximated to be a cylinder of length 40 mm and diameter 10 mm (the actual value depends on the shear wavelength and examination type). This volume is 200 times larger than a 20 mm long and 1 mm diameter biopsy specimen.

Main limitations of Fibroscan® are the presence of ascites and obesity. Actually shear waves do not propagate through liquids. Thus Fibroscan® examination fails in some patients with ascites. However this limitation is counter balanced by the fact that ascites is already in itself an indication of liver pathological state. Thick subcutaneous tissues can result in a strong aberration of ultrasound and/or shear waves. As a result, it may be impossible to acquire enough valid measurements with Fibroscan® in some obese patients. However, a new probe, called XL probe, is now available to overcome this limitation. XL probe measures 60 % of the patients not measured with M probe (de Ledinghen et al. 2010).

## 4. Applications in hepatology

A review of literature is made. In this review, the use of liver stiffness measured with Fibroscan® is studied for diagnosis, prognostic, prognosis and treatment follow-up purposes.

### 4.1 Repeatability and reproducibility

Several groups have reported that liver stiffness measurements using Fibroscan® are repeatable and reproducible. The intra operator variability has been assessed (Boursier et al. 2008; Fraquelli et al. 2007) with intra-class correlation coefficient of 0.94 and 0.98 on 20 and 200 patients, respectively. The same publications as well as (Huwart et al. 2006) also evaluated the inter operator reproducibility with intra-class correlation coefficient ranging from 0.93 to 0.98. It shows that liver stiffness measurement using Fibroscan® is not dependent of the operator once the latter has been properly trained.

### 4.2 Diagnosis of liver fibrosis

#### 4.2.1 Patients with chronic liver diseases

As shown in Fig. 10, liver stiffness increases with the fibrosis stage obtained using liver biopsy. Liver stiffness has been shown to be closely related to fibrosis stage assessed by liver biopsy in patients suffering from chronic hepatitis C (Shaheen et al. 2007) and B (Marcellin et al. 2009), chronic cholestatic diseases (Corpechot et al. 2006), alcoholic liver disease (Melin et al. 2005; Mueller et al. 2010; Nguyen-Khac et al. 2008) and, recently, non-alcoholic fatty liver disease (Musso et al.). The most complete meta-analysis on the diagnosis accuracy of liver stiffness measured with Fibroscan® to assess liver fibrosis in patients with chronic liver disease of various etiology using liver biopsy as the gold standard (Friedrich-Rust et al. 2008) compiled up to 38 studies (publications or abstracts) (Table 4). For the diagnosis of significant fibrosis, the average AUROC was 0.84 (0.82-0.86) (and 0.91 when adjusted for liver biopsy quality) with an optimal cut-off of 7.7 kPa. For the diagnosis of cirrhosis, the average AUROC was 0.94 (0.93-0.95) (and 0.99 when adjusted for liver biopsy quality) with an optimal cut-off of 13.0 kPa.

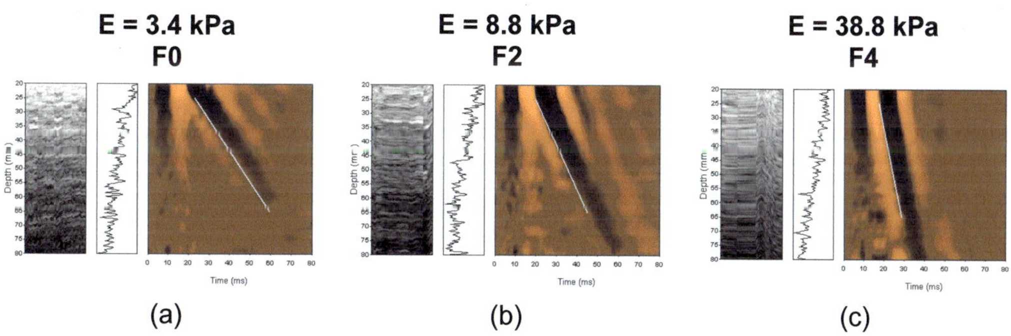


Fig. 10. The stiffer the liver the faster the shear wave (white line). From 3.4 kPa in a healthy subject to 8.8 kPa and 38.8 kPa in a F2 and a F4 patients, respectively. The slope given by the shear wave front gets steeper as the stiffness increases.

| Fibrosis grade | AUROC (confidence interval) | AUROC corrected for liver biopsy quality |
|---|---|---|
| F ≥ F2 | 0.84 (0.82 - 0.86) | 0.91 |
| F = 4 | 0.94 (0.93 - 0.95) | 0.99 |

Table 4. Diagnosis accuracy of liver stiffness measured with Fibroscan® to assess liver fibrosis in patients with chronic liver disease of various etiology using liver biopsy as the gold standard. Compilation of 38 studies (publications or abstracts).

#### 4.2.2 General population

Roulot (Roulot et al. 2010; Roulot et al. 2008) performed a study which aimed at detecting fibrosis in the general population. 1368 subjects attending a free check up in a medical center were measured. Liver biopsy was proposed to subjects (N=80) with stiffness values above 8 kPa. 28 subjects accepted to go through liver biopsy. Interestingly, all of them had fibrosis and cirrhosis was found in all subjects with stiffness above 14.6 kPa. Among the 72 subjects between 8 kPa and 14.6 kPa : 45 were overweight with metabolic syndrome, 18 were alcoholic, 5 had HCV and 4 had HBV.

### 4.3 Prognosis value

#### 4.3.1 Complication of cirrhosis

In addition to being related to portal hypertension assessed by HVPG measurement (Bureau et al. 2008; Carrion et al. 2006; Vizzutti et al. 2008), liver stiffness was shown to be related to other complications of cirrhosis. In a study (Foucher et al. 2006) on 144 patients with biopsy proven cirrhosis or bridging fibrosis, liver stiffness measurement had an AUROC of 0.90, 0.89, 0.71 and 0.88 for the detection of Child-Pugh score A versus BC, past history of ascites, presence of hepatocellular carcinoma and past history of ascites, respectively.

#### 4.3.2 Liver transplantation

Rigamonti et al (Rigamonti et al. 2008) reported that liver stiffness accurately predicts fibrosis progression in liver transplanted patients with recurrent hepatitis C, suggesting that protocol liver biopsy might be avoided in patients with improved or stable transient elastography values during follow-up..

#### 4.3.3 Survival

Vergniol et al (Vergniol et al.) followed 1457 patients (median 47.3 months) and demonstrated that the prognostic value of liver stiffness on survival was superior to that of liver biopsy. As a good predictive factor of survival, liver stiffness may help physician to evaluate earlier the severity of chronic liver diseases, to decide with stronger arguments of a liver transplantation or a portosystemic shunt and to evaluate more precisely the surgical risk of our cirrhotic patients.

### 4.4 Treatment follow-up

Fibroscan® was successfully used to assess liver fibrosis in patients during HCV or HBV therapy (Barreiro et al. 2006; Oliveri et al. 2008; Soriano et al. 2006). Ogawa et al (Ogawa et al. 2009) demonstrated that liver stiffness values measured by Fibroscan(r) may predict a progressively better clinical outcome for patients with successful virological and biochemical responses. Vergniol et al (Vergniol et al. 2009) suggested that Fibroscan(r) should be useful for assessing treatment efficacy in clinical trials of new drugs.
Recently, Berends et al (Berends et al. 2007) reported that Fibroscan(r) accurately predicted the absence of significant liver fibrosis in methotrexate users.

## 5. The pressure-stiffness-fibrosis sequence hypothesis

### 5.1 Factors influencing liver stiffness

As reported in the literature, liver stiffness is very well correlated with liver fibrosis. However studies showed that other factors influence liver stiffness. Several groups reported that liver stiffness significantly increases during inflammatory episodes (Arena et al. 2008; Oliveri et al. 2008; Sagir et al. 2008). They showed that during several months monitoring, liver stiffness values paralleled those of ALT in patients with hepatitis exacerbation and observed a progressive decrease during antiviral therapy. Millonig (Millonig et al. 2009; Millonig et al. 2008) reported that mechanical cholestasis drastically and reversibly increases liver stiffness and that liver stiffness is influenced by central venous pressure and thus liver congestion, for example due to cardiac insufficiency.

### 5.2 Physical point of view

From a physical point of view, liver stiffness is obviously mainly driven by the liver extracellular matrix which provides structural support to the liver. However, since the liver is self-contained in a non extensible Glisson's capsule, stiffness is definitively influenced by pressure that can be either hydrostatic or osmotic. The amount of collagen contained in the matrix yields a static stiffness. As shown in Fig. 11, on top of this static stiffness, hydrostatic and osmotic pressure effects will add a pressure-related stiffness term which results from body flood dynamics: blood flow, interstitial liquids, etc. On one hand, central venous pressure is directly related to hydrostatic pressure resulting from heart beating. On the other hand, flow of fluid from plasma to interstitial fluid is driven by osmotic pressure. During inflammatory episodes, accumulation of interstitial liquid and inflammatory infiltrate increases osmotic pressure.

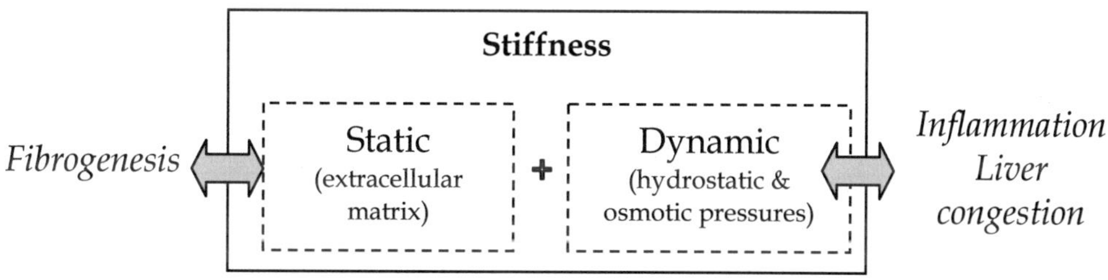


Fig. 11. Liver stiffness is composed of two components: static stiffness due to the extracellular matrix and dynamic stiffness linked to hydrostatic pressure and osmotic pressure.

### 5.3 Molecular mechanism

A study from Sakata (Sakata et al. 2004) supports the pressure-matrix-stiffness sequence hypothesis (Mueller & Sandrin 2010). Under this hypothesis, pressure results in increased mechanical stretching which induces transforming growth factor (TGF)-β synthesis in hepatic stellate cells, which is known to be highly expressed under profibrogenic conditions. Therefore, increased dynamic stiffness due to pressure induces mechanical stretches which stimulate the production of collagen (fibrotic tissue) which results in a static stiffness increase as if the liver was adapting its structure to inner body mechanical conditions.

Among the numerous questions that still need to be answered on this very exciting subject, one of the more interesting may be the understanding of the respective roles of portal fibrosis and perisinusoidal fibrosis in liver stiffness.

## 6. Discussion

Liver stiffness measurement using Fibroscan® has been studied in all major causes of chronic liver diseases: chronic hepatitis C, chronic hepatitis B, HIV - HCV co-infection, alcoholic liver disease (ALD), non alcoholic fatty liver disease (NAFLD), biliary disease, etc.

### 6.1 The keys of Fibroscan® success and its limitations

The success of liver stiffness measurement using Fibroscan® may be explained by several factors. First of al, it is a bedside procedure which lasts between 2 and 5 minutes and gives an immediate result. Second, the procedure is highly standardized with dedicated training which provides low operator dependence compared to ultrasound guided procedures, as an example. Third it offers new perspectives as liver stiffness is providing more information to physicians than fibrosis. Furthermore, it can be used for diagnosis, prognostic and follow-up.
As any other procedure, liver stiffness measurement using Fibroscan® is having limitations. Main physical limitation is linked to the presence of ascites as liquids prevent the propagation of shear waves. As a consequence, shear waves are stopped before they can enter liver. Another limitation is related to obesity and more specifically to a large skin to liver capsula distance. In this case, ultrasound and shear wave aberration may occur and significantly reduce the success rate of liver stiffness measurements. A new probe, XL probe, was released to overcome this issue and demonstrated a significant improvement of the measurement success in obese patients.

### 6.2 Liver stiffness is a clinically relevant parameter by itself

In 2003, liver stiffness measured using Fibroscan® was introduced as an alternative to liver biopsy in order to assess liver fibrosis non-invasively. Nowadays liver stiffness is considered as a novel objective physical parameter that will eventually be used like arterial pressure or temperature. Primarily related by liver fibrosis, liver stiffness is influenced by venous pressure, inflammation and mechanical cholestatis. It is now part of the tools a physician may use to diagnose liver diseases. For this purpose, it should obviously be interpreted in the full context of clinical, imaging and laboratory findings (Fig. 12).

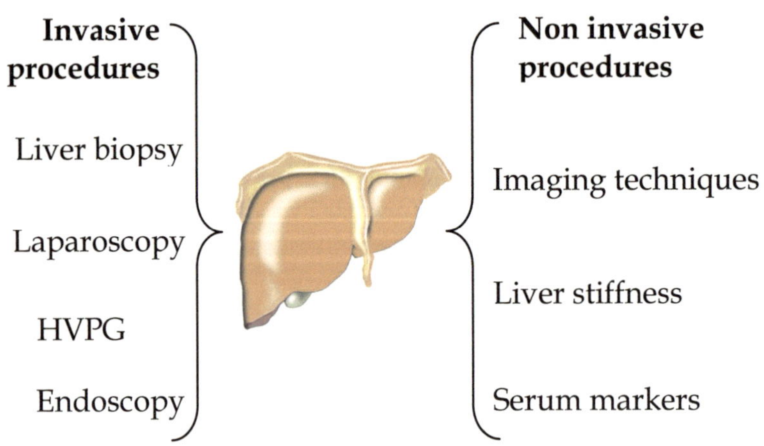


Fig. 12. Liver stiffness should always be interpreted in the context of clinical, imaging and laboratory findings.

As explained earlier in this chapter, liver stiffness is not only affected by the liver matrix but also by pressure increase which may be attributed to several factors from congestion to inflammation. Furthermore, there are very disruptive elements that suggest that liver stiffness may not only be the consequence fibrosis deposits within the liver but also one of the causes of fibrogenesis as it has been demonstrated that hepatic stellate cells tend to generate fibrosis when they are under mechanical stress. For these reasons liver stiffness shall not be considered as a secondary endpoint; liver stiffness is a clinically relevant parameter by itself.

### 6.3 Recent developments

Even though liver stiffness provides an alternative to liver biopsy for fibrosis staging, it can not yield very important histologic features such as macrovesicular steatosis, ballooned hepatocytes, inflammation, etc. Recently, a new parameter, Controlled Attenuation Parameter (CAP), was designed to quantify liver steatosis using Fibroscan®. This measurement is performed at the exact same location where liver stiffness is measured and showed good performances for steatosis quantification (Sasso et al. 2010).

The need for small animal non-invasive preclinical tools is growing. Obviously a Fibroscan® based instrumentation device adapted to small animal would have very interesting applications for the development of new drugs and for the study of drug-induced liver injury. Recently, Bastard (Bastard et al. 2011) demonstrated that VCTE™ can be adapted for small animal liver stiffness measurements.

## 7. Conclusion

Initially studied for its potential benefit for breast and prostate cancer, quantitative elastography eventually led to a promising diagnostic device in hepatology. The name Fibroscan® was invented at the time when liver stiffness measurement was intended to serve as an alternative to fibrosis staging using liver biopsy. Obviously, today the name Fibroscan® is misleading as liver stiffness has become a clinically relevant parameter by itself. Liver stiffness opened new possibilities in the field of hepatology: in routine and in research. These possibilities were made possible because of key advantages of non-invasive liver stiffness measurement with Fibroscan®. Among the important outcomes, the possible differentiation between early and advanced cirrhosis, the good prognostic value of liver stiffness on patient survival and the follow-up of patients undergoing treatments can be pointed out. Liver stiffness shall continue to be studied in many ways and will help physicians to better understand the natural history of liver diseases. With significant developments in the field of hepatology, for example the steatosis quantification, Fibroscan® may become the companion of hepatologists in their day to day clinical practice and research projects.

## 8. Acknowledgments

The authors are grateful to Anis Hadj Henni (RheoLution Inc) for providing useful data.

## 9. References

Abdi, W., Millan, J. C. & Mezey, E. (1979). Sampling variability on percutaneous liver biopsy, *Arch Intern Med,* Vol.139, No.6, (Jun), pp. 667-9

Arena, U., Vizzutti, F., Corti, G., Ambu, S., Stasi, C., Bresci, S., Moscarella, S., Boddi, V., Petrarca, A., Laffi, G., Marra, F. & Pinzani, M. (2008). Acute viral hepatitis increases liver stiffness values measured by transient elastography, *Hepatology,* Vol.47, No.2, (Feb), pp. 380-4

Barreiro, P., Labarga, P., Martin-Carbonero, L., Amor, A., Ruiz-Sancho, A., Castellares, C., Gonzalez-Lahoz, J. & Soriano, V. (2006). Sustained virological response following HCV therapy is associated with non-progression of liver fibrosis in HCV/HIV-coinfected patients, *Antivir Ther,* Vol.11, No.7, pp. 869-77

Bastard, C., Bosisio, M. R., Chabert, M., Kalopissis, A., Mahrouf-Yorgov, M., Gilgenkrantz, H., Mueller, S. & Sandrin, L. (2011). Transient micro-elastography: A novel approach to measure liver stiffness in mice, *World Journal of Gastroenterology,* Vol.17, No.8, pp. 968-975

Bedossa, P., Dargere, D. & Paradis, V. (2003). Sampling variability of liver fibrosis in chronic hepatitis C, *Hepatology,* Vol.38, No.6, (Dec), pp. 1449-57

Bercoff, J., Tanter, M. & Fink, M. (2004). Supersonic shear imaging: a new technique for soft tissues elasticity mapping, *IEEE Transactions on Utrasonics, Ferroelectrics, and Frequency Control,* Vol.51, No.4, pp. 374-409

Berends, M. A., Snoek, J., de Jong, E. M., Van Krieken, J. H., de Knegt, R. J., van Oijen, M. G., van de Kerkhof, P. C. & Drenth, J. P. (2007). Biochemical and biophysical assessment of MTX-induced liver fibrosis in psoriasis patients: Fibrotest predicts the presence and Fibroscan predicts the absence of significant liver fibrosis, *Liver Int,* Vol.27, No.5, (Jun), pp. 639-45

Boursier, J., Konate, A., Gorea, G., Reaud, S., Quemener, E., Oberti, F., Hubert-Fouchard, I., Dib, N. & Cales, P. (2008). Reproducibility of liver stiffness measurement by ultrasonographic elastometry, *Clin Gastroenterol Hepatol,* Vol.6, No.11, (Nov), pp. 1263-9

Bravo, A. A., Sheth, S. & Chpra, S. (2001). Liver biopsy, *The New England Journal of Medicine,* Vol.344, No.7, pp. 495-500

Bureau, C., Metivier, S., Peron, J. M., Selves, J., Robic, M. A., Gourraud, P. A., Rouquet, O., Dupuis, E., Alric, L. & Vinel, J. P. (2008). Transient elastography accurately predicts presence of significant portal hypertension in patients with chronic liver disease, *Aliment Pharmacol Ther,* Vol.27, No.12, (Jun), pp. 1261-8

Cadranel, J. F., Rufat, P. & Degos, F. (2001). Pratiques de la ponction-biopsie hépatique transpariétale en France, *Gastroenterologie Clinique et Biologique,* Vol.25, pp. 77-80

Carrion, J. A., Navasa, M., Bosch, J., Bruguera, M., Gilabert, R. & Forns, X. (2006). Transient elastography for diagnosis of advanced fibrosis and portal hypertension in patients with hepatitis C recurrence after liver transplantation, *Liver Transpl,* Vol.12, No.12, (Dec), pp. 1791-8

Castera, L., Vergniol, J., Foucher, J., Le Bail, B., Chanteloup, E., Haaser, M., Darriet, M., Couzigou, P. & de Ledinghen, V. (2005). Prospective comparison of transient elastography, Fibrotest, APRI and liver biopsy for the assessement of fibrosis in chronic hepatitis C, *Gastroenterology,* Vol.128, pp. 343-350

Corpechot, C., El Naggar, A., Poujol-Robert, A., Ziol, M., Wendum, D., Chazouilleres, O., de Ledinghen, V., Dhumeaux, D., Marcellin, P., Beaugrand, M. & Poupon, R. (2006). Assessment of biliary fibrosis by transient elastography in patients with PBC and PSC, *Hepatology,* Vol.43, No.5, (May), pp. 1118-24 de Ledinghen, V., Vergniol, J., Foucher, J., El-Hajbi, F., Merrouche, W. & Rigalleau, V. (2010). Feasibility of liver transient elastography with FibroScan using a new probe for obese patients, *Liver Int*, Vol.30, No.7, (Aug), pp. 1043-8

Fahey, B. J., Palmeri, M. L. & Trahey, G. E. (2006). Frame rate considerations for real-time abdominal acoustic radiation force impulse imaging, *Ultrason Imaging*, Vol.28, No.4, (Oct), pp. 193-210

Foucher, J., Castera, L., Bernard, P. H., Adhoute, X., Laharie, D., Bertet, J., Couzigou, P. & de Ledinghen, V. (2006). Prevalence and factors associated with failure of liver stiffness measurement using FibroScan in a prospective study of 2114 examinations, *European Journal of Gastroenterology & Hepatology*, Vol.18, No.4, (Apr), pp. 411-412

Fraquelli, M., Rigamonti, C., Casazza, G., Conte, D., Donato, M. F., Ronchi, G. & Colombo, M. (2007). Reproducibility of transient elastography in the evaluation of liver fibrosis in patients with chronic liver disease, *Gut*, Vol.56, No.7, (Jul), pp. 968-73

Friedrich-Rust, M., Ong, M. F., Martens, S., Sarrazin, C., Bojunga, J., Zeuzem, S. & Herrmann, E. (2008). Performance of transient elastography for the staging of liver fibrosis: a meta-analysis, *Gastroenterology*, Vol.134, No.4, (Apr), pp. 960-74

Huwart, L., Peeters, F., Sinkus, R., Annet, L., Salameh, N., ter Beek, L. C., Horsmans, Y. & Van Beers, B. E. (2006). Liver fibrosis: non-invasive assessment with MR elastography, *Nmr in Biomedicine*, Vol.19, No.2, (Apr), pp. 173-179

Klatt, D., Asbach, P., Rump, J., Papazoglou, S., Somasundaram, R., Modrow, J., Braun, J. & Sack, I. (2006). In vivo determination of hepatic stiffness using steady-state free precession magnetic resonance elastography, *Invest Radiol*, Vol.41, No.12, (Dec), pp. 841-8

Marcellin, P., Ziol, M., Bedossa, P., Douvin, C., Poupon, R., de Ledinghen, V. & Beaugrand, M. (2009). Non-invasive assessment of liver fibrosis by stiffness measurement in patients with chronic hepatitis B, *Liver Int*, Vol.29, No.2, (Feb), pp. 242-7

Melin, P., Dacon, A., Gauchet, A., Schoeny, M. & Diebold, M.-D. (2005). Dépistage non invasif de la fibrose : Intérêt du FibroScan en consultation d'alcoologie [Non-invasive detection of liver fibrosis: Value of FibroScan in alcohol consulting out-patients], *Alcoologie et Addictologie*, Vol.27, No.3, pp. 191-196

Millonig, G., Friedrich, S., Adolf, S., Fonouni, H., Golriz, M., Mehrabi, A., Stiefel, P., Poschl, G., Buchler, M. W., Seitz, H. K. & Mueller, S. (2009). Liver stiffness is directly influenced by central venous pressure, *J Hepatol*, Vol.52, No.2, (Feb), pp. 206-10

Millonig, G., Reimann, F. M., Friedrich, S., Fonouni, H., Mehrabi, A., Buchler, M. W., Seitz, H. K. & Mueller, S. (2008). Extrahepatic cholestasis increases liver stiffness (FibroScan) irrespective of fibrosis, *Hepatology*, Vol.48, No.5, (Nov), pp. 1718-23

Mueller, S., Millonig, G., Sarovska, L., Friedrich, S., Reimann, F. M., Pritsch, M., Eisele, S., Stickel, F., Longerich, T., Schirmacher, P. & Seitz, H. K. (2010). Increased liver stiffness in alcoholic liver disease: differentiating fibrosis from steatohepatitis, *World J Gastroenterol*, Vol.16, No.8, (Feb 28), pp. 966 72

Mueller, S. & Sandrin, L. (2010). Liver stiffness: a novel parameter for the diagnosis of liver disease, *Hepatic Medicine: Evidence and Research*, Vol.2, (May), pp. 49-67

Muller, M., Gennisson, J. L., Deffieux, T., Tanter, M. & Fink, M. (2009). Quantitative viscoelasticity mapping of human liver using supersonic shear imaging:

preliminary in vivo feasibility study, *Ultrasound Med Biol,* Vol.35, No.2, (Feb), pp. 219-29

Musso, G., Gambino, R., Cassader, M. & Pagano, G. Meta-analysis: Natural history of non-alcoholic fatty liver disease (NAFLD) and diagnostic accuracy of non-invasive tests for liver disease severity, *Ann Med,* (Nov 2), pp.

Muthupillai, R., Lomas, D. J., Rossman, P. J., Greenleaf, J. F., Manduca, A. & Ehman, R. L. (1995). Magnetic resonance elastography by direct visualization of propagating acoustic strain waves, *Science,* Vol.269, No.5232, (Sep 29), pp. 1854-7

Nguyen-Khac, E., Chatelain, D., Tramier, B., Decrombecque, C., Robert, B., Joly, J. P., Brevet, M., Grignon, P., Lion, S., Le Page, L. & Dupas, J. L. (2008). Assessment of asymptomatic liver fibrosis in alcoholic patients using fibroscan: prospective comparison with seven non-invasive laboratory tests, *Aliment Pharmacol Ther,* Vol.28, No.10, (Nov 15), pp. 1188-98

Nightingale, K., McAleavey, S. & Trahey, G. (2003). Shear-wave generation using acoustic radiation force: in vivo and ex vivo results, *Ultrasound Med Biol,* Vol.29, No.12, (Dec), pp. 1715-23

Ogawa, E., Furusyo, N., Toyoda, K., Takeoka, H., Maeda, S. & Hayashi, J. (2009). The longitudinal quantitative assessment by transient elastography of chronic hepatitis C patients treated with pegylated interferon alpha-2b and ribavirin, *Antiviral Res,* Vol.83, No.2, (Aug), pp. 127-34

Oliveri, F., Coco, B., Ciccorossi, P., Colombatto, P., Romagnoli, V., Cherubini, B., Bonino, F. & Brunetto, M. R. (2008). Liver stiffness in the hepatitis B virus carrier: a non-invasive marker of liver disease influenced by the pattern of transaminases, *World J Gastroenterol,* Vol.14, No.40, (Oct 28), pp. 6154-62

Palmeri, M. L. & Nightingale, K. R. (2004). On the thermal effects associated with radiation force imaging of soft tissue, *IEEE Trans Ultrason Ferroelectr Freq Control,* Vol.51, No.5, (May), pp. 551-65

Palmeri, M. L., Wang, M. H., Dahl, J. J., Frinkley, K. D. & Nightingale, K. R. (2008). Quantifying hepatic shear modulus in vivo using acoustic radiation force, *Ultrasound Med Biol,* Vol.34, No.4, (Apr), pp. 546-58

Poynard, T., Imbert-Bismut, F., Munteanu, M., Messous, D., Myers, R. P., Thabut, D., Ratziu, V., Mercadier, A., Benhamou, Y. & Hainque, B. (2004). Overview of the diagnostic value of biochemical markers of liver fibrosis (FibroTest, HCV FibroSure) and necrosis (ActiTest) in patients with chronic hepatitis C, *Comparative Hepatology,* Vol.3, No.1, (Sep 23), pp. 8

Rigamonti, C., Donato, M. F., Fraquelli, M., Agnelli, F., Ronchi, G., Casazza, G., Rossi, G. & Colombo, M. (2008). Transient elastography predicts fibrosis progression in patients with recurrent hepatitis C after liver transplantation, *Gut,* Vol.57, No.6, (Jun), pp. 821-7

Roulot, D., Costes, J. L., Buyck, J. F., Warzocha, U., Gambier, N., Czernichow, S., Le Clesiau, H. & Beaugrand, M. (2010). Transient elastography as a screening tool for liver fibrosis and cirrhosis in a community-based population aged over 45 years, *Gut,* (Nov 10), pp.

Roulot, D., Czernichow, S., Le Clesiau, H., Costes, J. L., Vergnaud, A. C. & Beaugrand, M. (2008). Liver stiffness values in apparently healthy subjects: influence of gender and metabolic syndrome, *J Hepatol,* Vol.48, No.4, (Apr), pp. 606-13

Rouviere, O., Yin, M., Dresner, M. A., Rossman, P. J., Burgart, L. J., Fidler, J. L. & Ehman, R. L. (2006). MR elastography of the liver: preliminary results, *Radiology,* Vol.240, No.2, (Aug), pp. 440-8

Sagir, A., Erhardt, A., Schmitt, M. & Haussinger, D. (2008). Transient elastography is unreliable for detection of cirrhosis in patients with acute liver damage, *Hepatology,* Vol.47, No.2, (Feb), pp. 592-5

Sakata, R., Ueno, T., Nakamura, T., Ueno, H. & Sata, M. (2004). Mechanical stretch induces TGF-beta synthesis in hepatic stellate cells, *Eur J Clin Invest,* Vol.34, No.2, (Feb), pp. 129-36

Sandrin, L., Cassereau, D. & Fink, M. (2004). The role of the coupling term in transient elastography., *Journal of the Acoustical Society of America,* Vol.115, pp. 73-83

Sandrin, L., Fourquet, B., Hasquenoph, J. M., Yon, S., Fournier, C., Mal, F., Christidis, C., Ziol, M., Poulet, B., Kazemi, F., Beaugrand, M. & Palau, R. (2003). Transient elastography: a new noninvasive method for assessment of hepatic fibrosis, *Ultrasound Med Biol,* Vol.29, No.12, (Dec), pp. 1705-13

Sandrin, L., Tanter, M., Catheline, S. & Fink, M. (2002). Shear modulus imaging with 2D transient elastography, *IEEE Transactions on Utrasonics, Ferroelectrics, and Frequency Control,* Vol.49, pp. 426-435

Sandrin, L., Tanter, M., Gennisson, J. L., Catheline, S. & Fink, M. (2002). Shear elasticity probe for soft tissues with 1-D transient elastography, *IEEE Trans Ultrason Ferroelectr Freq Control,* Vol.49, No.4, (Apr), pp. 436-46

Sarvazyan, A. P., Skovoroda, A. R., Emelianov, S. Y., Fowlkes, J. B., Pipe, J. G., Adler, R. S., Buxton, R. B. & Carson, P. L. (1995). Biophysical bases of elasticity imaging, *Acoustical Imaging,* Vol.21, pp. 223-240

Sasso, M., Beaugrand, M., de Ledinghen, V., Douvin, C., Marcellin, P., Poupon, R., Sandrin, L. & Miette, V. (2010). Controlled attenuation parameter (CAP): a novel VCTE guided ultrasonic attenuation measurement for the evaluation of hepatic steatosis: preliminary study and validation in a cohort of patients with chronic liver disease from various causes, *Ultrasound Med Biol,* Vol.36, No.11, (Nov), pp. 1825-35

Shaheen, A. A., Wan, A. F. & Myers, R. P. (2007). FibroTest and FibroScan for the prediction of hepatitis C-related fibrosis: a systematic review of diagnostic test accuracy, *Am J Gastroenterol,* Vol.102, No.11, (Nov), pp. 2589-600

Soriano, V., Nunez, M., Garcia-Samaniego, J., Labarga, P., Simarro, N., Martin-Carbonero, L., Romero, M., Ramos, B. & Barreiro, P. (2006). Chronic hepatitis C in HIV-infected patients: those who more need therapy are those who respond less, *Infect Disord Drug Targets,* Vol.6, No.1, (Mar), pp. 57-88

Vergniol, J., Foucher, J., Castera, L., Bernard, P. H., Tournan, R., Terrebonne, E., Chanteloup, E., Merrouche, W., Couzigou, P. & de Ledinghen, V. (2009). Changes of non-invasive markers and FibroScan values during HCV treatment, *J Viral Hepat,* Vol.16, No.2, (Feb), pp. 132-40

Vergniol, J., Foucher, J., Terrebonne, E., Bernard, P. H., Le Bail, B., Merrouche, W., Couzigou, P. & de Ledinghen, V. (2011). Non-Invasive Tests for Fibrosis and Liver Stiffness Predict 5-Year Outcomes of Patients with Chronic Hepatitis C, *Gastroenterology,* (Mar 1), pp.

Vizzutti, F., Arena, U., Rega, L. & Pinzani, M. (2008). Non invasive diagnosis of portal hypertension in cirrhotic patients, *Gastroenterol Clin Biol,* Vol.32, No.6 Suppl 1, (Sep), pp. 80-7

Ziol, M., Handra-Luca, A., Kettaneh, A., Christidis, C., Mal, F., Kazemi, F., de Ledinghen, V., Marcellin, P., Dhumeaux, D., Trinchet, J.-C. & Beaugrand, M. (2005). Non-invasive assessment of liver fibrosis by stiffness measurements: a prospective multicenter study in patients with chronic hepatitis C, *Hepatology,* Vol.41, No.1, pp. 48-54

# 20

# Virtual Reality Simulation of Liver Biopsy with a Respiratory Component

Pierre-Frédéric Villard[1,2], Piers Boshier[1],
Fernando Bello[1] and Derek Gould[3]
[1]*Imperial College, London,*
[2]*LORIA, Nancy University,*
[3]*Royal Liverpool Hospital, Liverpool,*
[1,3]*UK*
[2]*France*

## 1. Introduction

The use of simulation to train skills has grown exponentially in the last few decades, especially in medicine, where simulator models can provide a platform where trainees can practice procedures without risk or harm to patients. Potential advantages of computer based simulator models over other forms of medical simulators include: (i) anatomical fidelity; (ii) the ability to train in an environment wherein physiological behavior is observed, something that is not possible using in-vitro phantoms; (iii) variability of anatomy and pathology which is important to the acquisition of experience; (v) quantification of metrics relating to task performance that can be used to monitor trainee performance throughout the learning curve; and (vi) cost effectiveness.

The work described herein was conducted as part of the CRaIVE collaboration (Gould et al., 2004), the aim of which is to develop simulator models specific to interventional radiology (IR). Our use of the term 'interventional radiology' is intended to encompass all micro-surgical, minimally invasive procedures that use percutaneous needle access for biopsy or for guidewire and catheter introduction and manipulation, and where medical imaging (i.e. ultrasound, fluoroscopy, computed tomography) is used for intra-procedural guidance. A frequently performed, IR technique is liver biopsy, where a needle is inserted into the liver to acquire a tissue sample for histological diagnosis of conditions such as cancer, inflammation, cirrhosis etc.

In this chapter we present a detailed description of a simulator framework for liver biopsy using patient-specific data. Key features of this simulator include the incorporation of modifiable respiratory movements and real-rime haptic interaction. We first present an overview of the current state of the art of medical simulators. Subsequent sections are intended to provide a complete description of parameters required to design a medical simulator for liver biopsy, detailing methods used to produce a computer-based model of both patient respiration and haptic interaction, as well as their integration into the final simulator.

## 2. State of the art

Various simulators exist to train IR practitioners (interventional radiologists). In the case of liver biopsy, which has the added challenge of respiratory motion, only non computer-based simulators currently exist (Müller et al., 2007). As outlined in the introduction, there are, however particular benefits of using computer-based medical simulators. We focus below on different aspects in the literature that are considered to be integral to the accurate simulation of liver biopsy.

Although liver displacement due to respiratory motion has not been incorporated into existing liver biopsy simulators, previous authors have sought to model respiration for a range of applications, including animated entertainment (Zordan et al., 2004) and medical applications. These latter models described in the literature focus on medical augmented reality (Santhanam et al., 2007) and pre-procedural planning of radiological interventions (Didier et al., 2007; Hoestettler et al., 2008). For future simulators to find application within clinical practice, they must be able to offer a realistic real time depiction of anatomical structures and their dynamic interaction. Thus, our aim was a simulator that is fast enough to support real-time, or near real-time, computer graphics techniques and interaction, but realistic enough for the specific medical application.

To date, needle insertion simulators have been developed for a range of applications (Abolhassani et al., 2007). In one example, complex mechanical models are used to simulate needle insertion and soft-tissue behavior in the setting of pre-procedural training and planning (Chentanez et al., 2009). Experimental data has also been used by others to model the force evolution during needle manipulation (Maurin et al., 2004). The requirement for a liver biopsy simulator to incorporate respiratory motion does, however, limit us to a relatively simplistic needle model.

The incorporation of force feedback in simulators has been recently reviewed (Coles et al., 2010). Application of this technology is intended to enhance the user's immersion in a virtual reality environment. Commercial devices are already available for both basic laparoscopic tasks and interventional radiology procedures. Figure 1 illustrates two examples of these simulators: the LAP Mentor by Simbionix for laparoscopic procedures (www.simbionix.com) and the Mentice VIST for endovascular IR procedures (www.mentice.com). Increased access to commercial haptic devices has helped support the application of this technology in new simulators.

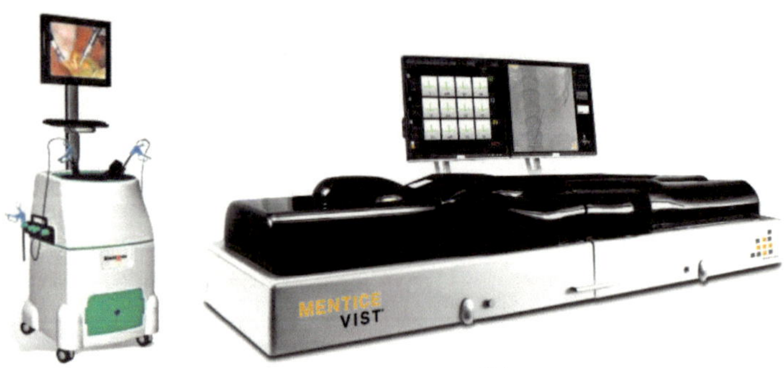


(a) (b)

Fig. 1. Existing micro-surgical simulators: (a) LAP Mentor by Simbionix, (b) VIST by Mentice.

## 3. Construction of the virtual patients

We now focus on the construction of the proposed virtual environment, defining the anatomy used in our simulation as well as the software framework, prior to detailing the simulation of organ behavior in a breathing patient during needle insertion.

### 3.1 Strategy and input data

The initial objective was to construct virtual patients for use in the proposed liver biopsy simulator. To achieve this, it was necessary to first construct a patient database for visualization of organ position and motion (graphic rendering), and subsequently to adapt this environment to support tool-tissue interactions within a collision detection loop (haptics rendering). This use of patient imaging data was passed by the local research ethics committee. A computer-based simulator was constructed based on the database, and depicting the anatomy of a virtual patient. In the current project we chose to extract this information from medical imaging of patients. Three-dimensional computed tomography (CT) scans of patients attending the Centre Léon Bérard (Lyon, France) and the Marie Curie Institute (Paris, France) were acquired. Scan parameters were as follows: size 512x512x$N_z$ with $N_z$ varying from 140 to 200, and voxel dimensions 0.976mm x 0,976mm x 2mm.
In addition to the liver, it is necessary to also include the ribcage and thoracic diaphragm, as they are essential to modeling respiratory motion. The strategy adopted for data acquisition was as follows: (i) retrieval of anonymized scan data for recruited patients after obtaining informed written consent; (ii) extraction of organ contours from scans; and (iii) computation of a more simplistic representation of organ geometry via a meshing process. Each of these steps is illustrated in Figure 2 using the ribcage as an example.

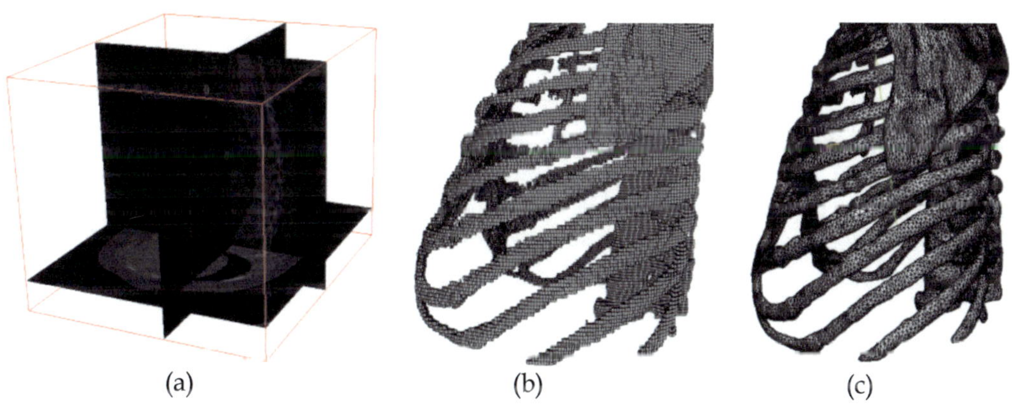


Fig. 2. Construction of the virtual patient using the ribcage as an example: (a) 3D CT scan showing the ribcage, (b) Voxels resulting from segmentation of the ribcage, (c) Polygonal mesh used in the simulation.

### 3.2 Segmentation

Contour data can be extracted from medical imaging either by automatic or manual segmentation. The current project utilized automatic segmentation for bony anatomy (spine and rib cage), and manual segmentation for the liver and diaphragm, where interpretation by a medical expert is required.

### 3.2.1 Bones, lungs and skin segmentation

All segmentation during the current project was performed using ITK-snap, an open-source program developed by the University of Pennsylvania (Yushkevich et al., 2005). Using this program, automatic segmentation is achieved by a process based on the level set technique. This method is divided into three steps: (i) bounded region is defined in order to drive the contour evolution. This boundary is given by the double-threshold image binarization method. (ii) Spherical seeds of different diameters are placed at different locations inside the previously defined boundaries, and (iii) an evolution function is applied to these seeds. This time-depending function, $\mathbf{C_t}$, is defined by equation (1).

$$C_t = (\delta g_I - \xi \mathrm{K})\vec{n} \tag{1}$$

where δ and ξ are tunable parameters that have been respectively set to 1.0 and 0.2; $\mathbf{g_I}$ is the force intensity based on the image gradient; **K** is the force intensity based on the contour curvature; and **n** is the contour normal.

Due to the high density of bone, segmentation of this tissue was performed using the automatic method with a double threshold (lower and upper) based on high Hounsfield density. The same method is used to segment the lungs. As the lungs are composed primarily of air, a double threshold based on low Hounsfield density is employed. The air-tissue interface at the skin can likewise be segmented by this method based on low Hounsfield density.

### 3.2.2 Liver segmentation

Segmentation of the liver by automated methods poses a far greater challenge, because of the difficulty in performing the initial step of the level set algorithm due to the similarity between the density of the liver and its surrounding organs and tissues. Whilst methods exist to overcome this problem (Chen et al., 2009; Foruzana et al., 2009; Rusko et al., 2009), they are seldom satisfactory. Consequently, manual segmentation of organs such as the liver, whilst time consuming, is preferred. Manual segmentation can be more reliably and easily performed by using graphic tablets, such as the Cintiq 21UX Tablet PC (Wacom Co Ltd., Saitama, Japan) that was used in the current project. Such tablets, used in combination with a pressure sensitive stylus, permit a trained expert performing the segmentation to trace, freehand, the border of the liver in consecutive CT scan images in the sagittal, coronal and axial view. As with automatic segmentation, manual segmentation was performed using the ITK-snap software.

### 3.2.3 Diaphragm segmentation

Due to its thickness, typically 3mm (1-2 pixels), it is often difficult to visualize the thoracic diaphragm in standard CT scan images. Moreover, the density of the fibro-muscular tissue which makes up the diaphragm is similar to that of other surrounding organs and tissues. Segmenting of this structure, therefore, presented a major challenge. The most effective way of manually segmenting the diaphragm was to isolate its boundaries with surrounding structures, namely the liver, lungs and thoracic wall. For the diaphragm, manual segmentation in the sagittal, coronal and axial planes is particularly desirable as it helps to ensure a smooth contour. Important anatomical relationships of the diaphragm include: (i) the spine in the region of the twelfth thoracic vertebra; diaphragmatic crura are demonstrable in the axial plane (see Figure 3.a); (ii) the inner aspect of the ribs and the costal margin; (iii) the overlying visceral and parietal pleura, including the potential space of the pleural reflection; (iv) the liver; (v) the heart / pericardium and lungs, (vi) stomach and (vii) spleen (See Figure 3.b and 3.c).

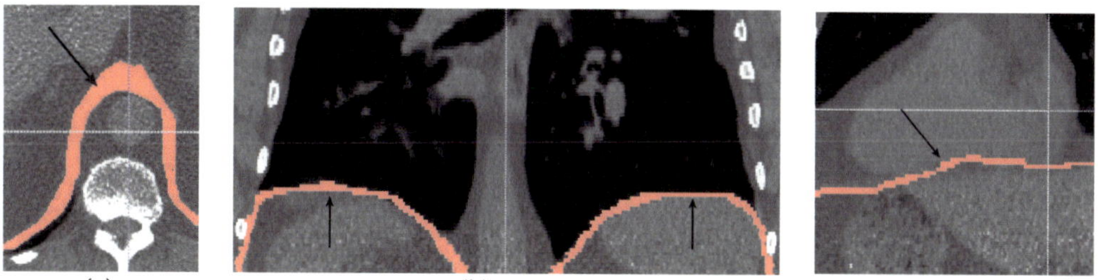


Fig. 3. Manual segmentation of the diaphragm: red line depicts (a) diaphragmatic crural attachments to the spine, (b) relationship to the lungs, pleura and ribs within the thorax, and (c) inferior aspect of the heart.

### 3.3 Meshing

For this project we have segmented scans from five patients with liver cancer, each with variation in both normal anatomy and tumour location. Data acquired from segmentation leads to the creation of 'stacks' of voxels that can be labeled according to the organ or structure they depict. These data are subsequently transformed into 3D models via a process of meshing, itself divided into three clear stages: (i) marching cubes algorithm; (ii) decimation; and (iii) smoothing. Marching cubes is a computer graphics algorithm for extracting a polygonal mesh of an isosurface from voxels. This isosurface comes directly from the label boundaries that are the result of segmentation. Decimation consists of replacing a large group of polygonal elements by a smaller group, given some constrains of curvature and position accuracy. The last technique, smoothing, is a methods used to diminish sharp edges within the model by "blurring" the angles between triangular elements.

### 3.4 Implementation

Once fully acquired and preprocessed, this 3D organ framework is implemented in object-oriented C++. We use the application programming interface H3D (SenseGraphics, 2008) as this environment combines both visual and haptic rendering. The H3D visual rendering is a superior layer to OpenGL, permitting the fast depiction of sets of triangles as organ meshes. The haptic rendering is also a superior layer to OpenHaptics, the software provided with the haptic device used in this project, the Phantom Omni (SensAble, Wilmington, USA). H3D uses the XML format called X3D to represent a scene or, in this particular instance, a set of organs, with different programmable behaviors. Figure 4 shows two examples of virtual patients that were developed within this framework.

The steps described up to this point have led to the creation of static models of the organs and tissues required for construction of the proposed liver biopsy simulator. Using a suitable deformation model, this static 3D representation of the organs and tissues can be manipulated without difficulty to allow deformation, either during breathing, or when there is interaction with a surgical instrument. In addition, it is required that force feedback is rendered to the user while inserting a needle through the body of the virtual patient. The next two sections of this chapter detail the methods used to achieve these goals.

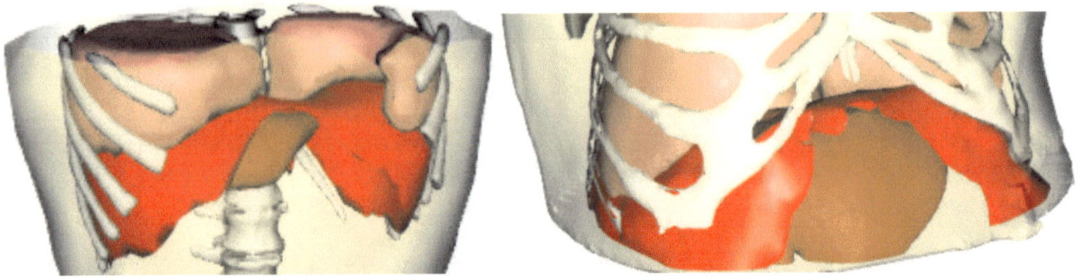

Fig. 4. Example of two virtual patients with transparent skin (light brown), lungs (pink), bones (white), liver (dark brown) and thoracic diaphragm (red)

## 4. Respiration simulation

In order to create a simulator which convincingly recreates conditions of liver biopsy, it is necessary to model liver displacement by respiration. In the current project this was achieved by applying dynamic behavior to previously segmented anatomy. This motion is defined by a sinusoidal curve that mimics normal tidal breathing in a patient. The curve **M(t)** modeled in equation (2), is used to defined the motion of respiratory muscles.

$$M(t) = A\sin(2\pi ft) \tag{2}$$

Where **A** is the muscle amplitude and **f** the respiration frequency. As is common during real liver biopsy, the clinician can instruct the virtual patient to perform an end tidal breath hold, whereupon motion due to respiration stops. In the following section we first introduce the mechanism of normal human respiration, and subsequently discuss details of the soft-tissue deformation technique that was used, as well as the handling of deformation for each organ.

### 4.1 Description of the natural respiration process

Respiration is a process consisting of the cyclical inflation and deflation of the lungs. The lungs are in effect passive organs whose motion is driven by muscles within the chest wall and diaphragm. The lungs are surrounded by the pleural cavity, bound by the visceral (lung surface) and parietal (chest wall and diaphragm) pleural membrane and containing a small volume of pleural fluid. Surface tension within the pleural fluid ensures close apposition of the lung surfaces with the chest wall and diaphragm, allowing for optional lung inflation. During inhalation, the active downwards contraction of the diaphragm and outwards motion of the chest wall (mainly due to contraction of the intercostal muscles) results in a negative pressure being generated within the thorax, which is in turn responsible for lung expansion. In comparison, exhalation, for the most part, is a passive process facilitated by relaxation of diaphragmatic and chest wall muscles.

The upper portion of the liver is attached to the diaphragm via a collection of ligaments (see Figure 5). The falciform ligament extends upwards on the anterior surface of the liver from a notch in the lower margin, as far back as the posterior surface. On the superior aspect of the liver, the falciform ligament extends medially as the left triangular ligament and laterally as the coronary ligament. The coronary ligament is formed of both an upper and lower layer which meet at the apex of the liver, where they form the right triangular ligament.

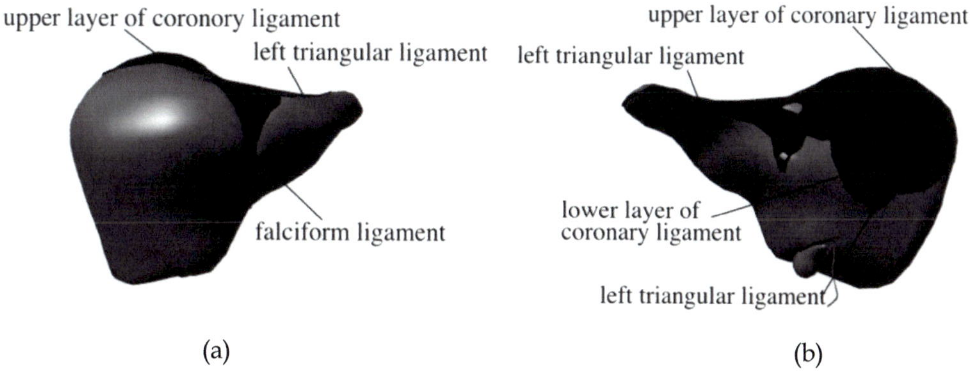


Fig. 5. Positions of liver ligaments; (a) anterior and (b) posterior views of the liver

The diaphragm is a sheet-like structure formed of both a tendinous (central) and a muscular (peripheral) part. During contraction, the diaphragm flattens, enlarging the volume of the thoracic cavity and causing the lungs to expand and inflate. When relaxed, the diaphragm is pulled upwards by the elastic recoil of the lung tissue. Due to its ligamentous attachments and close anatomical relationship, during normal respiration the liver follows the downwards and upwards motions of the diaphragm (Moore &Dalley, 2009).
The liver is also surrounded by the lower portion of the chest wall, which comprises ribs (bony elements) and costal cartilage (cartilaginous component of the rib cage), and associated muscle and other soft tissues. All twelve pairs of ribs are attached posteriorly to their respective thoracic vertebrae. Anteriorly, ribs 1 to 10 attach to the sternum via costal cartilage. Ribs 11 and 12 are considered 'floating ribs' as they have no anterior connection to the sternum. The rib cage, whilst rigid, is able to move in what is classically described as a combination of 'bucket handle' and 'pump handle' motions. Contraction of chest wall muscles generates an outwards and upwards motion of the anterior chest wall, causing expansion of the thoracic cavity. The attachments of the ribs to the thoracic vertebrae act as a pivot for this movement. Motions and deformations that are described from the diaphragm, ribcage and liver are shown in Figure 6.

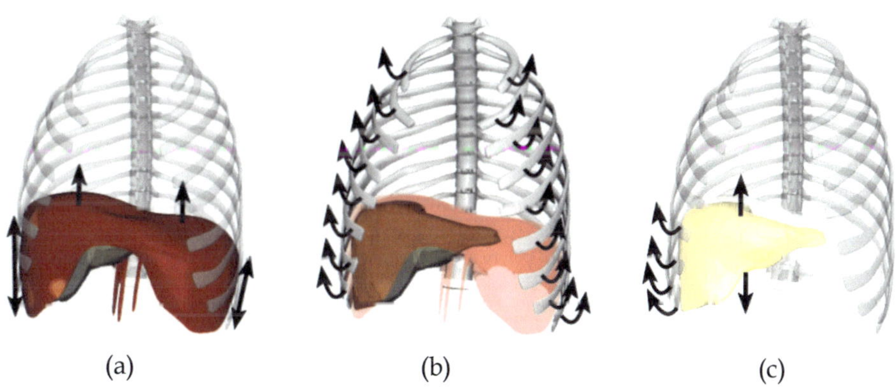


Fig. 6. Physiological behavior and motion of the: a) diaphragm, b) ribcage and c) liver. The **black arrows** represent the organ deformations during breathing.

Both the diaphragm and the ribcage are therefore independently involved in the process of normal respiration and, as such, their motions influence the position of the liver. Accordingly, a model of respiratory motion is essential to the development of a realistic simulation of liver biopsy.

### 4.2 Soft-tissue behavior simulation

Modeling soft-tissue behavior for computer-based simulators has been widely studied over the last few decades. Efforts have primarily focused on improving mechanical fidelity so as to best mimic reality. Some algorithms use, directly, the continuous mechanics equations that are adopted in the field of mechanical engineering, whilst others use the time-consuming finite element formulation (Bro-Nielsen, 1996). Algorithms that use fewer equations have also been developed, including the boundary element method (James & Pai, 1999) and the mass-tensor method (Cotin et al., 1998), but their computing time still remains high. Another approach that attempts to minimize computational time, requires that the object being modeled is no longer considered as a continuous body, but rather as one that is discretized. The most recognized example of such a model is the mass-spring method, which consists in linking discrete elements by springs and then using the proportional spring interaction law (Zordan et al., 2004). A similar method is the particle-system, where the elements are no longer connected, but are restricted by a repulsion/attraction law that helps to ensure the systems stability (Amrani et al., 2000). We have chosen to use the Chainmail (Meier et al., 2005) method as it is one of the fastest available for simulation of soft tissue behavior.

A full description of the Chainmail method can be found in (Gibson, 1997). The primary aim of this method is to simulate soft tissues as if they were a sheet of medieval chain mail, composed of small, interconnected metal rings. The expected behavior is as follows: when a chain element is moved, it may influence its neighbors; if the initial motion is too small, only the first element is moved but, if this motion is large enough, neighboring elements may also moved (see Figure 7).

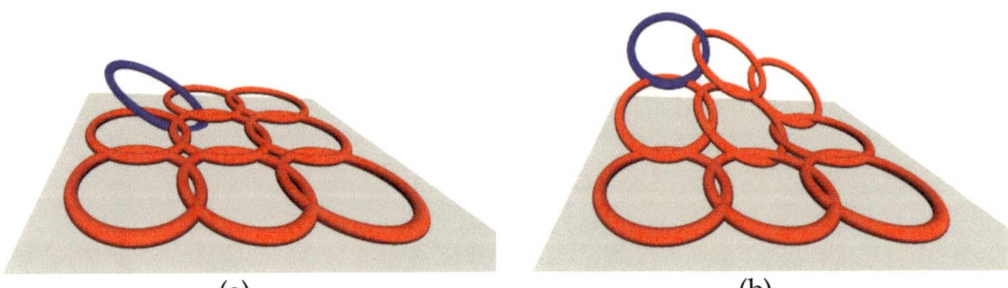

(a) (b)

Fig. 7. Chainmail behavior: the blue element is moved and the red elements may move depending on the first element displacement amplitude and direction. Element displacement that is (a) small enough to not influence its neighbors and (b) large enough to influence its neighbors.

Mathematically, this model can be described by the mechanical parameters of compression, $\gamma$; stretching, $\lambda$; and shearing, $\mu$. If we focus on an axis, $\mathbf{i}$, and on the motion of two elements along this axis, the second element will not move if the length between the elements remains below a quantity $\mathbf{i}_{max}$ and above a quantity $\mathbf{i}_{min}$ defined by $\gamma$, $\lambda$ and $\mu$. Consequently, compression is observed when the length becomes small enough *i.e.* $\mathbf{i}_{min}$ is equal to $\gamma$ times the initial length with $\gamma<1$. Stretching is observed when the length becomes high enough *i.e.* $\mathbf{i}_{max}$ is equal to $\lambda$ times the initial length with $\lambda>1$. Finally, shearing is observed when the combined displacement in the other axes becomes high enough *i.e.* $\mathbf{i}_{max}$ is equal to $\mu$ times the initial combined displacement with $\mu>1$. The behavior defined by the Chainmail algorithm is given by equations (3-8).

$$x_{min} = x_2 + (\gamma * |x_2 - x_1| - \mu * (|y_2 - y_1| + |z_2 - z_1|)) \tag{3}$$

$$x_{max} = x_2 + (\lambda * |x_2 - x_1| - \mu * (|y_2 - y_1| + |z_2 - z_1|)) \tag{4}$$

$$y_{min} = y_2 + (\gamma * |y_2 - y_1| - \mu * (|x_2 - x_1| + |z_2 - z_1|)) \tag{5}$$

$$y_{max} = y_2 + (\lambda * |y_2 - y_1| - \mu * (|x_2 - x_1| + |z_2 - z_1|)) \tag{6}$$

$$z_{min} = z_2 + (\gamma * |z_2 - z_1| - \mu * (|x_2 - x_1| + |y_2 - y_1|)) \tag{7}$$

$$z_{max} = z_2 + (\lambda * |z_2 - z_1| - \mu * (|x_2 - x_1| + |y_2 - y_1|)) \tag{8}$$

These equations give the minimum and maximum location of elements linked at a moving element, whose position goes from $(x_1, y_1, z_1)$ before displacement, to $(x_2, y_2, z_2)$ after displacement.

### 4.3 Rib cage simulation

Due to their rigid nature, it is not necessary to use soft-tissue deformation to model movement of the ribs. Their motion can instead be based on kinematics laws. Furthermore, we assume each rib to have only rotation and no translation, unlike the finite helical axis model used by previous authors (Didier et al., 2007). As this model is only defined by rotational motion, it is comparably simpler (Wilson et al., 2001). In this project, rotational parameters are independently defined for each rib; and are composed of a rotation center, two rotation axes, a minimal rotation angle and a maximal rotation angle. The first axis defines a ribs 'bucket handle' rotation (angle $\alpha$) and the second axis defines the 'pump handle' rotation (angle $\beta$), as seen in Figure 6. These angles have been previously defined by other authors (Wilson et al., 2001) using patient data. The statistical amplitude angles, $\alpha_{max}$ and $\beta_{max}$, are presented on Table 1.

| Rib number | $\alpha_{max}$ | $\beta_{max}$ |
|---|---|---|
| 2 | 14,3 | 13,7 |
| 3 | 11,4 | 13,3 |
| 4 | 10,7 | 10,1 |
| 5 | 9,6 | 8,9 |
| 6 | 9,4 | 6,9 |
| 7 | 7,9 | 6,6 |
| 8 | 7,9 | 6,2 |
| 9 | 6 | 6,3 |

Table 1. List of angle amplitude for each rib and in the two rotation plans

We have applied such methodology during the current project on datasets acquired from patient scans. To achieve this, we initially computed the rotation parameter during a preprocessing stage and chose to use a mechanical approach by computing the inertia matrix. This matrix, **M,** is defined by equation (9). It corresponds to integrations over the volume of each rib; **x**, **y** and **z** being the position of a within a rib.

$$M = \begin{pmatrix} \int y^2 + z^2 dv & \int xydv & \int xzdv \\ \int xydv & \int x^2 + z^2 dv & \int zydv \\ \int xzdv & \int zydv & \int y^2 + x^2 dv \end{pmatrix} \quad (9)$$

These moments of inertia represent the rigidity of a 3D object and are widely used in solid mechanics. The Eigen vectors of this matrix directly give the principal axes of the objects. The two highest Eigen values give the axis that contains the largest proportion of matter and is therefore of most interest to us. We define the 'rib plane' as that which is given by these two Eigen vectors (see Figure 8).

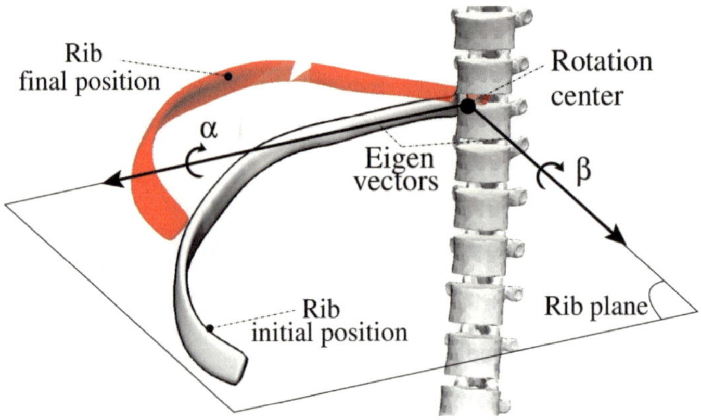


Fig. 8. Rib rotation algorithm. Inputs are: (i) Eigen vectors; (ii) rotation angles α and β; (iii) rotation center; and (iv) initial rib location. The output is the rib at its final position.

The rotation centers are found by a heuristic method. First, we compute the higher Eigen value of the spine inertia matrix, the associated axis gives the axial line of the spine. The rotation center is then given by the intersection between this line and the rib plane. From this pre-computation stage, we can determine for each rib the rotation center and the two axes. The next step is to apply a dynamic behavior to each rib based on these patient-customized parameters. At each time step, the new coordinates of the rib points are computed with Rodrigues' rotation formula (Koks, 2006). These two rotations are time-dependant and their angle values are derived from equation (2) taking α and β as parameters. The results are given by equations (10) and (11). Acquired behavioral data was stored and accessed in X3D format.

$$\alpha(t) = \alpha_{max} \sin(2\pi f t) \quad (10)$$

$$\beta(t) = \beta_{max} \sin(2\pi f t) \quad (11)$$

### 4.4 Diaphragm simulation

Diaphragmatic behavior has been modeled using various techniques, including geometrical methods based on external sensors (Hoestettler et al., 2008); Mass-spring systems with incompressibility constraints (Zordan et al., 2004); and nature-inspired tensegrity (Villard et al., 2008). These methods are time-consuming and their accuracy is beyond that which is required by the current application. Accordingly, we have developed a faster method that still reflects the physiological parameters discussed in section 4.1.

During normal inhalation, the peripheral muscular portion of the diaphragm contracts pulling downwards on the central tendon and increasing intrathoracic volume. In comparison, during exhalation, the central tendon of the diaphragm retracts upwards into the chest as the muscle relaxes. We have, however, proposed a model whereby the central tendon of the diaphragm assumes an active role, with a sinusoidal up and down motion derived from equation (2), whilst the muscular portion remains passive. As the central tendon of the diaphragm is naturally stiff, our model assumes it to be a rigid structure. The motion function, **T(t)**, of the model, where **t** is the time as given by equation (12). The translation amplitude, $\mathbf{d_{max}}$, was set at 2cm.

$$T(t) = d_{\max} \sin(2\pi f t) \tag{12}$$

In contrast, the muscle portion of the diaphragm follows an elastic behavior based on the Chainmail algorithm detailed in section 4.2. This also preserved the natural deformation of the muscle during the contraction-relaxation cycle. The portion of the diaphragm, which is attached to the spine, is programmed to remain motionless. Illustrations of diaphragm behavior, as programmed by our model, are presented in Figure 9.

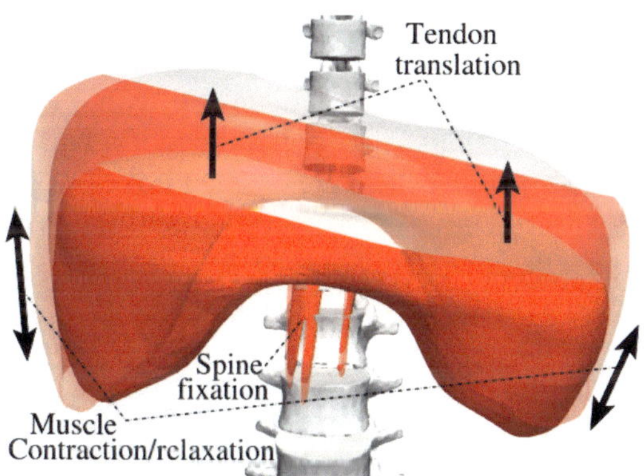


Fig. 9. Programmed diaphragmatic behavior: the central tendon of the diaphragm, presented here in white, is considered to have a stiff translation in the longitudinal plane. In comparison, the muscular portion (red), with the exception of regions directly attached to the spine, passively deform in response to tendon displacement. The initial and final positions of the diaphragm are depicted above by opaque and transparent boundaries respectively.

### 4.5 Liver simulation

The final organ whose behavior needs to be detailed is the liver. Whilst the liver is entirely passive during respiration, its upper border lies immediately adjacent to the diaphragm and is attached to its inferior surface via a series of ligaments (refer to details in section 4.1). To model this interaction we chose to apply coupling forces as opposed to displacement constrains, allowing continuous smooth deformation that would otherwise have been hard to reproduce. Coupling between the liver and diaphragm was characterized in a pre-computing step using X3D data. A threshold distance of 5mm was established, below which a connection force is applied. Internal deformations of the liver due to respiration were modeled by the Chainmail algorithm.

Our model also allowed deformation of the liver under the influence of an external force applied by the biopsy needle. This interaction primarily occurs between the tip of the needle and what is in real life a thin fibrous layer covering the liver, referred to as the liver capsule. This layer is deformed as the operator attempts to introduce the biopsy needle into the body of the liver. Once perforated, however, this layer no longer shows deformation. Again, we use the Chainmail algorithm to model this interaction by applying the needle tip displacement to the three closest points on the liver surface. In reality, the greatest influence on needle insertion is not the visual displacement of the liver capsule, but haptic interaction. In the next section we focus on the method used to render this important 'force feedback' experienced by the operator during needle insertion.

## 5. Haptic rendering

As in many simulators, we have attempted to enhance the user's immersion through the addition of haptic rendering. This is achieved by the operator interacting with the virtual environment through a haptic device that resembles tools used during the actual task. In this section we introduce the synchronization between the visual feedback and the haptic device, as well as explain the computation and rendering to the user of the physical forces.

### 5.1 Needle avatar

In this project a haptic device is used to simulate the liver biopsy needle. This device generates two important parameters used by our framework; namely, the position (**P**) and the direction (**D**) of the needle. The needle avatar is then linked to the stylus that the user is manipulating. At each time step, **P** and **D** are recorded and the needle is displayed. When the needle is inserted into the patient's body, a force feedback (**F**) is computed and rendered back to the user (see Figure 10).

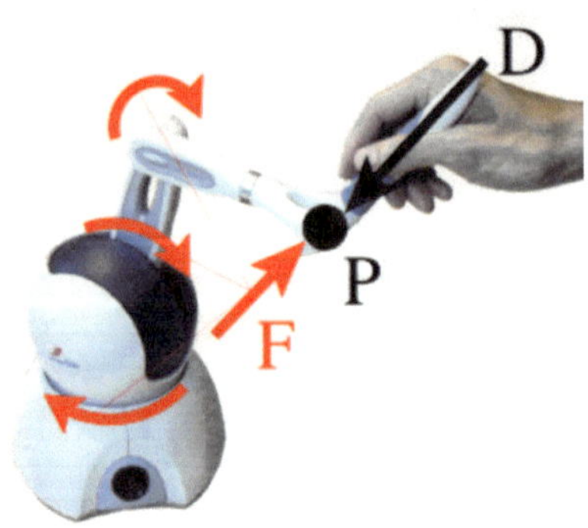


Fig. 10. Commercially available haptic device. The haptic device is driven by the position (**P**) and direction (**D**) of the stylus that are determined by the user's movements, and renders back a force (**F**) processed by the computer.

## 5.2 Soft-tissue force feedback

Haptic rendering is often based on collision detection and collision response algorithms. The combination of these methods could not, however, be directly applied during the current project as it would have resulted in a model that was too complex due to the number of organs and tissues potentially traversed by the needle. In addition, it would need haptic sub-layers, for example the organs inside the skin or the tumor inside the liver. Such an option is currently not fully supported by haptics APIs.

We chose instead the method implemented in (Vidal et al., 2008), where force is no longer dependent on collision detection, but is always computed while the needle is inside the patient's body and never while outside. In the same way, no classical collision response force algorithm is performed. Instead, force is computed using the initial 3D CT scan data, without the mesh environment information. As the biopsy needle is inserted into the virtual patient, it is possible to access the corresponding voxel Hounsfield densities, provided the medical image remains appropriately registered to the polygonal information. Longitudinal force is then determined on line by means of the voxel gradient as it is similar to matter density. The operator can therefore feel the boundaries between tissue planes as they are traversed by the advancing needle

Soft tissues are not only responsible for forces generated along the long axis of the needle (needle axial forces), they also apply a constraining force that inhibits lateral movement of the needle. Consequently, once the needle has been inserted more than a few millimeters into the virtual patient, lateral movement of needle is greatly constrained by the influence of the surrounding tissue(s), such that it is almost impossible to deviate from the initial trajectory. In our model we have added constraining forces in order to reproduce this phenomenon. The direction of the force ($\mathbf{F_a}$) acting upon the needle is computed from the initial position ($\mathbf{P_0}$) and direction ($\mathbf{D_0}$) of insertion and from current position ($\mathbf{P_t}$). Thus, the relationship describing the soft-tissue force feedback is given by equation (13).

$$F_a = (P_t - P_0) * \sin\left(\frac{D_0}{P_t - P_0}\right) \tag{13}$$

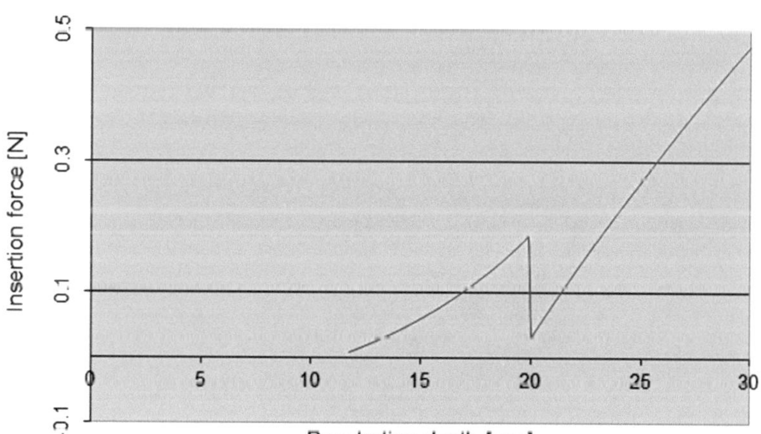


Fig. 11. Needle insertion force in Newtons with the penetration depth in millimeters (equation (14).

### 5.3 Liver force feedback

Haptic feedback is of particular importance during needle insertion into the substance of the liver. As was described in section 4.5, the liver is covered by a fibrous capsule that offers considerable resistance to continued passage of the needle. This resistance is, however, dramatically reduced at the moment of capsule penetration. Thereafter, continued needle insertion deeper into the liver is subjected to increasing resistance. In this project we have simulated this behavior by adding a needle axial force whose value is extracted from (Maurin et al., 2004). Experimental data were acquired with a force sensor during IR procedures (Karuppasamy et al., 2008) and fitted to a mathematical model. It defines the force, $\mathbf{F_n}$, varying with the penetration depth **d**. This force is defined piecewise, before and after penetration with two sets of parameters τ, ω, υ and φ that define equation (14). The corresponding curve is shown on Figure 11.

$$F_n(d) = (\nu + \varphi)e^{\tau(d-\omega)} + \varphi \quad (14)$$

## 6. Resulting simulator

The final simulator encompasses all of the elements described in the preceding sections: a collection of virtual patients and their organs, segmented from CT scans of actual patients and represented by meshes; cyclical deformation of theses meshes in accordance with a model of respiration; a virtual needle that can be manipulated with six degrees of freedom via the arm of a haptic device. As the needle passes through the different tissues, the operator is able to determine additional information about their nature through haptic feedback. Furthermore, as this needle is inserted into the capsule of the liver, deformation of the organ's surface can be observed and felt. The biopsy is triggered by the operator pressing one of the buttons in the Omni haptic interface. In the following sections we present a complete description of the final simulator, including patient-customised anatomy and physiology. We also add a module to measure the user performance. Finally, we present a review of feedback received from both expert and trainee interventional radiologists.

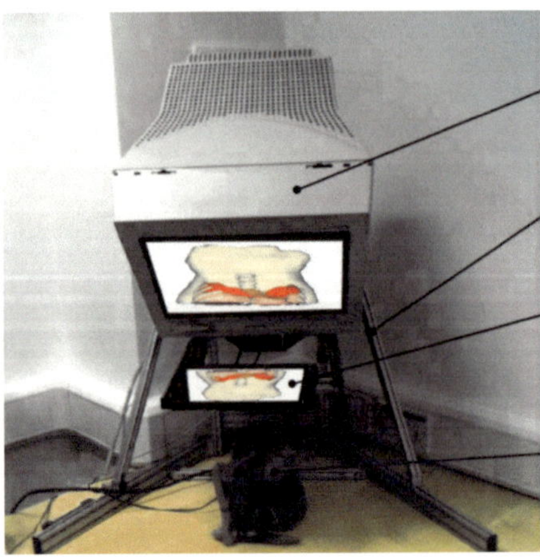


Fig. 12. Liver biopsy simulator using the Sensegraphics Immersive Workbench and Phantom Omni haptic device

### 6.1 Immersive Workbench

In developing this simulator particular emphasis was made on selecting algorithms that are suitably fast. This has, ultimately, allowed the simulator to be real time, offering 500Hz and 20Hz for haptic and graphic rendering respectively. To achieve a superior ergonomic and 3D immersive experience, the simulator framework has been integrated with the Sensegraphics Immersive Workbench[1] (see Figure 12). This system required active 3D glasses with a shuttering system synchronized with a CRT monitor to visualize the virtual environment in 3D. As is shown in Figure 12, the monitor is positioned at a 45° angle above a horizontal semi-transparent mirror. With this configuration, the user is able to view the 3D target object collocated with their hand and the haptic device.

### 6.2 Patient specific physiology

The final 3D simulator has been designed to take into account variability in the speed and strength of factors contributing to motion. This has allowed the simulator to match diaphragmatic or thoracic breathing patterns and the overlap that exists between these two dynamic processes (see Figure 13).

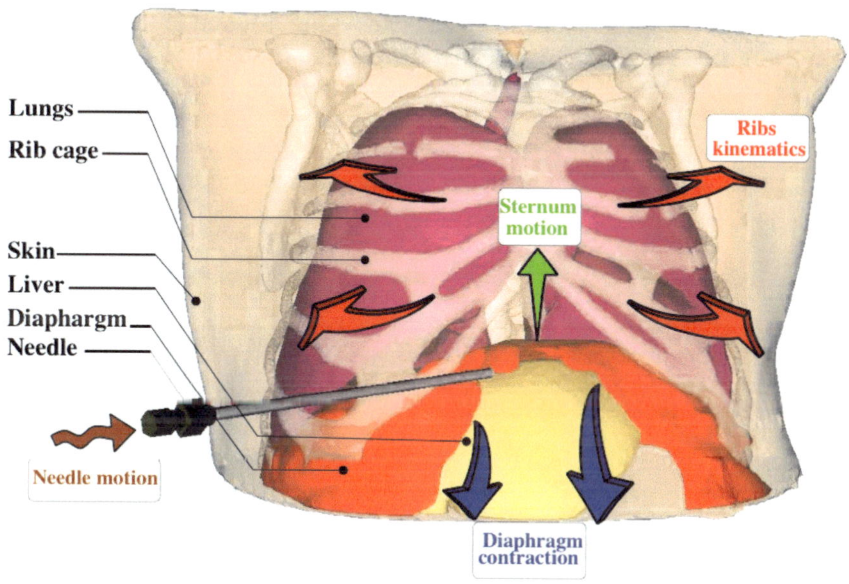


Fig. 13. Patient customized anatomy with inhalation motion and needle avatar controlled via a haptic device

The respiration is mathematically monitored by time-dependant functions defined by equations (10), (11) and (12). The breathing frequency could be changed by modifying the shared parameter **f**. The user can change from quiet breathing to hyperventilation. In the same way the influence of the diaphragm is linked to the $\mathbf{d_{max}}$ parameter of equation (12) and the thoracic behavior is tuned with a scalar value linked to the $\alpha_{max}$ and $\beta_{max}$ parameters of respectively equations (10) and (11). Figure 14.a shows the panel displayed to the user in order to set a respiration pattern.

[1] http://www.sensegraphics.com/

### 6.3 Performance metrics

As previously stated, simulators such as the one described here, provide a valuable and safe environment in which trainees may practice and be assessed. To support this application, a number of computer-based metrics are provided, including: time taken; number of times contact is made with designated 'no-go' areas (representing errors of needle tip location); number of attempted needle insertions; and biopsy accuracy (adequacy of tissue sample obtained). The time taken for the procedure begins when the task is initialized and finishes when the biopsy sample is acquired. The number of times voxels designated as 'no go' areas are crossed by the biopsy needle is also determined. 'No go' voxels include the lungs, costophrenic recess, colon, gallbladder, neurovascular bundles (located below the ribs), and bone. A further metric counts the number of attempted needle insertions; these are repeated whenever the operator perceives a failure to locate the biopsy target on the needle trajectory, as defined by the insertion point and the direction of the virtual needle. The final metric computed by the simulator was biopsy precision. In the current simulator, the tumor is modeled by a spherical body of 15mm. Four levels of precision are defined depending on the distance between the site of biopsy and the center of the tumor. Biopsy samples taken from within 5mm of the centre of the tumor are considered to contain "Necrotic debris", that is a feature of tumors as they outgrow their blood supply. Biopsies taken from within 5-10mm of the tumor centre are judged as being a "good specimen" because this is the region of actively growing tumour cells, whilst tissues 10-15mm from the center may contain "some tumor cells". Any biopsy that is >15mm from the centre of the tumor will contain normal cells and hence is regarded as "not pathologic". All metrics described are displayed to the operator on completion of the procedure, allowing objective assessment of their performance (see Figure 14.b)

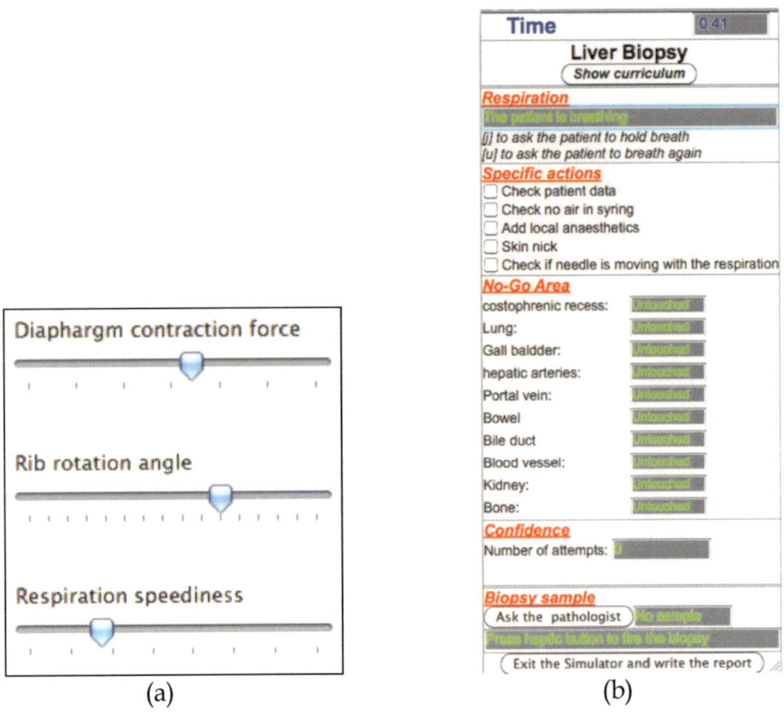


Fig. 14. Simulator user interface. a) Tuning of patient breathing pattern b) Metrics display.

### 6.4 Qualitative evaluation

In order to evaluate the simulator, we invited both expert and trainee interventional radiologists to use it to perform a number of tasks. A review of the main comments made by clinicians is presented below.

Feedback received for each module of the simulator was generally positive. Most clinicians reported that the inclusion of movement due to respiration was an important feature of the simulator and considered that the realism of the procedure was enhanced when this function was active. Many comments were made about the haptic rendering, which was considered to satisfactorily reflect the forces experienced during liver biopsy in patients.

It was suggested that the simulator was most suitable for first and second year trainees who generally have limited opportunity to practice and maintain their technical skills in this procedure. By using the simulator, clinicians felt that trainees would be able to acquire and maintain both core practical skills and confidence, within a safe environment, remote from patients. The general consensus of all clinicians was that simulators, such as this, are needed and that there is a place for them in training curricula. Indeed the Royal College of Radiologists and British Society of Interventional Radiologists in the UK are actively developing training opportunities using simulation

We also received a number of comments relating to potential improvement of the simulator. Several clinicians noted that, during this procedure, they would tend to rest their hands on the patients body, something that was not possible with a virtual patient. One clinician reported difficulty in pressing the button on the Omni haptic device used to trigger biopsy, whilst another found it difficult to manouvre the same device.

## 7. Future work

Future work must both address issues raised by clinicians during the evaluation stage, as well as modifying the existing framework to allow simulation of other interventional radiology procedures within the abdomen. We also intend to develop new methods of automatic segmentation that will aid in the isolation of anatomical structures, including the diaphragm. It is intended that this will enhance the retrieval of 3D data from CT scans, widening the application of this technology to allow patient specific pre-procedural training and planning. Finally, refinement of the respiratory model will allow the described framework to be used in other applications including the administration of targeted radiotherapy. Further thorough and systematic validation is also required and to this end a skills transfer study has recently commenced.

## 8. Conclusion

In conclusion, we have presented here a new framework of a liver biopsy simulator that includes respiratory motion. This framework is composed of 3D virtual organs extracted from patient data. In addition, organ motion due to respiration and haptic feedback during needle insertion is computed on-line and in real time within a virtual reality environment. An immersive workbench permits the operator to perform the procedure in a 3D environment that allows co-location of their hands with the virtual target. The feedback of experienced and trainee clinicians who were invited to use the simulator was obtained to evaluate the simulator's strengths and weaknesses. As a direct consequence of its efficacy, the simulator framework described here has been applied in two other medical simulators that are based on fluoroscopic (Villard et al., 2009) and ultrasound (Bello et al., 2009) image guidance.

## 9. Acknowledgment

The author would like to acknowledge the financial support of the UK Department of Health under the Health Technology Devices (HTD) Program during the course of this study.

## 10. References

Abolhassani, N., Patel, R. & Moallem, M. (2007). Needle insertion into soft tissue: A survey, Medical Engineering & Physics, Vol 29, Issue 4, Pages 413-431, ISSN 1350-4533.

Amrani, M., Jaillet, F. & Shariat B. (2000). Deformable Objects Modeling and Animation : Application to Organs'Interactions Simulation. Journal for Geometry and Graphics, Vol.4, No. 2, pp. 181-188.

Bello, F., Bulpitt, A.,. Gould, D.A,Holbrey,R., Hunt, C., John,N.W., Johnson, S., Phillips, R., Sinha, A., Vidal, F.P., Villard, P.-F. & Woolnough, H. (2009). ImaGiNe-S : Imaging Guided Needle Simulation. In*Eurographics 2009*, Munich, Germany, pp 5-8.

Bro-Nielsen, M. (1996). Surgery simulation using fast finite elements in: K.H. Bohme, R.Kikinis, Proceedings of the Visualization in Biomedical Computing (VBC : 4), Lecture Notes in Computer Science, vol. 1131, Springer, Berlin, 1996, pp.529-534.

Chen, Y., Wang, Z., Zhao, W. & Yang, X. (2009). Liver Segmentation from CT Images Based on Region Growing Method, in Proc. 3rd International Conference on Bioinformatics and Biomedical Engeneering (ICBBE), pp. 1-4.

Chentanez, N., Alterovitz, R., Ritchie, D., Cho, L., Hauser, K. K., Goldberg, K ., Shewchuk, J. R. & O'Brien, J. F. (2009). Interactive Simulation of Surgical Needle Insertion and Steering. In *Proceedings of ACM SIGGRAPH 2009*, pages 88:1–10.

Coles, T. R., Meglan, D. & John, N.W. (2010)."The Role of Haptics in Medical Training Simulators: A Survey of the State-of-the-art," IEEE Transactions on Haptics.

Cotin, S., Delingette, H. & Ayache N. (1998). Efficient linear Elastic Models of Soft Tissues for real-time surgery simulation, INRIA Technical Report RR-3510, 1998.

Didier, A., Villard, P-.F., Bayle, J., Beuve, M. & Shariat, B. (2007). Breathing Thorax Simulation based on Pleura Behaviour and RibKinematics. In IEEE, ed.: Information Visualisation - MediVis. (2007) 35-40

Foruzana, A. H., Zoroofia, R. A., Horib, M. & Satoc, Y. (2009).A knowledge-based technique for liver segmentation in CT data, in Computerized Medical Imaging and Graphics, vol. 33, pp. 567-587, 2009.

Gibson, S.F. (1997). 3D ChainMail: a Fast Algorithm for Deforming Volumetric Objects. Symposium on Interactive 3D Graphics ,pp 149 - ., 1997

Gould, D.A., Healey, A., Phillips, R., Ward, J.W., et al. (2004). Challenges in realising effective RadiologicalInterventional Virtual Environments - The CRaIVE approach, Proceedings of MedicineMeets Virtual Reality 2004, pp 127-9, IOS Press, January 14-17 2004, Newport Beach.

Hostettler, A., Nicolau, S.A.,Soler, L., Remond, Y. & Marescaux, J. (2008). A Real time predictive simulation of abdominal organ positions induced by free breathing Lecture Notes in Computer Science, Biomedical Simulation, 2008

James, D.L. & Pai, D.K. (1999). ArtDefo Accurate Real Time Deformable Objects, In SIGGRAPH pages 65-72, 1999.

Karuppasamy, K., Zhai, J., How, T.V. & Gould, D.A. (2008). Development and validation of an unobtrusive sensor for in-vivo force data collection during interventional procedures. In Proceedings, BSIR Annual Conference. Manchester. November 2008.

Koks, D. (2006) Explorations in Mathematical Physics, Springer Science+Business Media,LLC. ISBN 0-387-30943-8. Ch.4, pps 147 et seq. A Roundabout Route to Geometric Algebra

Li, Y. & Brodlie, K. (2003). Soft object modelling with generalised chainmail - extending the boundaries of webbased graphics. Comput. Graph. Forum 22, 4 (2003), 717-727.

Maurin, B., Bayle, Z., Gangloff, De Mathelin, Gangi, S. & Forgione, A. (2004). In Vivo Study of Forces During Needle Insertions. Proceedings of the Medical Robotics, Navigation and Visualisation Scientific Workshop 2004, 1-8.Remagen, Germany, March 2004.

Meier, U., Lopez, O., Monserrat, C., Juan, M.C. & Alcaniz, M. (2005). Real-time deformable models forsurgery simulation : a survey. Computer Methods and Programs in Biomedicine, 77 (3),pp. 183-197,2005.

Moore, K. & Dalley, A.F. (2009). Clinically Oriented Anatomy, 6th ed. Lippencott, Williams & Wilkins, 2009

Müller, SA, Maier-Hein, L, Mehrabi, A, Pianka, F, Rietdorf, U, Wolf, I, Grenacher, L, Richter, G, Gutt, CN, Schmidt, J, Meinzer, HP, & Schmied, BM. (2007). In *Med. Phys.* 34, 4605

Santhanam, A. P.,Imielinska, C., Davenport, P., Kupelian, P. & Rolland, J.P. (2007). Modeling realtime 3D lung deformations for medical visualization In *IEEE Transaction on information technology in Biomedicine.* p 257-270.

Rusko, L., Bekes, G. & Fidrich, M. (2009). Automatic segmentation of the liver from multi- and single-phase contrast-enhanced CT images, in Medical Image Analysis, vol. 13, pp. 871-882.

SenseGraphics AB. (2008). H3D OPEN SOURCE HAPTICS. "H3D API Manual (for version 2.0)". http://h3dapi.com

Vidal, F.P., John, N.W., Gould, D.A. & Healey, A.E. (2008). Simulation of Ultrasound Guided Needle Puncture using Patient Specific Data with 3D Textures and Volume Haptics. Comp. Anim. & Virt. Worlds, John Wiley & Sons. Vol 19 (2), pp. 111-127.

Villard, P.-F., Bourne, W & Bello, F. (2008). Modelling organ deformation using mass-springs and tensional integrity". In *4th International Symposium on Biomedical Simulation*, 5104:221-226,(LNCS). London (UK), July 2008.

Villard, P.-F., Vidal,F.P., Hunt, C., Bello,F., John, N.W., Johnson, S. & Gould, D.A. (2009). A prototype percutaneous transhepatic cholangiography training simulator with real-time breathing motion. In *Int. Jour. of Computer Assisted Radiology and Surgery* (November 2009), Springer. Volume 4, Issue 6, pp. 571-578.

Wilson, T. A., Legrand, A., Gevenois, P.-A. & Troyer A. (2001). Respiratory effects of the external and internal intercostal muscles in humans. J. Physiol. (Lond.) 530, 2 (2001), 319-330.

Yushkevich, P.A., Piven, J., Cody, H., Ho, S., Gee, J.C. & Gerig, G. (2005). User-Guided Level Set Segmentation of Anatomical Structures with ITK-SNAP, Insight Journal, Special Issue on ISC/NA-MIC/MICCAI Workshop on Open-Source Software, Nov 2005.

Zordan, V. B., Celly, B., Chiu, B. & Dilorenzo, P.C. (2004). Breathe easy : Model and control of simulated respiration for animation. In Proc. ACM SIGGRAPH/ Eurographics SCA (2004), pp. 29-37.

# 21

# Acoustic Radiation Force Impulse Elastography: A Non-Invasive Alternative to Liver Biopsy

Hirokazu Takahashi[1] et al.*

[1]*Department of Internal Medicine, Saga Medical School, Nabeshima, Saga, Japan*

## 1. Introduction

The prognosis of chronic liver disease depends on the progression of liver fibrosis. Liver biopsy is recommended as the gold standard method for determining fibrosis stage, prognosis and therapeutic indications in patients with chronic liver disease. However, liver biopsy is an invasive procedure associated with a risk of potentially serious complications. Approximately 1–3% of patients require hospitalization for complications, and a quarter of them report pain after percutaneous liver biopsy. The diagnostic accuracy of liver biopsy for assessing liver fibrosis is influenced by the quality of the biopsy samples. In addition, there are several absolute or relative contraindications to liver biopsy, including severe coagulopathy. A safe and non-invasive alternative to liver biopsy is therefore needed for assessing liver fibrosis in daily clinical practice.

## 2. Principle of acoustic radiation force impulse

Acoustic radiation force impulse (ARFI) imaging is a radiation force based imaging method that is provided by conventional B-mode ultrasonography (Acuson S2000; SIEMENS Medical Solutions) (Fig. 1). ARFI imaging involves transmission of an initial ultrasonic pulse at diagnostic intensity levels to obtain a baseline signal for later comparison. A short-duration (approximately 0.3 s), high-intensity acoustic 'pushing pulse' is then transmitted by the same transducer, followed by a series of diagnostic intensity pulses, which are used to track the displacement of the tissue caused by the pushing pulse (Nightingale et al., 2001, Palmeri et al., 2005, Dahl et al., 2007). The response of the tissue to the radiation force is observed using conventional B-mode imaging pulses, and it is possible to display the quantitative shear-wave velocity (Vs; m/s) of ARFI displacement. This velocity (m/s) is proportional to the square root of tissue elasticity. Because the velocity of the shear wave depends on tissue stiffness, it is possible to apply ARFI technology to elastography. This

* Naofumi Ono[2], Yuichiro Eguchi[1], Toshihiko Mizuta[1], Keizo Anzai[1], Atsushi Miyoshi[3], Masato Yoneda[4], Atsushi Nakajima[4] and Kazuma Fujimoto[1].

1 *Department of Internal Medicine, Saga Medical School, Nabeshima, Saga, Japan,*

2 *Department of Clinical Gastroenterology, Eguchi Hospital, Mikazuki, Ogi, Saga, Japan,*

3 *Department of Surgery, Saga Medical School, Nabeshima, Saga, Japan,*

4 *Division of Gastroenterology, Yokohama City University Hospital, Yokohama, Japan.*

technology was named "Virtual Touch Tissue Quantification" by SIEMENS. Previous reports have also referred to it as ARFI elastography or ARFI elastometry. In this chapter, we use the term ARFI elastography.

## 3. Protocol of ARFI elastography

ARFI imaging involves targeting an anatomic region to be examined for its elastic properties using a region-of-interest (ROI) cursor measuring 10×5 mm at the same time as or after performing real-time B-mode imaging (Fig. 2). This enables a comprehensive range of tissue strain analytic parameters to be assessed, allowing quantitative values of the mechanical stiffness (elasticity) properties of tissues to be measured. In general, the stiffer a region of tissue, the greater the shear-wave speed as it travels through this region. ARFI elastography is performed using a curved array at 4 MHz for B-mode imaging. The right lobe of the liver is examined through the intercostal space with the patient lying in the dorsal decubitus position, with their right arm maximally abducted. A measurement depth of 2–3 cm below the liver capsule is chosen to standardize the examination. No consensus has yet been reached regarding the ROI position and the approach point on the body surface, but our experience indicates that measurement at 2–3 cm depth from the right intercostals seems to produce stable results. According to a recent report, there was no significant difference in ARFI measurements between the intercostal and abdominal approaches; however, the intercostal approach had the highest success rates (Popescu et al., 2011). Although different values of ARFI measurements were reported for each depth under the liver capsule, the differences were not significant (Sporea et al., 2010). Boursier et al. reported that the reproducibility of measurements in the right lobe was high, but measurements in the left lobe included cases with outliers (Boursier et al., 2010). Further studies are needed to determine the depth of ROI for the appropriate stratification of liver fibrosis stages. The Acuson S2000 has a memory capability, and more than five successful acquisitions should thus be performed for each patient; the median or mean value can then be calculated to produce a reliable measurement.

## 4. Reproducibility of ARFI elastography

According to previous reports, ARFI elastography has high reproducibility. Boursier et al. reported that the interobserver reproducibility of ARFI was excellent (interclass correlation coefficient = 0.91) and no training effect was observed in terms of ARFI measurements (Boursier et al., 2010). Friedrich-Rust et al. found 87% agreement regarding ARFI elastography-derived stages between two examiners (Friedrich-Rust et al., 2009).

## 5. ARFI elastography in normal healthy subjects

Several studies have determined the normal range of ARFI measurements for healthy subjects. Popescu et al. reported a mean shear-wave velocity of 1.15 ± 0.21 m/s (Popescu et al., 2011). The study by Takahashi et al. included 25 healthy controls, and found a mean shear-wave value of 1.08 ± 0.13 m/s (Takahashi et al., 2010). The mean shear-wave velocity in the study by Horster et al., which included 68 healthy volunteers with a mean age of 28 years, was 1.19 m/s (range, 0.77–1.63 m/s) (Horster et al., 2010), while Goertz et al. obtained a mean value of 1.09 m/s (range, 0.79–1.32 m/s) in 20 healthy subjects. Kim et al. included 133 subjects with normal livers in their series and derived a mean value of 1.08 ± 0.15 m/s (Goertz et al., 2010, Kim et al., 2010). No correlations between ARFI values and age, gender or body mass index (BMI) have been identified.

## 6. Diagnostic accuracy for liver fibrosis

Ultrasonography-based evaluation offers several advantages, including ready availability, real-time examination, relatively low cost and lack of ionizing radiation. Recent studies have indicated the clinical feasibility of ARFI elastography for assessing liver fibrosis (Table 1). The results demonstrated that shear-wave velocity measured by ARFI elastography offers a reliable and non-invasive method for estimating liver fibrosis in chronic liver diseases. In particular, liver stiffness assessed by shear-wave velocity was significantly correlated with liver fibrosis according to the pathological scoring system. Furthermore, the staging of liver fibrosis in chronic liver diseases could be accurately classified based on shear-wave velocity. Friedrich-Rust et al. reported that the area under the receiver operating characteristic curve for the accuracy of ARFI elastography was 0.91 for the diagnosis of both moderate fibrosis ($F \geq 2$) and cirrhosis, respectively. According to their report, the cut-off value for liver cirrhosis was 1.75 m/s in all subjects, and 1.75 m/s in subjects with hepatitis C virus (HCV) infection (Friedrich-Rust et al., 2009). Other reports have identified variable cut-off values for cirrhosis, ranging from 1.6–1.95 m/s (Table 1). In the studies by Takahashi et al. and Sporea et al., which included 47 (85%) and 54 (76%) HCV-positive subjects, respectively, the cut-off value for cirrhosis was 1.8 m/s (Takahashi et al., 2010, Sporea et al., 2010). The study by Yoneda et al. included subjects with non-alcoholic fatty liver disease (NAFLD), and found a cut-off value for cirrhosis of 1.9 m/s, which was higher than in other studies (Yoneda et al., 2010). It is possible that differences in background chronic liver diseases might account for the variations in cut-off values. In addition, different distributions of fibrosis stages among subjects in different studies may affect the results of ROC analysis, and direct comparison of cut-off values among studies should therefore be avoided. The Obuchowski measure, which allows for differential penalization of more serious misdiagnoses, was recently reported (Obuchowski et al., 2005). This method allows the diagnostic accuracy of ARFI elastography among studies with different distributions of fibrosis stages to be compared (Lambert et al., 2008). However, because the Obuchowski measure is statistically technical, analysis with commercially based medical statistical software might be difficult. Further studies on the correlations between different liver disease etiologies and the results of ARFI elastography are needed, as are standardized measurement protocols and statistical methods. Nonetheless, ARFI elastography appears to offer good diagnostic accuracy for staging liver fibrosis.

| | | AUROC | | | Cut-off for cirrhosis |
|---|---|---|---|---|---|
| Author | Subjects | FS 0–1vs FS 2–4 | FS 0–2 vs. FS 3–4 | FS 0–3 vs. FS 4 | (m/s) |
| Friedrich-Rust et al. | HCV, HBV | 0.84 | 0.91 | 0.91 | 1.75 |
| Takahashi et al. | HCV, HBV, NASH | 0.94 | 0.94 | 0.96 | 1.8 |
| Yoneda et al. | NAFLD | - | 0.97 | 0.98 | 1.9 |
| Sporea et al. | HCV, HBV | 0.65 | | 0.87 | 1.8 |
| Goertz et al. | HCV, HBV | 0.85 | 0.92 | 0.87 | - |
| Fierbinteanu-Braticevici et al. | HCV | 0.92 | 0.99 | 0.99 | 1.95 |
| Rifai et al. | HCV, HBV, NAFLD | - | - | 0.82 | 1.6 |

Table 1. Diagnostic accuracy of ARFI for liver fibrosis

AUROC, area under the receiver operating characteristic curve; FS, fibrosis stage; HCV, hepatitis C virus; HBV, hepatitis B virus; NAFLD, non-alcoholic fatty liver disease. Fibrosis stage was assessed using the Metavir scoring system, except in the case of Yoneda et al., who used the method of Brunt.

## 7. Factors influencing ARFI elastography measurements

The degree of liver fibrosis is the most significant factor determining shear-wave velocity. However, several other factors can affect shear-wave velocity. Rifai et al. reported that shear-wave velocity was faster in patients with significant liver inflammation compared with those with no significant inflammation (Rifai et al., 2011). They suggested that liver and spleen sizes were positively correlated with the results of ARFI elastography measurements. Takahashi et al. reported that serum aspartate aminotransferase and alanine aminotransferase levels as well as pathological liver inflammation were positively correlated with ARFI elastography measurements (Takahashi et al., 2010). These results suggest that pathological and serological liver inflammation might affect shear-wave velocity. However, it should be noted that significant proportions of patients in those studies had viral hepatitis, and the severity of pathological fibrosis has been shown to correlate with pathological inflammation in viral hepatitis. Further studies including larger sample sizes are needed to evaluate the impact of inflammation on ARFI elastography measurements in patients with the same severities of fibrosis stage.

Pathological liver steatosis is a significant factor affecting ARFI elastography measurements in NAFLD. Yoneda et al. suggested that shear-wave velocity in NAFLD with no fibrosis was slower than in healthy controls. Additionally, NAFLD with mild liver fibrosis was associated with almost normal shear-wave velocities (Yoneda et al., 2010, Palmeri et al., 2011). They suggested that steatosis might make the liver softer because of fat deposition in the liver parenchyma. Palmeri et al. showed that hepatocyte ballooning and inflammation in NAFLD had no significant effects on shear-wave velocity (Palmeri et al., 2011).

## 8. Comparison with other non-invasive methods

Several scoring systems or indexes based on serum biochemical markers have been proposed for the non-invasive prediction of liver fibrosis in chronic liver disease. Additionally, transient elastography (FibroScan) has recently been developed as a non-invasive method for the evaluation of liver fibrosis, by assessing liver stiffness based on a mechanical wave generated by vibration. The diagnostic accuracy of ARFI has been shown to be comparable with that of previously reported non-invasive scoring systems such as AST to Platelet Ratio Index (APRI), Fib-4 and Forn's index (Takahashi et al, 2010). Several studies have reported both ARFI and FibroScan measurements. The results of ARFI elastography were highly correlated with those of FibroScan measurements, though the success rate of ARFI measurements was higher than that for FibroScan. To the best of our knowledge, few reports have compared the diagnostic accuracies of ARFI and FibroScan, based on the gold standard of liver biopsy. Sporea et al. suggested that the accuracy of ARFI elastography was acceptable but lower than that of FibroScan (Sporea et al., 2010), while Friedrich-Rust et al. and Rifai et al. found no significant differences in diagnostic accuracy between the two techniques (Table 2) (Friedrich-Rust et al., 2009, Rifai et al., 2011). It thus remains unclear which form of elastography is more reliable; however, a prospective multicenter study and meta-analysis are currently underway. Nonetheless, ARFI elastography appears to be useful because of its fewer limitations and the integration of elastography and conventional B-mode ultrasonography.

| | | FS 0–1 vs. FS 2–4 | | FS 0–3 vs. FS 4 | |
|---|---|---|---|---|---|
| Author | Subjects | ARFI | FibroScan | ARFI | FibroScan |
| Friedrich-Rust et al. | HCV, HBV | 0.82 | 0.84 | 0.91 | 0.91 |
| Sporea et al. | HCV, HBV | 0.65 | 0.73 | 0.87 | 0.94 |
| Rifai et al. | HCV, HBV, NAFLD | - | - | 0.82 | 0.84 |

Table 2. Diagnostic accuracy of ARFI and FibroScan for liver fibrosis

AUROC, area under the receiver operating characteristic curve; FS, fibrosis stage; HCV, hepatitis C virus; HBV, hepatitis B virus; NAFLD, non-alcoholic fatty liver disease. Fibrosis stage was assessed using the Metavir scoring system, except in the case of Yoneda et al., who used the method of Brunt.

## 9. Limitations and possible contraindications of ARFI elastography

No significant limitations or contraindication of ARFI elastography for liver assessment have been reported to date. However, the Japan Society of Ultrasonics in Medicine recommends that ARFI elastography should be avoided after contrast-enhanced ultrasonography with some kinds of contrast agents, because of the risk of cavitation. The limitations of transient elastography, such as narrow intercostal spaces, ascites and obesity, do not appear to apply to the use of ARFI elastography, according to our data and the results of previous reports. However, the success rate of ARFI measurements in subjects with a BMI >40 kg/m$^2$ was reportedly only 58% (Palmeri et al., 2011). Further studies are needed to allow more precise evaluation of the limitations of ARFI elastography.

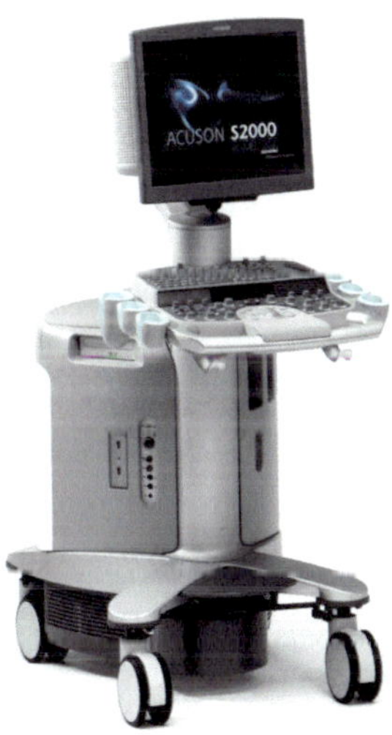


Fig. 1. SIEMENS Acuson S2000

Acoustic radiation force impulse (ARFI) is a radiation force-based impulse that is provided by conventional B-mode ultrasonography, using an Acuson S2000. The ARFI method can be used for elastography. The technology was named "Virtual Touch Tissue Quantification" by SIEMENS.

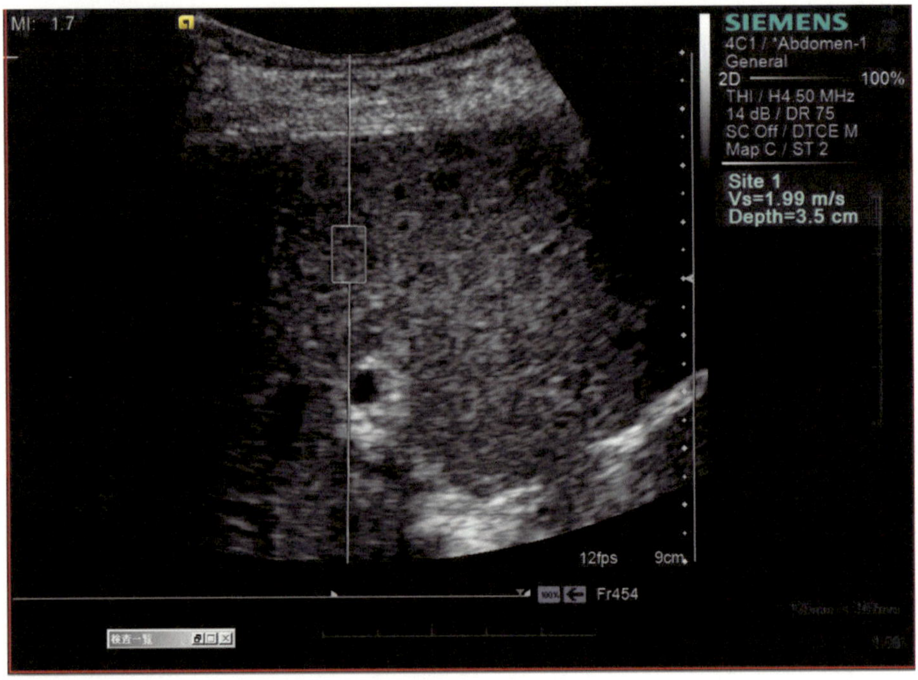


Fig. 2. Measurement window for ARFI elastography

## 10. Conclusion

In conclusion, the novel, non-invasive ultrasonic ARFI elastography technique, coupled with conventional ultrasonography, could offer a reliable method for the assessment of liver fibrosis in patients with chronic liver diseases. ARFI elastography could be useful for real-time evaluation of liver fibrosis as an alternative to liver biopsy.

## 11. Acknowledgments

The authors would like to thank Ms Yukie Watanabe, Ms Chieko Ogawa, all the staff at Saga Medical School Hospital and Yokohama City University Hospital, and Ritsuko Fukusima at Mochida SIEMENS Medical Systems, Japan, for their assistance and excellent advice.

## 12. References

Boursier J, Isselin G, Fouchard-Hubert I, Oberti F, Dib N, Lebigot J, Bertrais S, Gallois Y, Calès P, Aubé C. Eur J Gastroenterol Hepatol. 2010;22:1074-84. Acoustic radiation force impulse: a new ultrasonographic technology for the widespread noninvasive diagnosis of liver fibrosis.

Dahl JJ, Pinton GF, Palmeri ML, Agrawal V, Nightingale KR, Trahey GE.. A parallel tracking method for acoustic radiation force impulse imaging. *IEEE Trans Ultrason Ferroelectr Freq Control.* 2007;54:301–12.

Fierbinteanu-Braticevici C, Andronescu D, Usvat R, Cretoiu D, Baicus C, Marinoschi G. Acoustic radiation force imaging sonoelastography for noninvasive staging of liver fibrosis. *World J Gastroenterol.* 2009;15:5525-32.

Friedrich-Rust M, Wunder K, Kriener S, Sotoudeh F, Richter S, Bojunga J, Herrmann E, Poynard T, Dietrich CF, Vermehren J, Zeuzem S, Sarrazin C. Liver fibrosis in viral hepatitis: noninvasive assessment with acoustic radiation force impulse imaging versus transient elastography.*Radiology.* 2009;252(2):595-604.

Goertz RS, Zopf Y, Jugl V, Heide R, Janson C, Strobel D, Bernatik T, Haendl T. Measurement of liver elasticity with acoustic radiation force impulse (ARFI) technology: an alternative noninvasive method for staging liver fibrosis in viral hepatitis. *Ultraschall Med.* 2010;31:151-55.

Horster S, Mandel P, Zachoval R, Clevert DA. Comparing acoustic radiation force impulse imaging to transient elastography to assess liver stiffness in healthy volunteers with and without valsalva manoeuvre. *Clin Hemorheol Microcirc.* 2010;46:159-68.

Kim JE, Lee JY, Kim YJ, Yoon JH, Kim SH, Lee JM, Han JK, Choi BI. Acoustic radiation force impulse elastography for chronic liver disease: comparison with ultrasound-based scores of experienced radiologists, Child-Pugh scores and liver function tests. *Ultrasound Med Biol.* 2010;36:1637-43.

Lambert J, Halfon P, Penaranda G, Bedossa P, Cacoub P, Carrat F. How to measure the diagnostic accuracy of noninvasive liver fibrosis indices: the area under the ROC curve revisited. *Clin Chem.* 2008;54:1372–8.

Nightingale KR, Palmeri ML, Nightingale RW, Trahey GE. On the feasibility of remote palpation using acoustic radiation force. *J Acoust Soc Am* 2001.110: 625–34.

Obuchowski NA. Estimating and comparing diagnostic tests' accuracy when the gold standard is not binary. *Acad Radiol.* 2005;12:1198–204.

Palmeri ML, Frinkley KD, Zhai L, Gottfried M, Bentley RC, Ludwig K, Nightingale KR. Acoustic radiation force impulse (ARFI) imaging of the gastrointestinal tract. *Ultrason Imaging.* 2005;27:75–88.

Palmeri ML, Wang MH, Rouze NC, Abdelmalek MF, Guy CD, Moser B, Diehl AM, Nightingale KR.Noninvasive Evaluation of Hepatic Fibrosis using Acoustic Radiation Force-Based Shear Stiffness in Patients with Nonalcoholic Fatty Liver Disease. *J Hepatol.* 2011 Jan 20 (Epub ahead of print. URL: http://www.sciencedirect.com/science/article/pii/S0168827811000079).

Popescu A, Sporea I, Sirli R, Bota S, Focşa M, Dănilă M, Nicoliță D, Martie A, Sendroiu M, Juchiş A.The mean values of liver stiffness assessed by Acoustic Radiation Force Impulse elastography in normal subjects. *Med Ultrason.* 201;13:33-7.

Rifai K, Cornberg J, Mederacke I, Bahr MJ, Wedemeyer H, Malinski P, Bantel H, Boozari B, Potthoff A, Manns MP, Gebel M. Clinical feasibility of liver elastography by acoustic radiation force impulse imaging (ARFI).*Dig Liver Dis.* 2011;43:491-7.

Sporea I, Sirli R, Popescu A, Danilă M. Acoustic Radiation Force Impulse (ARFI)--a new modality for the evaluation of liver fibrosis. *Med Ultrason.* 2010;12:26-31.

Takahashi H, Ono N, Eguchi Y, Eguchi T, Kitajima Y, Kawaguchi Y, Nakashita S, Ozaki I, Mizuta T, Toda S, Kudo S, Miyoshi A, Miyazaki K, Fujimoto K. Evaluation of acoustic radiation force impulse elastography for fibrosis staging of chronic liver disease: a pilot study. *Liver Int*. 2010;30:538-45.

Yoneda M, Suzuki K, Kato S, Fujita K, Nozaki Y, Hosono K, Saito S, Nakajima A. Nonalcoholic fatty liver disease: US-based acoustic radiation force impulse elastography. *Radiology*. 2010;256:640-7.

# 22

# Comparison of Five Liver Fibrosis Indexes with Serum Levels of Laminin and N Terminal Peptide of Procollagen Type III in Chronic Hepatitis Patients

Hadi Parsian[1,2], Mohammad Nouri[3], Ali Rahimipour[4], Mohammad Hossein Somi[3] and Durdi Qujeq[1,2]
[1]*Department of Biochemistry and Biophysics, Babol University of Medical Sciences, Babol,*
[2]*Cellular and Molecular Biology Research Centre, Babol University of Medical Sciences, Babol,*
[3]*Liver and Gastrointestinal Diseases Research Centre, Tabriz University of Medical Sciences, Tabriz,*
[4]*Department of Clinical Biochemistry, Shahid Beheshti University of Medical Sciences, Tehran, Iran*

## 1. Introduction

Different types of disease for example viral hepatitis, ethanol and biliary tract disease can produce liver fibrosis (Stalnikowitz & Weissbrod AB, 2003). Liver fibrosis can be divided into those diseases in which the fibrosis is portal based and those that are central based. Chronic viral hepatitis (viral and autoimmune), chronic cholestatic diseases and hemochromatosis are the major portal based diseases and steatohepatitis and chronic venous outflow obstruction of any cause can causes central based diseases (Benyon & Arthur, 2001). Chronic viral hepatitis (especially hepatitis B and C) and autoimmune hepatitis are the major causes of liver fibrosis, especially in developing countries.

The hepatitis B virus (HBV) belongs to the Hepadnaviridae family (Marco et al, 1999) and it is estimated worldwide HBV infection prevalence is to be around 350 million chronic carriers (Kao & Chen, 2002). Infection with the hepatitis C virus (HCV) in the general population varies from 0.2% to 18% (Neighbors, 2007). HCV can infect liver cells and is able to cause severe inflammation of the liver with serious complications. Autoimmune hepatitis (AIH) similar to the above mentioned diseases, is a chronic disease that is associated with some autoantibodies such as antinuclear antibodies (ANA), liver-kidney microsomal antibodies (LKM), anti mithochondial antibody (AMA), soluble liver antigen (SLA), smooth muscle antibodies (SMA) and hypergammaglobulinemia. The prevalence of this disesesis is between 0.1 and 1.2 cases per 100,000 in Western Europe and North America but only 0.08–0.015 cases per 100,000 in Japan (Manna & Strassburg, 2001).

### 1.1 Hepatic fibrosis

In response to liver injury, because of any cause, accumulation of extracellular matrix (ECM) proteins (collagen types, proteoglycans, fibronectin and laminin) will occur. The ECM scaffold is taken down by some special matrix proteinases while activated stellate cells (SC) undergo apoptosis and try to restore the normal tissue structure. Hepatic SC will produce matrix metalloproteinases (MMPs) to regulate the extracellular degradation of matrix proteins. Ultimately, as a result of an imbalance between fibrogenesis and fibrolysis, collagen deposition will occurs and scar will form. When scarring progressed, architectural distortion, liver fibrosis and ultimately cirrhosis will occur (Stalnikowitz & Weissbrod, 2003). Figure 1 illustrates this phenomenon.

### 1.2 Hepatic inflammation

After liver cell injury, recruitment of leukocytes will takes place (Marra, 1999). Leukocytes together with kupffer cells will produce compounds that modulate stellate cell behavior. Nitric oxide (NO) and inflammatory cytokines, such as tumor necrosis factor α (with stimulatory ability on the stellate cell for collagen synthesis) will produce by monocytes and macrophages. In addition, kupffer cells can stimulate matrix synthesis by stellate cells through the actions of transforming growth factor β (TGF-β) and reactive oxygen species (ROS) (Stalnikowitz & Weissbrod, 2003; Granger & Kubes, 1994) –Figure 1.

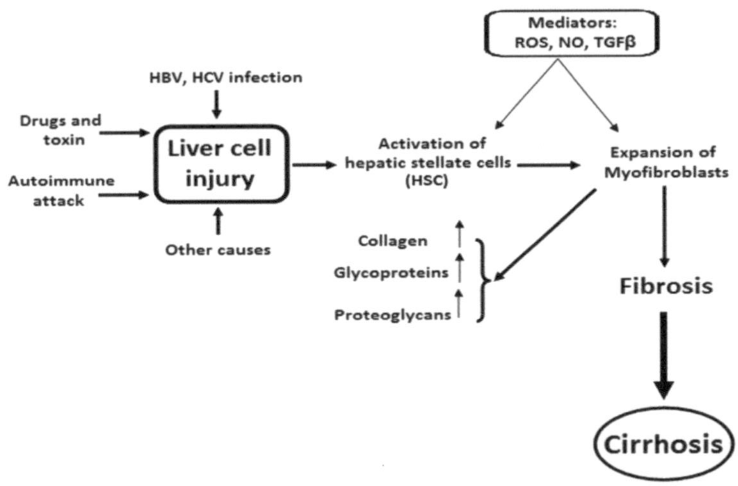


Fig. 1. Proposed mechanism of activation of hepatic stellate cells leading to fibrosis and cirrhosis. ROS, reactive oxygen species; NO, nitric oxide; TGFβ, transforming growth factor β (resulted from Gressner et al., 2007).

### 1.3 Assessment of severity of liver fibrosis

Now, the gold standard for assessment of liver fibrosis is liver biopsy. For scoring liver fibrosis, several systems have been proposed that all of them are based on visual assessment of collagen staining of liver biopsy samples. These are including the histology activity index (HAI), the modified Knodell score, the Ishak score and the Metavir score (Marcellin et al, 2002). Recently a newly scoring system is proposed and named modified Knodell score system. The grading of liver inflammation injuries was scored from 0 to 18. The staging of liver fibrosis was scored from 0 to 6 and is according to the Table 1 (Knodell et al., 1981; Ishak et al., 1995).

| Score | Fibrosis stage |
|---|---|
| 0 | No fibrosis |
| 1 | Fibrous expansion of some portal areas, with or without short fibrous septa |
| 2 | Fibrous expansion of most portal areas, with or without short fibrous septa |
| 3 | Fibrous expansion of most portal areas with occasional portal to portal (P-P) bridging |
| 4 | Fibrous expansion of portal areas with marked bridging [portal to portal (P-P) as well as portal to central (P-C)] |
| 5 | Marked bridging (P-P and/or P-C) with occasional nodules (incomplete cirrhosis) |
| 6 | Cirrhosis, probable or definite |

Table 1. Modified Knodell score system for liver fibrosis staging (Knodell et al., 1981).

Liver biopsy, as a clinical tool, has some major limitations (Rossi et al., 2007). Most famous limitations of liver biopsy are: fibrosis staging systems (with this assumption that there is a linear increase in the severity of fibrosis between stages) (Rosenberg et al., 2004), sampling error (a 10–15 mg sample of tissue represents a tiny fraction of an organ weighing 1500 g) (Regev et al., 2002) and inter-observer variation amongst pathologists in categorizing the degree of fibrosis (Westin et al., 1999).
For assessment of liver fibrosis, in addition to invasive method (liver biopsy), there are some serum-based noninvasive markers individually or in an algorithm-based score. Noninvasive markers in assessment of liver necroinflammatory injuries are the best markers, because they can analyze frequently during the treatment protocol of liver fibrosis and also for highlighting the efficacy of treatment.
The most famous individual markers for assessment of liver fibrosis are: liver function tests (aspartate aminotransferase: AST and alanine aminotransferase: ALT) that reflect hepatocyte damage, bilirubin and alkaline phosphatase that show biliary obstruction and albumin and prothrombin time (PT) that reveal biosynthetic function of liver. These tests only provide information about important aspects of liver function but they do not assess severity of liver fibrosis or cirrhosis (Rossi et al., 2007). Other serum markers such as α-2-Macroglobulin (Naveau et al., 1994), apolipoprotein A1 (Poynard et al., 1991), haptoglobin (Bismut et al., 2001), matrix metalloproteinases (MMPs) and their tissue inhibitors (TIMPs) (Leroy et al., 2004), hyaluronic acid, collagen markers, aminoterminal propeptide of type III procollagen (PIIINP) and laminin (LN) are proposed, too, as surrogate indices instead of liver biopsy (Gressner et al., 2007). New researches indicated that these individuals' serum markers have limited accuracy in predicting hepatic fibrosis and proposed that the individual markers are useful for establishing the presence, but not absence, of fibrosis. Due to the limitations of individual markers to assess liver fibrosis, algorithms or indices combining the results of panels of markers have been studied which reportedly improve diagnostic accuracy. The serum marker panels have been proposed as an alternative to liver biopsy (Crockett et al., 2006; Castera & Pawlotsky, 2005).

Some of the available serum marker panels include HCV FibroSURE, ASH FibroSURE, NASH FibroSURE, FIBROSpect II, Hepascore, Forns score, APRI, AAR, AP, SHASTA, Fibro Q and FIB4 index and European Liver Fibrosis Group (ELFG) algorithm. Some are beyond the scope of this chapter; however five of them that evaluated in this study, briefly are discussed here. In this study the serum levels of LN and PIIINP, in addition to the five serum marker panels of liver necroinflammatory injury and the histologicall evaluation of liver biopsies according to the modified Knodell score system were studied.

### 1.3.1 Laminin (LN)

One of the main glycoproteins of the basement membrane is laminin (LN). This molecule participates in a series of biological events such as the maintenance of the cytoskeleton (Rosa & Parise, 2008). Hpatocytes and sinusoidal cells are able to synthesis of LN (Rosa & Parise, 2008; Gressner et al., 2007). Deposition of LN and collagen determine the formation of a true basement membrane along sinusoids in the liver. Increased in production of LN in the liver and a lack of degradation of this glycoprotein by liver endothelial cells, are the major causes of elevated serum levels of this protein in fibrotic and cirrhotic liver. It is proposed that laminin serum concentration is a sensitive screening test for hepatic fibrotic disease (Rosa & Parise, 2008).

### 1.3.2 Aminoterminal propeptide of type III procollagen: PIIINP

During the processing of type III procollagen, the PIIINP molecule is produced by a specific N-proteinase. There are evidences that proposed purified preparations of the PIIINP molecule will degrade by scavenger receptors located on the liver endothelial cells. In various clinical situations such as liver fibrosis, metabolism of type III collagen will alter, therefore measurement of PIIINP concentration in serum will has some clinical application. Some studies revealed that there is a significantly increased serum level of PIIINP in patients with liver fibrosis and cirrhosis. It proposed that these increased serum levels are related to increased hepatic synthesis of connective tissue components and also a decreased in hepatic clearance ability (Smedsr et al., 1990).

### 1.3.3 Serum marker panels/models

#### 1.3.3.1 Age-platelet (AP) index

AP index is a simple index that derived from age and platelet counts and is calculate as follow:

Age (years) $<30 = 0$; $30\text{-}39 = 1$; $40\text{-}49 = 2$; $50\text{-}59 = 3$; $60\text{-}69 = 4$; $\geq 70 = 5$,

Platelets counts ($10^9/l$): $\geq 225 = 0$; $200\text{-}224 = 1$; $175\text{-}199 = 2$;
$150\text{-}174 = 3$; $125\text{-}149 = 4$; $<125 = 5$

The sum of age and platelet counts scores according to the above mentioned scoring system, named AP index (Poynard et al,. 1997).

#### 1.3.3.2 AST to platelet ratio index (APRI)

Several studies have suggested that the APRI may be a useful noninvasive marker of hepatic fibrosis in patients with chronic liver disease. APRI Score was initially described by Wai et al (Wai et al., 2003) and calculated by this formula:

$$APRI = ((AST / \text{upper limit of normal}) / \text{platelet count } (10^9 / L)) \times 100)$$

#### 1.3.3.3 AAR index

Another simple index that used for evaluation of liver fibrosis is AAR index. One can calculate this index by dividing the levels of AST to ALT (Williams et al., 1988).

#### 1.3.3.4 Fibro Q

Fibro Q is another index that dependent to age (years), AST level, platelet count and also PT International Normalized Ratio (INR) and can be calculating by the following formula (Hsieh et al., 2009).

$$\text{Fibro Q} = [(10 \times \text{age (years)} \times AST \times PT\ INR)/ (PLT \times ALT)].$$

#### 1.3.3.5 FIB4

FIB-4 is an index that is dependent to age (years), AST and ALT levels (U/L) and platelet count (Sterling et al., 2006). It can be calculated simply by the following formula.

$$\text{FIB-4} = [\text{age (year)} \times AST\ (U/L)] / [PLT\ (10^9/L) \times ALT\ (U/L))^{1/2}).$$

The aim of this study was identify the efficiency of the extracellular matrix components i.e. LN and PIIINP in comparison with five noninvasive fibrosis models (AP, APRI, AAR, Fibro Q and FIB4 index) and to recognize the most important model for discrimination of patients with liver fibrosis (chronic hepatitis B, C and auto immune hepatitis (AIH) patients) vs. control and also for discrimination of patients with severe liver fibrosis (stage≥3) vs. mild liver fibrosis (stage≥2).

## 2. Methods

### 2.1 Study population

Sixty-two patients; (35 men and 27 women, mean ± SD: 35.4 ± 11.3 years) were enrolled in this study. Among these patients 35 patients had hepatitis B, 14 had hepatitis C and 13 were autoimmune hepatitis (AIH). The patients were selected from the persons who referred to Liver and Gastrointestinal Disease Research Center of Tabriz, Babol and Gorgan (Gonbad) University of Medical Sciences for diagnosis of the disease.

Control sera for the determination of LN and PIIINP were obtained from 20 healthy volunteer's person who referred to the Tabriz University of Medical Sciences (10 women and 10 men, mean ± SD: 42 ± 14.7 years). Control groups had normal serum levels of aminotransferases and alkaline phospahtase. None of the controls had a history of gastrointestinal bleeding and chronic liver disease, smoking (never smoker), alcohol intake (never drinker), a family history of hepatitis and liver disease, active intravenous drug abuse and a liver transplantation, according to the information's gathered in the questionnaire form. Persons who smoked (>1 cigarette/day) and drunk alcohol (>1 gr/day), were classified as smoker and alcohol drinker.

All of the subjects were informed about the study and their consents were taken. This study was approved by Tabriz Medical University Ethical Committee.

#### 2.1.1 Inclusion criteria

Patients were included in the study, if they were positive for serum hepatitis B surface antigen (HBs-Ag) or HCV antibodies, and having persistently elevated serum aminotransferases greater than 1.5 times the upper limit of the reference range for at least six months. AIH patients were diagnosed according to the International Autoimmune Hepatitis Group Report protocol (Manna & Strasburg, 2001). For assessment of liver fibrosis scores, all patients underwent liver biopsy as part of the normal diagnostic procedure and were subsequently sub-classified according to the score for the histological activity index (HAI).

### 2.1.2 Exclusion criteria

Patients with a history of gastrointestinal bleeding and other chronic liver disease (such as Wilson's disease, hemochromatosis, alpha1-antitrypsin deficiency, biliary disease, hepatocellular carcinoma), active intravenous drug abuse, and liver transplantation were excluded.

## 2.2 Blood collection and sample preparation

Blood samples (7ml) were collected after an overnight fast. After analyzing cell blood counts (CBC) on aliquots of whole blood, on remainder the samples, serum was separated (at 2500 g for 5 minutes) within one hour of blood collection. Standard LFT, including AST and ALT and hepatitis serology were performed on aliquots of each sample and recorded. Routine LFT and hepatitis serology was assayed using commercial available kits. Briefly AST and ALT were measured by colorimetric test (Ziestchem kit, Iran) with 2, 4 DNPH (2, 4 dinitrophenylhydrazone) with Apel spectrophotometer (PD303S, Japan).

The hepatitis serology markers were analyzed by an ELISA reader (Norahan Fajr, Iran) and the following Kits. The AIH serology markers that analyzed were: antinuclear antibody (ANA; Biazyme ELISA kit, Birmingham, UK) and anti-LKM-1 (LKM-1: type 1 liver and kidney microsomes, Euroimmun ELISA kit, Germany), hepatitis B serology markers were: hepatitis B surface antigen (HBsAg; Diakey, shinjin Medics Inc. ELISA kit, Korea), hepatitis B Surface Antibody (HBsAb; Diakey, shinjin Medics Inc. ELISA kit, Korea) and hepatitis B Core Antibody (HBcAb; Dia-Pro ELISA kit, Italy) and hepatitis C serology marker was: HCV antibody (HCVAb; Diakey, shinjin Medics Inc. ELISA kit, Korea). HCV RNA was assayed using a PCR kit (Roche Diagnostics, Mannheim, Germany) by an Eppendorf Thermocycler (Mastercycler Personal) according to the manufacturer's instructions. Two primers (Sinagene, Tehran, Iran) with the following sequences were used: first primer sequence 5′-GCA GAA AGC GTC TAG CCA TGG CGT-3′ and second primer sequence 5′-CTC GCA AGC ACC CTA TCA GGC AGT-3′.

The rest of the blood samples were stored at –20°C. The controls were dealt with in the same manner.

## 2.3 Determination of serum LN and PIIINP

### 2.3.1 LN assay

Serum LN concentrations were assayed using a LN EIA Kit (Takara Bio, product number: MK107) on an ELISA reader (BDSL, Immunoscan, Lab System, Switzerland) and the amount of LN was determined by a standard curve. The intra assay and inter-assay variability (CV) of the procedure according to the manufacturer, were 4.0 -5.7% and 0.3-5.0%, respectively.

### 2.3.2 PIIINP assay

Serum PIIINP levels were assayed by a PIIINP ELISA Kit (USCN life and technology company, product no: E0573h) on an ELISA reader (BDSL, Immunoscan, Lab System,

Switzerland). Briefly, a monoclonal antibody specific for PIIINP had been precoated onto a microplate. Standards and samples were pipetted into the wells and any PIIINP present was bound by the immobilized antibody. An enzyme-linked polycolonal antibody specific for PIIINP was added to the wells. Following a wash to remove any unbound antibody-enzyme reagent, a substrate solution was added to the wells and color developed in proportion to the amount of PIIINP bound in the initial steps. The color development was stopped and the intensity of the color was measured and ultimately the amount of PIIINP was determined by a standard curve. The intra assay variability (CV) of the procedure according to the manusfacturer declares was 4-5-5.0%.

### 2.4 Histological assessment of liver damage

Sixty-two patients underwent a percutaneous liver biopsy with a Trucut needle number 16 guided by B type ultrasound for assessing the presence and severity of liver disease. The biopsy fragments were fixed in a 10% formalin solution for 12 hours and embedded in paraffin. Sections were stained with hematoxylin-eosin, Masson's trichrome and reticulin stain. Specimens were graded and staged according to the modified Knodell scoring system (Knodell et al., 1981) by a pathologist who was blinded to the results of serum indices in the study subjects. The grading system was scored from 0 to 18 and was based on sum of four indices:

1. Periportal or periseptal interface hepatitis (piecemeal necrosis, score 0-4)
2. Confluent necrosis (score 0-6)
3. Focal (spotty) lytic necrosis, apoptosis, and focal inflammation (score 0-4)
4. Portal inflammation (score 0-4).

The fibrosis score were determined on the basis of the table 1.

### 2.5 Statistical analysis

The SPSS 12.0 statistical package (SPSS for Windows 12.0, SPSS, Chicago, IL, USA) was used on statistical analysis. Data were expressed as mean ± SD, and P less than 0.05 was considered statistically significant. The mean patient serum LN and PIIINP levels between different types of chronic hepatitis and healthy controls were compared with analysis of variance (ANOVA). Five serum markers panels were calculated as mentioned in the introduction section 1.3.3. To assess the diagnostic accuracy of LN and PIIINP and also five serum marker panels for discrimination chronic hepatitis patients with severe liver fibrosis from healthy individuals, and also discrimination of patients with severe liver fibrosis vs. mild liver fibrosis, we plotted the receiver operating characteristic curve (ROC). Receiver operating characteristic curves were generated by plotting the relationship of the true positivity (sensitivity) and the false positivity (1- specificity) at various cut-off points of the tests. An AUC of 1.0 is characteristic of an ideal test, whereas 0.5 indicates a test of no diagnostic value (Zweig & Campbell, 1993). Taking sensitivity and specificity into account, the cut-off points were selected according to max number of sensitivity add specificity. The diagnostic accuracy, sensitivity, specificity, positive predictive values (PPV) and negative predictive values (NPV) also were calculated.

## 3. Results

Histological examination of liver for fibrosis scoring revealed that 10, 19, 11, 9, 8, 4 and 1 patient were at stages 0, 1, 2, 3, 4, 5 and 6 of liver fibrosis, respectively. In the other hand,

35% of patients to be suffering from significant fibrosis (stage ≥3). In addition 32.2% of patients had liver inflammation grades ≥5. Hepatitis serology revealed that 56.4% of the patients were suffering from chronic hepatitis B, 22.5% from chronic hepatitis C and 20.9% from autoimmune hepatitis. In table 2 characteristics of chronic hepatitis patients and controls are shown. The results of laboratory tests showed that the serum levels of AST and ALT in patients groups were significantly higher than in the control group (p<0.001) but the differences in platelet count and prothrombin time were not significant.
The results also showed increased serum LN and PIIINP levels in patients, as compared with the healthy controls (p<0.001).

| Variables | Patients (n=62) | Controls (n=20) | P value |
|---|---|---|---|
| Male/Female (n) | 35 / 27 | 10 / 10 | - |
| Age in years | 35.4 ± 11.3 | 42.0 ± 14.7 | - |
| Platelet count ($10^9$/L) | 225.7± 122.4 | 179.7± 25.5 | 0.051 |
| Prothrombin time (s) | 13.56± 1.65 | 13.15± 1.47 | 0.345 |
| ALT, IU/L | 143.0 ± 145.6 | 27.3 ± 6.4 | <0.001 |
| AST, IU/L | 101.1 ± 143.1 | 28.3 ± 6.5 | <0.001 |
| Laminin, ng/ml | 91.9 ± 20.9 | 46.1 ± 10.1 | <0.001 |
| PIIINP, ng/ml | 6.8 ± 1.7 | 4.5 ± 1.1 | <0.001 |

Table 2. Characteristics of the patient and control groups included in the study.

The mean serum LN and PIIINP concentrations in patients with HBV, HCV, AIH and healthy controls are presented in Table 3. These results showed statistically increased serum LN and PIIINP levels in patients as compared with healthy controls (P < 0.001).
The patient's serum LN and PIIINP levels in different stages of liver fibrosis are presented in Table 4. Almost in all stages of hepatic fibrosis, the serum levels of LN and PIIINP, were higher than those of the healthy group (p<0.05). In stage 0 of liver fibrosis the LN and PIIINP serum concentrations did not differ compare from the healthy controls. In fibrosis stage 6, which was represented by only one patient, the serum levels of LN and PIIINP are presented.

| Disease | LN | PIIINP |
|---|---|---|
| HBV | 92.0 ± 20.1* | 6.6 ± 1.9* |
| HCV | 92.8 ± 24.1* | 7.4 ± 1.5* |
| AIH | 90.6 ± 18.4* | 6.8 ± 1.4* |
| Total | 91.9 ± 20.9* | 6.8 ± 1.7* |
| Healthy controls | 46.1 ± 10.1 | 4.5 ± 1.1 |

* P value ≤ 0.001.

Table 3. Comparison of LN and PIIINP serum concentration in different types of chronic hepatitis and control group. Data are presented as Mean ± SD (ng/ml).

Figure 2 (a and b), are illustrated scatter plots for serum LN and PIIINP level (ng/ml) in hepatitis patients in various grades of inflammation. According to these figures, patients in higher grades of liver inflammation had higher serum concentrations of LN and PIIINP and the highest level were observed in grades of 5-12 of liver inflammation. We had no patient in inflammation grades of 13-18.

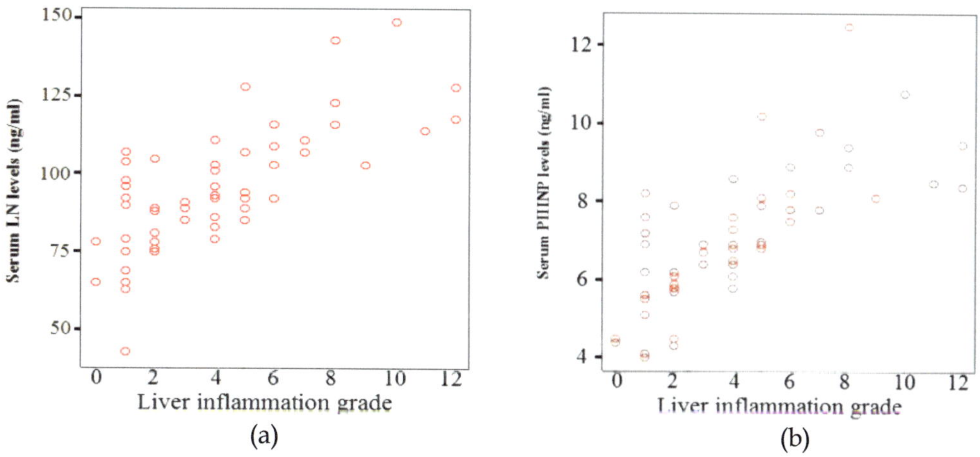


Fig. 2. Scatter plots for serum LN (a) and PIIINP (b) level (ng/ml) in patients at various grades of inflammation.

| Stage | LN | PIIINP |
|---|---|---|
| 0 | 63.0 ±12.1 | 4.5 ± 0.5 |
| 1 | 85.7 ± 6.3* | 6.1 ± 0.9* |
| 2 | 94.0 ± 10.2** | 7.0 ± 0.8* |
| 3 | 100.6 ± 8.6** | 7.7 ± 0.6** |
| 4 | 104.2 ± 20.2** | 8.0 ± 1.5** |
| 5 | 130.2 ± 13.7** | 9.8 ± 0.8** |
| 6† | 143.0 | 12.5 |
| Total | 91.9 ± 20.9** | 6.8 ± 1.7** |

† There was only one patient in stage 6 of liver fibrosis.
* P value ≤ 0.05
** P value ≤ 0.001

Table 4. Serum concentrations (ng/ml) of LN and PIIINP in various stages of liver fibrosis Data are presented as Mean ± SD (ng/ml).

A cut-off point of 52.0 ng LN/ml and 5.0 ng PIIINP/ml for the discrimination of patients with liver fibrosis from those without liver fibrosis showed a good accuracy, AUC, sensitivity, specificity, PPV and NPV (Table 5).

| Marker | AUC | P | Sen | Sp | PPV | NPV | Accu |
|---|---|---|---|---|---|---|---|
| AAR | 0.907 | 0.001 | 86 | 76 | 77 | 69 | 85 |
| AP | 0.632 | 0.179 | 68 | 55 | 64 | 45 | 59 |
| APRI | 0.818 | 0.001 | 79 | 82 | 78 | 69 | 79 |
| FIB4 | 0.754 | 0.001 | 77 | 81 | 76 | 65 | 76 |
| FibroQ | 0.957 | 0.001 | 89 | 90 | 85 | 79 | 87 |
| LN | 0.974 | 0.001 | 94 | 78 | 91 | 86 | 89 |
| PIIINP | 0.873 | 0.001 | 85 | 70 | 89 | 60 | 81 |

(AUC, area under the ROC curve; Sen, sensitivity; Sp, specificity; PPV, positive predictive value ;NPV, negative predictive value; Accu, accuracy).

Table 5. Accuracy of tests for discrimination of patients with liver fibrosis vs. control.

We selected other cut-off points (92.5 ng LN/ml and 8.9 ng PIIINP/ml) for the discrimination of patients with mild fibrosis (stage 0-2) from severe fibrosis (stage 3-6) and the results are presented in Table 6. For comparison of the AUC of the serum marker panels (i.e. AP, AAR, APRI, FIB4 and FiroQ) with the AUC of the serum HA and LN levels, the AUC of these parameters were also calculated and the results are presented in table 5 and 6, too.

| Marker | AUC | P | Sen | Sp | PPV | NPV | Accu |
|---|---|---|---|---|---|---|---|
| AAR | 0.491 | 0.947 | 45 | 44 | 32 | 56 | 54 |
| AP | 0.518 | 0.137 | 56 | 50 | 45 | 39 | 59 |
| APRI | 0.268 | 0.107 | 29 | 22 | 31 | 28 | 33 |
| FIB4 | 0.232 | 0.110 | 27 | 28 | 26 | 31 | 29 |
| FibroQ | 0.491 | 0.997 | 44 | 45 | 33 | 55 | 56 |
| LN | 0.879 | 0.005 | 86 | 71 | 87 | 69 | 82 |
| PIIINP | 0.911 | 0.002 | 89 | 72 | 85 | 71 | 83 |

(AUC, area under the ROC curve; Sen, sensitivity; Sp, specificity; PPV, positive predictive value ;NPV, negative predictive value; Accu, accuracy).

Table 6. Accuracy of tests for discrimination of patients with severe liver fibrosis vs. mild liver fibrosis.

Figures 3 and 4 are illustrated the results of ROC analysis of LN (a) and PIIINP (a) for discrimination of patients with liver fibrosis vs. control and also for discrimination of patients with severe liver fibrosis vs. mild liver fibrosis, respectively.

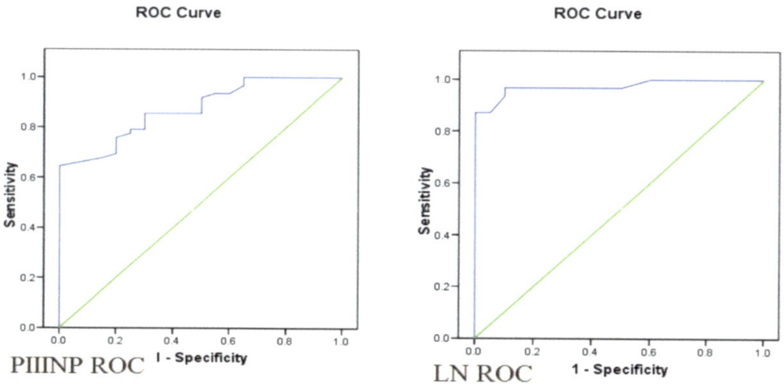


a b

Fig. 3. ROC analysis of LN (a) and PIIINP (b) for discrimination of patients with liver fibrosis vs. control.

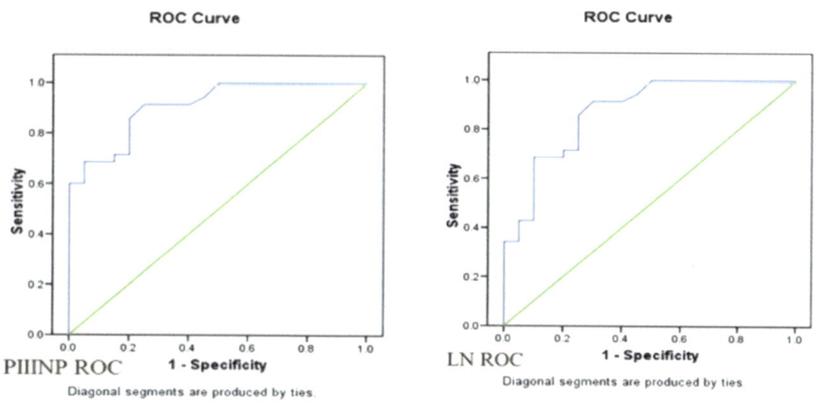


a b

Fig. 4. ROC analysis of LN (a) and PIIINP (b) for discrimination of patients with severe liver fibrosis vs. mild liver fibrosis.

## 4. Discussion

Mean serum LN and PIIINP levels in chronic hepatitis B, C and auto immune hepatitis were significantly higher than in healthy controls ($p < 0.001$). Patients with higher stages of liver fibrosis had higher serum LN and PIIINP concentrations and the correlations between serum LN and PIIINP concentrations with liver fibrosis stages were linear and strong (data not presented). Also, the mean serum LN and PIIINP concentrations in the stages 2, 3, 4 and 5 of the liver fibrosis showed statistically significant differences as compared with the healthy group. We didn't observe such a statistically differences in the stage 0 of liver fibrosis. In fibrosis Stage 6, which was represented by only one patient, we could not compare this single patient with the control group.
In addition, we observed that patients who had greater inflammation grades had higher serum LN and PIIINP concentrations (according to the figure 2) and the correlation of serum

LN and PIIINP with the inflammation grades were linear (correlation data not presented). These findings suggest that patients with higher serum LN and PIIINP concentrations might have higher liver fibrosis stage and inflammation grade. Therefore we can conclude that when liver damage develops, the liver more poorly metabolized the LN and PIIINP. Patients in early stage of liver fibrosis possibly metabolized better LN and PIIINP in the liver than those with advanced liver fibrosis stages.

A cut-off point of 52.0 ng LN/ml and 5.0 ng PIIINP/ml for the discrimination of patients with liver fibrosis from those without liver fibrosis showed a good AUC (0.974 and 0.873, respectively), accuracy, sensitivity, specificity, PPV and NPV. Also serum marker panels in selected cut points (cut points not presented) showed reasonably good AUC (AP: 0.632, AAR: 0.907, APRI: 0.818, FIB4: 0.754 and Fibro Q: 0.957), accuracy, sensitivity, specificity, PPV and NPV. It means that all of these serum markers, individually or in a panel model, can discriminate between persons with liver fibrosis and healthy individuals.

A cut-off point of 92.5 ng LN/ml and 8.9 ng PIIINP/ml for discrimination of patients with mild fibrosis from those with severe fibrosis showed the AUCROC (p-value) of 0.879 (0.005) and 0.911 (0.002), respectively. It means that LN and PIIINP can discriminate between patients with mild fibrosis from those with severe fibrosis. But the AUCROC (p-value) of serum panel markers for discrimination of severe liver fibrosis (stage≥3) than mild liver fibrosis (stage≥2) revealed a different pattern as follows: AAR=0.491 (0.947), AP=0.518 (0.137), APRI=0.268 (0.107), FIB-4=0.232 (0.110) and Fibro Q=0.491 (0.997). It seems only the LN and PIIINP performed better at excluding advanced fibrosis than mild fibrosis.

The reported researches about these markers is controversial, but in recent years there is increasing evidences that show these markers can be used for assessing the liver fibrosis stages (Gressner et al.,2007). Serum level of LN, have been used by several authors as a non-invasive marker to assess liver fibrosis in patients with viral hepatitis. LN determination together with PIIINP, hydroxyproline, prothrombin activity, and AST/ALT ratio has been used in the diagnosis of advanced fibrosis in chronic hepatitis C patients (Rosa & Parise et al., 2008). Serum levels of PIIINP were studied in viral hepatitis patients and studies showed strong correlation between its levels and histological stage of hepatic fibrosis. Also PIIINP levels were in correlation with aminotransferase levels (Bensen et al., 1987).

Murawaki reported that differences in serum ALT and PIIINP levels between stage F0 (no fibrosis), F1 (mild fibrosis), F2 (moderate fibrosis) and F3 (severe fibrosis) in patients with chronic hepatitis C were statistically significant (P-value: <0.005, <0.0002, respectively) (Murawaki et al., 2001). In a study by Attallah, mean level of PIIINP and LN in severe liver fibrosis stages were greater than mild liver fibrosis stages (Attallah et al., 2007). As well in additional reports, LN concentrations were increased in early stages of chronic liver disease and the highest concentrations were in active cirrhosis and chronic active hepatitis (Castera et al., 2000). 84).

The grater serum markers, in higher liver inflammation grades, reported by others (Parsian et al., 2009, Parsian et al., 2010). Zheng reported that serum fibrosis indices (PIIINP and LN) increased as the grade of inflammation aggravated (Zheng et al., 2002). Cai reported that LN was in correlation with liver histopathopathological injuries and inflammation grades (Cai et al., 2004). Also increased serum level of PIIINP and its association with the severity of liver necroinflammation in other studies reported (Murawaki et al., 1994).

Reported diagnostic criteria are not reliable and to some extent are controversial. There is some studies reported that PIIINP has reached a limited clinical application, but no widespread acceptance (Collazos & Diaz, 1994). Sensitivities of about 76.0–78.0% and specificities of 71.0–81.0% have been reported, which can be increased up to 88.0%, if combined with additional collagen fragment markers.

Zheng reported that in ROC curves analysis the AUC of PIIINP and LN was 0.800 and 0.463, respectively. The analysis also showed that PIIINP have greater diagnosis performances than LN according to fibrosis staging (Zheng et al., 2002). Guechot reported that PIIINP and HA serum concentrations correlated with the histological grades of liver fibrosis in untreated patients with chronic viral hepatitis C (P <0.001). In addition, ROC curves showed that serum HA had greater diagnostic performance than PIIINP both for discriminating patients with extensive liver fibrosis from those with no or mild fibrosis (AUC: 0.864 vs. 0.691, P <0.001) or for discriminating patients with cirrhosis from those without cirrhosis (AUC: 0.924 vs. 0.734, P <0.001) (Guechot et al., 1996).

There are various studies about the efficiency of serum marker panels. In a retrospective study, Snyder reported that APRI (with AUROC=0.887) is a simple biochemical index that has been shown to be useful and accurate in about 50% of patients with HCV (Snyder et al., 2007). Yilmaz reported that the APRI had an acceptable accuracy for the assessment of liver fibrosis in patients with chronic hepatitis C (CHC), but not in those with chronic hepatitis B (CHB) (Yilmaz et al., 2011). Wai evaluated the APRI in a cohort of 270 patients with CHC and reported that the AUCROC of the APRI for predicting significant fibrosis and cirrhosis were 0.80–0.88 and 0.89–0.94, respectively and concluded that the APRI can obviate liver biopsy in approximately 50% of patients (Wai et al., 2003).

In another study it has been shown that the AUCROC of the APRI for predicting significant fibrosis and cirrhosis were 0.76 and 0.82, respectively (Shaheen et al., 2008). The results of our study showed that APRI had sensitivity of 79.0% and specificity 82.0% for discrimination of patients with liver fibrosis vs. control and sensitivity of 29.0% and specificity 22.0% for discrimination of patients with severe liver fibrosis vs. mild liver fibrosis. In a study by Hsieh, the authors evaluated 140 patients with chronic viral hepatitis and calculated the APRI, AAR, and FibroQ for assessment of liver fibrosis (Hsieh et al., 2009). They concluded that FibroQ performed better than APRI, but was equal to AAR, in the prediction of significant fibrosis: [AUCROC (p-value): 0.783 vs 0.631 (0.02) and 0.783 vs 0.733 (p = 0.26), respectively] and cirrhosis [AUCROC (p-value): 0.791 vs 0.634 (p = 0.03), and 0.791 vs 0.782 (p =0.47), respectively). Liu demonstrated a low accuracy of APRI and AAR for predicting significant fibrosis in viral hepatitis C carriers with persistently normal ALT levels. The AUCROC in differentiating significant fibrosis were only 0.673 for APRI and 0.504 for AAR (Liu et al., 2006). In a study by Martinez, the performances of APRI and FIB-4 index were validated in 340 patients who underwent antiviral therapy (Martinez et al., 2011). APRI and FIB-4 showed comparable diagnostic accuracies for significant fibrosis (AUROC: 0.83 and 0.85, respectively). To identify cirrhosis, FIB-4 index showed a significantly better performance over APRI score (AUROC: 0.89 vs. 0.83).

In another study Zhang assessed the diagnostic value of FIB-4 in 212 chronic hepatitis B by comparing their results with histological features (Zhang et al., 2010). The AUCROC (p-value) of FIB-4 for significant fibrosis, extensive fibrosis and cirrhosis were 0.733 (< 0.01), 0.746 (< 0.01), 0.756 (< 0.01), respectively. They concluded that the FIB-4 index is an accurate and inexpensive method to assess liver fibrosis in chronic hepatitis and may reduce the need for liver biopsy. Ladep compared the diagnostic validity of AP, APRI and AAR index to histology fibrosis stage among 90 CHB patients (Ladep et al., 2007). The PPV of AAR, API and APRI scores were 52%, 63% and 54%, with sensitivities of 60, 11 and 96%, respectively and interestingly the diagnostic accuracy of AAR for cirrhosis was 100%. They concluded non-invasive fibrosis markers are not as sensitive for diagnosing significant fibrosis in chronic hepatitis B compared to hepatitis C patients and might have a limited utility for use in hepatitis B endemic populations.

Lackner evaluated diagnostic accuracies of AAR, AP and APRI index in 211 patients with chronic hepatitis C and observed that diagnostic accuracy of APRI for prediction of significant fibrosis was superior to that of AAR and AP (Lackner et al., 2005). Fujii calculated AAR, AP, APRI indices in 100 patients with HCV. The AUC of the AAR, AP and APRI index for predicting cirrhosis were respectively 0.555, 0.652 and 0.761. They concluded that these indices are good as noninvasive laboratory tests to predict cirrhosis in patients with HCV (Fujii et al., 2009).

Mahassadi conducted a prospective cohort study to determine the diagnostic accuracy of APRI, AAR, AP and FIB-4 index for the prediction of significant fibrosis or cirrhosis in 117 patients with CHB. APRI and FIB-4 index ruled out significant fibrosis with high specificity of 84.7% and 86.1%, respectively and NPV of 78.2% and 72.9%, respectively. More accurately, APRI or FIB-4 index ruled out cirrhosis with high sensitivity of 94.4% and 88.9% and high NPV of 98.1% and 96.3%, respectively in another cut points. They suggested that APRI and FIB-4 index are simple readily available indices for assessment of liver fibrosis in CHB patients (Mahassadi et al., 2010).

Kim determined the clinical performances of AAR, AP and APRI index for the prediction of liver fibrosis in chronic viral liver diseases in 225 patients with chronic viral liver diseases (180 with hepatitis B virus, 43 with hepatitis C virus, and 2 with hepatitis B+C virus) that underwent a liver biopsy procedure. The AUCROC for APRI, ARR were 0.822, 0.756, 0.642, respectively, for predicting significant fibrosis and were 0.691, 0.711 and 0.794, respectively, for predicting extensive fibrosis. They concluded these serum markers were useful for predicting significant or extensive liver fibrosis in chronic viral liver diseases and APRI was most useful for the prediction of significant fibrosis (Kim et al., 2009).

As it is clear, numerous researchers have attempted to validate these findings, but the results were conflicting. Some researches as mentioned earlier, found a good AUCROC of these serum marker panels for discrimination between patients with mild fibrosis and those with severe fibrosis, but we didn't observe. The differences in patient populations, including the prevalence of significant fibrosis, differences in the reference ranges for AST, differences in the etiology and cause of liver fibrosis and also the pattern of the studies may in part explain these discrepancies (Yilmaz et al., 2011).

In summary, we observed that all serum markers including AAR, AP, APRI, FIB-4, FibroQ, LN, and PIIINP were useful for predicting liver fibrosis in chronic hepatitis patients compared with the healthy control, But we didn't observe such a similar pattern for discrimination between patients with mild fibrosis and those with severe fibrosis and only LN and PIIINP performed better at excluding advanced fibrosis than mild fibrosis and patients with liver fibrosis than healthy individuals. Therefore serum LN and PIIINP measurement together with these tests could be used for predicting of liver fibrosis as alternate to liver biopsy, when liver biopsy is damaging.

## 5. Conclusions

Our findings suggest that measurement of serum LN and PIIINP concentrations can discriminate between patients with liver fibrosis and healthy individuals and between patients with mild fibrosis and those with severe fibrosis. An increase in serum LN and PIIINP concentrations above the predictive value is associated with liver fibrosis. In addition, the values of the AAR, AP, APRI, FIB-4 and FibroQ score and serum LN and PIIINP levels for discrimination between patients with liver fibrosis and healthy individuals are in the same order, but there is not such a similar pattern for discrimination between patients with mild fibrosis and those with severe fibrosis. It seems only the extracellular matrix components i.e. LN and PIIINP performed better at excluding advanced fibrosis than mild fibrosis and patients with liver fibrosis than healthy individuals. Therefore, serum LN and PIIINP levels together with the AAR, AP, APRI, FIB-4 and FibroQ score could be an additional non-invasive tool for evaluation of liver fibrosis, when liver biopsy is contraindicated. These indices may also be used for the assessment of therapeutic efficiency in chronic hepatitis patients, if liver biopsy cannot be performed.

## 6. Acknowledgments

The authors gratefully acknowledge the financial support from the Liver and Gastroenterology Research Centre, Tabriz University of Medical Sciences, Tabriz, Iran.

## 7. References

Attallah AM, Toson EA, Shiha GE, Omran MM, Abdelaziz MM, El-Dosoky. (2007). Evaluation of serum procollagen aminoterminal propeptide III, laminin, and hydroxyproline as predictors of severe fibrosis in patients with chronic hepatitis C.*J Immunoassay Immunochem*, 28, 199-211.

Bensen KD, Petersen K, Junker P. (1987). Serum aminoterminal procollagen type III in acute viral hepatitis. A long term follow-up study. *Liver*,7, 96-105.

Benyon D, Arthur MJP. (2001). Extracellular matrix degradation and the role of stellate cells. *Semin Liver Dis*, 21,373-384.

Bismut F, Ratziu V, Pieroni L, Charlotte F, Benhamou Y, Poynard T. (2001). Multivirc Group.Biochemical markers of liver fibrosis in patients with hepatitis C virus infection: aprospective study. *Lancet*, 357, 1069–75.

Cai WM, Zhang BB, Weng HL, Hu ZR, Lv J, Zheng M, Liu RH. (2004). The diagnostic value of eight serum indices for liver fibrosis. Zhonghua Gan Zang Bing Za Zhi., 12,4, 219-22.

Castera L, Hartmann DJ, Chapel F, Guettier C, Mall F, Lons T, et al. (2000). Serum laminin and type IV collagen are accurate markers of histologically severe alcoholic hepatitis in patients with cirrhosis. *J Hepatol*, 32,3, 412–418.

Castera L, Pawlotsky JM. (2005). Noninvasive diagnosis of liver fibrosis in patients with chronic hepatitis C. *MedGenMed*. Nov 9,4, 39.

Collazos J, Diaz F. (1994). Role of the measurement of serum procollagen type III N-terminal peptide in the evaluation of liver diseases. *Clin Chim Acta*, 227, 37–43.

Crockett SD, Kaltenbach T, Keeffe EB. (2006). Do we still need a liver biopsy? Are the serum fibrosis tests ready for prime time? *Clin Liver Dis*. 10, 3, 513 31.

Fujii H, Enomoto M, Fukushima W, Ohfuji S, Mori M, Kobayashi S, Iwai S, Morikawa H,Tamori A, Sakaguchi H, et al. (2009).Noninvasive laboratory tests proposed for predicting cirrhosis in patients with chronic hepatitis C are also useful in patients with non-alcoholic steatohepatitis. *Journal of Gastroenterology*,44, 6, 608-614.

Granger DN, Kubes P. (1994). The microcirculation and inflammation modulation of leukocytre- endothelial cell adhesion. *J Leukocyte Biol*, 55, 662–675.

Gressner OA, Weiskirchen R, Gressner AM. (2007). Biomarkers of liver fibrosis: Clinical translation of molecular pathogenesis or based on liver-dependent malfunction tests. *Clinica Chimica Acta*, 381, 107–113.

Guechot J, Laudat A, Loria A, Serfaty L, Poupon R, Giboudeau J. (1996). Diagnostic accuracy of hyaluronan and type III procollagen amino terminal peptide serum assays as markers of liver fibrosis in chronic viral hepatitis C evaluated by ROC curve analysis. *Clin Chem*, 42,558–63.

Hsieh YY, Tung SY, Lee IL, Lee K, Shen CH, Wei KL, Chang TC, Chuang CS, Wu CS, Lin YH. (2009). FibroQ: An Easy and Useful Noninvasive Test for Predicting Liver Fibrosis in Patients with Chronic Viral Hepatitis. *Chang Gung Med J* 32, 6, 614-622.

Ishak K, Baptista A, Bianchi L, Callea F, Groote J, Gudat F, et al. (1995). Histologic grading and staging of chronic hepatitis. *J Hepatol*, 22, 696-699.

Kao JH, Chen DS. (2002). Global control of hepatitis B virus infection. *Lancet Infect Dis*, 2, 7,,395-403.

Kim SM, Sohn JH, Kim TY, Roh YW, Eun CS, Jeon YC, Han DS, Oh YH. (2009). Comparison of various noninvasive serum markers of liver fibrosis in chronic viral liver disease. *Korean J Hepato*, 15(4):454-63.

Knodell RG, Ishak KG, Black WC, Chen TS, Craig R, Kaplowilz N, et al. (1981). Formulation and application of a numerical scoring system for assessing histological activity in symptomatic chronic active hepatitis. *Hepatology*, 1, 431 - 5.

Lackner C, Struber G, Liegl B, Leibl S, Ofner P, Bankuti C, Bauer B, Stauber RE. (2005).Comparison and Validation of Simple Noninvasive Tests for Prediction of Fibrosis in Chronic Hepatitis C. *Hepatology*, 41,6,1376-82.

Ladep NG , Okeke EN, Umar MS, Echejoh G, Malu AO. (2007). Comparison of Simple Non-Invasive Tests for Liver Fibrosis with Histology of Chronic Hepatitis B Patients of African Descent. *Hungarian Medical Journal* 4, 469–476.

Leroy V, Monier F, Bottari S. (2004). Circulating matrix metalloproteinases 1, 2, 9 and their inhibitors TIMP-1 and TIMP-2 as serum markers of liver fibrosis in patients with chronic hepatitis C: comparison with PIIINP and hyaluronic acid. *Am J Gastroenterol*, 99, 271–9.

Liu CH, Lin JW, Tsai FC, Yang PM, Lai MY, Chen JH, Kao JH, Chen DS. (2006). Noninvasive tests for the prediction of significant hepatic fibrosis in hepatitis C virus carriers with persistently normal alanine aminotransferases. *Liver Int*,26, 1087-94.

Mahassadi AS, Attia AF, Bathaix FMY, Agbé1 NB, Doffou S, Kissi1 HY, Diomandé IM, Cales P, Ndri-Yoman T. (2010). Diagnostic accuracy of biochemical markers of fibrosis in black African patients with chronic hepatitis B. *Health*, 2, 1413-1420.

Manna MP, Strassburg CP. (2001). Autoimmune Hepatitis: Clinical Challenges. *Gastroenterol*, 120, 1502–1517.

Marcellin P, Asselah T, Boyer N. (2002). Fibrosis and Disease Progression in Hepatitis C. *Hepatology*, 36, S47- -56.

Marco V, Iacono O, Camma C, Vaccaro A, Giunta M, Martorana G, et al. (1999). The long-term course of chronic hepatitis B. *Hepatology*, 30, 257-64.

Marra F. (1999). Hepatic stellate cells and the regulation of liver inflammation. *J Hepatol*, 31, 1120–1130.

Martinez SM, Fernández-Varo G, González P, Sampson E, Bruguera M, Navasa M, Jiménez W, Sánchez-Tapias JM, Forns X. (2011). Assessment of Liver Fibrosis before and after Antiviral Therapy by Different Serum Marker Panels in Patients with Chronic Hepatitis C. *Alimentary Pharmacology & Therapeutics*, 33,1,138-148

Murawaki Y, Ikuta Y, Koda M, Kawasaki H. (1994). Serum type III procollagen peptide, type IV collagen 7S domain, central triplehelix of type IV collagen and tissue inhibitor of metalloproteinases in patients with chronic viral liver disease: relationship to liver histology. *Hepatology*, 20, 780–7.

Murawaki Y, Ikuta Y, Okamoto K, Koda M, Kawasaki H. (2001). Diagnostic value of serum markers of connective tissue turnover for predicting histological staging and grading in patients with chronic hepatitis C. *J Gastroenterol*, 36, 399–406

Naveau S, Poynard T, Benattar C, Bedossa P, Chaput JC. (1994). Alpha-2-macroglobulin and hepatic fibrosis. Diagnostic interest. *Dig Dis Sci*, 39, 2426–32.

Neighbors J. (2007). The Diagnosis and Management of Hepatitis C: The Role of the Physician Assistant. *The Internet Journal of Academic Physician Assistants*, 5, 2, 25-37.

Parsian H, Nouri M, Soumi MH, Rahimipour A, Qujeq D. (2009). Attenuation of serum laminin concentrations upon treatment of chronic hepatitis, N *Z J Med Lab Sci*, 63, 12-7.

Parsian H, Rahimipour A, Nouri M, Somi MH, Qujeq D, Fard MK, Agcheli K. (2010). Serum hyaluronic acid and laminin as biomarkers in liver fibrosis, *J Gastrointestin Liver Dis*, 19, 169-74.

Poynard T, Aubert A, Bedossa P, et al. (1991). A simple biological index for detection of alcoholic liver disease in drinkers. *Gastroenterol*, 100, 1397–402.

Poynard T, Bedossa P. (1997). Age and platelet count: a simple index for predicting the presence of histological lesions in patients with antibodies to hepatitis C virus. METAVIR and CLINIVIR Cooperative Study Groups. *J Viral Hepatol*,4, 199-208

Regev A, Berho M, Jeffers LJ, et al. (2002). Sampling error and intraobserver variation in liver biopsy in patients with chronic HCV infection. *Am J Gastroenterol*, 97, 2614–8.

Rosa h, Parise ER. (2008). Is there a place for serum laminin determination in patients with liver disease and cancer? *World J Gastroenterol*, 21; 14, 3628-3632.

Rosenberg WM, Voelker M, Thiel R, et al. (2004). Serum markers detect the presence of liver fibrosis: a cohort study. *Gastroenterol*, 127, 1704–13.

Rossi E, Adams LA, Bulsara M, Jeffrey GP. (2007). Assessing Liver Fibrosis with Serum Marker Models. *Clin Biochem Rev*, 28, 1, 3–10.

Shaheen AA, Myers RP .(2008). Systematic review and meta-analysis of the diagnostic accuracy of fibrosis marker panels in patients with HIV/hepatitis C coinfection. *HIV Clin Trials*, 9,1,43-51.

Smedsr B, Perotoft H, Gustsfson S and Laurent B. (1990). Review article. Scavenger functions of the liver endothelial cell. *Biochem J*, 266, 313-327.

Snyder N, Nguyen A, Gajula L, Soloway R, Xiao SY, Lau DT, Petersen J. (2007). The APRI may be enhanced by the use of the FIBROSpect II in the estimation of fibrosis in chronic hepatitis C. *Clin Chim Acta*. ,381,2,119-23.

Stalnikowitz DK, Weissbrod AB. (2003). Liver fibrosis and inflammation. A review. *Annals of Hepatology*, 2, 4, 159-163.

Sterling RK, Lissen E, Clumeck N, Sola R, Correa MC, Montaner J, et al. (2006). Development of a simple noninvasive index to predict significant fibrosis in patients with HIV/HCV coinfection. *Hepatology*, 43, 1317-1325.

Wai CT, Greenson JK, Fontana RJ, Kalbfleisch JD, Marrero JA, Conje evaram HS, et al. (2003). A simple noninvasive index can predict both significant fibrosis and cirrhosis in patients with chronic hepatitis C. *Hepatology*, 38,2, 518-26.

Wai CT, Greenson JK, Fontana RJ, Kalbfleisch JD, Marrero JA, Conjeevaram HS, et al.(2003). A simple noninvasive index can predict both significant fibrosis and cirrhosis in patients with chronic hepatitis C. *Hepatology*, 38, 2, 518-26.

Westin J, Lagging LM, Wejstal R, Norkrans G, Dhillon AP. (1999). Interobserver study of liver histopathology using the Ishak score in patients with chronic hepatitis C virus infection. *Liver*, 19, 183–7.

Williams AL, Hoofnagle JH. (1988). Ratio of serum aspartate to alanine aminotransferase in chronic hepatitis Relationship to cirrhosis. *Gastroenterology*, 95, 734-9.

Yilmaz Y, Yonal O, Kurt R Bayrak M, Aktas B, Ozdogan O. (2011). Noninvasive assessment of liver fibrosis with the aspartate transaminase to platelet ratio index (APRI): Usefulness in patients with chronic liver disease. *Hepat Mon*, 11, 2, 103-107.

Zhang YF, Shi H, Chen LB, Xu QH. (2010). Value of FIB-4 for the diagnosis of liver fibrosis in chronic hepatitis B. *Zhonghua Shi Yan He Lin Chuang Bing Du Xue Za Zhi*, 24,3, 215-7.

Zheng M, Cai W, Weng H, Liu HR. (2002). ROC curves in evaluation of serum fibrosis indices for hepatic fibrosis. *World J Gastroenterol*, 8,6, 1073-1076.

Zweig MH, Campbell G. (1993). Receiver-operating characteristic (ROC) plots: a fundamental evaluation tool in clinical medicine. *Clin Chem*, 39, 4, 561–577.

# Part 3

## Complications of Liver Biopsy

# 23

# Complications of Liver Biopsy

Abdullah Saeed Gozai Al-Ghamdi
*Gastroenterology Unit, Medical Department, King Fahad General Hospital, Jeddah, Saudi Arabia*

## 1. Introduction

Determination of the extent of progress of hepatic fibrosis and inflammation is important in clinical practice, where it may reflect the severity of liver disease and predict response to treatment. Percutaneous liver biopsy is the gold standard for grading and staging of liver disease which has been used for more than hundred years. The aim of this review is to know the safety and the complications related to such procedure in clinical practice. From experience and review of literatures, liver biopsy is frequently cited as a simple and safe procedure that may be performed at the bedside and as outpatient. Complications were more often experienced by those with relative contraindications and increased number of passes and if performed by less-experienced individuals. (1)

The complications after liver biopsy were reported to be more frequent in the presence of vascular liver lesions, biliary radical dilatation and in the presence of ascites.

Ultrasonography is a simple technique and recommended to detect vascular liver lesions, cystic lesions in the liver like echinococcal, biliary tree anatomy and to exclude presence of massive ascites which all is considered to be contraindications to liver biopsy and to determine the most suitable biopsy site. (2, 3)

Before biopsy the patient should understand the whole procedure and the possible complications and to sign the consent form and also need to be cooperative during the procedure.

The history before the procedure is very important, like history of unexplained bleeding and family history of bleeding tendencies or blood diseases like hemophilia and the patient should be off medications that increase bleeding tendencies for certain time, like acetylsalicylic acid, non steroidal anti-inflammatory drugs and colpidogrel. (3) The operator should know about the coagulation profiles and platelets level of the patient before the procedure.

1-5% of patients require hospitalization for complications and approximately 60% of complications occur within the first 2 hours following the procedure, and 96% within the first 24 hours. (3, 4, 5)

The morbidity and mortality related to liver biopsy was reported to be 0.08-0.34% and 0-0.19% respectively. (?)

Liver biopsy can be obtained by different techniques other than percutaneous, like Fine needle aspiration, trsnsjugular and laparoscopic especially if there are relative contraindications to percutaneous liver biopsy.

## 2. Percutaneous liver biopsy complications

### 2.1 Pain

The most common complication is pain at biopsy site and shoulder and usually dull, mild and brief. A study using the visual analogue scale confirmed that the procedure is distinctly unpleasant, with 20% of the patients indicating that they experienced severe pain and approximately 1-5 % of the patients requiring admission from pain and most recover with only supportive measures. Ongoing, severe pain in the abdomen should alert the physician to the possibility of a more serious complication, such as bleeding or peritonitis. (3, 6, 7, 8, 9, 10)

The overall frequency of pain requiring analgesics appears to be around 30-50% in patients not receiving prebiopsy medications. (7, 10)

Outside of frank trauma to adjacent organs or severe bleeding, the mechanism of postbiopsy pain is uncertain and the biopsy site pain is likely to be a nociceptive pain that originates from the skin, the nociceptive innervated liver capsule, or both and high anxiety levels have been shown to exacerbate acute postoperative pain. (10, 11, 12)

The right-shoulder pain after liver biopsy is well known but has never been fully characterized. In other words, pain in the right shoulder begins, reaches its peak, and subsides together with the biopsy site pain. This may indicate that the right-shoulder pain is likely to be a viscerosomatic referred pain, rather than an indication of a severe complication, such as intraabdominal bleeding. (13)

It has been noticed in 2 studies that women tended to report higher pain level than men at all time points tested, the cause for the sex differences in pain perception is unknown. (13, 14)

Analgesia before liver biopsy is usually avoided due to worries of masking pain that might indicative of abdominal symptoms and complications and still no consensus as to pain prevention and treatment for patients undergoing liver biopsy.

The practice of conscious sedation is variable, the midazolam-treated patients had a numerically lower mean pain score and significantly lower mean memory score than the untreated patients. (15)

It was noticed in the study by Brouillette DE et al, that patients receiving midazolam admitted to experiencing less discomfort during the biopsy procedure and had less memory for the procedure. More importantly, 79% of those receiving midazolam stated they would have little or no trouble undergoing a subsequent percutaneous liver biopsy as compared to 55% of those given saline. These data suggest that midazolam reduces subject anxiety and perceived discomfort before and during percutaneous liver biopsy produces partial amnesia for the biopsy experience and thereby may improve patient acceptance of follow-up liver biopsies. (16)

One possible way to improve pain control is to assess the anxiety level before the procedure, to adjust the dose of the anxiolytic drug accordingly, to add conscious sedation to those who are at a high level of stress, to infiltrate the biopsy site with long-acting local anesthetics, and to administer adequate analgesics for as long as needed. (13)

### 2.2 Bleeding

Of the serious complications, bleeding post liver biopsy is considered to be the most common cause. Bleeding is usually presented as subcapsular or parenchymal hematoma, free intraperitoneal hemorrhage, hemobilia or rarely hemothorax.

Most complications and, in particular, hemorrhage and bile peritonitis, will be recognized within 4 hr after biopsy. Delayed bleeding has been reported as late as 15 days after biopsy. (17)

It has been reported in two large studies of patients post liver biopsy that bleeding occur in 0.32 - 0.35% with morbidity related to hemorrhage of 0.24 % and around 0.11% had mortality from severe bleeding. (5, 18)

It has been found in some series that malignancy, cirrhosis, older age, and more than three passes were predictable risk factors for postbiopsy bleeding. (5, 8, 18)

Subclinical bleeding in the form of subcapsular or intrahepatic hematomas can be seen in up to 23% of patients and this is usually detectable by ultrasound 24 hours after biopsy. These hematomas are generally small and are not associated with significant hemodynamic compromise. (11)

The initial indications of bleeding are right upper quadrant abdominal pain that require analgesia and changes in vital signs with drop in blood pressure and rise in pulse rate.(19)

Most cases of fatal hemorrhage especially free intraperitoneal resulted from perforation of portal or hepatic veins or aberrant arteries. It may also occur as a result of a tear in the liver when the patient breathes deeply during the biopsy. (20, 21) Free intraperitoneal hemorrhage can occur in 0.32% and this can be suspected clinically when the patient experienced abdominal pain, hypotension and tachycardia and can be confirmed by ultrasound or computed tomography. (22)

Hemorrhage usually stops spontaneously and patient is managed by measures to improve the hemodynamic status with intravenous fluids and blood products if needed. If bleeding is severe, selective angiography of the hepatic artery, besides establishing the diagnosis also provides the opportunity for embolisation or balloon occlusion of the segmental artery involved. (21)

Surgical exploration is indicated if hemodynamic instability persists despite the above measures and the laparotomy rate amongst patients who bled range from 6% to 25%. (21, 23, 24)

The least common of the hemorrhagic complications is hemobilia and in one study by Piccinino F, et al reported 4 patients with hemobilia out of 86,276 liver biopsies.

Hemobilia is a term first used in 1946 by Sandblom to describe bleeding into the bile ducts.(22)

Hemobilia usually suspected when a post procedure fall in hemoglobin is associated with the classic triad of abdominal pain, hyperbilirubinemia, and unexplained gastrointestinal bleeding with average onset of approximately five days after biopsy. (3, 5, 25)

The bleeding is usually arterial in origin and can be venous in patients with portal hypertension. Biopsy can induce hematoma or pseudoaneurysm into bile duct and delayed bleeding can occur from gradual dissolution of that clot, while acute bleeding which is less common is secondary to simultaneous perforation of intrahepatic bile ducts and blood vessels. (25) Clinical presentation ranges from chronic anemia to rapid massive bleeding with hematemsis and/or melena and rarely patient may present with only hematochezia.

Diagnosis is usually suspected in patients with history of recent liver biopsy and most of endoscopic and radiological modalities including angiography can help in diagnosis.

Hemobilia can stop spontaneously and if patient still have continuous or intermittent bleeding then immediate selective angiography needed as diagnostic and therapeutic and considered to be the cornerstone of management. (26)

### 2.3 Biliary peritonitis

Biliary peritonitis is the second most frequent serious complication after hemorrhage and can occur in 0.03%-0.22% and usually occur in the presence of biliary obstruction and can be in other patients secondary to gallbladder perforation. [24, 27] The patient is usually presented with severe abdominal pain and vasovagal hypotension immediately postbiopsy and this may be followed by fever, leukocytosis and ileus. Painless bile collection in the peritoneal cavity has been described. Radiolgical investigations like ultrasonography or computed tomography scan may identify an intra-abdominal collection of bile, and bile leaks may be demonstrated by ERCP. Conservative management is recommended with intravenous fluids, antibiotics and pain control and in case of clinical deterioration surgery may be needed. [27]

### 2.4 Pulmonary complications

Pulmonary complications post liver biopsy is considered to be rare and this can occur if needle biopsy passed in the costophrenic angle above the reflection of between the parietal and the visceral pleura. The patients can develop pneumothorax and hemothorax and also hydrothorax can be developed in cirrhotic patient with ascites by passage of ascitic fluid through the puncture site on diaphragm. [20, 21] The incidence of pneumothorax and/or pleural effusion occur in the range of 0.08 - 0.28% and the symptoms usually mild and pulmonary collapse not exceeding 10%. [28] Hemothorax post liver biopsy is also rare with incidence of 0.18%-0.49% and this can be managed conservatively and rarely need thoracotomy. [28, 29, 30]

There is no role for angiogram with embolisation of diaphragmatic vessel for the treatment of hemothorax, as blood supply to the parietal diaphragm arises from vessels from the chest wall and abdominal wall. [31]

### 2.5 Sepsis

Sepsis and septic shock post liver biopsy is considered to be rare and can develop occasionally in patients with biliary obstruction. Inconsequential transient bacteremia has been reported in 5.8 to 13.48% of patients, therefore prophylactic antibiotics are not recommended for the routine use in patients undergoing liver biopsy, including those with risk factor for endocarditis. [28, 32, 33]

### 2.6 Other complications

Other rare complications after percutaneous liver biopsy include perforation of abdominal organs which is well tolerated and not require specific treatment, subphrenic abscess, and pancreatitis secondary to hemobilia. Needle track seeding following biopsy of malignant tumor of liver have been reported and some authors recommend liver biopsy only for patients who are not a candidate for surgical resection. [21, 34, 35]

## 3. Fine needle aspiration

Fine needle aspiration (FNA) is a technique used under ultrasound or CT scan guidance in those patients with focal hepatic lesions and at risk of bleeding. The diagnosis accuracy range from 80 - 95% and the cytologic findings that are negative for cancer do not rule it out. An important precaution is to choose the path of the needle in which normal tissue is interposed between the liver capsule and the lesion and to make as few needle passes as possible. FNA biopsy is generally a very safe procedure, even in patients with hemangiomas and echinococcal cysts and is associated with a low risk of seeding of the needle tract with malignant cells. (3, 36, 37, 38, 39)

## 4. Transjugular liver biopsy

Transjugular liver biopsy was first described experimentally in 1964 and in human subjects at 1967 and usually through transjugular catheterization of the hepatic veins. Liver tissue is obtained from within vascular system and this minimizes the risk of bleeding. (40, 41) It is performed in a vascular catheterization laboratory with video fluoroscopy equipment and cardiac monitoring because of the risk of cardiac arrhythmia as the catheter passes through the right atrium. The duration of the procedure is between 30 and 60 minutes and adequate specimen was obtained in 97%. (3, 42) Although not easy, this technique is safe and preferable in the management of selected patients with coagulopathy and risk of bleeding, moderate to severe ascites, massive obesity, small cirrhotic liver and patients with suspected vascular tumor. (43)

The total complication rate in 7469 transjugular liver biopsies reported in 62 series published between 1978 and 2006 was 7.1%, 3.5% were related to liver puncture while 3.3% were not. (13) The major complications of transjugular liver biopsy are rare and occur between 0.01 to 0.2% and may include large hepatic hematoma, intraperitoneal hemorrhage, inferior vena cava perforation, renal vein perforation, ventricular arrhythmia, pneumothorax and respiratory arrest. The patients may also get some minor complications like pyrexia, abdominal pain, neck hematoma, transient Horner's syndrome, transient dysphonia, subclinical capsular perforation, formation of a fistula from the hepatic artery to the portal vein or the biliary tree and all these complications can occur in 0.01 - 1.6%. Deaths can occur in 0.1% of patients mainly secondary to intraperitoneal hemorrhage or ventricular arrhythmia. (43)

## 5. Laparoscopic liver biopsy

A laparoscopic liver biopsy is another method for obtaining liver tissue and may be done solely or may be part of another operative procedure and this allows direct inspection of the liver surface prior to the biopsy, demonstrate cirrhosis in almost all patients and allow direct compression of the biopsy site if bleeding is excessive. (44)

It has also been used in centers where access to transjugular liver biopsy is not available, for patients with abnormal clotting parameters, and also in patients who have a combination of a focal liver lesion and a coagulopathy where a histological diagnosis is essential in the management of that patient. (42) The complications of laparoscopic liver biopsy include vasovagal reaction, seizure, abdominal wall hematoma, abdominal viscus perforation, hemobilia, splenic laceration, bleeding and prolonged abdominal pain. (45)

## 6. Conclusion

We conclude that in properly selected patients and after exclusion of risk factors for complications, liver biopsy is considered to be safe outpatient procedure and still the gold standard method and definitive diagnostic test for difficult cases of liver diseases.

## 7. References


[1] Perrault J, McGill DB, Ott BJ, et al. liver biopsy: complications in 1000 inpatients and outpatients. Gastroenterology 74 (1), 1978.

[2] Froehlich F, Lamy O, Fried M, Gonvers JJ. Practice and complications of liver biopsy. Results of a nationwide survey in Switzerland. *Dig Dis Sci.* Aug 1993;38 (8):1480-4

[3] Bravo, AA, Sunil GS, Chopra S. Liver biopsy. NEJM 344 (7), 2001.

[4] van Leeuwen DJ, Wilson L, Crowe DR. Liver biopsy in the mid-1990s: questions and answers. Semin Liver Dis 1995;15:340-59.

[5] Piccinino F, Sagnelli E, Pasquale G, Giusti G. Complications following percutaneous liver biopsy: a multicentre retrospective study on 68,276 biopsies. J Hepatol 1986;2:165-73.

[6] Crockett SD, Kaltenbach T, Keeffe EB. Do we still need a liver biopsy? Are the serum fibrosis tests ready for prime time? Clin Liver Dis 2006;10:513-34.

[7] Castera L, Negre I, Samii K, Buffet C. Pain experienced during Percutaneous liver biopsy. Hepatology 1999;30:1529-30.

[8] Janes C.H., Lindor K.D.. Outcome of patients hospitalized for complications after outpatient liver biopsy. Ann Intern Med 1993; 118:96-98.

[9] Perrault J., McGill D.B., Ott B.J., Taylor W.F. Liver biopsy: Complications in 1000 inpatients and outpatients. Gastroenterology 1978;74:103-106.

[10] Caldwell S H. Controlling pain in liver biopsy, or "we will probably need to repeat the biopsy in a year or two to assess the response". A J Gastroenterol 96 (5), 2001.

[11] Minuk G.Y., Sutherland L.R., Wiseman D.A., et al. Prospective study of the incidence of ultrasound-detected intrahepatic and subcapsular hematomas in patients randomized to 6 or 24 hours of bed rest after percutaneous liver biopsy. Gastroenterology 1987;92:290-293.

[12] Hartmann H, Beckh K. Nerve supply and nervous control of liver function. In: Mclntyre N, Benhamou JP, Bircher J, eds. Oxford textbook of clinical hepatology. Vol 1, sections 1–13. Oxford: Oxford University Press, 1993:93.

[13] Eisenberg E , Konopniki M , Veitsman E , et al. Prevalence and characteristics of pain induced by percutaneous liver biopsy . *Anesth Analg* . 2003;96:1392–1396.

[14] Cadranel J, Rufat P, Degos F. Practices of liver biopsy in France: results of a prospective nationwide survey. Hepatology 2000;32:477–80.

[15] Alexander JA, Smith BJ. Midazolam sedation for Percutaneous liver biopsy. Dig Dis Sci 1993;38:2209–11.

[16] Brouillette DE, Yoo YK, Chien MC, et al. Use of midazolam for percutaneous liver biopsy. Dig Dis Sci 1989;34:1553–8.

[17] Jacobs W H; Goldberg S B. Statement on outpatient percutaneous liver biopsy. Digestive diseases and sciences 1989;34 (3):322-3.

[18] McGill DB, Rakela J, Zinsmeister AR, Ott BJ. A 21-year experience with major hemorrhage after percutaneous liver biopsy. Gastroenterology 1990; 99:1396-400.

[19] Mahal AS, Knauer CM, Gregory PB. Bleeding after liver biopsy. West J Med. 1981 Jan;134 (1):11–14.

[20] Zamcheck N, Sidman RI.. Liver biopsy I. Its use in clinical and investigative medicine. N Engl J Mcd 1953; 249: 1020.

[21] Chuah SY. Liver biopsy—past, present and future. *Singapore Med J* 1996;37:86–90.

[22] Sandblom P. Hemorrhage into the biliary tract following trauma-"traumatic hemobilia". Surgery 1948; 24:571-86.
[23] Lindner H. Grenzen und Gefuhren der perkutanen Leberbiopsie mit der Menghini-Nadel. Erfahrungen bei 80,000 leberbiopsien. Dtsch Med Wochenschr 1967; 39: 1751-7.
[24] Terry R. Risks of needle biopsy of the liver. Br Med J 1952; 1:1102-5.
[25] Lichtenstein DR, Kim D, Chopra S. Delayed massive hemobilia following percutaneous liver biopsy: treatment by embolotherapy. Am J Gastroenterol 1992;87:1833-8.
[26] Dang S, Neelima V, Atiq M, Olden KW, Aduli F: Hemobilia after Percutaneous Liver Biopsy Presenting as Hematochezia: A Rare Complication of a Commonly Performed Procedure. Chir Gastroenterol 2008;24:313-315.
[27] Ruben, RA, Chopra, S. Bile peritonitis after liver biopsy: Nonsurgical management of a patient with an acute abdomen: A case report with review of the literature. Am J Gastroenterol 1987; 82:265.
[28] Campbell MS, Jeffers LJ, Reddy KR. Liver biopsy and laparoscopy. In: Schiff L, Schiff ER. eds. Diseases of the Liver. 10th ed. Lippincott William & wikins. 2007: 62-83.
[29] Majid AA. Hemorrhage from the diaphragm: an unusual cause of hemothorax after liver biopsy. Am J Gastroenterol 1990;85:104-5.
[30] Chahal PS, Ready J. Hemothorax after percutaneous liver biopsy: an unusual complication. Am J Gastroenterol 2002; 97:1068-9.
[31] Yeo WT, Tan LK, Dan YY, et al (2008) Delayed bleeding after liver biopsy: a dreaded complication. Singapore Med J. 49: 76–80.
[32] McClosky RV, Gold M, Waser E. Bacteremia after liver biopsy. Arch Intern Med 1973;132:213–215.
[33] LeFrock JL, Ellis CA, Turchik JB, et al. Transient bacteremia associated with percutaneous liver biopsy. J Infect Dis 1975;131:S105–S107.
[34] John TG,Garden OJ. Needle track seeding of primary and secondary liver carcinoma after percutaneous liver biopsy. IIPB Surg 1993; 6:199-203.
[35] Evans GH, Harries SA, Hobbs KE.Safety of and necessity of needle biopsy of liver tumou rs.Heuer ]. Lancet 1987; i: 620.
[36] General principles. In: Lee RG. Diagnostic liver pathology. St. Louis: Mosby–Year Book, 1994:1-21.
[37] Eisenberg PJ, Bolland GW, Mueller PR. Introduction. In: Pitman MB, Szyfelbein WM, eds. Fine needle aspiration biopsy of the liver: a color atlas. Boston: Butterworth-Heinemann, 1994:3-5.
[38] Smith EH. Complications of percutaneous abdominal fine-needle biopsy: review. Radiology 1991;178:253-8.
[39] Drinkovic I, Brkljacic B, Two cases of lethal complications following ultrasound-guided percutaneous fine-needle biopsy of the liver. Cardiovasc Intervent Radiol. 1996; 19 (5):360-3.
[40] Dotter CT. Catheter biopsy. Experimental technique for transvenous liver biopsy. Radiology 1964;82:312–314.
[41] Hanafee W, Weiner M. Transjugular percutaneous cholangiography. Radiology 1967;88:35-9.
[42] Grant A, Neuberger J (1999) Guidelines on the use of liver biopsy in clinical practice. British Society of Gastroenterology. *Gut* 45 Suppl 4: IV1-IV11.

[43] Kalambokis G, Manousou P, Vibhakorn S, et al. Transjugular liver biopsy—indications, adequacy, quality of specimens, and complications—a systematic review. *Journal of Hepatology.* 2007;47 (2):284–294
[44] Pagliaro L, Rinaldi F. Craxi A, Di Piazza S, Filippazzo G, Gatto G, et al. Percutaneous blind biopsy versus laparoscopy with guided biopsy in diagnosis of cirrhosis: a prospective randomized trial. Dig Dis Sci 1983; 28: 39-43.
[45] Vargas C, Jeffers LJ, Bernstein D, et al. Diagnostic laparoscopy: a 5-year experience in a hepatology training program. Am J Gastroenterol 1995;90:1258-62.

# 24

# Complications of Liver Biopsy

Daren Subar[1], Ali Khan[2] and Derek O'Reilly[1,3]
[1]Department of Hepatopancreaticobiliary Surgery,
North Manchester General Hospital, Crumpsall, Manchester
[2]Department of Radiology,
North Manchester General Hospital, Crumpsall, Manchester
[3]Cancer Studies Research Group, The University of Manchester,
Manchester Academic Health Science Centre, Manchester
UK

## 1. Introduction

The liver is the second largest organ in the body after the skin and has important storage, detoxification and synthetic functions. Liver diseases encompass a multitude of pathologies and the management of these diseases involves diagnostic and therapeutic investigations and interventions; some of which are invasive. Histological assessment of the liver and lesions within via liver biopsies are an important tool in the armamentarium of invasive investigations for liver diseases of both a surgical and non-surgical nature.

Liver biopsy has been used for over 100 years in the assessment of liver diseases (Valori and Elias 1989). Paul Ehrlich performed one of the first percutaneous liver biopsies in the late 19$^{th}$ century in Germany to assess glycogen levels in the liver of a diabetic patient (Grant and Neuberger 1999). However, the procedure did not really gain popularity until Menghini refined the technique in the mid 20$^{th}$ century(Menghini 1958). In the last fifty years the techniques for liver biopsy has been continuously refined and although today there are several biochemical and imaging techniques to assess liver disease biopsy remains important in assessment. Today, widespread application allows for blind, open and image guided liver biopsies, although ultrasound guided biopsies are considered superior (Younossi, Teran, Ganiats and Carey 1998). Image guided percutaneous liver biopsies remains the mainstay of this procedure while open biopsies may be undertaken as an adjunct to laparoscopic or other open surgical procedures. There are presently various techniques and equipment for percutaneous liver biopsies and this procedure is performed by both gastroenterologists/hepatologists and radiologists. The choice of technique and equipment is however operator dependent.

## 2. Indication

In the past the indications for liver biopsies and the practice thereof varied significantly between institutions. This was born out in an audit conducted by the British society of Gastroenterology and the Royal College of Physicians of London (Gilmore, et al. 1995). Subsequent to this the British Society of Gastroenterology published guidelines on the use of liver biopsy in an attempt to standardize indications and technique for this procedure

(Grant, et al. 1999). Similar guidelines have since been published by the American Association for the Study of Liver Diseases (Rockey, Caldwell, Goodman, Nelson and Smith 2009). These indications are beyond the remit of this chapter and can be sourced from the guidelines.

## 3. Methods

There are various methods for performing liver biopsies. In the main most liver biopsies are performed percutaneously. In the UK this method is performed by radiologists under image guidance. In support of image guided biopsies Vautier et al suggests that the ideal liver biopsy is one that is performed under ultrasonic guidance (Vautier, Scott and Jenkins 1994). However there are still some clinicians who practice liver biopsies without image guidance. In a survey conducted by Muir et al about current practice of liver biopsy 53.2% of clinicians still performed liver biopsies without image guidance (Muir and Trotter 2002). Guided liver biopsies are undertaken with real time imaging using ultrasound or CT scans. Real time imaging allows for accurate biopsy of lesions and avoidance of major vascular, biliary or bowel structures and thus reduce the incidence of complications. This can be via the transthoracic or the subcostal route and may be plugged or unplugged. Plugged percutaneous liver biopsies involves the injection of a gelatin substance into the biopsy cavity after withdrawal of the specimen. It reduces the complication of bleeding and can be used in patients with impaired coagulation (Fandrich, Davies and Hall 1996). In patients with coagulopathy in whom a percutaneous biopsy is considered inappropriate a transvenous (transjugular or transfemoral) approach can be used (Lebrec, Goldfarb, Degott, Rueff and Benhamou 1982, Sawyerr, et al. 1993). Laparoscopic liver biopsy is used in centres where expertise in the transvenous approach is unavailable for patients with a bleeding coagulopathy. A general anaesthetic is necessary where the laparoscopic approach is contemplated. In many instances it is undertaken when a liver lesion is found incidentally during diagnostic or staging laparoscopy. It can also be used in assessing the degree of cirrhosis of the future liver remnant in patients who are undergoing staging laparoscopy for consideration of liver resection for hepatocellular carcinoma. Laparoscopic liver biopsy allows direct visualisation of the area to be biopsied and immediate control of any haemorrhage. The complications of this procedure includes those associated with the anaesthesia, the laparoscopy and the biopsy. In our institution, we believe that all percutaneous liver biopsies should be image guided. As a result of the associated risks our patients are admitted for post biopsy observation for 6 hours as per the British society of Gastroenterology and the American Gastroenterological Association guidelines(Grant, et al. 1999, Rockey, et al. 2009). In other centres in the USA percutaneous liver biopsy is performed as an outpatient procedure with one of the stipulations being the patient is able to return to the hospital within 30 minutes if symptoms of a complication develop(Jacobs and Goldberg 1989).

## 4. Complications

The complications of liver biopsy can be divided into those in the immediate, early or late period (Table 1). The overall reported complication rate varies significantly (Galati, et al. 1994, Gilmore, et al. 1995, Grant, et al. 1999). These can range from minor complications such as pain and transient hypotension to major complications such as visceral perforation or significant bleeding which may lead to death. The incidence of major complications was reported to be as high as 4% with a mortality rate ranging from 0.01% to 0.33%(McGill, Rakela, Zinsmeister and Ott 1990). Differences in complication rate has been reported between blind and ultrasound guided liver biopsies with ultrasound guided biopsies proving superior for both accuracy and risk of complications(Riley 1999, Al Knawy and Shiffman 2007).

| Immediate | Early(within 24 hours) | Late |
|---|---|---|
| Death | Death | Needle tract seeding of Tumour cells |
| Pain | Pain | Biliary fistula |
| Bleeding | Bleeding | Septicaemia |
| Septicaemia | Septicaemia | Biloma |
| Perforation of nearby organs | Biliary peritonitis | Pleural effusion |
| Pneumothorax Haemothorax | Haemobilia | Intrahepatic arterio-venous fistula |
| Needle fracture | | |

Table 1. Complications of Liver Biopsy

In addition, it is well documented that the risk of complications increases with the increase in the number of needle passes necessary for sampling(McGill, et al. 1990). Blind biopsies require more needle passes than ultrasound guided biopsies and have been statistically proven to increase the risk of complications(Cadranel, Rufat and Degos 2000, Mayoral and Lewis 2001). The issue of the relationship of needle size or type to complication rate remains controversial. McGill et al compared a 1.6mm diameter needle to a 1.9mm needle and found no difference in the incidence of of haematomas(McGill, et al. 1990). The same is true for the study by Forsell et al (Forssell, Bonkowsky, Anderson and Howell 1981). However prior to this, the multicentre retrospective study conducted by Piccinino suggested a higher incidence of bleeding with cutting type needles (Piccinino, Sagnelli, Pasquale and Giusti 1986).

Finally, as with most invasive procedures the most significant factor in the incidence of complications associated with liver biopsy is operator experience. In the nationwide survey conducted in Switzerland on the practice and complications of liver biopsy Froelich et al reported that no complications occurred with internists performing more than 50 biopsies a year but a 1.68% complication rate with internists performing less than 12 biopsies a year (Froehlich, Lamy, Fried and Gonvers 1993). The national audit of percutaneous liver biopsy conducted in England and Wales confirms Froelich's findings. It was found that the frequency of complications was 3.2% for biopsies performed by operators with less than 20

previous biopsy procedures. In contrast, it was only 1.1% when performed by those who had conducted more than 100 biopsies(Gilmore, et al. 1995).
From the large retrospective study conducted by Piccinino it was reported that 61% of complications occurred within the first 2 hours after biopsy and 96% in the first 24 hours (Piccinino, et al. 1986). Arturo et al suggests that up to 3% of patients may require hospitalization for complications of liver biopsy, more so if the procedure is performed with a tru-cut needle(Bravo, Sheth and Chopra 2001). For the purpose of this chapter we are going to focus on the complications associated with percutaneous liver biopsy as this is the commonest method in use. The specific complications associated with other methods will be briefly discussed at the end.

### 4.1 Mortality

Liver biopsy associated mortality is reportedly related to haemorrhage or biliary peritonitis (Vautier, et al. 1994, Shah, Mayberry, Wicks, Rees and Playford 1999). The reported incidence of mortality varies (Grant, et al. 1999) and to date the true incidence is not known. Three month post biopsy mortality rate is reported to be as high as 19%(Gilmore, et al. 1995). This is probably a result of the primary indication for the liver biopsy; i.e. liver failure and malignancy and not necessarily a result of the biopsy itself. Although logic would suggest that image guided biopsy would result in a statistically lower mortality rate compared to blind biopsies, this has actually never been born out in published reports. Griffiths et al(Griffiths, Viiala and Olynyk 2002) and others reported the mortality associated with liver biopsies to range from 0.01% to 0.1%(Piccinino, et al. 1986, McGill, et al. 1990). However, this is for both blind and guided biopsy.
Other authors have also refuted the claim that image guided biopsies reduces mortality rates. Centinkaya et al published a retrospective study of 205 patients who had either blind or guided biopsies of the liver and no difference was found in the incidence of mortality(0% in each group) (Züleyha Akkan Çetinkaya 2010). Indeed, most of the published data on mortality is from retrospective studies. In 1991 the national audit undertaken in England and Wales looked at the outcome of 1504 liver biopsies. Two patients died as a result of blind biopsy whereas there were no directly related deaths in the image guided cohort. This was not statistically significant however(Gilmore, et al. 1995). In 2010 West and Card published an epidemiological study on the mortality rates in elective percutaneous liver biopsy(West and Card 2010). Again this was a study based on restrospective data analysis. In it the all cause seven day mortality was 0.2% but mortality directly related to liver biopsy was 1 in 10,000.
In effect, the true incidence of biopsy related mortality and the effect of image guidance on the incidence of mortality is not known. Vautier et al(Vautier, et al. 1994) suggested that a large study involving an estimated 10,000 patients would be needed to demonstrate any statistical difference.

### 4.2 Pain

Pain is the most common complication after percutaneous liver biopsy. The incidence of pain during liver biopsy is reported to be as high as 84%(Eisenberg, et al. 2003). This pain can be acute and can last for more than 24 hours after the procedure(Castera, Negre, Samii and Buffet 1999). Eisenberg et al reported that 40% of patients in their prospective study experienced pain 24 hours after the procedure. Indeed, if the pain is due to hepatic friction rub the pain may last for a few weeks (Chuah 1996). The intensity of this pain is mainly mild to moderate(Farrell, et al. 1999, Cadranel, et al. 2000) but can be severe. In a study conducted by Christine Janes in 1993, of the four hundred and five patients who had liver biopsies as outpatients, five of the thirteen patients (1.2%) requiring post-procedure hospitalization was as a result of pain(Janes and Lindor 1993). A similar figure of 1.2% was quoted for the experience of severe pain by Christopher Pokorny in his study of radiologically guided liver biopsy, however none of these patients were admitted to hospital(Pokorny and Waterland 2002). The pain can be localized to the site of the biopsy or commonly be referred to the right shoulder tip. There is also a distinct sex difference in the experience of pain. The intensity of pain is reportedly higher in women although the cause of this is unknown (Cadranel, et al. 2000). In addition, Eisenberg et al demonstrated that there was a linear correlation between the level of pre-biopsy anxiety and the intensity of the experienced pain. It is possible that there is a positive correlation between levels of anxiety and gender but this has yet to be assessed and reported.

The etiology of post liver biopsy pain is thought to be multi-modal. Pain can indicate post biopsy peritoneal irritation if bleeding or peritoneal soiling from biliary leakage of visceral perforation occurs. However, pain at the biopsy site may emanate from stimulation of nocioceptive fibres in the skin and liver capsule. In contrast, shoulder tip pain may be viscerosomatic in origin(Hederstrom, Forsberg, Floren and Prytz 1989). The use of ultrasound guided biopsy has been reported to decrease the incidence of post biopsy pain. In the study conducted by Lindor et al nine patients required post biopsy hospitalization when ultrasound was not used compared to two patients in the biopsy under ultrasound guidance group. More importantly, of the nine patients, seven were hospitalized for pain(Lindor, et al. 1996). This view is supported by the review of the literature on blind versus ultrasound guided biopsy by Knawy et al. They found that ultrasound guidance resulted in a 10.9% decrease in biopsy pain ($P<0.0001$) and a decrease in pain related morbidity (1.8% vs 7.7%) (Al Knawy, et al. 2007).

Interestingly, both local anaesthetic with or without conscious sedation has been used in an attempt to control pain and in spite of this pain continues to be the commonest complication of liver biopsy. Conscious sedation has however shown some promise in reducing pain during and after liver biopsy. It is also possible that the administration of anxiolytics pre-biopsy may alleviate some of the pain experienced. Despite pain being a significant issue there is no published data on the optimization of pain control in patients undergoing liver biopsy.

### 4.3 Bleeding

Bleeding after percutaneous liver biopsy is a well documented complication second only to pain(Chuah 1996). This can be minor or be significant enough to warrant intervention. The reported incidence of bleeding varies significantly (Piccinino, et al. 1986, Chuah, Moody, Wicks and Mayberry 1994, Thampanitchawong and Piratvisuth 1999) and is the main cause of mortality after biopsy(Froehlich, et al. 1993). McGill reports it to be between 2%-4% in their 21 year experience with a mortality rate of 0.01%-0.03%(McGill, et al. 1990). The admission of those with bleeding is about 0.2%. The fatalities are usually due to inadvertent perforation of the hepatic or portal vein or aberrant hepatic artery. It may also result from a laceration in the liver if the biopsy needle is intrahepatic while the patient inhales deeply(Chuah 1996).

The risk is reportedly increased with the presence of ascites (Grant, et al. 1999) probably as a result of the dilutional effect of the ascitic fluid on clotting factors however the incidence is not affected by the use of ultrasound (Stone and Mayberry 1996). Like the use of ultrasound, the risk of haemorrhage is not related to needle diameter or type (Froehlich, et al. 1993). However, the relationship between coagulopathy and bleeding remains controversial. In the United States the conventional approach is to withhold percutaneous biopsy if the INR is greater than 1.5 (Rockey, et al. 2009). The survey conducted by Chuah et al suggested that coagulopathy should be corrected prior to biopsy (Chuah, et al. 1994). This is supported by other studies. Caldwell et al reviewed 2740 percutaneous liver biopsies in patients with hepatitis C. They recorded 16 out of 29 adverse events caused by severe bleeding. Statistically, the factors that were associated with increased bleeding included a platelet count of less than 60,000, INR greater than 1.3, the presence of varices and low albumin (Caldwell and Northup 2010). They suggested that the increase in bleeding with low albumin and varices is likely to be due to the changes in hepatic vasculature and not a clotting abnormality.

Although one other study has corroborated the cut off value of platelet count as 60,000 (Sharma, McDonald and Banaji 1982) there are other studies that suggest otherwise. Sherlock et al reports a cut off platelet count of 80,000 and Sue et al a cut off count of 50,000 (Grant, et al. 1999). In the retrospective study conducted by Pornpen et al they found that coagulopathy was related to bleeding complications and death (Thampanitchawong, et al. 1999). The bleeding complication rate increased from 3.6% to 10.5% and the death rate increased from 1% to 7% when the thrombin time increased by greater than 3 seconds over control and the prothrombin time increased by more than 10 seconds over control. The same was true for patients with a platelet count of greater than 70,000. However, platelet count was the only independent variable on logistic regression analysis. In effect, the absolute cut off point is unknown. In addition to this it is thought that platelet function also plays a more important role in the risk of bleeding after biopsy than platelet number (Tripodi, et al. 2006). Other risk factors include multiple passes with the biopsy needle, the presence of cirrhosis (Janes, et al. 1993) and the use of cutting needles (Piccinino, et al. 1986).

In contrast, Ewe et al and others demonstrated no effect of bleeding abnormalities on the risk of bleeding with either laparoscopic or percutaneous liver biopsy (Ewe 1981, McVay and Toy 1990, Dillon, Simpson and Hayes 1994). Even in Caldwell's study three of the patients with haemorrhagic complications after biopsy had a platelet count of over 150,000. Finally, the question of ultrasound reducing the risk of haemorrhage remains unanswered. Several studies have demonstrated that ultrasound reduces the incidence of complications, none of these studies reported any specific difference in haemorrhage(Lindor, et al. 1996, Stone, et al. 1996, Manolakopoulos, et al. 2007). In our unit, we accept a platelet count of greater than 80,000 and an INR of less than 1.5 in order to proceed to biopsy.

The haemorrhage associated with percutaneous liver biopsy can present as intraperitoneal bleeding, intrahepatic bleeding, haemobilia and subcapsular haematoma(Figure 1) (Caldwell, et al. 2010). Intraperitoneal bleeding although rare, when clinically significant generally becomes apparent within the first 2-3 hours after biopsy(Van Thiel, Gavaler, Wright and Tzakis 1993) and is usually heralded by a drop in haemoglobin of greater than 2g/dL or haemodynamic instability(Knauer 1978). If intraperitoneal haemorrhage is suspected the patient should be resuscitated, have imaging studies (CT or ultrasound) to confirm this and if resuscitation fails then angiography and embolisation or less commonly surgery to halt bleeding. Intrahepatic or subcapsular haematomas tend to be asymptomatic(Raines, Van Heertum and Johnson 1974) and occurs in about 23% of patients(Minuk, Sutherland, Wiseman, MacDonald and Ding 1987). However, large haematomas can present with pain or signs of intravascular depletion i.e hypotension and tachycardia(Van Thiel, et al. 1993). In the main these haematomas can be treated conservatively with resuscitation and correction of coagulopathy or thrombocytopenia if it exists.

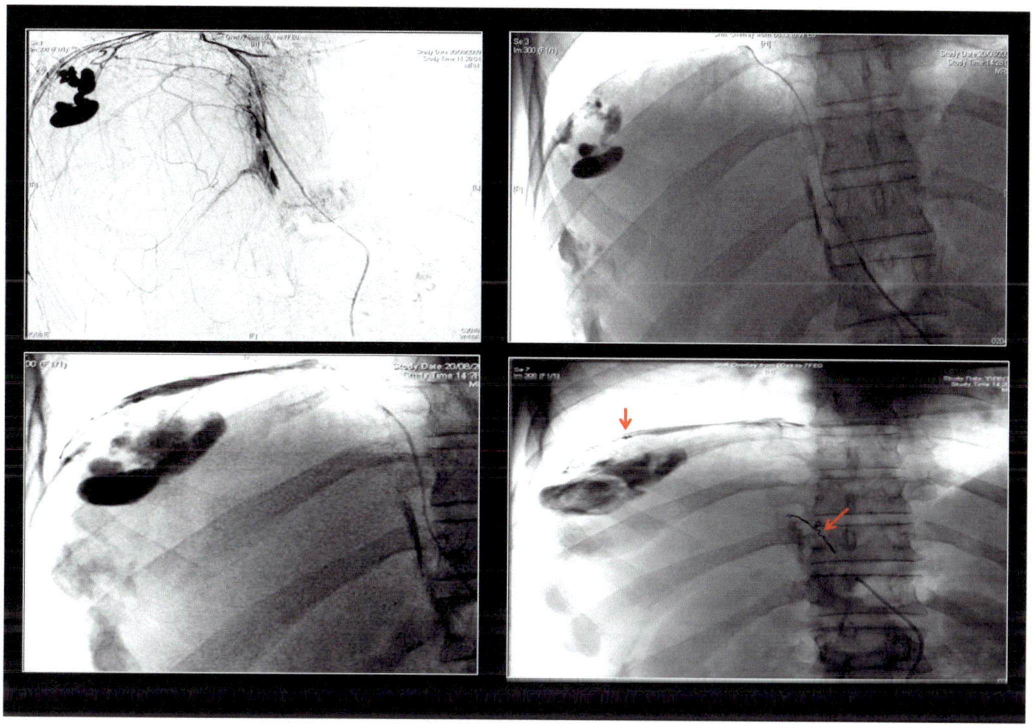

Fig. 1. This patient with hepatitis C became haemodynamically unstable following a percutaneous liver biopsy. A superselective angiogram of the liver shows a subcapsular bleed, which was embolized with microcoils (red arrows).

Although post biopsy haemorrhage usually presents itself within the fist 2-3 hours there have been reports of delayed bleeding (Reichert, Weisenthal and Klein 1983) Yeo et al described a case of a patient who was hepatitis C positive with haemophilia who presented 10 days after an image guided percutaneous liver biopsy(Yeo, Tan, Dan and Wai 2008). He presented to the emergency department complaining of hypochondrial pain and investigations demonstrated a haemothorax and subcapsular haematoma. He decompensated and had an emergency resuscitative thoracotomy In another case a 46 year old gentleman who represented 4 days after percutaneous biopsy with right hypochondrial pain. He was diagnosed with a bleeding pseudoaneurysm of the right hepatic artery which was embolised. Subsequently, he continued to bleed and had a laparotomy which demonstrated a right hepatic lobe laceration (Ren, Piao and Jin 2006). Although this is very rare there have been other reports of post biopsy pseudoaneurysm formation(Figure 2 a & b)(Kowdley, Aggarwal and Sachs 1994, Own, Balzer and Vogl 2005). Surprisingly, Terjung et al reported the incidence of delayed bleeding in their series to be 70%(Terjung, et al. 2003). In their series they defined delayed bleeding as occurring after 24 hours. This is a particularly high incidence and it may well reflect the definition criteria or the enthusiasm with which patients are investigated for haemorrhage. There may well be a large cohort of post biopsy delayed haemorrhage who are asymptomatic and therefore the true incidence is not known.

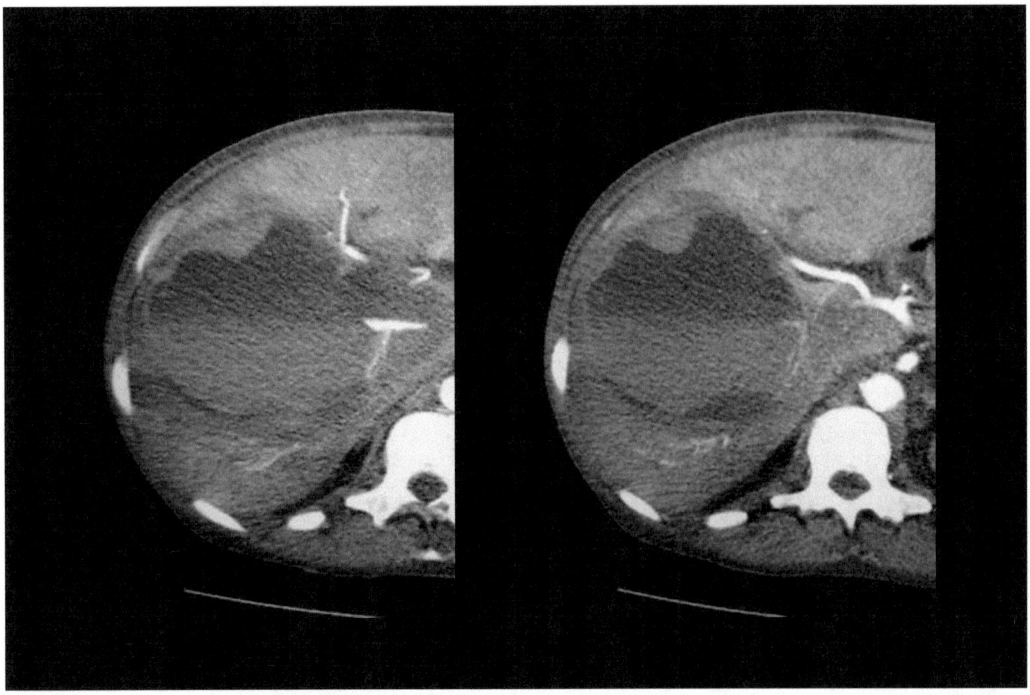

(a) (b)

Fig. 2. (a & b) CT scans on a patient with a past history of a percutaneous liver biopsy showing a ruptured pseudoaneurysm with active bleeding.

Haemobilia is a rare complication of liver biopsy and was first reported by in 1967 by Cox (Cox 1967). In 1991 Merrell and Schneider described the evolution of haemobilia and suggested a lag time between biopsy and presentation to be about 5 days. Interestingly, haemobilia after biopsy has been associated with acute pancreatitis(Pena, Horn and Cross 2009). It is thought that the pancreatitis is induced in the same manner as gallstones; impairment of pancreatic drainage. The treatment required is ERCP and sphincterotomy. Angiography has also been used to stem the bleeding but only in a few cases.

### 4.4 Septicaemia

Septicaemia is a result of bacteraemia during needle biopsy. It can also result from the development of intrahepatic abscesses (Figure 3). The incidence of bacteraemia is reported to be as high as 13 % (McCloskey, Gold and Weser 1973, Le Frock, Ellis, Turchik, Zawacki and Weinstein 1975). However more commonly the figure is quoted to be less than 1% (Larson, et al. 1997). It is more common in patients with biliary abnormalities including biliary obstruction, cholangitis and those who have had biliary bypass(Bubak, Porayko, Krom and Wiesner 1991, Larson, et al. 1997, Bravo, et al. 2001). However, one of these studies was in patients who had liver transplant and therefore may be immunosuppressed and at higher risk of infections. McCloskey et al reported an incidence of liver biopsy related septicaemia of 2.9%. They suggested that in patients with liver disease there is a defect in the defence mechanisms related to a deficiency of complement and inhibition of chemotaxis among others (McCloskey, et al. 1973). In those with septicaemia the commonest organism cultured from the blood is E. Coli (Moreira Vicente, Hernandez Ranz, Ruiz Del Arbol and Bouza 1981) although polymicrobial organism infection has been reported (Dhawan, Thadepalli, Ulmer and Akhtar 1983) including klebsiella and streptococcus.

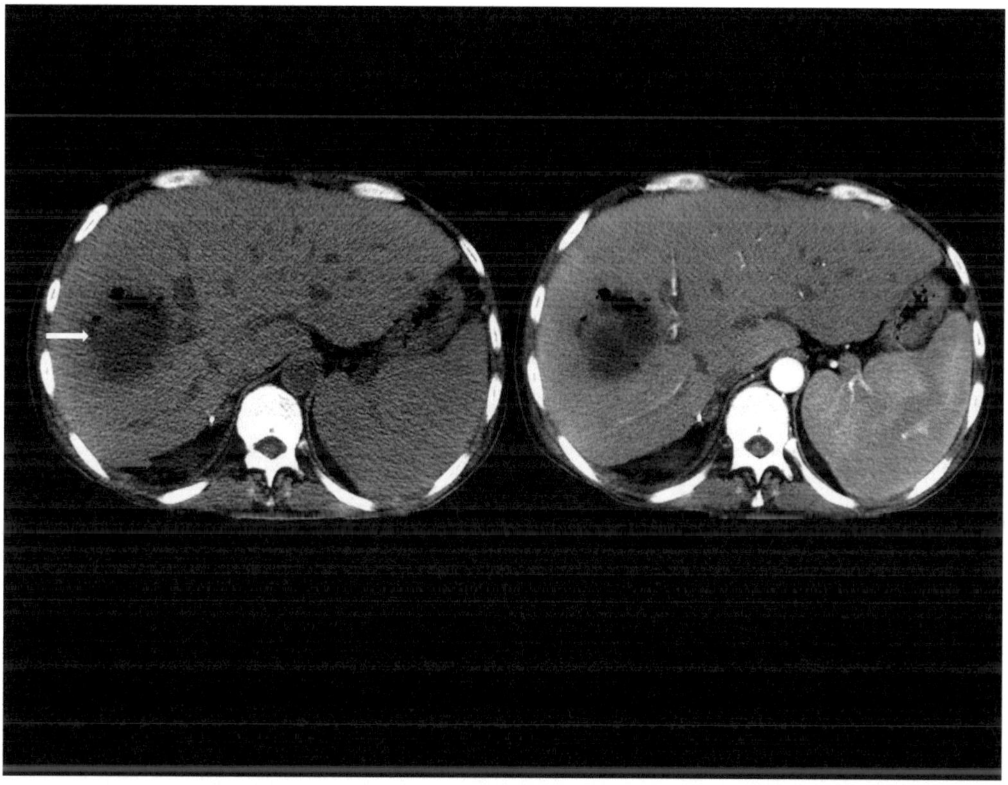

Fig. 3. This patient presented with right upper quadrant pain and pyrexia 4 days following a percutaneous liver biopsy. Note the liver mass associated with air within and surrounding the mass. The patient was treated for a liver abscess. Note echogenic contents within the pleural sac indicative of blood or pus (arrow).

Although bacteraemia with or without septicaemia is a rare but recognized complication of liver biopsy the question of whether prophylactic antibiotics is warranted remains unanswered. This is mainly because there are no randomized trials examining this and most of the reported data are either case reports or retrospective studies. It is probably worthwhile in patients who are immunocompromised (e.g transplant patients). It would be considered prudent to delay this invasive procedure if possible in patients who have confirmed sepsis. In addition, patients with obstructive jaundice or who are considered at risk should also probably have prophylactic antibiotics.

### 4.5 Pulmonary complications

The transthoracic approach traverses the pleural space. The incidence of complications was reported to be 25% in the Swiss survey (Froehlich, et al. 1993). Hydrothorax occurs as a result of leakage of ascitic fluid via the biopsy tract into the pleural cavity (Zamcheck and Sidman 1953). Pneumothoraces tend to occur in about 0.35% of cases (Piccinino, et al. 1986) (Figure 4). In addition, haemothoraces are also possible but rare with a reported incidence of 0.018% (Piccinino, et al. 1986). It is thought to be a result of injury to the diaphragmatic vessels (Majid 1990) and the event usually declares itself early on.

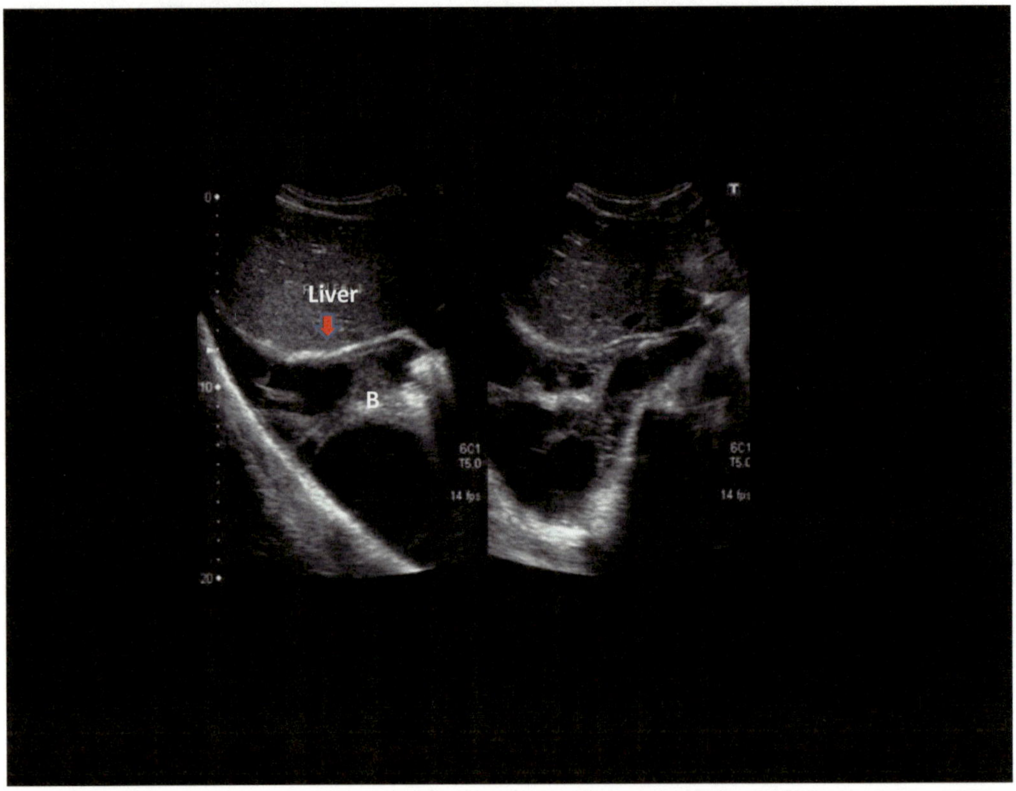


Fig. 4. Attempted liver biopsy on a 36-year old female with non-specific hepatic dysfunction. The needle entered the pleural cavity. Ultrasound examination shows blood in the pleural sac (B) at various stages of organization. The diaphragm is marked by a red arrow.

### 4.6 Visceral perforation

Visceral perforation includes puncture of the colon, kidney, lung or gallbladder. Piccinino et al reported the incidence of visceral perforation to be between 0.01%-0.1%(Piccinino, et al.

1986). This is supported by others (van der Poorten, et al. 2006). These complications can resolve with conservative management or can result in peritonitis requiring surgery.

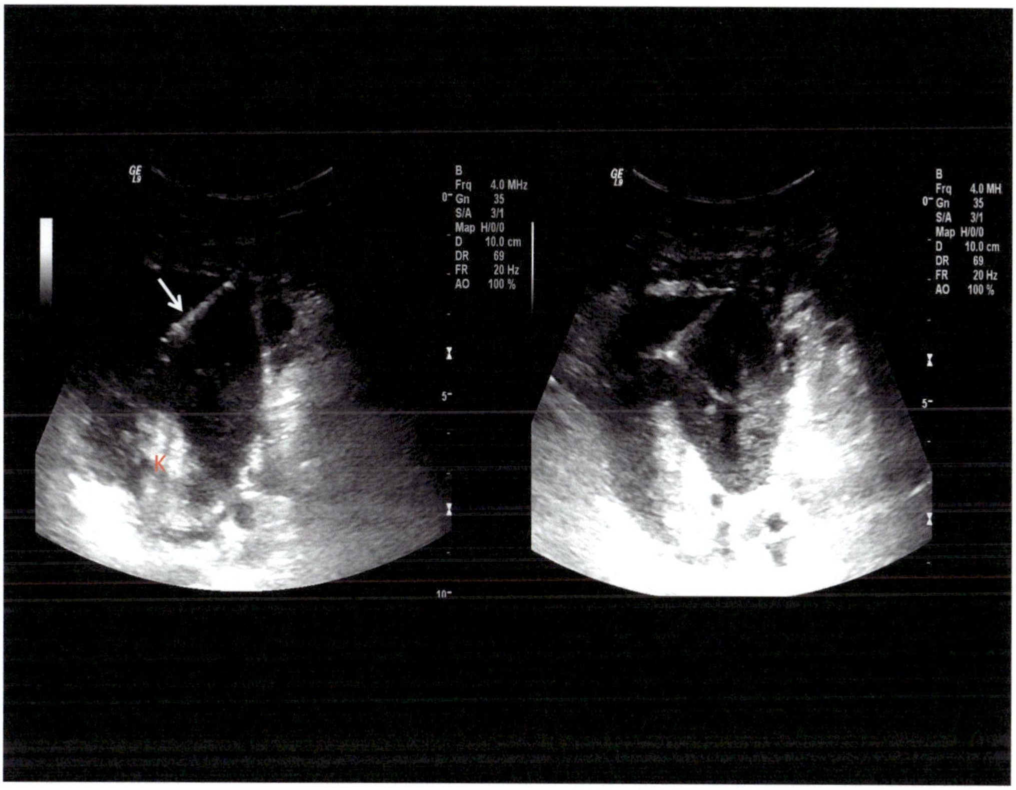


Fig. 5. Attempted liver on a 16 year old with a Riedle's lobe. The needle has entered the kidney (white arrow) the kidney is labelled K. The patient subsequently developed intractable haematuria and had to have several blood transfusions.

### 4.7 Needle fracture

Fracture of the needle is a very rare complication. Robert Peters reported a case of a Menghini needle fracture during liver biopsy in 1968 leaving the distal end in the patient's chest wall (Peters 1968). Subsequent to that Purow et al in 1977 and Lazar et al in 1978 reported this as a complication of liver biopsy (Grant, et al. 1999). It is thought to be a result of thrusting the needle onto the rib in the transthoracic approach. However, there have only been a few reported cases of needle fracture. Indeed, a search of the literature has not resulted in any reported cases in the last decade. This is probably due to the increasing expertise in those carrying out liver biopsies and possibly the use of image guidance.

### 4.8 Arteriovenous fistula

Traumatic arteriovenous fistulas in relation to the biliary vasculature has been described as early as 1952(Strickler, Lufkin and Rice 1952). The incidence is reported to be as high as 50% if an angiogram is performed within one week of the biopsy (Hellekant 1976). A number of other authors have quoted a much lower incidence(Okuda, et al. 1978). This is probably a function of the fact that these lesions are not investigated unless the patients are symptomic and they tend to resolve spontaneously(Hurwitz and Thompson 2002). These patients tend to present as delayed haemorrhage in the form of frank intraperitoneal haemorrhage with shock, intrahepatic haematoma with pain and anaemia or haemobilia (Ormann, Starck and Pausch 1991). However, late presentations occur in the form of portal hypertension for arterio-portal fistulas and congestive cardia failure in the case of hepatic arteriovenous fistulas(Wallace, Medellin and Nelson 1972). The occurrence of fistulas is not isolated to percutaneous liver biopsy. Guarkuqi et al described a case of fatal haemobilia after transjugular liver biopsy in a patient with alcoholic cirrhosis 1 day after biopsy(Gurakuqi, et al. 2008). The haemobilia itself can cause pancreatitis(Machicao, Lukens, Lange and Scolapio 2002) and may result from an arteriovenous fistula(Cacho, et al. 1996) or a portobiliary or arteriobiliary fistula. Interestingly, arteriovenous fistulas after liver biopsy have been described elsewhere. In 1975 Satava et al described a case of an arteriovenous fistula of the omentum after liver biopsy. Whatever the presentation of the fistula, the main components of treatment is resuscitation, investigation and treatment. Treatment in the form of embolisation is usually successful and if not then surgery with the aim of ligation of the arterial component is the next best step.

### 4.9 Tumour seeding

Advances in imaging, operative procedures and chemotherapeutic agents has increased the pool of patients suitable for Liver resection of primary and secondary liver cancers and the long term survival. Needle track seeding is well documented in the literature (Davies, Tulgan, Parkinson, Goel and Budnitz 1968, Evans, Harries and Hobbs 1987)(Figure 6). This has been reported in both biopsies for primary or secondary liver tumours(Park, et al. 1989, Smith 1991, Vergara, Marucci, Marcarino, Brunello and Capussotti 1993, Jones, Rees, John, Bygrave and Plant 2005). It is thought that needling a tumour could implant up to 100,000 tumour cells along the tract(Ryd, Hagmar and Eriksson 1983). The occurrence of needle track seeding after tumour biopsy is known to result in poorer long term survival(Cresswell, Welsh and Rees 2009) and convert a potentially resectable lesion to being unresectable. In spite of this there are still reported incidences of patients undergoing biopsy of liver lesions before being referred to a specialist unit (Al-Leswas, O'Reilly and Poston 2008). The incidence of tumour seeding has been reported to be has high as 19% and in one study significantly reduced 4-year survival from 46.7% to 32.5% (Jones, et al. 2005). The same holds true for hepatocellular carcinoma. The meta-analysis and systematic review by Silva et al reported a seeding rate 2.7% in biopsy of hepatocellular carcinoma(Silva, et al. 2008). In addition, the long term survival is also significantly affected with 5 year survival reported to decrease from 52% to 24%(Young, et al. 2007).

It is clear that modern day practice of surgery dictates that all patients with liver lesions should be referred to a specialist centre for investigation and management. The advances in MRI, PET and CT along with ultrasound and measurement of tumour markers without histology have reported accuracies of over 97% and should provide enough information in the majority of cases for management decisions to be made(Torzilli, et al. 2004). The only real indication for biopsy of suspicious liver lesions would be in patients who are considered to be irresectable by a specialist centre and a histological diagnosis is necessary to determine consideration for chemotherapy.

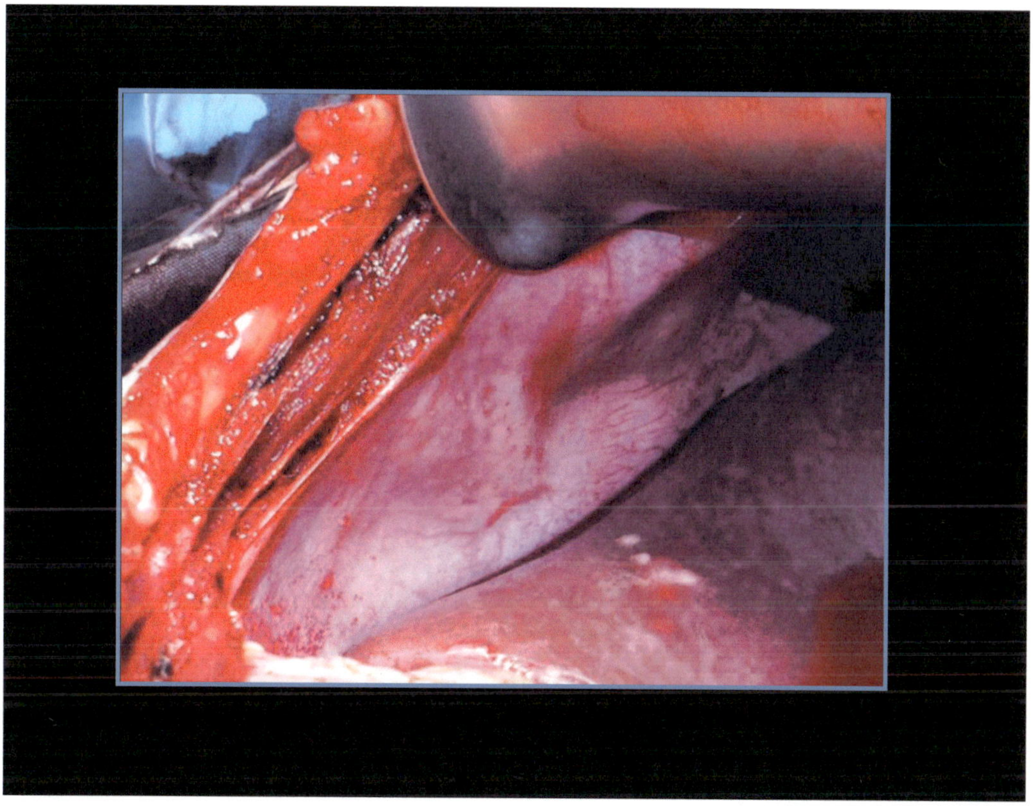

Fig. 6. This patient with a colorectal cancer had a small subcapsular lesion shown on a CT. At laparoscopy the subcapsular lesion was biopsied, which was positive for a metastasis. The patient had a laparotomy 3 weeks latter. The picture shows multiple tiny serosal deposits

#### 4.10 Biliary fistulas

Biliary fistulas are a rare complication of liver biopsy. They can be divided into intenal or external fistulas. Internal fistulas occur between the biliary tree and an adjacent sturcture. These include arterio-biliary or bilio-venous fistulas. These patients can present with haemobilia or pancreatitis. In one large series percutaneous liver biopsy has been reported to cause haemobilia in 4 out of 68,276 patients (Piccinino et al 1986). The reported incidence of this is between 0 to 1% (Rossi et al 2002) and can usually be managed by embolisation of the vessel. More rarely, biliovenous fistulas can present as bile pulmonary embolism with fatal consequences (Brown and Walsh 1952). Fistulas can also develop between the biliary tree and an adjacent organ or cavity such as a bronchobiliary or pleurobiliary fistula (Ferguson and Thomas 1967). They can present as bilioptysis and can be managed conservatively by ERCP to decompress the biliary tree and allow preferential flow of bile into the duodenum or, failing that, surgical intervention (Chong et al. 2008). Biliary fistulas can also present bilio-cutaneous fistulas (Hatzidakis et al 2006). The true incidence is not known. The management of these fistulas also varies and will depend on the underlying pathology. The options for management include conservative, allow the fistula to heal spontaneously, radiological by embolisation of the fistula tract (Hatzidakis et al) or surgical.

## 5. Transvenous liver biopsy

Transvenous liver biopsy can be undertaken via the femoral or the more commonly described transjugular route. It was first described by Dotter in 1964(Dotter 1964) but the first major series was reported by Rosch et al in 1973(Rosch, Lakin, Antonovic and Dotter 1973). The transvenous route was introduced as an alternative to the percutaneous route when there are concerns about coagulopathy or significant ascites and in those with morbid obesity(Rockey, et al. 2009). The transjugular route has the added advantage of being able to measure the hepatic venous wedge pressure where necessary. The basic principle of the procedure is the same for both techniques. The procedure is usually performed by a radiologist under fluoroscopic guidance. The inferior vena cava(IVC) is cannulated and via this one of the hepatic veins (usually the right) is entered and a biopsy is taken from within the liver. The technical failure rate is reported to be 3.2% (Kalambokis, et al. 2007).

The reported complication for the transjugular is as high as 20% (Grant, et al. 1999) with major complications occurring between 1.3 to 2.7% (Gamble, Colapinto, Stronell, Colman and Blendis 1985, McAfee, Keeffe, Lee and Rosch 1992). However, the most recent review of the literature reports a complication rate of 6.7% in adult series, comparable to complication rates reported in other series(Thampanitchawong, et al. 1999). The complications were described as both liver puncture related and non-liver puncture related and the incidence for both were similar. The non-liver puncture related complications are associated with the process of cannulating the jugular or hepatic vein or technical failure. In their retrospective study Soyer et al suggests that the complications associated with cannulation of the jugular vein can be minimized by the use of ultrasonic guidance(Soyer, Fargeaudou, Boudiaf and Rymer 2008). These include skin haematoma, pneumothorax, Horner's syndrome, dysphonia, cholangitis and cardiac arrhythmias. One particular risk associated with this route is perforation of the liver capsule and intraperitoneal haemorrhage(McAfee, et al. 1992). Even if the procedure was attempted via the femoral route capsular perforation was still a noted complication(Khosa, et al. 2003). Khosa suggested that this complication could be avoided if biopsies were taken within a central area of the liver and biplane fluoroscopy was used. The same would probably hold true for the transjugular route. In addition, Papatheodoridis et al suggested that capsular penetration was more frequent with the Menghini needle as a result of difficulty in controlling the depth of penetration (Papatheodoridis, Patch, Watkinson, Tibballs and Burroughs 1999). In their series capsular penetration only resulted in minor complications. The mortality rate is about 0.09% and like percutaneous liver biopsy was due to haemorrhage. In contrast, some deaths with transjugular biopsy were also related to ventricular arrhythmias as a result of manipulation of the catheter through the right atria and ventricle.

One of the few comparative studies between transjugular and percutaneous biopsy was reported in 1994 by Hong-Chaing Meng et al. In this study the complication rate for the transjugular route was 7% and 9% for the percutaneous route suggesting that transjugular biopsy was at least as safe as percutaneous liver biopsy and re-affirmed the idea that it is a safe alternative in patients in whom percutaneous biopsy is contra-indicated. Interestingly, Atar et al reported a comparative study of plugged percutaneous liver biopsy and transjugular biopsy and found no difference in major complications in either group(Atar, et al. 2010). They suggested that the plugged percutaneous biopsy technique should be used instead of the transjugular route when available.

The use of the transvenous route for liver biopsy is well established. However, this technique is only practiced in a few centres mainly by radiologists or hepatologists with significant experience in the technique. The indications for this procedure is restricted and as yet the percutaneous route is still the procedure of choice as it is simpler, requires less specialized equipment and is therefore cheaper.

## 6. Laparoscopic liver biopsy

Laparoscopic liver biopsy is a well established method. It is usually undertaken when liver lesions are found incidentally during laparoscopy for diagnostic or staging purposes. In addition, staging of patients with cirrhosis and hepatocellular carcinoma who are being considered for resection can have a biopsy of the future liver remnant. Laparoscopic liver biopsy had the added advantage of direct view of the liver which reduces sampling errors and bleeding after biopsy allowing better control(Denzer, et al. 2007). This is supported by Nord et al who reported a significant decrease in sampling errors of laparoscopic biopsy compared to the percutaneous route in cirrhotic patients(Tobkes and Nord 1995).

The risks of laparoscopic liver biopsy can be divided into the risks of any laparoscopic procedure and the risks of liver biopsy. Beckmann et al did a comparative study with laparoscopic, transjugular and percutaneous liver biopsy. They found that the complication rate was similar for all groups (2.7%, 2.9% and 3% respectively)(Beckmann, et al. 2009). However, in their study the transjugular route had a low success rate and they suggested that the laparoscopic route as an alternative especially in patients with severe coagulopathy (Denzer, Helmreich-Becker, Galle and Lohse 2003). The only randomized study comparing laparoscopic with percutaneous biopsy was reported by Denzer et al(Denzer, et al. 2007). This study was undertaken in cirrhotics but found a slightly higher but not significant difference in total complication rate between the groups (8.8% vs 5.8%).

The main risks that we divulge to our patients specific to any laparoscopic procedure are bowel or aortic/inferior vena cava perforation, bleeding, post-operative shoulder tip pain and port-site pain and hernias. Specifically for laparoscopic liver biopsy our unit informs patients of the risk of bleeding or biliary leak. As a general rule we do not undertake laparoscopic biopsies of possible malignant lesions unless we know that the tumour is inoperable and a histological diagnosis is needed prior to starting chemotherapy

## 7. Conclusion

The role of liver biopsy in the investigation of liver disease has changed over time. This is due to the advances in other non-invasive imaging techniques providing adequate information for diagnosis. It is still however a very important investigative tool in certain circumstances. These indications have been laid out in the American Association for the study of Liver Disease and the British Society of Gastroenterology. It is mainly carried out under image guidance although some centres still practice blind biopsies. Importantly, it is not without its risks and complications that both physicians and surgeons should be aware of. The role of bleeding parameters and other adopted protocols may not necessarily be rooted in good quality evidence and there is scope for well designed randomized trials in certain aspects of this procedure. Finally, any patient discovered to have a lesion in the liver either from radiological investigation or during surgery should be referred to a specialist hepato-biliary unit for further evaluation.

## 8. References

Al-Leswas, D., O'Reilly, D. A., and Poston, G. J. (2008), "Biopsy of Solid Liver Tumors: Adverse Consequences," *Hepatobiliary Pancreat Dis Int*, 7, 325-327.

Al Knawy, B., and Shiffman, M. (2007), "Percutaneous Liver Biopsy in Clinical Practice," *Liver Int*, 27, 1166-1173.

Atar, E., et al. (2010), "A Comparison of Transjugular and Plugged-Percutaneous Liver Biopsy in Patients with Contraindications to Ordinary Percutaneous Liver Biopsy and an "in-House" Protocol for Selecting the Procedure of Choice," *Cardiovasc Intervent Radiol*, 33, 560-564.

Beckmann, M. G., et al. (2009), "Clinical Relevance of Transjugular Liver Biopsy in Comparison with Percutaneous and Laparoscopic Liver Biopsy," *Gastroenterol Res Pract*, 2009, 947014.

Bravo, A. A., Sheth, S. G., and Chopra, S. (2001), "Liver Biopsy," *N Engl J Med*, 344, 495-500.

Brown, C.Y, Walsh, G.C., (1952),"Fatal bile embolism folowing liver biopsy" *Ann Intern Med* 36, 1529-1533

Bubak, M. E., Porayko, M. K., Krom, R. A., and Wiesner, R. H. (1991), "Complications of Liver Biopsy in Liver Transplant Patients: Increased Sepsis Associated with Choledochojejunostomy," *Hepatology*, 14, 1063-1065.

Cacho, G., et al. (1996), "Arterioportal Fistula and Hemobilia with Associated Acute Cholecystitis: A Complication of Percutaneous Liver Biopsy," *Hepatogastroenterology*, 43, 1020-1023.

Cadranel, J. F., Rufat, P., and Degos, F. (2000), "Practices of Liver Biopsy in France: Results of a Prospective Nationwide Survey. For the Group of Epidemiology of the French Association for the Study of the Liver (Afef)," *Hepatology*, 32, 477-481.

Caldwell, S., and Northup, P. G. (2010), "Bleeding Complication with Liver Biopsy: Is It Predictable?," *Clin Gastroenterol Hepatol*, 8, 826-829.

Castera, L., Negre, I., Samii, K., and Buffet, C. (1999), "Pain Experienced During Percutaneous Liver Biopsy," *Hepatology*, 30, 1529-1530.

Chuah, S. Y. (1996), "Liver Biopsy--Past, Present and Future," *Singapore Med J*, 37, 86-90.

Chuah, S. Y., Moody, G. A., Wicks, A. C., and Mayberry, J. F. (1994), "A Nationwide Survey of Liver Biopsy--Is There a Need to Increase Resources, Manpower and Training?," *Hepatogastroenterology*, 41, 4-8.

Chong, C.F., Chong,V.H., Jahilal, A., Mathews,L (2008), "Bronchobiliary fistula successfully treated surgically," *Singapore Med J* 49,e208-11

Cox, E. F. (1967), "Hemobilia Following Percutaneous Needle Biopsy of the Liver," *Arch Surg*, 95, 198-201.

Cresswell, A. B., Welsh, F. K., and Rees, M. (2009), "A Diagnostic Paradigm for Resectable Liver Lesions: To Biopsy or Not to Biopsy?," *HPB (Oxford)*, 11, 533-540.

Davies, W. J., Jr., Tulgan, H., Parkinson, A. T., Goel, V. G., and Budnitz, J. (1968), "Subcutaneous Tumor Implantation after Percutaneous Liver Biopsy," *JAMA*, 205, 700-702.

Denzer, U., et al. (2007), "Prospective Randomized Comparison of Minilaparoscopy and Percutaneous Liver Biopsy: Diagnosis of Cirrhosis and Complications," *J Clin Gastroenterol*, 41, 103-110.

Denzer, U., Helmreich-Becker, I., Galle, P. R., and Lohse, A. W. (2003), "Liver Assessment and Biopsy in Patients with Marked Coagulopathy: Value of Mini-Laparoscopy and Control of Bleeding," *Am J Gastroenterol*, 98, 893-900.

Dhawan, V. K., Thadepalli, H., Ulmer, D. D., and Akhtar, A. (1983), "Polymicrobial Septicemia after Liver Biopsy," *West J Med*, 139, 376-378.

Dillon, J. F., Simpson, K. J., and Hayes, P. C. (1994), "Liver Biopsy Bleeding Time: An Unpredictable Event," *J Gastroenterol Hepatol*, 9, 269-271.

Dotter, C. T. (1964), "Catheter Biopsy. Experimental Technic for Transvenous Liver Biopsy," *Radiology*, 82, 312-314.

Eisenberg, E., et al. (2003), "Prevalence and Characteristics of Pain Induced by Percutaneous Liver Biopsy," *Anesth Analg*, 96, 1392-1396, table of contents.

Evans, G. H., Harries, S. A., and Hobbs, K. E. (1987), "Safety of and Necessity for Needle Biopsy of Liver Tumours," *Lancet*, 1, 620.

Ewe, K. (1981), "Bleeding after Liver Biopsy Does Not Correlate with Indices of Peripheral Coagulation," *Dig Dis Sci*, 26, 388-393.

Fandrich, C. A., Davies, R. P., and Hall, P. M. (1996), "Small Gauge Gelfoam Plug Liver Biopsy in High Risk Patients: Safety and Diagnostic Value," *Australas Radiol*, 40, 230-234.

Farrell, R. J., et al. (1999), "Guided Versus Blind Liver Biopsy for Chronic Hepatitis C: Clinical Benefits and Costs," *J Hepatol*, 30, 580-587.

Ferguson, T. B., Burford, T.H. (1967), "Pleurobiliary and Bronchobiliary fistulas," *Archives of Surgery* 95, 380-386

Forssell, P. L., Bonkowsky, H. L., Anderson, P. B., and Howell, D. A. (1981), "Intrahepatic Hematoma after Aspiration Liver Biopsy. A Prospective Randomized Trial Using Two Different Needles," *Dig Dis Sci*, 26, 631-635.

Froehlich, F., Lamy, O., Fried, M., and Gonvers, J. J. (1993), "Practice and Complications of Liver Biopsy. Results of a Nationwide Survey in Switzerland," *Dig Dis Sci*, 38, 1480-1484.

Galati, J. S., et al. (1994), "The Nature of Complications Following Liver Biopsy in Transplant Patients with Roux-En-Y Choledochojejunostomy," *Hepatology*, 20, 651-653.

Gamble, P., Colapinto, R. F., Stronell, R. D., Colman, J. C., and Blendis, L. (1985), "Transjugular Liver Biopsy: A Review of 461 Biopsies," *Radiology*, 157, 589-593.

Gilmore, I. T., et al. (1995), "Indications, Methods, and Outcomes of Percutaneous Liver Biopsy in England and Wales: An Audit by the British Society of Gastroenterology and the Royal College of Physicians of London," *Gut*, 36, 437-441.

Grant, A., and Neuberger, J. (1999), "Guidelines on the Use of Liver Biopsy in Clinical Practice. British Society of Gastroenterology," *Gut*, 45 Suppl 4, IV1-IV11.

Griffiths, A., Viiala, C. H., and Olynyk, J. K. (2002), "Liver Biopsy in the 21st Century: Where and Why?," *Med J Aust*, 176, 52-53.

Gurakuqi, G. C., et al. (2008), "Fatal Hemobilia Resulting from an Iatrogenic Arteriobiliary Fistula as a Rare Complication of Transjugular Liver Biopsy," *Eur J Gastroenterol Hepatol*, 20, 83-86.

Hatzidakis,A.,Petrakis,I.,Mantatzis,M.,Chamalakis,C.,Chalkiadakis,G., Gourtsoyiannis,N. (2006) "Bilio-cutaneous fistula formation after percutaneous liver mass biopsy: embolization of the tract with a gelatin matrix." *Int Surg* 91,341-4

Hederstrom, E., Forsberg, L., Floren, C. H., and Prytz, H. (1989), "Liver Biopsy Complications Monitored by Ultrasound," *J Hepatol*, 8, 94-98.

Hellekant, C. (1976), "Vascular Complications Following Needle Puncture of the Liver. Clinical Angiography," *Acta Radiol Diagn (Stockh)*, 17, 209-222.

Hurwitz, L. M., and Thompson, W. M. (2002), "Calcified Hepatic Arteriovenous Fistula Found after Biopsy of the Liver: Unusual Cause of Calcification in the Right Upper Quadrant," *AJR Am J Roentgenol*, 179, 1293-1295.

Jacobs, W. H., and Goldberg, S. B. (1989), "Statement on Outpatient Percutaneous Liver Biopsy," *Dig Dis Sci*, 34, 322-323.

Janes, C. H., and Lindor, K. D. (1993), "Outcome of Patients Hospitalized for Complications after Outpatient Liver Biopsy," *Ann Intern Med*, 118, 96-98.

Jones, O. M., Rees, M., John, T. G., Bygrave, S., and Plant, G. (2005), "Biopsy of Resectable Colorectal Liver Metastases Causes Tumour Dissemination and Adversely Affects Survival after Liver Resection," *Br J Surg*, 92, 1165-1168.

Kalambokis, G., et al. (2007), "Transjugular Liver Biopsy--Indications, Adequacy, Quality of Specimens, and Complications--a Systematic Review," *J Hepatol*, 47, 284-294.

Khosa, F., et al. (2003), "Transvenous Liver Biopsy Via the Femoral Vein," *Clin Radiol*, 58, 487-491.

Knauer, C. M. (1978), "Percutaneous Biopsy of the Liver as a Procedure for Outpatients," *Gastroenterology*, 74, 101-102.

Kowdley, K. V., Aggarwal, A. M., and Sachs, P. B. (1994), "Delayed Hemorrhage after Percutaneous Liver Biopsy. Role of Therapeutic Angiography," *J Clin Gastroenterol*, 19, 50-53.

Larson, A. M., et al. (1997), "Infection Complicating Percutaneous Liver Biopsy in Liver Transplant Recipients," *Hepatology*, 26, 1406-1409.

Le Frock, J. L., Ellis, C. A., Turchik, J. B., Zawacki, J. K., and Weinstein, L. (1975), "Transient Bacteremia Associated with Percutaneous Liver Biopsy," *J Infect Dis*, 131 Suppl, S104-107.

Lebrec, D., Goldfarb, G., Degott, C., Rueff, B., and Benhamou, J. P. (1982), "Transvenous Liver Biopsy: An Experience Based on 1000 Hepatic Tissue Samplings with This Procedure," *Gastroenterology*, 83, 338-340.

Lindor, K. D., et al. (1996), "The Role of Ultrasonography and Automatic-Needle Biopsy in Outpatient Percutaneous Liver Biopsy," *Hepatology*, 23, 1079-1083.

Machicao, V. I., Lukens, F. J., Lange, S. M., and Scolapio, J. S. (2002), "Arterioportal Fistula Causing Acute Pancreatitis and Hemobilia after Liver Biopsy," *J Clin Gastroenterol*, 34, 481-484.

Majid, A. A. (1990), "Hemorrhage from the Diaphragm: An Unusual Cause of Hemothorax after Percutaneous Liver Biopsy," *Am J Gastroenterol*, 85, 104-105.

Manolakopoulos, S., et al. (2007), "Ultrasound-Guided Liver Biopsy in Real Life: Comparison of Same-Day Prebiopsy Versus Real-Time Ultrasound Approach," *J Gastroenterol Hepatol*, 22, 1490-1493.

Mayoral, W., and Lewis, J. H. (2001), "Percutaneous Liver Biopsy: What Is the Current Approach? Results of a Questionnaire Survey," *Dig Dis Sci*, 46, 118-127.

McAfee, J. H., Keeffe, E. B., Lee, R. G., and Rosch, J. (1992), "Transjugular Liver Biopsy," *Hepatology*, 15, 726-732.

McCloskey, R. V., Gold, M., and Weser, E. (1973), "Bacteremia after Liver Biopsy," *Arch Intern Med*, 132, 213-215.

McGill, D. B., Rakela, J., Zinsmeister, A. R., and Ott, B. J. (1990), "A 21-Year Experience with Major Hemorrhage after Percutaneous Liver Biopsy," *Gastroenterology*, 99, 1396-1400.

McVay, P. A., and Toy, P. T. (1990), "Lack of Increased Bleeding after Liver Biopsy in Patients with Mild Hemostatic Abnormalities," *Am J Clin Pathol*, 94, 747-753.

Menghini, G. (1958), "One-Second Needle Biopsy of the Liver," *Gastroenterology*, 35, 190-199.

Minuk, G. Y., Sutherland, L. R., Wiseman, D. A., MacDonald, F. R., and Ding, D. L. (1987), "Prospective Study of the Incidence of Ultrasound-Detected Intrahepatic and Subcapsular Hematomas in Patients Randomized to 6 or 24 Hours of Bed Rest after Percutaneous Liver Biopsy," *Gastroenterology*, 92, 290-293.

Moreira Vicente, V. F., Hernandez Ranz, F. M., Ruiz Del Arbol, L., and Bouza, E. P. (1981), "Septicemia as a Complication of Liver Biopsy," *Am J Gastroenterol*, 76, 145-147.

Muir, A. J., and Trotter, J. F. (2002), "A Survey of Current Liver Biopsy Practice Patterns," *J Clin Gastroenterol*, 35, 86-88.

Okuda, K., et al. (1978), "Frequency of Intrahepatic Arteriovenous Fistula as a Sequela to Percutaneous Needle Puncture of the Liver," *Gastroenterology*, 74, 1204-1207.

Ormann, W., Starck, E., and Pausch, J. (1991), "[Arterial Embolization of an Arteriovenous Fistula with Hemobilia after Blind Liver Puncture]," *Z Gastroenterol*, 29, 153-155.

Own, A., Balzer, J. O., and Vogl, T. J. (2005), "Bleeding Hepatic Pseudoaneurysm Complicating Percutaneous Liver Biopsy with Interventional Treatment Options," *Eur Radiol*, 15, 183-185.

Papatheodoridis, G. V., Patch, D., Watkinson, A., Tibballs, J., and Burroughs, A. K. (1999), "Transjugular Liver Biopsy in the 1990s: A 2-Year Audit," *Aliment Pharmacol Ther*, 13, 603-608.

Park, Y. M., et al. (1989), "A Case of Subcutaneous Seeding of Hepatocellular Carcinoma after Fine Needle Aspiration Biopsy," *Korean J Intern Med*, 4, 96-100.

Pena, L. R., Horn, T. L., and Cross, C. B. (2009), "Acute Pancreatitis Secondary to Hemobilia after Percutaneous Liver Biopsy," *Therap Adv Gastroenterol*, 2, 165-168.

Peters, R. S. (1968), "Fracture of Menghini Needle in Liver Biopsy," *JAMA*, 206, 1575-1576.

Piccinino, F., Sagnelli, E., Pasquale, G., and Giusti, G. (1986), "Complications Following Percutaneous Liver Biopsy. A Multicentre Retrospective Study on 68,276 Biopsies," *J Hepatol*, 2, 165-173.

Pokorny, C. S., and Waterland, M. (2002), "Short-Stay, out-of-Hospital, Radiologically Guided Liver Biopsy," *Med J Aust*, 176, 67-69.

Raines, D. R., Van Heertum, R. L., and Johnson, L. F. (1974), "Intrahepatic Hematoma: A Complication of Percutaneous Liver Biopsy," *Gastroenterology*, 67, 284-289.

Reichert, C. M., Weisenthal, L. M., and Klein, H. G. (1983), "Delayed Hemorrhage after Percutaneous Liver Biopsy," *J Clin Gastroenterol*, 5, 263-266.

Ren, F. Y., Piao, X. X., and Jin, A. L. (2006), "Delayed Hemorrhage from Hepatic Artery after Ultrasound-Guided Percutaneous Liver Biopsy: A Case Report," *World J Gastroenterol*, 12, 4273-4275.

Riley, T. R., 3rd. (1999), "How Often Does Ultrasound Marking Change the Liver Biopsy Site?," *Am J Gastroenterol*, 94, 3320-3322.

Rockey, D. C., Caldwell, S. H., Goodman, Z. D., Nelson, R. C., and Smith, A. D. (2009), "Liver Biopsy," *Hepatology*, 49, 1017-1044.

Rosch, J., Lakin, P. C., Antonovic, R., and Dotter, C. T. (1973), "Transjugular Approach to Liver Biopsy and Transhepatic Cholangiography," *N Engl J Med*, 289, 227-231.

Rossi, P., Sileri, P., Gentileschi, P., Sica, G.S.,Ercoli, L.,Coscarella,G.,De Majo, A., Gaspari,A.L. (2002) "Delayed symptomatic hemobilia after ultrasound-guided liver biopsy: a case report." *Hepatogastroenterology* 49,1659-62

Ryd, W., Hagmar, B., and Eriksson, O. (1983), "Local Tumour Cell Seeding by Fine-Needle Aspiration Biopsy. A Semiquantitative Study," *Acta Pathol Microbiol Immunol Scand A*, 91, 17-21.

Sawyerr, A. M., et al. (1993), "A Comparison of Transjugular and Plugged-Percutaneous Liver Biopsy in Patients with Impaired Coagulation," *J Hepatol*, 17, 81-85.

Shah, S., Mayberry, J. F., Wicks, A. C., Rees, Y., and Playford, R. J. (1999), "Liver Biopsy under Ultrasound Control: Implications for Training in the Calman Era," *Gut*, 45, 628-629.

Sharma, P., McDonald, G. B., and Banaji, M. (1982), "The Risk of Bleeding after Percutaneous Liver Biopsy: Relation to Platelet Count," *J Clin Gastroenterol*, 4, 451-453.

Silva, M. A., et al. (2008), "Needle Track Seeding Following Biopsy of Liver Lesions in the Diagnosis of Hepatocellular Cancer: A Systematic Review and Meta-Analysis," *Gut*, 57, 1592-1596.

Smith, E. H. (1991), "Complications of Percutaneous Abdominal Fine-Needle Biopsy. Review," *Radiology*, 178, 253-258.

Soyer, P., Fargeaudou, Y., Boudiaf, M., and Rymer, R. (2008), "Transjugular Liver Biopsy Using Ultrasonographic Guidance for Jugular Vein Puncture and an Automated Device for Hepatic Tissue Sampling: A Retrospective Analysis of 200 Consecutive Cases," *Abdom Imaging*, 33, 627-632.

Stone, M. A., and Mayberry, J. F. (1996), "An Audit of Ultrasound Guided Liver Biopsies: A Need for Evidence-Based Practice," *Hepatogastroenterology*, 43, 432-434.

Strickler, J. H., Lufkin, N., and Rice, C. O. (1952), "Hepatic Portal Arteriovenous Fistula; a Case Report," *Surgery*, 31, 583-589.

Terjung, B., et al. (2003), "Bleeding Complications after Percutaneous Liver Biopsy. An Analysis of Risk Factors," *Digestion*, 67, 138-145.

Thampanitchawong, P., and Piratvisuth, T. (1999), "Liver Biopsy:Complications and Risk Factors," *World J Gastroenterol*, 5, 301-304.

Tobkes, A. I., and Nord, H. J. (1995), "Liver Biopsy: Review of Methodology and Complications," *Dig Dis*, 13, 267-274.

Torzilli, G., et al. (2004), "Indication and Contraindication for Hepatic Resection for Liver Tumors without Fine-Needle Biopsy: Validation and Extension of an Eastern Approach in a Western Community Hospital," *Liver Transpl*, 10, S30-33.

Tripodi, A., et al. (2006), "Thrombin Generation in Patients with Cirrhosis: The Role of Platelets," *Hepatology*, 44, 440-445.

Valori, R., and Elias, E. (1989), "How to Perform a Percutaneous Liver Biopsy," *Br J Hosp Med*, 42, 408-410.

van der Poorten, D., et al. (2006), "Twenty-Year Audit of Percutaneous Liver Biopsy in a Major Australian Teaching Hospital," *Intern Med J*, 36, 692-699.

Van Thiel, D. H., Gavaler, J. S., Wright, H., and Tzakis, A. (1993), "Liver Biopsy. Its Safety and Complications as Seen at a Liver Transplant Center," *Transplantation*, 55, 1087-1090.

Vautier, G., Scott, B., and Jenkins, D. (1994), "Liver Biopsy: Blind or Guided?," *BMJ*, 309, 1455-1456.

Vergara, V., Marucci, M., Marcarino, C., Brunello, F., and Capussotti, L. (1993), "Metastatic Involvement of the Pancreas from Renal Cell Carcinoma Treated by Surgery," *Ital J Gastroenterol*, 25, 388-390.

Wallace, S., Medellin, H., and Nelson, R. S. (1972), "Angiographic Changes Due to Needle Biopsy of the Liver," *Radiology*, 105, 13-18.

West, J., and Card, T. R. (2010), "Reduced Mortality Rates Following Elective Percutaneous Liver Biopsies," *Gastroenterology*, 139, 1230-1237.

Yeo, W. T., Tan, L. K., Dan, Y. Y., and Wai, C. T. (2008), "Delayed Bleeding after Liver Biopsy: A Dreaded Complication," *Singapore Med J*, 49, 76-80.

Young, A. L., et al. (2007), "Large Hepatocellular Carcinoma: Time to Stop Preoperative Biopsy," *J Am Coll Surg*, 205, 453-462.

Younossi, Z. M., Teran, J. C., Ganiats, T. G., and Carey, W. D. (1998), "Ultrasound-Guided Liver Biopsy for Parenchymal Liver Disease: An Economic Analysis," *Dig Dis Sci*, 43, 46-50.

Zamcheck, N., and Sidman, R. L. (1953), "Needle Biopsy of the Liver. I. Its Use in Clinical and Investigative Medicine," *N Engl J Med*, 249, 1020-1029; contd.

Züleyha Akkan Çetinkaya, M. S., Fatih Güzelbulut, Yusuf Ziya Benek, Selvinaz Özkara, Yasemin Gökden, Bülent Yaşar, Oya Övünç Kurdaş (2010), "Liver Biopsy: Ultrasonography Guidance Is Not Superior to the Blind Method" *Journal of Gastrointestinal and Liver Diseases*, 19, 49-52.

# 25

# Complications of Liver Biopsy - Risk Factors, Management and Recommendations

Norman Oneil Machado
*Sultan Qaboos University Hospital*
*Oman*

## 1. Introduction

The role of liver biopsy (LB), the traditional gold standard for assessing liver disease, continues to evolve[1-4]. Fewer biopsies are being done for diagnosis as noninvasive tests such as new imaging techniques and accurate serological tests can now be done instead in many cases[2-4]. Most biopsies are currently performed for parenchymal disease not to make specific diagnosis but to assess the liver damage (the degree of inflammation, fibrosis) or the response to therapy[5]. In contrast to past when nearly all biopsies were done for diagnostic purpose, presently more than 50% are being done for staging versus 15% for diagnosing the parenchymal liver disease[5]. In addition, biopsies are often done to help in guiding the management of hepatitis C and nonalcoholic steatohepatitis and to assess the response to therapy[2, 3]. The increased use of liver transplantation as standard treatment of end stage liver disease of diverse etiologies has led to more biopsies being performed to differentiate the cause of graft dysfunction and to assess the suitability of potential liver donors for transplantation[1-3]. The dramatic increase in obesity, diabetes, hyperlipidaemia and hypertension (the metabolic syndrome) in western societies and its accompanying fatty liver problems are requiring liver biopsy for histological assessment[2]. Evaluation of liver histology remains very important as LB is reported to change the clinical diagnosis in 8-14%, management in 12-18% and frequency of liver test monitoring in 36% of cases[5]. Hence the main indication are a) chronic hepatitis- for grading, staging, establishing a therapeutic strategy and monitoring therapy, b)unexplained abnormal liver function tests or hepatomegaly and c) follow up of patients after liver transplantation. However no liver biopsy is free of risk as it is an invasive procedure. Rational assessment of overall risk in LB however is hampered by the wide variation in the indication and its outcome reported in the existing literature.

## 2. Factors that may influence the risk of complication following liver biopsy

Several factors my influence the risk of complication following liver biopsy and are listed in table 1

*Uncooperative patient-* The risk of bleeding is enhanced in an uncooperative patient who may inadvertently move when the biopsy needle is in the liver leading to tear or laceration[1-4]. In such uncooperative patients if liver biopsy was required it could be achieved by performing the procedure under moderate or deep sedation or under general anaesthesia[6, 7]. A transjugular approach is an alternative option[8]. Conscious sedation for LB are performed using midazolam and fentanyl or mepverdine[6,7]. This adds to small risk and the cost of conscious sedation to the procedure. However patients are found to be remarkably cooperative and usually breathe somewhat superficially and will hold their breath if instructed[6,7]. However while sedation may allay anxiety and pain there is no strong evidence to suggest that it either increases or reduces the risk of major complications. It however makes an uncooperative patient cooperative[1].

| Factors that may influence the risk of complication following liver biopsy |
|---|
| Patient cooperation |
| Coagulation status / bleeding disorders |
| Operator experience |
| Advanced age |
| Certain pathologies (liver cirrhosis, amyloidosis, malignancy, renal failure) |
| Use of image guidance |
| ascites |
| Type of technique (percutaneous / transvenous) |
| Number of needle passes |
| Needle diameter (large needle) |
| Type of needle (cutting or Automatic) |
| Blind technique |

Table 1.

*Ascites-*_Moderate to severe ascites_is likely to make it difficult to hit the liver via the standard intercostal approach. In such patients, options would include total therapeutic paracentesis performed immediately prior to palpation /percussion guided transcutaneous biopsy or transvenous or laparoscopic biopsy[9].There are however reports of successful LB under CT scan or US guidance without increasing the risk of bleeding[9].

*Mass lesion-* Although LB in patients with mass lesion is generally safe, biopsy of known vascular lesion should be avoided[10]. Similarly biopsy of potentially malignant lesion should be avoided because it is believed that tumour vessels are more likely to bleed. However with the use of ultrasound colour Doppler to guide the site of biopsy, large tumour vessels and liver vessels can be identified and avoided[1,11,12]. Biopsy of malignant lesion is also associated with a risk of tumour spread usually along the biopsy tract. The risk is estimated to be around 0 to 0.13%[12] and the risk decreases with use of co-axial approach (i.e. utilization of a 17 gauze introducer and 18 gauze biopsy needle introduced along a co-axial plane[13].

*Impaired haemostasis-* Standard percutaneous liver biopsy is often withheld in patients with a PT-INR above 1.5[1-4]. However while alteration in haematological parameters are of utmost importance when considering the risk associated with liver biopsy, strict cutoffs for PT-INR may not be prudent in light of the risk associated with plasma infusion[1-4]. While it is often presumed that abnormal increase in the PT-INR correlates with an increased risk of bleeding and that correcting the abnormal PT-INR with plasma replacement therapy or agents such as recombinant activated factor V11 will reduce or eliminate the risk of bleeding, the available data in the literature are not sufficient to support this presumption particularly in mild coagulopathy defined as INR of less than 2.0[14-15]. Hence it is not clear whether prolongation of the INR in chronic liver disease while of prognostic significance actually represents a net diathesis or not[2]. Thus better tests are needed to more acutely define the net

bleeding risks in these patients. A new measure of coagulation in liver disease has recently been introduced, the $INR_{Liver}$[16,17]. It recalculates the international sensitivity index from a reference point of patients with liver disease rather than Coumadin –treated patients as has been the convention[16,17]. Whether this test will provide a reliable measure of bleeding risk remains to be determined. Therefore a large randomized controlled trial of plasma replacement therapy in patients undergoing invasive therapy appears to be warranted[1].
There are however several conditions which are more definitely associated with enhanced risk of bleeding and therefore warrant additional caution. These include patients with factor V11 (FV11) or 1X (F1X) deficiency, von Willebrand's disease, other hereditary bleeding disorders and those with sickle cell anaemia[17]. Patients with known underlying coagulopathy requiring liver biopsy represents a challenge but liver biopsy can be performed in these patients with definitive factor replacement. Nonetheless the risk benefit ratio must be carefully considered on a case by case basis

### 2.1 Ultrasound guided LB

This has been done to reduce the risk of both minor and major complications by avoiding large intra-hepatic vessels and other structures in the vicinity (gall bladder, colon, lung) and by decreasing the passes to sample a good specimen[18-21]. Ultrasound (US) may influence in selecting the site of puncture as was noted in 15% of cases in one study[19]. The main causes for the change in site were due to ascites or small liver. US guided liver biopsy is reported to be performed in 56% of cases in France and in 76% of cases in USA[20,21]. This could either be performed as US guided or US assisted LB. US guided LB is particularly reserved for small liver, interposition of colon or lung, focal liver lesion (Haemangioma or cysts) or in patients with increased risk of bleeding[19-21].

## 3. Post biopsy care and complications

Rate of complications vary in different case series and relate in part to operator experience although the most experienced clinician still will encounter complications[1-4]. The risk of major complications is listed in table 2. Intraoperative needle biopsy observation indicates that almost all patients have transient bleeding from the capsular puncture site[1,2]. Following outpatient LB the period of observation varies among different institution but usually does not exceed 6 hours[1-4]. Patients who have had uneventful single pass biopsy may be discharged after 3 hours observation and if patients require analgesia may need observation for at least 4 hours[2-4]. The majority of major complications requiring hospitalization have been shown in prospective observational series to occur within 3 hours of biopsy, although later complication can occasionally ensue[1-4].

### 3.1 Complications

*Pain-* Pain is the most common complication of percutaneous liver biopsy and is seen in up to 84% of patients including those with mild discomfort[22]. Often pain can be managed with small amounts of narcotics typically codeine[1-4]. The pain immediately after the procedure at times can be very distressing and some patients remember the procedure as a very unpleasant experience. Moderate to severe pain however is seen in 1-5% of the patients and should raise the possibility of a complication such as active bleeding or trauma to adjacent structures like gall bladder[23]. The mechanism of pain following percutaneous biopsy is most likely a result of bleeding or perhaps bile extravasation from the liver puncture wound with subsequent capsular swelling although the exact mechanism for the pain remains uncertain in most cases[2-4]. The site of biopsy (intercostal or subcostal) did not influence the incidence of pain[24]. However the use of US guidance, premedication with midazolam and fenatnyl and self delivering of mixture of $N_2o$ and oxygen via mask decreased significantly the incidence of post biopsy pain and anxiety[24,25]. For LB performed with US guidance the incidence of pain decreased from 47% to 35%. The 2 factors that were demonstrated to be associated with increased use of post procedure analgesics are, cutting biopsy needles and less experienced operator[25,26]. Other controversial factors associated with more pain are larger needle, increasing number of biopsy passes, hepatitis C infection, younger age and history of intravenous drug abuse[27]. The use of automatic cutting needles are associated with a low incidence of postbiopsy pain with a reported incidence 31.4 to 34.3% in comparison to hand held needles( 40.6 to 52.6%)[25,26].Besides the above factors the patient characteristics play an important role in pain medication requirement after LB . Thus previous intravenous drug abusers and those with significant anxiety prior to LB are associated with 9 and 4 fold increase in post biopsy analgesia respectively[27].

| *Scenario* | *Reported frequency (%)* |
|---|---|
| Pain at biopsy site or right shoulder (pleuritic, peritonel, diaphragmatic) | 0.056-22 |
| Haemorrhage | |
| -intraperitoneal | 0.03-0.7 |
| -intrahepatic or subcapsular | 0.59 -0.23 |
| -haemobilia | 0.058-0.2 |
| Bile peritonitis | 0.03-0.22 |
| Pneumothorax and /or pleural effusion | 0.08-0.28 |
| Haemothorax | 0.18-0.49 |
| Arteriovenous fistula | 5.4 |
| Anaesthetic reaction | 0.029 |
| Biopsy of adjacent organs | 0.001-0.044 |
| lung | -0.001- 0.014 |
| gall bladder | -0.034- 0.117 |
| kidney | -0.029- 0.096 |
| colon | -0.0038- 0.0044 |
| Reaction to anaesthetic agent | 0.029 |
| Breakage of needle | 0.02- 0.059 |
| Death | 0.0083-0.03 |

Table 2. Potential complications and the range in reported frequencies

A decision about when to investigate with imaging and or to hospitalize the patient for observation due to pain should be made on a case by case basis[1-4]. When pain is severe enough to require hospitalization radiological evaluation is usually warranted. While some would prefer the use of ultrasound as an initial investigation due to the ease with which it can be performed , others would perform an abdominal CT with contrast to be more definitive[1-4](figure 1).

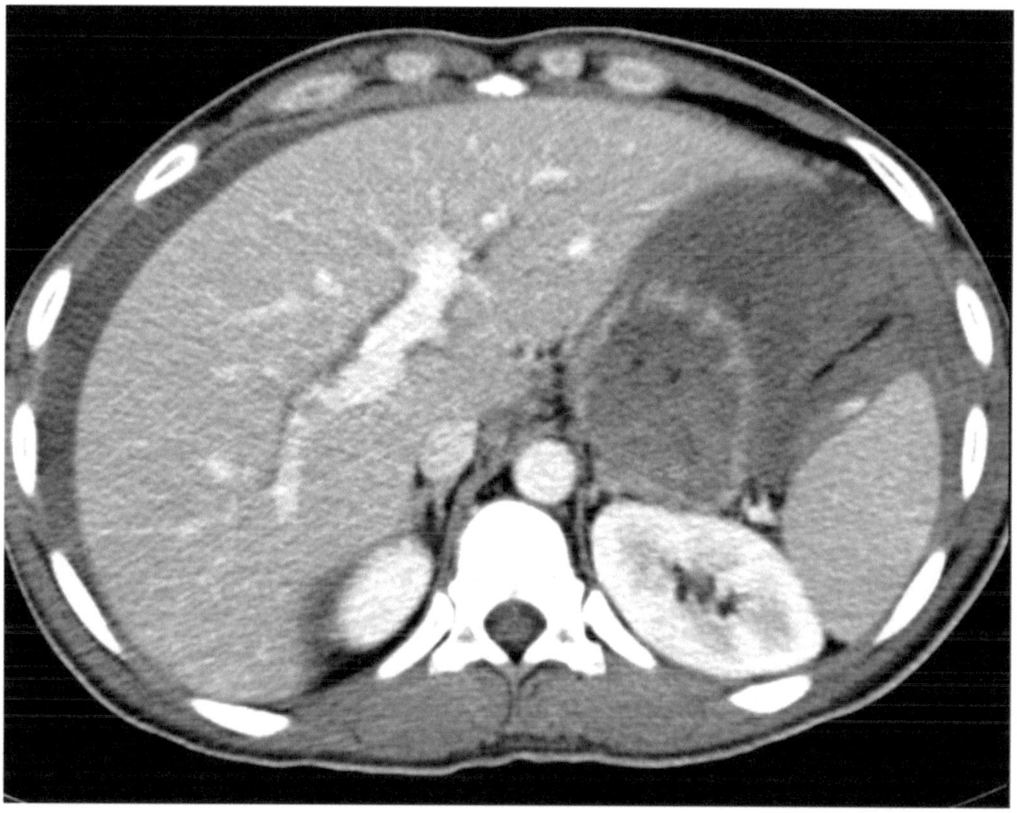

Fig. 1. CT scan revealing intraperitoneal bleeding following subcostal percutaneous liver biopsy. The bleeding was successfully managed conservatively

*Bleeding*- Bleeding could either be major or minor. The risk of major bleeding is reported to be around 0.16%[1 1,28 30]. Major bleeding is severe bleeding defined clinically by change in vital signs with radiographic evidence of intraperitoneal bleeding that requires hospitalization with the likelihood of transfusion or even radiologic intervention or surgery. Such bleeding has been estimated to occur in between 1 in 2500, to 1 in 10,000 biopsies after intercostal percutaneous approach for diffuse nonfocal liver disease[23,31-33]. Minor bleeding is less severe bleeding which is characterized by pain or reduced blood pressure or tachycardia but not requiring transfusion or intervention and occurs in approximately in 1 in 500 biopsies. About 18 to 20% of intrahepatic and perihepatic bleeding is also detected on ultrasonography[28]. Severe bleeding is usually clinically evident within 2 to 4 hours but late haemorrhage can occur even up to one week after biopsy[34]. Premature clot dissolution due to liver disease associated with hyperfibrinolysis has been proposed to play a role in some patients especially those with delayed bleeding, although this has not been extensively studied[35]. Some degree of bleeding occur after all percutaneous liver biopsies based on observation made on laparoscopy.

Bleeding can manifest as haemoperitoneum(0.3 to 0.7%), intrahepatic haematoma(0.59 to 0.23%) or haemobilia(0.058- 0.2%) [28-30](figure 1). Bleeding into peritoneal cavity produces pain, hypotension or less frequently may be asymptomatic. Intrahepatic haemtoma occurs in 1 to 23% of cases and are localized to intrahepatic or subcapsular region[28,29]. Usually they are small and asymptomatic but larger haematomas may cause pain from stretching of the liver capsule, hypotension or a delayed decrease in haematocrit[28,29]. The incidence of haematoma after LB seems to be high after LB with larger needles[30]. Conservative treatment of haematoma together with a close follow up by US is generally sufficient[1-2,36]. The least common of the haemorrhagic complications is haemobilia which presents with the classical triad of upper gastrointestinal bleeding, pain and jaundice[4,18,36]. It may appear acutely following simultaneous perforation of adjacent intrahepatic bile ducts and blood vessels or more commonly much later following the erosion of haematoma or psuedoaneurysm into a bile duct[37]. This occurs typically 5 days following the biopsy[31]. Haemobilia is a very rare event with a frequency of 0.0006 to 0.023% in large series[31,37,38]. If bile is checked routinely after LB, haemobilia may be detected in 10% of cases[31,37,38]. Large volume of haemobilia may cause acute pancreatitis, although this is a very rare event with only 5 cases being reported in the literature[39].

The risk of bleeding is influenced by several factors including bleeding disorders, advanced age, ascites, high number of passages, large needle size, blind technique and certain liver pathologies including liver cirrhosis , amyloidosis, malignancy and renal failure[1-4,28,31]. The factors that are also related to the risk of bleeding include arterial bleeding and operator experience. Whether cutting needle(eg Trucut and automated variants) have a different risk than aspiration needles(eg, Menghini or Jamshidi) is unknown although some retrospective data suggest that cutting needle may be associated with slightly greater risk[31]. At particular risk for bleeding are patients with chronic renal failure, those with underlying coagulopathy due to congenital abnormalities in coagulation parameter (such as haemophilics) and those with cirrhosis who may have acquired abnormalities in coagulation parameter. Use of DDAVP immediately before liver biopsy (0.3ug/kg ) body weight in patients with renal failure undergoing invasive procedure is useful[40,41]. In patients on chronic renal replacement therapy, dialysis is often performed prior to liver biopsy[1,2]. Although platelet count less than 60,000/cmm, INR greater than 1.3 and bleeding time > 10 minutes are well known practical contraindication to percutaneous LB, bleeding from liver does not correlate with the indices of peripheral coagulation when these are mildly impaired thus making bleeding an unpredictable event[42,43]. The accurate prediction of bleeding based on coagulation indices is problematic as the available data suggest poor relationship between bleeding and common laboratory tests (such as platelets, PT-NR etc)[42,43]. As a result there is wide variation in "acceptable" prebiopsy coagulation parameter[44]. Whether the use of prophylactic blood products alters the risk of bleeding is currently unknown[1-3]. Furthermore because of the conventional parameter of coagulation correlate poorly with risk of bleeding, recommendation regarding correction of coagulation indices is limited and tempered by the risk of blood product exposure[42,43].

Transvenous liver biopsy (typically with jugular approach) is often recommended in patients with known or suspected bleeding diathesis because it is commonly perceived to be safer[8]. However a recent systematic review reported minor and major complication in 6.5% and 0.6% respectively among the 7649 patients who underwent transvenous biopsy and may be related to capsular piercing with subsequent haemorrhage[32]. However as this study was retrospective, there may have been a selective bias (i.e. it is highly likely that patients suspected to be at risk of bleeding would have been preferred for transvenous rather than percutaneous biopsy).

### 3.2 Miscellaneous
A number of other complications have been reported after liver biopsy. These include pneumothorax, hemothorax, perforation of any of the several viscous organs, bile peritonitis, infection (bacteraemia. abscess, sepsis), haemobilia, intrahepatic arteriovenous fistula, neuralgia and rare complication such ventricular arrhythmias with transvenous biopsy[1-4].

#### 3.2.1 Infective complications
Transient bacteraemia which has been reported in 5.8 to 13.5% of patients after LB, is in most cases harmless[31]. Intrahepatic abscess, septicaemia and septic shock are much rare events occurring only in patients with biliary obstruction and cholangitis or when the colon is incidentally punctured[18]. Infectious complication appear to be increased in post transplant patients who underwent choledochojejunostomy during liver transplantation[45]. There is however no recommendations of prophylactic antibiotics in patients scheduled for LB except in those with valvular heart disease

#### 3.2.2 Complications in the thorax
Haemothorax, pneumothorax, leakage of ascites in the pleural cavity, subcutaneous emphysema occur after injury of pleura or lung or right diaphragm[18,31,46]. Haemothorax can occur even in US assisted LB when the patient changes his position or takes a deep inspiration after the site of puncture was set, the cause of bleeding being an injury to a diaphragmatic vessel[46] . Pneumothorax is critical to recognize immediately after biopsy in presence of reduced breath sounds and typical radiographic findings because it can lead to immediate catastrophic outcome if not promptly recognized and treated[18,31].

#### 3.2.3 Puncture of other viscera
This occurs rarely (0.01 to0.1%) and involves usually gall bladder, colon, and right kidney. The incidence is significantly reduced when LB is performed under US guidance[49,48] . Bile peritonitis , formation of bilioma or bilious pleural effusion occur mainly in patients with biliary obstruction although they are reports of them occurring even in patients without biliary obstruction or when the gall bladder is incidentally punctured[48,49].
Other very rare complications include reaction to the anaesthetic agents, breakage of the needle and arterioportal fistula, neuralgia and ventricular arrythmias [42,45].
*Death-* Is very uncommon after percutaneous biopsy but precise figure vary widely in the literature ranging from 0.009% to 0.11% .and is usually related to haemorrhage[10,20,24,31,41,45,49]. Mortality after transvenous biopsies was 0.0009% (9 in 10,000) in a recent report of 7649 transvenous biopsies but again may reflect the selection of higher risk patients for this intervention[40]. The main cause of death after LB is intraperitoneal bleeding mainly occurring in patients with malignancy or cirrhosis[45]. The incidence of fatal complications can be significantly reduced by careful post biopsy observation with prompt recognition of bleeding and aggressive subsequent therapy which may involve transfusion followed by therapeutic embolisation or laparotomy[10]

### 3.3 Management
The most critical aspect of management of complications such as bleeding, pneumothorax and visceral perforation is to recognize that one these complications has occurred.

Suspicion of a potential complication should be high when the patient complains of pain that is out of proportion to the clinical events that surrounded the biopsy and is associated with drop in blood pressure and tachycardia and is then confirmed by radiological investigation. All complications are supported by initial resuscitation. Bleeding is most often managed expectantly with placement of wide bore intravenous cannula, volume resuscitation and blood transfusion as necessary. Angiographic embolisation and surgery may be required in some of these patients with persistent bleeding. Pneumothorax may be self limiting but may require more aggressive intervention depending on the severity of symptoms. Visceral perforation is usually managed expectantly in most situations. Observation is all that may be required although occasionally surgical intervention may be needed in the case of gall bladder puncture with persistent bile leak or in case of secondary peritonitis

## 4. Recommendations

1. The person who performs the LB should be acutely aware of the multiple potential complications (including death) that may occur after liver biopsy and it is of outmost importance to discuss these appropriately with the patient's beforehand (class 1. Level C evidence)
2. Percutaneous liver biopsy with or without image guidance is appropriate only in cooperative patients and this technique should not be utilized in uncooperative patients(claas 1 level C)
3. Uncooperative patients who require liver biopsy should undergo the procedure under general anaesthesia or via transvenous route(class 1 level C)
4. In patients with clinically evident ascites requiring a liver biopsy a transvenous approach is generally recommended although percutaneous biopsy (after removal of ascites) or laparoscopic biopsy are acceptable alternatives(class 1 level C)
5. Haematological abnormalities particularly low platelet count (levels less than 50,000-60,000/ml) should be dealt with platelet transfusion prior to the procedure. This applies for both percutaneous and transvenous approach
6. The use of prophylactic or rescue strategies such as plasma, fibrinolytic inhibitors or recombinant factors should be considered in specific situations although their effectiveness remains to be established.(class 11a, level C)
7. In patients with renal failure or on hemodialysis , desmopressin(DDAVP) may be considered, although its use is necessary in patients on stable dialysis regimen(class 11a, level B)
8. Patients on chronic haemodialysis should be well dialysed prior to liver biopsy and heparin should be avoided if at all possible(class 1, level C)

## 5. Conclusion

The indications for liver biopsy are evolving. While liver biopsy may play a major role in management of some of the hepatic disorders, it is not without risk. Mild pain following the procedure is not uncommon however persistent and severe pain should warrant further investigation to rule out significant intraperitoneal bleed. Liver biopsy performed under ultrasound guidance and premedication is reported to significantly reduce complications including pain. The risk of major bleeding post liver biopsy is low but is of serious consequence as it is the main cause of a rare event of death. Among the various factors that may influence complication risk, patients coagulation status and operator experience are of outmost importance. The coagulation status should be optimized to the extent possible with platelet and coagulation factor infusion and the use of DDAVP and haemodialysis in patients with renal failure. The most critical aspect of management of these complications is to be acutely aware of it and to promptly treat it.

## 6. References


[1] Ghent CN. Percutaneous liver biopsy : Reflections and refinements . Can J Gastroenterol. 2006;20(2):75-9

[2] Rockey DC, Caldwell SH, Goodman ZD, Nelson RC, Smith AD. Liver biopsy. Hepatology. 2009;49(3):1017-1044

[3] Siegel CA, Silas AW, Suriawinata AA, van Leeuwen DJ. Liver biopsy 2005: When and how ? Cleve Clin J Med.2005;72(3):199-224

[4] Friedman LS. Controversies in liver biopsy: who, where, when, how, why?. Curr Gastroenterol Rep.2004;6(1):30-36

[5] Sheela H, Seela S, Caldwell C, Boyer JL, Jain D. Liver biopsy: evolving role in the new millennium. J Clin Gastroenterol.2005;39:603-10

[6] Alexander GA, smith BJ, Midazolam sedation for percutaneous liver biopsy. Dig Dis Sci. 1993;38(12):2209-2211

[7] Cartera I, Negre I, Samii K, Buffer C. Patient administration nitrous oxide/ oxygen inhalation provides safe and effective analgesics for percutaneous liver biopsy: a randomized placebo

[8] Lebrec D, Goldfar G, Degott C, Rueff B, Benhamou JP. Transvenous liver biopsy :an experience based on 1000 hepatic tissue sampling with this procedure. Gastroenterology. 1982;83:338-40

[9] Little AF, Ferris JV, Dodd GD 3rd, Baron RL. Image- guided percutaneous hepatic biopsy: effect of ascites on the complication rate. Radiology.1996;199(1):79-83

[10] McGill DB, Rakela J, Zinsmeister AR, Ott BJ. A 21 year experience with major haemorrhage after percutaneous liver biopsy. Gastroenterology.1990;99(5):1396-1400

[11] Chang S, Kim SH, Lim HK, Lee WJ, Choi D, Lim JH. Needle tract implantation after sonographically guided percutaneous biopsy of hepatocellular carcinoma: evaluation of doubling time, frequency and features on CT. AJR Am J Roentgenol.2005;185(2):400-5

[12] Tung WC, Huang YJ, Leung SW, Kuo FY, Tung HD, Wang JH et al. Incidence of needle tract seeding and response of soft tissue metastasis by hepatocellular carcinoma post radiotherapy. Liver Int.2007;27(2):192-200

[13] Maturen KE, Nghiem HV, Marrero JA, Hussain HK, Higgins EG, Fox GA et al. Lack of tumour seeding of hepatocellular carcinoma after percutaneous needle biopsy using co-axial cutting needle technique. AJR Am J Roentgenol.2006;187(5):1184-87

[14] Segal JB, Dzik WH. Paucity of studies to support that abnormal coagulation test results predict bleeding in the setting of invasive procedures: an evidence based review. Transfusion.2005;45:1413-25

[15] Stanworth SJ, Brunskill SJ, Hyde CJ, McClelland DB, Murphy MF. Is fresh frozen plasma clinically effective? A systematic review of randomized controlled trials. Br J Haematol.2004;126(1):139-52

[16] Bellest L, Eschwege V, Poupon R, Chazouilleres O, Robert A. A modified international normalized ratio as an effective way of prothrombin time standardization in hepatology. Hepatology .2007;46(2):528-34

[17] Theodore D, Fried MW, Kleiner DE, Kroner BL, Goedert JJ, Eyster ME et al. Liver biopsy in patients with inherited disorders of coagulation and chronic hepatitis C. Haemophilia.2004;10(5):413-21

[18] Grant A, Neuberger J. Guidelines on the use of liver biopsy in clinical practice. Gut.1999.45(suppl 1V):1V1- 1V11

[19] Cadranel JF, Rufat P, Degos F. practices of liver biopsy in France. Results of a prospective nationwide survey. For the group of epidemiology of the French association for the study of liver. Hepatology.2000;32:477-81

[20] Riley TR 3rd. How often does ultrasound marking change the liver biopsy site ? Am J Gastroenetrol. 1999;94(11):3320-22

[21] Angtuaco TL, Lal SK, Banaad-Omiotek GD, Zaidi SS, Howden CW. Current liver biopsy practices for suspected parenchymal liver diseases in the united states: the evolving role of radiologists. Am J Gastroenetrol.2002;97(6):1468-71

[22] Eisenberg E, Konopniki M, Veitsman E, Kramskay R, Gaintini D, Baruch Y. Prevalence and characteristics of pain induced by percutaneous liver biopsy. Anaesth Analg.2003;96(5):1392-96

[23] Janes CH, Lindor KD. Outcome of patients hospitalized for complications after outpatient liver biopsy. Ann intern Med.1993;118(2):96-98

[24] Tan KT, Rajan DK, Kachura JR, Hayeems E, Simons ME, Ho CS. Pain after percutaneous liver biopsy for diffuse hepatic disease: a randomized trial comparing subcostal and intercostal approaches. J Vas Interv Radiol.2005;16(9):1215-19

[25] Lindor KD, Bru C, Jorgensen RA , Rakela J, Bordas JM, Gross JB et al. The role of ultrasonography and automatic needle biopsy in outpatient percutaneous liver biopsy. Hepatology.1996;23(5):1079-83

[26] Chevallier P, Ruitor TF, Denys A et al. Significance of operator experience in diagnostic accuracy of biopsy gun procedures. Eur Radiol.1994;4:430-33

[27] Riley TR 3rd. Predictors of pain medication use after percutaneous liver biopsy. Dig Dis Sci.2002;47(10):2151-53

[28] Minuk GY, Sutherland LR, Wiseman DA, MacDonald FR, Ding DL. Prospective study of the incidence of ultrasound detected intrahepatic and subcapsular haematoma in patients randomized to 6 or 24 hours of bed rest after percutaneous liver biopsy. Gastroenetrology.1987;92(2):290-93

[29] Lankisch PG, Thiele E, Mahlke R, Lubbers H. Riesner K. Prospective study of the incidence of ultrasound detected hepatic haematomas 2 to 24 hours after percutaneous liver biopsy. Z Gastroenterol.1990;28(5):247-50

[30] Sugano S, Sumino Y, Hatori T, Mizugami H, Kuwafuni T, Abei T. incidence of ultrasound detected intrahepatic haematoma due to trucut needle liver biopsy. Dig Dis Sci.1991;36(9):1229-33

[31] Piccinino F, Sagnelli E, Pasquale G, Giusti G. complications following percutaneous liver biopsy. A multicentre retrospective study on 68,276 biopsies . J Hepatol.1986;2(1):165-73

[32] Kalambokis G, Manousou P, Vibhakron S, Marelli I, Cholongetas E, Senzolo M et al. Transjugualr liver biopsy: indications , adequacy , quality of specimen and complications. a systematic review . J Hepatol.2007;47:284-94

[33] Perrault J, McGill DB, Ott BJ, Taylor WF. Liver biopsy complications in 1000 inpatients and outpatients. Gastroenetrology.1978;74:103-106

[34] Reicher CM, Weisenthal LM, Kleen HG. Delayed haemorrhage after percutaneous liver biopsy. J Clin Gastroenterol. 1983;5:263-66

[35] Caldwell SH, Hoffman M, Lisman T, Macik BG, Northup PG, Reddy KR. Coagulopathies disorders and hemostasis in liver disease pathophysiology and critical assessment of current management . Hepatology.2006;44.1039-1046

[36] Bravo AA, Sheth SG, Chopra S. liver biopsy . N Engl J Med.2001;344(7):495-500

[37] Hodgson RS, Taylor- Robinson SD, Jackson JE. Haematochezia in Crohn's disease caused by late onset haemobilia following percutaneous liver biopsy . Eur J Gastroenterol Hepatol.2004;16(2):229-32

[38] Lin CL, Chang JJ, Lee TS, Lui KW, Yen CL. Gall bladder polyp as a manifestation of haemobilia caused by arterial portal fistula after percutaneous liver biopsy: a case report. World J Gastroenterol.2005;14:11(2):305-307

[39] Machicao VI, Lukens FJ, Lange SM, Scolapio JS. Arterioportal fistula causing acute pancreatitis and haemobilia after liver biopsy. J Clin Gastroenetrol.2002;34(4):481-84

[40] Mannucci PM, Remuzzi G, Pusineri F, Lombordi R, Valsecchi C, Mecca G et al. Deamino-8-D-arginine vasopressin shortens the bleeding time in uraemia. N Engl J Med. 1983;308(1):8-12

[41] DiMichele DM, Hathaway WE. Use of DDAVP in inherited and acquired platelet dysfunction. Am J Haematol. 1990;33(1):39-45

[42] McVay PA, Toy PT. lack of increased bleeding after liver biopsy in patients with mild hemostatic abnormalities. Am J Clin Pathol.1990;94(6):747-53

[43] Dillon JF, Simpson KJ, Hayes PC. Liver biliary bleeding time: an unpredictable event. J Gastroenterol Hepatol.1994;9(3):269-71

[44] Sue M, Caldwell SH, Dickson RC, Macalindong C, Rourk RM, Charles C et al. Variations between centers in technique and guidelines for liver biopsy. Liver 1996;16(4):267-70

[45] Bubak ME, Porayko MK, Krom RA, Wiesner RH, Complications of liver biopsy in liver transplant patients: increased sepsis associated with choledochojejunostomy. Hepatology.1991:14(6);1063-1065

[46] Myers RP, Fong A, Shaheen AA. Utilization rates, complications and costs of percutaneous liver biopsy ; a population based study including 4275 biopsies . liver Int.2008;28(5):705-12

[47] Chahal PS, Ready J. Haemothorax after percutaneous liver biopsy: an unusual complications. Am J Gastroentrol.2002;97:1068-9

[48] Ahluwalia JP, LaBrecque DR. A large bilioma causing gastric outlet obstruction after a percutaneous liver biopsy. J Clin Gastroenterol.2004;38(6):535-39

[49] Lublin M, Danforth DN. Iatrogenic gall bladder perforation: conservative management by percutaneous drainage and cholecystectomy. Am Surg.2001;67(8):760-63